Encyclopedia of Head and Neck Cancer

ncyclopedia of Head nd Neck Cancer

dited by **Kimball Cho**

hayle medical

New York

Published by Hayle Medical,
30 West, 37th Street, Suite 612,
New York, NY 10018, USA
www.haylemedical.com

Encyclopedia of Head and Neck Cancer
Edited by Kimball Cho

International Standard Book Number: 978-1-63241-165-5 (Hardback)

Printed in China.

Contents

Preface

This book has been a concerted effort by a group of academicians, researchers and scientists, who have contributed their research works for the realization of the book. This book has materialized in the wake of emerging advancements and innovations in this field. Therefore, the need of the hour was to compile all the required researches and disseminate the knowledge to a broad spectrum of people comprising of students, researchers and specialists of the field.

Head and neck cancer is a severe disease basically described as the cancer that arises in the head or neck region. This book presents an interesting and extensive outline of major features of head and neck cancer including an introduction of the disease, basic science characteristics pertaining to the disease, diagnosis, treatment and result for patients with this disease. This book is a collective effort of renowned specialists from across the world. It encompasses the complete domain of head and neck oncology and also discusses regional disparity, improvements in basic science understanding, developments in radiotherapy, chemotherapy and targeted agents. It also emphasizes on reconstruction, prostheses, and characteristics of quality of life and health results. This book will surely come in handy and expansive for physicians engaged in the treatment of this complicated disease.

At the end of the preface, I would like to thank the authors for their brilliant chapters and the publisher for guiding us all-through the making of the book till its final stage. Also, I would like to thank my family for providing the support and encouragement throughout my academic career and research projects.

Editor

Part 1

Squamous Cell Carcinoma of the Head and Neck

1

Hypopharyngeal Cancer

Valentina Krstevska
Department of Head and Neck Cancer,
University Clinic of Radiotherapy and Oncology, Skopje
Republic of Macedonia

1. Introduction

Hypopharyngeal cancers arise from the mucosa of one of the three anatomical subsites of the hypopharynx and are characterised by advanced disease at presentation mainly because the hypopharynx, laying outside the glottis and being a silent area, allows tumours to grow for a substantial period of time before symptoms occur (Elias et al., 1995; Sewnaik et al., 2005). Hypopharyngeal cancers are relatively rare neoplasms and have one of the most unfavourable prognosis among all cancers of the upper aerodigestive tract (Prades et al., 2002; Samant et al., 1999). The reasons for the remarkably poor prognosis of hypopharyngeal cancers is their aggressive behaviour represented by strong tendency for submucosal spread, early occurrence of nodal metastatic involvement, propensity for direct invasion of adjacent structures in the neck and high incidence of distant metastases (Elias et al., 1995; Johansen et al., 2000).

Treatment options for early stage hypopharyngeal cancer include conservation or radical surgery or radiotherapy, whereas total laryngectomy with partial or total pharyngectomy followed by postoperative radiotherapy have been the standard form of treatment for advanced stage disease. Over the past two decades, organ preservation strategies with either altered fractionation radiotherapy or combination of chemotherapy and radiotherapy have been used for the treatment of advanced hypopharyngeal cancers. Progressive tumour-related dysphagia prior to diagnosis, associated tobacco and alcohol use, commonly older age, medical comorbidities and social issues present in most of the patients, unequivocally contribute to additional challenges for employment of aggressive treatment management, and increase the risk of morbidity and mortality following therapy. The complex management of these tumours creates an essential need for multidisciplinary team approach involving a head and neck surgeon, radiation oncologist, medical oncologist, radiologist, pathologist, nutritionist, speech and swallow therapist, and social worker. This chapter will review the epidemiology and etiology, clinical presentation, diagnosis, prognosis, treatment modalities for early and locally-regionally advanced resectable hypopharyngeal cancer, management of unresectable disease, and treatment of recurrent and metastatic disease.

2. Epidemiology and etiology

Hypopharyngeal cancer is a rare disease representing about 0.5% of all human malignancies with an incidence of less than 1 per 100,000 population and constituting only 3% - 5% of all head and neck cancers (Cooper et al., 2009; Hoffman et al., 1998; Johansen et al., 2000). Hypopharyngeal cancers are more common in men than in women. Increased incidence in males of over 2.5:100,000 is seen in India, Brazil, Central and Western Europe and decreased incidence under 0.5:100,000 in Eastern Asia, Africa and Northern Europe. The incidence in women is as high as 0.2:100,000 in the majority of the countries, except for India (1:100,000) (Popescu et al., 2010). These tumours typically occur in individuals who are older than 50 years of age, with a peak incidence in the sixth and seventh decades and their occurrence is extremely rare in children (Siddiqui et al., 2003). The most common site of origin of hypopharyngeal cancer is the pyriform sinus (66%-75%), followed by the posterior pharyngeal wall, and postcricoid area (20%-25%) (Carpenter & DeSanto, 1977). There are differences in the geographical distribution of the hypopharyngeal cancer with regard to tumour location and patient gender, with postcricoid lesions showing a consistent moderate female preponderance particularly in Scandinavia (Farrington et al., 1986; Kajanti & Mantyla, 1990; Lederman, 1962; Popescu et al., 2010; Tandon et al., 1991). Pyriform sinus and posterior pharyngeal wall lesions demonstrate typical male predominance in North America and especially in France (Vandenbrouck et al., 1987).

Excessive tobacco and alcohol consumption contribute to the development of squamous cell carcinomas in the upper aerodigestive tract (Flanders & Rothman, 1982; Jayant et al., 1977). Tobacco and alcohol represent the major risk factors for the development of hypopharyngeal cancer with more than 90% of patients presenting with a history of tobacco use (Hoffman et al., 1997). Risk increases with both the quantity and duration of tobacco and alcohol use (Menvielle et al., 2004; Tuyns et al., 1988). An increased smoking rate in women resulted in narrowing the gap between genders in some countries (Llatas et al., 2009; Popescu et al., 2010). Also, the early introduction of smoking in the individual habits could be considered as a factor contributing to a downward readjustment of the age of appearance of hypopharyngeal cancer (Lefebvre & Chevalier, 2004). The high rate of synchronous and metachronous primary tumours identified in patients with hypopharyngeal cancer and the concomitant mucosal dysplasia frequently found surrounding primary tumours appear to relate to a field cancerisation effect, which is consistent with widespread exposure to carcinogens (Shah et al., 2008; Slaughter et al., 1953; Van Oijen & Slootweg, 2000).

The importance of the role of genetic factors for the development of head and neck cancer is not fully understood at the present time. Abnormalities of the tumour suppressor gene p53 are common in hypopharyngeal cancer, occurring in up to 70% of patients (Somers et al., 1992). The association between tobacco use and p53 mutations is found in a much larger percentage of smokers and drinkers than that of nonsmokers and nondrinkers (Brennan et al., 1995; Koch et al., 1999; Sorensen et al., 1997). Also, the overexpression of oncogenes at the 11q13 locus appears to be more frequent in hypopharyngeal cancers compared with other head and neck cancer (Muller et al., 1997; Williams et al., 1993). The loss of heterozygosity at 9p and abnormalities in chromosome 11 present in histologically normal mucosa adjacent to hypopharyngeal cancers further support the field cancerisation effect hypothesis (Van der Riet et al., 1994). Mutations in the p21 gene have also been identified in hypopharyngeal cancers (Ernoux-Neufcoeur et al., 2011).

The role of human papilloma virus (HPV) as a contributing factor to carcinogenesis in head and neck squamous cell carcinomas represent an area of active investigation (Fakhry & Gillison, 2006). Although the association of HPV with head and neck cancer, especially with oropharyngeal tumours has been supported by epidemiologic and molecular biology studies (Franceschi et al., 1996; McKaig et al., 1998), HPV in the carcinogenesis of hypopharyngeal cancer is less well defined. Studies have demonstrated rates of detection of HPV DNA in patients with hypopharyngeal cancer ranging from 20% to 25% (Mineta et al., 1998). However, the clinical implications of the presence of the genome of the oncogenic high-risk HPV types in hypopharyngeal cancer are yet to be defined.

The development of hypopharyngeal cancers in the postcricoid area in women aged 30 to 50 without a history of tobacco or alcohol use is associated with previous Plummer-Vinson syndrome, also termed Patterson-Brown-Kelly syndrome (Goldstein et al., 2008; Kajanti & Mantyla, 1990; Stell et al., 1978). This syndrome is characterised by hypopharyngeal webs, dysphagia, weight loss, and iron-deficiency anemia. Its early diagnosis and treatment with supplemental iron were shown to be effective in stooping further cancer development (Pfister et al., 2009).

A substantial proportion of hypopharyngeal cancers could be attributable to occupational exposures (Menvielle et al., 2004). Possible environmental carcinogens that have been implicated in hypopharyngeal cancer include asbestos and welding fumes (Gustavsson et al., 1998; Marchand et al., 2000; Shangina et al., 2006).

3. Anatomy of the hypopharynx

The hypopharynx is the part of the pharynx that is contagious superiorly with the oropharynx and is situated posterior and lateral to the larynx. The hypopharynx extends from the superior border of the epiglottis and the pharyngoepiglottic folds from the level of the hyoid bone superiorly to the lower border of the cricoid cartilage inferiorly where it narrows and becomes continuous with the esophagus (Gale et al., 2006; Moore et al., 2010). It is divided into three primary anatomic subsites: the pyriform sinuses, the postcricoid area, and the posterior pharyngeal wall.

The pyriform sunuses are analogous to an inverted pyramids situated lateral to the larynx with their base located superiorly and with the anterior, lateral, and medial walls narrowing inferiorly to form the apices with their tips extending slightly below the cricoid cartilage. It is separated from the laryngeal inlet by the aryepiglottic fold. The superior limit of the base is the pharyngoepiglottic fold and the free margin of the aryepiglottic fold. The lateral wall of the pyriform sinus is formed by the inferior constrictor muscles and the internal branches of the superior laryngeal neurovascular bundle. Its superior aspect is bordered by the thyrohyoid membrane. Inferiorly, it is bounded by the thyroid cartilage. Its medial boundary is the lateral surface of the aryepiglottic fold, arytenoids, and lateral aspect of the cricoid cartilage. The median wall is formed by the lateral surface of the aryepiglottic fold, arytenoids, and lateral aspect of the cricoid cartilage (Moore et al., 2010).

The postcricoid area includes the mucosa that overlies the cricoid cartilage and represents the anterior surface extending from the superior aspect of the arytenoid cartilages to the inferior border of the cricoid cartilage. Inferiorly, it is contagious with the cervical esophagus. Its important relations are the arytenoids, the cricoarytenoid joints, the intrinsic laryngeal muscles, and inferiorly, below the cricoid, the trachealis muscle and recurrent laryngeal nerves.

Posterior pharyngeal wall extends superiorly from the horizontal level of the floor of the vallecula (the level of the hyoid bone) to the inferior border of the cricoid inferiorly and laterally from the apex of one pyriform sinus to the other being contagious with the lateral wall of the pyriform sinus. The posterior pharyngeal wall is predominantly comprised of mucosa covering the middle and inferior pharyngeal constrictor muscles. Posteriorly, it is related to the bodies of the third through sixth cervical vertebra. It is separated from the prevertebral fascia by retropharyngeal space. The posterior pharyngeal wall is contagious with the lateral wall of the pyriform sinus.

There is a rich network of lymphatic channels within the hypopharynx. The first echelon of lymphatic drainage is represented by the upper and midjugular (level II and III) nodes. Lymphatic channels from the pyriform sinuses drain through the thyrohyoid membrane following the superior laryngeal artery to the jugulodigastric, midjugular (level II and III), and retropharyngeal nodes. The lymphatics of the postcricoid area may drain directly to local lymph nodes, may ascend with the lymphatic drainage of the pyriform sinus (levels II and III), but mainly tend to follow the retropharyngeal lymph nodes to the paratracheal, paraesophageal, and lower jugular nodes (level IV and VI), or may occasionally drain down into the superior mediastinum (Clayman & Weber, 1996). Lymphatics of the posterior pharyngeal wall may drain bilaterally, passing to the lateral retropharyngeal nodes including the most cephalad retropharyngeal nodes of Rouviere, or to the upper jugular nodes (level II).

The sensory innervation of the hypopharynx is by the glossopharyngeal and vagus nerves via the pharyngeal plexus, superior laryngeal nerves, and recurrent laryngeal nerves (Moore et al., 2010). The common origin of the auricular nerve of Arnold from the synapsis of the internal branch of the superior laryngeal nerve and the vagal branches from the middle ear in the jugular ganglion results in the phenomenon of referred otalgia seen in patients presenting with hypopharyngeal cancer (Clayman & Weber, 1996). Motor innervation of the hypopharynx is from the pharyngeal plexus and recurrent laryngeal nerves. The arterial supply is derived from the superior laryngeal, lingual, and ascending pharyngeal collateral arteries (Standring, 2004).

4. Patterns of spread and clinical presentation

4.1 Patterns of spread

Hypopharyngeal cancers, particularly those arising in the postcricoid area, have a strong tendency for extensive submucosal spread. The extent of subclinical spread beyond the macroscopic tumour edge is greatest in the inferior direction ranging between 5 and 30 mm (Davidge-Pitts & Mannel, 1983; Hong et al., 2005). The presence of submucosal tumour extension frequently demonstrated in surgical specimens can result in inaccuracy in the estimation of tumour volume. Therefore, the submucosal spread as a characteristic feature for hypopharyngeal cancer should be taken into consideration during the treatment being either surgery or radiotherapy. Pyriform sinus cancers with lateral extension can invade the thyroid cartilage (Kirchner, 1975), but cricoid cartilage and thyroid gland involvement is also possible by the extension through the cricothyroid membrane. Medial extension is associated with invasion of the aryepiglottic folds, preepiglottic and paraglottic space, and intrinsic laryngeal muscles that results in a loss of vocal cord mobility (Kirchner, 1975; Tani

& Amatsu, 1987). Superior tumour extension beyond the lateral pharyngoepiglottic fold into the vallecula can involve the base of the tongue and inferior tumour extension beyond the apex can involve the thyroid gland. Postcricoid tumours tending to grow circumferentially frequently involve the cricoid cartilage, arytenoids and intrinsic laryngeal muscles with resultant vocal cord fixation. Involvement of the recurrent laryngeal nerve can also result in vocal cord immobility. The inferior tumour spread can lead to invasion of cervical esophagus and trachea. Posterior pharyngeal wall tumours with their superior spread may invade the base of the tonsil and the oropharyngeal wall, while inferior extension may be associated with invasion of the postcricoid hypopharynx. These tumours may also invade through the posterior wall to involve the prevertebral fascia and the vertebral bodies.

Lymph node metastases in the neck are associated with even the earliest stages of hypopharyngeal cancer. Metastases in the neck lymph nodes are already present in approximately 70% of patients at the time of presentation with levels II and III being the most frequently affected sites (Lefebvre et al., 1987; Vandenbrouck et al., 1987). Metastases in paratracheal and paraesophageal nodes (level VI) are most commonly present in patients with cancers in the postcricoid area (De Bree et al., 2011; Joo et al., 2010; Timon et al., 2003; Weber et al., 1993). Retropharyngeal lymph node metastases are most frequently present in patients with cancers of the posterior pharyngeal wall and the postcricoid area, but can also be present in those patients who have positive nodes in other levels in the neck (Amatsu et al., 2001; Hasegawa & Matsuura, 1994; Kamiyama et al., 2009). Apart from the high incidence of clinically apparent regional spread, another striking problem is the presence of occult nodal disease in high percentage of patients with hypopharyngeal primaries. Thus, in patients with clinically positive neck, the incidence of bilateral occult lymph node metastases is at least 50% (Byers et al., 1988; Buckley & MacLennan, 2000). The reported percentage of occult contralateral neck metastases in patients with pyriform sinus cancer and ipsilateral metastatic neck nodes involvement is 77% (Aluffi et al., 2006). Bilateral occult lymph node metastases in patients with clinically negative neck are most frequently associated with cancers of the pyriform sinus (Buckley & MacLennan, 2000; Koo et al., 2006). The risk of occult lymph node metastases at levels IV and V in patients with clinically negative neck is low, whereas in patients with clinically positive neck is more than 20% (Byers et al., 1988; Buckley & MacLennan, 2000; Gregoire et al., 2000). Occult nodal disease in ipsilateral paratracheal lymph nodes has been reported in 20% of patients with tumours arising from postcricoid area or pyriform sinus apex presenting with clinically negative neck (Buckley & MacLennan, 2000).

Distant metastases at presentation are more common in hypopharyngeal cancers than in other head and neck cancers. At the time of clinical diagnosis distant metastatic disease is present in approximately 17% of hypopharyngeal cancers (Hsu & Chen, 2005; Spector, 2001). The frequency of distant metastatic development in patients with hypopharyngeal cancer during the course of the disease is also among the highest of all head and neck cancers. In the ten years experience of treatment for advanced hypopharyngeal cancer reported by Hirano et al. (Hirano et al., 2010), approximately half of the recurrences was distant metastatic disease. The most common site for distant metastases is the lung. According to Spector et al. (Spector et al., 2001), development of distant metastases at some time following initial treatment is associated with tumour recurrence at the primary site, or neck metastases.

4.2 Clinical presentation

Early hypopharyngeal cancers produce a mild, nonspecific sore throat or vague discomfort on swallowing. In these patients, globus sensation can be the only complaint with normal clinical findings (Tsikoudas et al., 2007). However, the majority of patients with cancers of the hypopharynx presents with advanced local and/or regional disease and provide a history of significant tobacco or alcohol use. Most patients have also poor dentition and halitosis. Predominating symptoms are those related to the locoregional disease spread including sore throat, odynophagia and dysphagia, weight loss, and a mass in the neck. Referred otalgia (external auditory canal pain) frequently present in patients with pyriform sinus cancers may be referred via the superior laryngeal nerve through the auricular branch of the vagal nerve (Arnold's nerve). Development of hoarseness (vocal cord paralysis) may be a result of either direct invasion of the larynx or involvement of recurrent laryngeal nerve indicating more advanced disease. A "hot potato" voice may be due to the involvement of the base of the tongue. Approximately 50% of patients present with palpable neck lymphadenopathy as the only complaint on initial clinical examination (Keane, 1982; Uzcudun et al., 2001).

5. Diagnosis, staging, and prognosis

5.1 Diagnosis

Pretreatment diagnostic workup of hypopharyngeal cancer starts with a complete medical history with attention paid to disease-related signs and symptoms, and continues with clinical examination and endoscopy including indirect mirror exam and fiberoptic endoscopy under local anesthesia. Clinical and endoscopic assessment should be focused on determining the extent of the primary tumour and laryngeal mobility. Endoscopy can often easily reveal tumours arising in the upper pyriform sinus and the posterior pharyngeal wall, whereas for tumours located in the apex of the pyriform sinus and obscured by pooled secretions, and for those arising in postcricoid area and causing significant arytenoid edema, the visualisation of the tumour during endoscopy is much more difficult. Panendoscopy under general anesthesia allows the physician a thorough evaluation of the entire upper aerodigestive tract with consequent precise assessment of the macroscopic extent of the primary tumour as well as detection of synchronous primary tumours. Detection of regional disease is obtained by careful examination of both sites of the neck.

Imaging studies including computed tomography (CT) and/or magnetic resonance imaging (MRI) and/or positron emission tomography (PET)/CT of the head and neck region are required to define the extent of the disease at the primary site in surrounding structures, such as the paralaryngeal space, preepiglottic space, laryngeal cartilages, extralaryngeal soft tissue, prevertebral space, and parapharyngeal space, and also to evaluate the extent of the disease in regional lymph nodes. Imaging studies are primarily helpful for staging the primary tumour and neck, but may also help in determining mediastinal spread and distant metastatic disease in the lung and can also inform on possible synchronous tumours in the upper aerodigestive tract. Fluorodeoxyglucose-PET (FDG-PET) scans, although not routinely indicated, may be helpful in the evaluation of locally advanced hypopharyngeal cancer. Histological confirmation is mandatory for the diagnosis of hypopharyngeal cancer.

Biopsy of primary tumour site is usually performed during endoscopic examination under anesthesia. If a neck adenopathy is present, ultrasound with a fine-needle aspiration or core biopsy is performed obtaining sufficient tumour to confirm diagnosis of suspicious metastatic lymph node. More than 95% of hypopharyngeal malignancies are squamous cell carcinomas which are often poorly differentiated. Uncommon nonsquamous cell malignancies include adenocarcinoma, composing the majority of the remaining 5% of the primary hypopharyngeal tumours, as well as lymphoma, and other rare neoplasms such as malignant fibrous histiocytoma, liposarcoma, fibrosarcoma, chondrosarcoma, and mucosal malignant melanoma.

Pretreatment evaluations should also include routine laboratory studies (a complete blood count, basic blood chemistry, liver function tests, and renal function tests), chest x-ray, and liver ultrasound. Swallowing and nutrition status should be also evaluated. When radiotherapy planned, preventive dental care and dental extractions should be dealt with 10 to 14 days prior to treatment commencement.

5.2 Staging

The accepted standard for staging of hypopharyngeal squamous cell carcinoma is represented by the American Joint Committee on Cancer (AJCC) Tumour Node Metastasis (TNM) staging system (Edge & Byrd, 2009) (Table 1). Clinical staging is based on data from medical history, clinical examination, endoscopy, and imaging studies. Regarding the primary tumour, the AJCC staging system does not differentiate the specific tumour subsite. Regional lymph nodes staging and stage grouping is identical to other sites within the oral cavity and pharynx with exception of nasopharynx. Pathologic staging is based on findings from clinical staging and data included in the report of histopathological analysis for resected specimen including the type, size, and grade of the primary tumour, the pattern of invasion, the minimum resection margin, the regional lymph nodes status, and the presence of nodal extracapsular extension.

5.3 Prognostic factors

Overall stage grouping (anatomic stage), stage of primary tumour (T stage), and stage of regional lymph nodes (N stage) are important prognostic factors for cancer of the hypopharynx. Regarding the data from literature concerning prognostic factors for hypopharyngeal cancer, it is apparent that the results of the analysis of different authors are not consistent. Thus, some authors showed nodal staging as the most important independent prognostic factor (Keane et al., 1983; Pivot et al., 2005; Sakata et al., 1998), whereas other authors confirmed the statistical significance of T stage (Toita et al., 1996; Tsou et al., 2006). According to some authors, overall stage grouping remains the most important determinants of outcome (Barzan et al., 1990; Gupta et al., 2009a), while other authors revealed T stage and N stage as dominant prognostic factors in hypopharyngeal cancer (Hall et al., 2009; Johansen et al., 2000; Spector et al., 1995; Wygoda et al., 2000).

Age and gender have been also shown to have prognostic significance in hypopharyngeal cancer with increased age and male gender negatively influencing patients' outcome (Nishimaki et al., 2002; Rapoport & Franco, 1993; Spector et al., 1995).

Primary tumour (T)	
TX:	Primary tumour cannot be assessed
T0:	No evidence of primary tumour
Tis:	Carcinoma in situ
T1:	Tumour limited to one subsite of hypopharynx and/or 2 cm or less in greatest dimension
T2:	Tumour invades more than one subsite of hypopharynx or an adjacent site, or measures more than 2 cm, but not more than 4 cm in greatest dimension without fixation of hemilarynx
T3:	Tumour more than 4 cm in greatest dimension or with fixation of hemilarynx or extension to esophagus
T4a:	Moderately advanced local disease. Tumour invades thyroid/cricoid cartilage, hyoid bone, thyroid gland, or central compartment soft tissue*
T4b:	Very advanced local disease. Tumour invades prevertebral fascia, encases carotid artery, or involves mediastinal structures
**Note:*	Central compartment soft tissue includes prelaryngeal strap muscles and subcutaneous fat
Regional lymph nodes (N)	
Nx:	Regional lymph nodes cannot be assessed
N0:	No regional lymph node metastasis
N1:	Metastasis in a single ipsilateral lymph node, 3 cm or less in greatest dimension
N2:	Metastasis in a single ipsilateral lymph node, more than 3 cm but not more than 6 cm in greatest dimension; or in multiple ipsilateral lymph nodes, not more than 6 cm in greatest dimension; or in bilateral or contralateral lymph nodes, not more than 6 cm in greatest dimension
N2a:	Metastasis in a single ipsilateral lymph node more than 3 cm but not more than 6 cm in greatest dimension
N2b:	Metastasis in multiple ipsilateral lymph nodes, not more than 6 cm in greatest dimension
N2c:	Metastasis in bilateral or contralateral lymph nodes, not more than 6 cm in greatest dimension
N3:	Metastasis in a lymph node, more than 6 cm in greatest dimension
Distant metastasis (M)	
M0:	No distant metastasis
M1:	Distant metastasis
Anatomic stage/prognostic groups	
0:	Tis N0 M0
I:	T1 N0 M0
II:	T2 N0 M0
III:	T3 N0 M0, T1-T3 N1 M0
IVA:	T4a N0 M0, T4a N1 M0, T1-T3 N2 M0, T4a N2 M0
IVB:	Any N M0, Any T N3 M0
IVC:	Any T Any N M1

Table 1. American Joint Committee on Cancer (AJCC) TNM classification of hypopharyngeal cancer

Several pathologic factors have been demonstrated to impact upon outcome in surgical treatment of hypopharyngeal cancer (Hall et al., 2009; Lee et al., 2008; Mochiki et al., 2007). Several studies reported the adverse impact of advanced stage, (Dinshaw et al., 2005; Hall et al., 2009; Lee et al., 2008; Mochiki et al., 2007), nodal extracapsular extension (Vandenbrouck et al., 1987; Lee et al., 2008), perineural invasion (Bova et al., 2005), and lymphovascular invasion (Bova et al., 2005; Mochiki et al., 2007). Increasing pathological nodal stage (Chu et al., 2008; Hall et al., 2009; Mochiki et al., 2007), and quality of tumour clearance were also revealed as significant prognostic factors (Gupta et al., 2010; Nishimaki et al., 2002).

Tumour volume is the most important prognostic factor of treatment outcome for patients with advanced hypopharyngeal cancer treated with concurrent chemoradiotherapy and should always be taken into consideration in treatment planning (Plataniotis et al., 2004; Tsou et al., 2006). Thus, confirming the significance of gross tumour volume as the only independent prognostic factor for treatment outcome, Chen et al. (Chen et al., 2009) concluded that pretreatment CT-based gross tumour volume measurements could be considered as strong predictor of local control and survival in patients with advanced stage hypopharyngeal cancers treated with concurrent chemoradiotherapy. For this patients category, low pretreatment hemoglobin level (Lee et al., 1998; Prosnitz et al., 2005) and age older than 70 years (Pignon et al., 2009) were revealed as negative prognostic factors.

6. Treatment of hypopharyngeal cancer

6.1 Treatment of small lesions (T1N0-1 and small T2N0)

Early-stage hypopharyngeal cancers include most T1N0-1 and small T2N0 cancers that do not require total laryngectomy. Patients with small lesions of the hypopharynx constitute approximately 20% of all patients presenting with hypopharyngeal cancer (Spector et al., 2001). Conservation surgery or radiotherapy alone are considered effective treatment modalities for patients who present with T1N0-1 and selected T2N0 obtaining satisfactory rates of local control while optimising functional outcome (Allal, 1997; Jones et al., 1994; Jones & Stell, 1991). However, discrepancies exist among different authors in the choice of treatment approach for early hypopharyngeal lesions. Thus, some authors advocate conservation surgery with or without postoperative radiotherapy whereas other authors advocate radiotherapy alone. The study conducted by Groupe d'Etude des Tumeurs de la Tête et du Cou (GETTEC) (Foucher et al., 2009), supported conservation surgery procedures in patients with T1 or T2N0 hypopharyngeal lesions showing that transoral approach or partial pharyngolaryngectomy led to completely satisfactory results in terms of survival and locoregional control. Comparing the effect of surgery or radiotherapy in the treatment of postcricoid carcinoma, Axon et al. (Axon et al., 1997) recommended surgery as a better method of improving survival, especially in patients with no nodal disease. El Badawi et al. (El Badawi et al., 1982) reviewing patients with cancer of the pyriform sinus treated with radiotherapy, surgery, or surgery and postoperative radiotherapy, concluded that superficial lesions without vocal cord mobility impairment were suitable for definitive radiotherapy. Similar conclusion regarding the effectiveness of radiotherapy alone in the management of small tumours in the postcricoid area with no clinical evidence of neck lymph node metastasis was drawn by Stell et al. (Stell et al., 1982). Levebvre & Lartigau (Levebvre & Lartigau, 2003), considering surgery and radiotherapy as approaches comparable in terms of local control and functional results in early hypopharyngeal cancer, emphasized that the impressive improvement in radiotherapy techniques unequivocally enabled the acceptance of radiotherapy as an indisputable alternative to surgery. Furthermore, additional arguments supporting definitive radiotherapy as a treatment of choice for small hypopharyngeal tumours are the expected superior functional outcome (Freeman et al., 1979; Marks et al., 1978), the necessity for postoperative radiotherapy because of positive resection margin or extracapsular spread of nodal disease with its related morbidity following conservation surgery, and the need for elective irradiation of the lymph nodes in the neck when elective dissection had not been performed during the surgical procedure. The selection of patients for conservation surgical procedures or radiotherapy as a primary treatment modality must be carefully accomplished. Because of the lack of studies that analyse and compare the results of conservation surgery and definitive radiotherapy in terms of local control and functional outcome in patients with early hypopharyngeal cancers, the decision for adoption of one of these two treatment modalities should incorporate a complex assessment of the extent and volume of tumour and expected response to treatment modalities, patient age and physical status, patient preference including occupational considerations, patient compliance, prior head and neck malignancy, risk for second head and neck primary cancer, the ability to deliver an adequate radiotherapy, or the expertise of the surgical team to effectively realise conservation surgery, treatment cost, and physician and institutional bias.

6.1.1 Surgery

Summarising the results of surgery reported in published series, Levebvre (Levebvre, 2000) revealed that the treatment of early hypopharyngeal cancers with properly selected conservation surgical procedure provides a 5-year local control ranging between 90% and 95% with a 5-year larynx function preservation ranging between 85% and 100%. For the small lesions of the pyriform sinuses, partial pharyngectomy or partial pharyngolaryngectomy should be considered. The indications for conservation surgery are represented by the absence of gross tumour involvement and impaired mobility of vocal cords and arytenoids, as well as by the absence of thyroid cartilage invasion and involvement of the apex of the pyriform sinus and postcricoid area (Freeman et al., 1979; Marks et al., 1978). Additionally, attention must be paid to the possible caudal, contralateral, and extralaryngeal extension, and soft tissue invasion. In selected patients with T1 and T2 lesions of the medial wall of the pyriform sinus a supracricoid hemilaryngopharyngectomy is advocated (Freeman et al., 1979; Laccourreye et al., 1987). In patients with T1 and T2 lesions of the lateral wall of the pyriform sinus, partial pharyngectomy through a lateral approach is indicated. Partial pharyngectomy through a transhyoid pharyngotomy, posterior pharyngectomy, or lateral pharyngotomy are conservation surgery procedures that allow the excision of T1 and small T2 lesions confined to the posterior wall of the hypopharynx. The lateral pharyngotomy as an approach that allows access to all subsites of the hypopharynx is also very suitable for small tumours of the posterior pharyngeal wall. Median labiomandibular glossotomy and transoral approach can also be employed for small lesions of the posterior pharyngeal wall. The reconstruction following excision of larger posterior wall lesions involves a free vascularised graft (Jol et al., 2003; Schwager et al., 1999). Tumours arising in the postcricoid area are usually presented as advanced lesions. Surgical excision followed by postoperative radiation is the treatment of choice for cancers not amenable to a conservation protocol (i.e., tumours destroying cartilage, tumours too bulky for control with primary radiation). The minimum operation recommended is total laryngectomy and partial pharyngectomy and pharyngoesophagectomy with reconstruction if extension into the esophagus is present. In several studies analysing the results obtained with partial surgery in patients with early cancer of the pyriform sinus the reported 5-year survival rates range between 47% and 83% (Barton, 1973; Chevalier et al., 1997; Laccourreye et al., 1993; Makeieff et al., 2004; Marks et al., 1978). Partial pharyngolaryngectomy also resulted in a 5-year local recurrence rate bellow 5% (Chevalier et al., 1997; Laccourreye et al., 1993). In the retrospective study of Vandenbrouck et al. (Vandenbrouck et al., 1987), the reported rate of locoregional control was 89% in patients with T1 and T2 cancers of the pyriform sinus treated with conservation surgery. In the retrospective study of Pene et al. (Pene et al., 1978), primary surgery and postoperative radiotherapy in patients with early lesions of posterior pharyngeal wall (T1 and T2) resulted in 5-year survival rate of 30%. In the study of Jones et al. (Jones et al., 1995), the results of surgery and radiotherapy alone in patients with carcinoma of the postcricoid area showed no significant difference in the observed tumour-specific five-year survival rates between surgery and radiotherapy group.

The transoral laser ednoscopic resection is a new conservation surgical approach suitable for T1 and T2 exophytic, highly differentiated squamous cell carcinomas of the upper part of the hypopharynx without extension to the apex of the pyriform sinus or to the postcricoid area (Glanz, 1999; Rudert & Hoft, 2003; Vilaseca et al., 2004). Few non-randomised studies evaluating transoral laser surgery in hypopharyngeal cancer reported 5-year overall survival rate of approximately 70% (Foucher et al., 2009; Rudert et al., 2003; Steiner et al., 2001), and local control rate at 5 years ranging between 82% and 90% (Foucher et al., 2009; Steiner et al., 2001).

Hypopharyngectomy by transoral robotic surgery as a procedure proposed to minimise the treatment-related morbidity following conventional surgical approaches for T1 or T2 lesions arising in the pyriform sinus analysed in terms of efficacy and feasibility has been also shown to be a safe technique for the treatment of early hypopharyngeal cancer (Park et al., 2010).

6.1.2 Radiotherapy

The use of radiotherapy as a single treatment approach for small hypoharyngeal lesions (T1N0-1 and small T2N0) offers treatment for both the primary tumour and the neck, thereby obviating the need for neck dissections and their associated morbidity. Definitive radiotherapy could be considered as treatment of choice for non-circumferential postcricoid lesions allowing organ preservation and a reasonable probability of cure and restoration of swallow. Additionally, definitive radiotherapy could be effectively employed in patients who refuse surgery or who are poor surgical candidates because of underlying medical conditions.

Several non-randomised controlled trials exploring the role of definitive radiotherapy in the treatment of early hypopharyngeal cancer, reported local control rates for T1 lesions arising from pyriform sinus ranging between 60% and 100% (Bataini et al., 1982; Mendenhall et al., 1987a; Million & Cassisi, 1981). However, in the reported update of the University of Florida experience with early pyriform sinus cancer, the involvement of the apex of the pyriform sinus and the high probability for early cartilaginous involvement was shown to significantly reduce local control for T1 lesions (Amdur et al., 2001). The rates of local control also decrease in bulky T2 lesions and in those larger than 2.5 cm (Pameijer et al., 1998; Mendenhall et al., 1987b). The published data for hypopharyngeal sites other than pyriform sinus are more limited. Most of the studies reporting results of definitive radiotherapy in patients with carcinoma of the pharyngeal wall included lesions arising from both hypopharynx and oropharynx, and there is also a lack of randomised controlled trials exploring the role of definitive radiotherapy in early hypopharyngeal cancer arising in the postcricoid area. In the study of Fein et al. (Fein et al., 1993), the achieved 2-year local control rates for T1 and T2 pharyngeal wall cancer treated with definitive radiotherapy using conventional fractionation were 100% and 67%, respectively. Meoz-Mendez et al. (Meoz-Mendez et al., 1978) analysing the results of irradiation in the treatment of cancers of the pharyngeal walls emphasized that the recurrence rate at the primary site was associated with increasing T stage, while Talton et al. (Talton et al., 1981) considered radiotherapy as the most effective treatment in the posterior wall lesions. In a series of Farrington et al. (Farrington et al., 1986), a significant survival rate decrease in lesions of the postcricoid area more than 2 cm in length was observed following radiotherapy alone. The disease-free survival in patients who completed radiotherapy was 66% and 21% in stages I and II, respectively. In the study of Garden et al. (Garden et al., 1996), the observed 2-year local control rates in patients with early stage hypopharyngeal cancer from all sites treated with definitive radiotherapy were 89% for T1 lesions and 77% for T2 lesions. Nakamura et al. (Nakamura et al., 2006) reported 5-year local control rates of 85% and 65% for T1 and T2 hypopharyngeal lesions. The observed overall survival at 5 years for stage I and II hypopharyngeal cancer from all sites treated by radiotherapy alone ranged between was 40% and 78% (Pingree et al., 1987; Van Mierlo et al., 1995). In summary, primary conventionally fractionated radiotherapy for T1-2 hypopharyngeal cancers results in a 2-year local control rate of 89-100% for T1 tumours and 60-70% for T2 tumours (Fein et al., 1993; Garden et al., 1996; Van Mierlo et al., 1995). In order to improve local control rates in patients with early hypopharyngeal lesions treated with definitive radiotherapy, altered fractionation regimens were also explored by several authors. It was shown that hyperfractionation and accelerated fractionation significantly improve the local control of hypopharyngeal cancers of T2 or greater, and possibly also for T1 tumours. (Fu et al., 2000; Garden et al., 1996 ; Niibe et al., 2003 ; Parsons et al., 1984 ; Rosenthal & Ang, 2004).

The employment of postoperative radiotherapy is recommended in the presence of microscopically involved surgical margins being a pathological feature predicting a high-risk for local recurrence (Cooper et al., 1998). Postoperative concurrent chemoradiotherapy is recommended in the presence of multiple high-risk factors represented by close or positive margins of resection, lymphatic and vascular embolism, perineural infiltration, and cartilage invasion (Bernier et al., 2004; Cooper et al., 2004).

6.1.3 Neck management

Neck management in patients with early hypopharyngeal cancer is also indicated because of the high risk of lymph node metastases (Layland & Sessions, 2005). Elective neck irradiation and elective neck dissection including retropharyngeal nodes are equally and highly effective in managing subclinical neck disease providing regional control of more than 90% (Ambrosch et al., 2001; Bataini, 1993; Pillsbury et al., 1997). Neck lymph node dissection should be performed according to the definitions of the American Academy of Otolaryngology Head and Neck Surgery (AAOHNS) (Robbins et al., 2008). In patients with clinically negative neck, ipsilateral selective neck dissection for lateralised lesions or bilateral selective neck dissection for midline lesions of levels II, III, IV is performed. Neck dissection in clinically N0 patients represents a procedure that has therapeutic value by removal of occult metastatic disease. Neck dissection identifies subclinical nodal disease and, based on pathologic staging, allows the selective use of postoperative concurrent chemoradiotherapy in cases with pathologically proven multiple metastases or nodal extracapsular extension (Pillsbury et al., 1997; Clayman & Frank, 1998). Nodal disease in patients with clinically positive neck (N1) is treated with ipsilateral or bilateral radical neck dissection that refers to the removal of all lymph nodes from levels I through V. Retropharyngeal nodes could be also resected at the time of partial pharyngectomy in patients with radiographic evidence of metastases in this lymph node group. Investigating the significance of dissection of retropharyngeal nodes in hypopharyngeal cancer, Kamiyama R et al. (Kamiyama et al., 2009) concluded that in order to improve prognosis, this dissection should be recommended at the time of primary surgical treatment in cancers whose primary subsites are posterior wall or pyriform sinus.

Patients with clinical N0 disease are eligible for elective radiotherapy of the neck encompassing bilateral lymph nodes in levels II, III and IV. Elective treatment of level VI is indicated for patients with cancer of the pyriform sinus (particularly those located in the apex) and postcricoid area, and for those with esophageal involvement. Elective treatment of the retropharyngeal lymph nodes is indicated for cancer of the posterior pharyngeal wall or postcricoid area, and for those with invasion of the posterior pharyngeal wall from other sites (Gregoire et al., 2003). The determination of the target volume of elective radiotherapy of the neck should follow the consensus guidelines developed by the European Organization for Research and Treatment of Cancer/Radiation Therapy Oncology Group/Danish Head and Neck Cancer Group (EORTC/RTOG/DAHANCA) (Gregoire et al., 2003). According to the recommendations given by Gregoire et al. (Gregoire et al., 2006) for selection and delineation of the levels of lymph nodes for elective irradiation in patients with clinically positive neck and in those with positive neck nodes determined in the surgical specimen following neck dissection, the levels that should be electively treated are I, II, III, IV, V and retropharyngeal nodes, and level VI for esophageal extension. Retrostyloid space should be also included in cases with positive lymph node in Level II whereas supraclavicular fossa should be electively irradiated if there were positive nodes in level IV or V. Given the radiotherapy as primary treatment approach in patients with positive lymph node smaller than 3 cm (N1), it should be mentioned that although there are data from the literature showing that using conventional fractionation, regional control could be achieved in 75%-90% of cases (Bataini et al., 1990; Mendenhall et al., 1984; Taylor et al., 1991), some authors reported lower rates of regional control observed in their studies. Thus, in the study of Johansen et al. (Johansen et al., 2000), definitive radiotherapy resulted in 5-year regional control of 36% for N1 disease. Similar results were found in the retrospective review of patients with hypopharyngeal cancers treated with definitive radiotherapy performed by Gupta et al. (Gupta et al., 2009a) with 3-year locoregional control rate of 41% in patients with N1 disease.

6.2 Surgery and postoperative radiotherapy in locally-regionally advanced resectable lesions

In order to improve outcome in patients with advanced stage resectable hypopharyngeal cancer (T2N1-3M0, T3-4N0-3M0), the role of postoperative radiotherapy following nonconservation surgery became a subject of analysis in many single-institution studies. An improvement in overall and disease-free survival was obtained in patients with locally-regionally advanced hypopharyngeal cancer if combined treatment modality with radical surgery consisting of total laryngectomy, total or partial pharyngectomy and unilateral or bilateral neck dissection followed by radiotherapy was used. Thus, in the 1970s and 1980s, surgery (i.e., total laryngectomy and pharyngectomy with or without neck dissection) followed by postoperative radiotherapy was the standard form of therapy for advanced stage disease (Arriagada et al., 1983; Mirimanoff et al., 1985) with reported 5-year survival rates varying between 19% and 48% (Elias et al., 1995; Kim et al., 2001; Kraus et al., 1997; Lajtmam & Manestar, 2001; Pingree et al., 1987). Comparing the results of total pharyngolaryngectomy, neck dissection, and postoperative radiotherapy in patients with squamous cell carcinoma of the pyriform sinus with those obtained by surgery alone, El Badawi et al. (El Badawi et al., 1982) showed an increased locoregional recurrence rate after surgery alone (39%) as opposed to that following combined therapy (11%). In the analysis of Frank et al. (Frank et al., 1994) surgery and postoperative radiotherapy was found to improve survival in patients with advanced hypopharyngeal cancer. Survival rates at five years for postoperative radiotherapy group and for surgery alone group were 48% and 18%, respectively. Lee et al. (Lee et al., 2008) reported that total laryngectomy with partial or total pharyngectomy with unilateral or bilateral radical neck dissection and postoperative radiotherapy resulted in 3-year local control, disease-free survival, and overall survival rate of 44%, 44%, and 39%, respectively. However, there are some conflicting data in the literature regarding the role of adjuvant radiotherapy. Thus, Yates et al. (Yates et al., 1984), analysing the impact of addition of adjuvant radiotherapy following surgery on survival of patients with squamous cell carcinoma of the pyriform sinus, found that the surgery alone group demonstrated the best results with 5-year survival rate of 56% as compared to 33% for the groups treated with pre- or postoperative radiotherapy. Worse outcome in patients with hypopharyngeal cancer treated with surgery and postoperative radiotherapy as compared with those treated with surgery or radiotherapy alone was also found in the study of Pingree et al. (Pingree et al., 1987). The reported 5-year survival rates for surgery alone, surgery and postoperative radiotherapy, and radiotherapy alone were 40%, 32%, and 11%, respectively.

The prognosis of patients with primary hypopharyngeal tumour and extensive and/or large lymph node metastases is highly determined by the N stage. Radiotherapy or surgery alone in the treatment of advanced nodal disease (N2-3) resulted in poor rates of regional control and survival (Gupta et al., 2009a; Johansen et al., 2000; Lou et al., 2008). In 1988, Teshima et al. (Teshima et al., 1988), analysing the results of radiotherapy in hypopharyngeal cancer with special attention paid to the nodal control, pointed out the role of postoperative radiotherapy in obtaining an effective nodal control for patients with clinically positive nodes. The use of postoperative radiotherapy following neck lymph node dissection is recommended for patients with N2 and N3 disease. Data from literature show improved regional control even in patients with very advanced nodal disease when postoperative radiotherapy was used following radical neck dissection (Ambrosch et al., 2001; Lundahl et al., 1998; Richards & Spiro, 2000; Smeele et al., 2000). Postoperative radiotherapy in patients with resectable locally and/or regionally advanced hypopharyngeal cancer should be prescribed to the entire operative bed and draining nodes. The determination of the target volume of elective radiotherapy of the neck should follow the proposal for delineation of the nodal clinical target volume in the node positive and postoperative neck by Gregoire et al. (Gregoire et al., 2006) (see section 6.1.3). According to the European Society for Medical Oncology (ESMO) clinical recommendations for treatment of squamous cell carcinoma of the head and neck, the standard option for advanced resectable hypopharyngeal cancers is represented by surgery and postoperative radiotherapy in patients without high-risk pathological features found at surgery (Pivot & Felip, 2008). However, despite such radical therapy leading to the loss of natural speech function and impairment of swallowing ability with a consequent negative impact on the quality of life, cure rates for advanced disease remained low with reported 5-year survival rates varying between 20% and 50% (Beauvillain et al., 1997; Hoffman et al., 1998; Johansen et al., 2000; Kim et al., 2004; Lajtmam & Manestar, 2001).

The confirmed negative influence of high-risk pathological features represented by surgical margins microscopically involved, extracapsular extension in positive lymph node, two or more positive lymph nodes, vascular embolism and perineural infiltration on patients outcome following surgery and postoperative radiotherapy (Ang et al., 2001), emerged the need for investigation of different treatment approaches including concomitant use of chemotherapy. Two similar, large-scale, postoperative randomised independent trials designed by the EORTC and RTOG were conducted to evaluate the role of high dose concurrent chemoradiotherapy in the postoperative treatment of high risk head and neck tumours (Bernier et al., 2004; Cooper et al., 2004). Both trials evaluated the role of concomitant cisplatin given every 3 weeks (100 mg/m^2 on days 1, 22, 43) during radiotherapy course (Table 2). Retrospective analysis of data from both trials, revealed that extracapsular extension of nodal disease and/or microscopically involved surgical margins were the only risk factors for which the impact of concurrent chemoradiotherapy was significant in both trials (Bernier & Cooper, 2005). In 2004, National Cancer Institute (NCI) level I evidence for recommendation was established, because both studies demonstrated that adjuvant concurrent chemoradiotherapy was more efficacious with respect to radiotherapy alone in terms of locoregional control and disease-free survival (Bernier & Cooper, 2005). Currently, concurrent chemoradiotherapy with single agent platinum should be the gold standard for those patients found at surgery to have high-risk features (extracapsular extension and positive margins of resection) (Pivot et al., 2008).

Based on the assumption that surgery may be a trigger of accelerated proliferation of remaining tumour cells, two phase III trials conducted to investigate the role of accelerated fractionation in the postoperative setting compared to conventionally fractionated postoperative radiotherapy (Ang et al., 2001; Sanguineti et al., 2005) failed to demonstrate any significant improvement of locoregional control and survival with accelerated postoperative radiotherapy. However, when in a phase III trial a weekendless continuous accelerated hyperfractionation postoperative radiotherapy (CHARTWEL) was employed in advanced squamous cell carcinoma of the oral cavity, larynx and hypopharynx who underwent radical surgery, the overall treatment time was shortened to only 12 days compared with conventionally fractionated radiotherapy (Awwad et al., 2002). The data from this trial revealed significantly better 3-year locoregional control rate in the accelerated fractionation group than in the conventional fractionation group (88% and 57%, respectively) suggesting that accelerated proliferation could be considered an important determinant of treatment outcome.

Trial	DFS	OS	LRFR
Bernier et al. (Bernier et al., 2004), (EORTC 22931)	(5-year estimates)	(5-year estimates)	(5-year estimates)
Experimental arm:	47% (p=0.04)	53% (p=0.02)	17% (p=0.007)
Control arm:	36%	40%	31%
Cooper et al. (Cooper et al., 2004), (RTOG 9501)	(2-year estimates)	(2-year estimates)	(2-year estimates)
Experimental arm:	54% (p=0.04)	64% (p=0.19)	18% (p=0.01)
Control arm:	45%	57%	28%

EORTC: European Organization for Research and Treatment of Cancer; DFS: disease-free survival; OS: overall survival; LRFR: locoregional failure rate; RTOG, Radiation Therapy Oncology Group

Table 2. Comparative analysis of treatment outcome in EORTC trial 22931 and RTOG trial 9501

6.3 Definitive treatment for anatomic and functional organ preservation in locally-regionally advanced resectable lesions

Primary definitive therapy in patients with advanced resectable hypopharyngeal cancers requiring total laryngectomy and partial or total pharyngectomy can also be realised with treatment modalities allowing organ preservation. Strategies employed to increase locoregional control and survival attempting at the same time to achieve anatomic and functional organ preservation include concurrent chemoradiotherapy, altered fractionation radiotherapy, intensified radiotherapy regimens in combination with chemotherapy, induction chemotherapy followed by radiotherapy, and targeted therapy using cetuximab. Concurrent drug-enhanced radiotherapy i.e. concurrent chemoradiotherapy (in relatively healthy patients) and altered fractionation radiation regimens (in relatively unfit patients), are considered best established as organ preservation approaches for cancers arising from hypopharynx and other sites in the head and neck region (Adelstein et al., 2000; Forastiere et al., 2001a; Fu et al., 2000; Koch et al., 1995; Pignon et al., 2000).

6.3.1 Concurrent chemoradiotherapy

Concurrent chemoradiotherapy as definitive treatment for advanced head and neck cancers including those arising from the hypopharynx has been studied in the past 15 years. However, due to the low incidence, hypopharyngeal cancers grouped with other head and neck cancers usually represented only smaller subgroups with details of their treatment being rarely specifically reported (Tai et al., 2008; Robson, 2002). The rarity of this disease, and the time needed for data collection could be accepted as an explanation for the absence of multicenter randomised clinical trials undertaken to evaluate the role of concurrent chemoradiotherapy in the treatment of advanced hypopharyngeal cancer. In 1990 Sanchiz et al. (Sanchiz et al., 1990) reported the results of a prospective randomised trial on 859 patients with advanced head and neck cancer including those having hypopharynx as a primary site. Patients were randomly assigned to receive conventionally fractionated radiotherapy, radiotherapy with standard fractionation with concomitant use of 5-fluorouracil or hyperfractionated radiotherapy. Significant improvement in survival compared with the group treated with conventional fractionation was obtained in groups treated either with concurrent chemoradiotherapy or altered fractionation (Table 3). Adelstein et al. (Adelstein et al., 2000) reported a single institution trial that enrolled 100 patients with stages III and IV squamous cell head and neck carcinoma. Patients were randomly assigned to receive conventionally fractionated radiotherapy alone or with concurrent chemotherapy consisting of two cycles of cisplatin and 5-fluorouracil. Planned neck dissection was encountered for patients with N2 and N3 disease. A significant improvement in the rates of local control (77% vs. 45%, $p < 0.001$), distant metastasis-free survival (84% vs. 75%, $p = 0.09$), and 5-year recurrence-free survival (62% vs. 51%, $p = 0.04$) was obtained with concurrent chemoradiotherapy (Table 3). The superiority of concurrent chemoradiotherapy in the improvement of overall survival in patients with advanced head and neck cancer has been confirmed in several meta-analyses (Browman et al., 2001; El-Sayed & Nelson, 1996; Munro, 1995; Pignon et al., 2000). The results of meta-analysis reported by Munro (Munro, 1995), and the results of meta-analysis of El-Sayed and Nelson (El-Sayed & Nelson, 1996) showed a statistically significant improvement in survival for chemotherapy given concurrently with radiotherapy. The largest meta-analysis performed by the Meta-Analysis of Chemotherapy on Head and Neck Cancer (MACH-NC) Collaborative Group and published by Pignon et al. (Pignon et al., 2000) in 2000, evaluated individual patient data from 63 randomised trials excluding trials on nasopharyngeal carcinoma. This meta-analysis confirmed the superiority of the overall use of chemotherapy with 5% improvement in 5-year overall survival with highest increase in survival with use of concurrent chemoradiotherapy (8% at 5-years; $p < 0.0001$). There was also an evident benefit when cisplatin was used in the combined approach. In patients over 70 years the benefit was less evident. In the updated meta-analysis published in 2004 (Bourhis et al., 2004), 24 new trials, most of them on concurrent chemoradiotherapy, were included totalising 87 trials and 16,000 patients. The update confirmed survival benefit of 8% at 5 years ($p < 0.0001$) of concurrent chemoradiotherapy. This updated analysis also confirmed the higher magnitude of the benefit for platinum-based chemotherapy. A decreasing effect of chemotherapy with age was also shown ($p = 0.01$). The overall survival gain was better for concurrent chemoradiotherapy with altered fractionation compared with concurrent chemoradiotherapy with conventional fractionation, indicating that alteration of fractionation might boost the effect of chemoradiotherapy. In the meta-analysis conducted by Browman et al. (Browman et al., 2001), only platinum-based chemotherapy given concomitantly with radiotherapy was found highly significant in overall survival improvement ($p < 0.0001$). The German meta-analysis suggested that, considering only concurrent chemoradiotherapy without prolonged overall treatment time, an absolute survival gain of 13% to 15% at 2 years with respect to conventional radiotherapy can be obtained (Budach et al., 2006). The extensive research of the influence of the addition of chemotherapy to radiotherapy on overall survival resulted in confirmation that only concurrent chemoradiotherapy as definitive treatment for patients with locoregionally advanced head and neck cancer including those with advanced hypopharyngeal cancer has succeeded to improve outcomes. Thus, evidence based medicine has shown that concurrent chemoradiotherapy without prolongation of overall treatment time and including cisplatin only or cisplatin-5-fluorouracil should be considered the treatment of choice for patients who fit chemotherapy (National Cancer Institute [NCI] level 1 of evidence supporting recommendation) (Corvo, 2007).

Authors	*Number of patients*	*Therapy regimens*	*Treatment results*	*Complications*
Chemotherapy given concurrently with conventionally fractionated radiotherapy regimens				
Sanchiz et al. (Sanchiz et al., 1990)	N=859, Arm A=277, Arm B=282, Arm C=300 Nh=119, Arm A=37, Arm B=36, Arm C=46	Arm A: 60 Gy given with 2.0 Gy/fx/d, 5 fx /wk vs. Arm B: 70.4 Gy given in 2.2 Gy/fx/twice daily vs. Arm C: 60 Gy given with 2.0 Gy/fx/d, 5 fx /wk plus 5-FU 250 mg/m^2 given i.v. on alternate days	5-year OS, 31% in Arm A vs. 59% in Arm B vs. 63% in Arm C Arm A vs. Arm B (p<0.001); Arm A vs. Arm C (p<0.001); Arm B vs. Arm C (n.s.)	Grade 3 mucositis, 6% in Arm A vs. 4% in Arm B vs. 10% in Arm C; no significant difference in acute and late toxic effects
Adelstein et al. (Adelstein et al., 2000)	N=100, Arm A=50, Arm B=50 Nh=16, Arm A=9, Arm B=7	Arm A: 66-72 Gy given with 1.8-2.0 Gy/fx/d, 5 fx /wk vs. Arm B: same RT regimen plus concurrent 5-FU 1000 mg/m^2/d and cisplatin 20 mg/m^2/d both given as continuous infusion over 4 days beginning on days 1 and 22 of RT	5-year LRC, 45% in Arm A vs. 77% in Arm B (p<0.001); 5-year RFS, 51% in Arm A vs. 62% in Arm B (p=0.04); 5-year DMFS, 75% in Arm A vs. 84% in Arm B (p=0.09) 5-year OS, 34% in Arm A vs. 42% in Arm B (p=0.004)	Significantly more acute toxicity in Arm B (Grade 3 or 4 neutropenia, thrombocytopenia, cutaneous reactions, and mucositis); no significant difference in late toxic effects.
Adelstein et al. (Adelstein et al., 2003)	N=271, Arm A=95, Arm B=87, Arm C=89 Nh=50, Arm A=19, Arm B=17, Arm C=14	Arm A: 70 Gy given with 2.0 Gy/fx/d, 5 fx /wk vs. Arm B: same RT regimen plus concurrent cisplatin 100 mg/m^2 i.v. on days 1, 22 and 43 vs. Arm C: same RT regimen with 3 courses of a 4-day continuous infusion of 5-FU 1,000 mg/m^2/d, with cisplatin bolus injection of 75 mg/m^2 on day 1, given every 4 weeks	3-year DSS, 33% in Arm A vs. 51% in Arm B vs. 41% in Arm C Arm A vs. Arm B (p=0.01); Arm A vs. Arm C (n.s.) 3-year OS, 23% in Arm A vs. 37% in Arm B vs. 27% in Arm C Arm A vs. Arm B (p=0.014); Arm A vs. Arm C (n.s.); Arm B vs. Arm C (n.s.)	Grade 3 or worse acute toxic effects, 52% in Arm A vs. 89% in Arm B (p<0.0001); late toxic effects not reported
Chemotherapy given concurrently with intensified radiotherapy regimens				
Brizel et al. (Brizel et al., 1998)	N=116, Arm A=60, Arm B=56 Nh=23, Arm A=10, Arm B=13	Arm A: 75 Gy as 1.25 Gy/fx/twice daily vs. Arm B: 70 Gy given with 1.25 Gy/fx/twice daily (7-10 days break after 40 Gy) plus cisplatin 12 mg/m^2/d and 5-FU 600 mg/m^2/d in week 1 and 6	3-year LRC, 44% in Arm A vs. 70% in Arm B (p=0.01); 3-year RFS, 41% in Arm A vs. 61% in Arm B (p=0.08); 3-year OS, 34% in Arm A vs. 55% in Arm B (p=0.07)	Similar mucositis; increased enteral feeding and sepsis with combination therapy; no difference in late toxic effects
Wendt et al. (Wendt et al., 1998)	N=270, Arm A=140, Arm B=130 Nh=97, Arm A=50, Arm B=47	Arm A: 70.2 Gy given with 1.8 Gy/fx/twice daily in 3 courses with 10-day break vs. Arm B: same RT regimen plus cisplatin 60 mg/m^2, 5-FU 350 mg/m^2 by i.v. bolus, and LV 50 mg/m^2 by i.v. bolus given on day 2, and 5-FU 350 mg/m^2/24 hour by continuous infusion and LV 100 mg/m^2/24 hours by continuous infusion given from day 2 to 5 starting on days 22 and 44	3-year LRC, 17% in Arm A vs. 36% in Arm B (p<0.004); 3-year OS, 24% in Arm A vs. 48% in Arm B (p<0.0003)	Grade 3-4 acute mucositis, 16% in Arm A vs. 38% in Arm B (p<0.001); no significant difference in late toxic effects

Authors	*Number of patients*	*Therapy regimens*	*Treatment results*	*Complications*
Jeremic et al. (Jeremic et al., 2000)	N=130, Arm A=65, Arm B=65 Nh=21, Arm A=11, Arm B=10	Arm A: 77 Gy given in 1.1 Gy/fx/twice daily vs. Arm B: same RT regimen plus cisplatin 6 mg/m²/d	5-year LRPFS, 36% in Arm A vs. 50% in Arm B (p=0.04); 5-year PFS, 25% in Arm A vs. 46% in Arm B (p=0.007); 5-year DMFS, 57 in Arm A % vs. 86% in Arm B (p=0.001); 5-year OS, 25% in Arm A vs. 46% in Arm B (p=0.008)	No significant difference in acute toxic effects with exception to leucopenia grade 3/4 (0% in Arm A vs. 12%, in Arm B [p=0.006]); no difference in late toxic effects
Staar et al. (Staar et al., 2001)	N=240, Arm A=127, Arm B=113 Nh=62, Arm A=26, Arm B=36	Arm A: 69.9 Gy over 5,5 weeks (1.8 Gy/fx/d for 3.5 weeks, then, individual fx of 1.8 Gy and 1.5 Gy daily for 2 weeks plus carboplatin 70 mg/m²/d and 5-FU (600 mg/m²/d) for 2 cycles of 5 days vs. Arm B: same RT regimen alone	2-year LRC, 51% in Arm A vs. 45% in Arm B (p=0.14) 1-year SLC, 58% in Arm A vs. 44% in Arm B (p=0.05); 2-year OS, 48% in Arm A vs. 39% in Arm B (p=0.09)	Grade 3-4 mucositis, 68% in Arm A vs. 52% in Arm B (p=0.01); feeding tube dependency, 51% in Arm A vs. 25% Arm B (p=0.02)
Huguenin et al. (Huguenin et al., 2004)	N=224, Arm A=112, Arm B=112 Nh=55, Arm A=27, Arm B=28	Arm A: 74.4 Gy given in 1.2 Gy/fx/twice daily vs. Arm B: same RT regimen plus cisplatin 20 mg/m²/d on 5 days of weeks 1 and 5	5-year LRC, 33% in Arm A vs. 51% in Arm B (p=0.039); 5-year OS, 32% in Arm A vs. 46% in Arm B (p=0.15)	Grade 3 mucositis, 61% in Arm A vs. 59% in Arm B; no significant differences in acute and late toxic effects
Budach et al. (Budach et al., 2005)	N=384, Arm A=194, Arm B=190 Nh=124, Arm A=62, Arm B=62	Arm A: 14 Gy given with 2.0 Gy/fx/d, followed by 1.4 Gy/fx/twice daily to a total dose of 77.6 Gy vs. Arm B: 30 Gy given with 2.0 Gy/fx/d, followed by 1.4 Gy/fx/twice daily to a total dose of 70.6 Gy concurrently with 5-FU 600 mg/m² given as continuous infusion and mitomycin 10 mg/m² given on days 5 and 36	5-year LRC, 37.4% in Arm A vs. 49.9% in Arm B (p=0.001); 5-year OS, 23.7% in Arm A vs. 28.6% in Arm B (p=0.023); 5-year PFS, 26.6% in Arm A vs. 29.3% in Arm B (p=0.009)	Grade 3-4 mucositis, 65.7% in Arm A vs. 75.7% in Arm B (p=0.045); grade 3 skin reaction 29.6% in Arm A vs. 46.3% in Arm B (p=0.002); no difference in late toxic effects

Nh: number of patients with hypopharyngeal cancer; fx: fraction, d: day, wk: per week; 5-FU: 5-fluorouracil; i.v.: intravenously; OS: overall survival; n.s.: not significant; RT: radiotherapy; LRC: locoregional control; RFS: recurrence-free survival; DMFS: distant metastases-free survival; DSS: disease-specific survival; LV: leucovorin; LRPFS: locoregional progression-free survival; PFS: progression-free survival; SLC: survival with local control

Table 3. Randomised studies comparing concurrent chemoradiotherapy with radiotherapy alone in patients with advanced head and neck cancer

Regarding the question about the number of drugs that can be added to radiotherapy and the timing of drug delivery once must be admitted that the optimum regimen is not yet known. The most common method used was delivery of drugs every 3 weeks (Adelstein et al., 1997; Adelstein et al., 2000) with the most frequently used regimen being the one proposed by Adelstein et al. (Adelstein et al., 2003) based on three courses of cisplatin every 3 weeks (100 mg/m² on days 1, 22, and 43) (Table 3). Weekly (Gupta et al., 2009b), or daily (Jeremic et al., 1997; Jeremic et al., 2000) administration of single-agent cisplatin has been also studied. According to the results of the meta-analysis of the MACH-NC Collaborative Group, platinum-based chemotherapy was more effective than non-platinum containing regimens, but multiagent therapy was not better than single agent. The superiority of platinum-based chemotherapy has been also confirmed in the meta-analysis of Browman et al. (Browman et al., 2001). According to Pignon et al. (Pignon et al., 2005), clinical benefit might be obtained even with a total dose of cisplatin of only 200 mg given in different timing concurrently with radiotherapy. Preliminary results from Radiation Therapy Oncology Group (RTOG) 97-03 three-arm randomised phase II trial enrolling patients with stage III or IV squamous carcinoma of the oral cavity, oropharynx, or hypopharynx revealed that concurrent radiotherapy and two-drug chemotherapy using either paclitaxel plus cisplatin, 5-fluorouracil plus cisplatin, or hyroxiurea plus 5-fluorouracil was feasible (Garden et al., 2004a). However, there was no phase III trial performed to show taxane-based concurrent chemoradiotherapy to be superior to radiotherapy alone, and no randomised trial has demonstrated a taxane, either as a single agent or in combination with other drugs to be superior to single-agent, platinum-based concurrent chemoradiotherapy.

6.3.2 Altered fractionation radiotherapy

Another approach focused on improvement of locoregional control and organ preservation in patients with locally advanced head and neck cancer was the investigation of modification of conventionally fractionated radiotherapy. Two prototypes of altered radiation fractionation regimens (hyperfractionation and accelerated fractionation) have been tested in retrospective and randomised trials for the last three decades. Promising improvements in locoregional control with the use of altered fractionated radiation schedules in the treatment of advanced head and cancer were demonstrated in several single-institution studies (Parsons et al., 1993; Wang et al., 1985). On the contrary, a retrospective study of Garden et al (Garden et al., 1995) did non reveal statistically significant differences in local control rates and survival rates between patients with carcinoma of the larynx or hypopharynx treated with conventional fractionation and those irradiated with hyperfractionation. However, only small number of studies referred on the role of altered fractionation exclusively in patients with advanced hypopharyngeal cancer. In one of those studies in which conventional radiotherapy was compared with hyperfractionated radiotherapy, multivariate analysis showed that twice-daily fractionation was the most important treatment-related variable in patients with squamous cell carcinoma of the pharyngeal wall (Fein et al., 1993). Retrospectively analising the results of definitive radiotherapy in patients with hypopharyngeal cancer, Antognoni et al (Antognoni et al., 1991) did not show any impact of fractionation regimen on patients outcome. On the contrary, in the retrospective study on 52 patients with hypopharyngeal carcinoma, significantly better 5-year survival rate was obtained with accelerated hyperfractionation (44%) than with conventional fractionation (12%) (Akimoto et al., 1996).

The largest prospective randomised trial undertaken to compare standard fractionation radiotherapy against hyperfractionation and accelerated fractionation with split course and accelerated radiotherapy with concomitant boost in the management of patients with advanced head and neck squamous cell carcinoma was RTOG trial 9003 (Fu et al., 2000). The results of this four-arm trial of 1073 patients with locally advanced head and neck cancer, showed that the locoregional control was significantly increased by increase of the total dose without changing the overall time using hyperfractionation (2-year locoregional control 54.4% with hyperfractionation vs. 46% with conventional fractionation, $p = 0.045$) without increase in overall survival. The results also revealed that accelerated fractionation with concomitant boost yielded a significantly better locoregional control than standard radiotherapy (2-year locoregional control 54.5% with accelerated fractionation with concomitant boost vs. 46% with conventional fractionation, $p = 0.05$) and a trend toward improved disease-free survival (2-year disease-free survival 39% with accelerated fractionation with concomitant boost vs. 32% with conventional fractionation, $p = 0.054$). Concerning the treatment related toxicity, hyperfractionation induced more severe acute mucositis compared to the conventional fractionation arm, and accelerated fractionation with concomitant boost-arm had significantly higher grade 3 or worse acute side effects ($p < 0.0001$) and significantly increased grade 3 or worse late side effects ($p < 0.011$). It should be pointed out that this most important randomised trial was not site specific to the hypopharynx. Results of recently published randomised controlled clinical study of accelerated fractionation performed by the national Swedish group including 750 patients with squamous cell carcinoma of the oral cavity, oropharynx, larynx and hypopharynx did not prove that accelerated radiotherapy was more efficacious compared with conventional radiotherapy in terms of both locoregional control and overall survival (Zackrisson et al., 2011). This randomised trial was also not site specific to the hypopharynx.

Meta-analysis undertaken by Meta-Analysis of Radiotherapy in Carcinomas of the Head and Neck (MARCH) Collaborative Group (Bourhis et al., 2006) and aimed to assess whether different types of altered fractionated radiotherapy in head and neck squamous cell carcinoma could improve survival compared with conventional radiotherapy, included findings of 15 trials with 6,515 patients. This meta-analysis of updated individual patient data showed an improvement of 6.4% of locoregional control (from 46% to 53%, $p < 0.0001$), and an improvement of 3.4% of overall survival (from 36% to 39%, $p < 0.03$) with altered fractionation. The benefit in overall survival was significantly higher with hyperfractionation regimen (8% at 5 years) than with accelerated radiotherapy. The advantage of hyperfractionation was also confirmed in the German meta-analysis by Budach et al (Budach et al., 2006). The findings of this meta-analysis based on published data suggested that, among different types of altered radiotherapy, hyperfractionation obtained better 2-year overall survival than conventional radiotherapy with a significant benefit of 12 months ($p < 0.001$). According to the results of randomised trials exploring altered fractionation regimens and considering the results of the two meta-analyses, evidence based medicine showed that acceleration of radiation of one week without dose reduction and hyperfractionation are consistently better than conventional fractionation for locoregional control of intermediate to advanced carcinomas without an increase in late toxic effects (National Cancer Institute [NCI] level 1 of evidence supporting recommendation).

6.3.3 Intensified radiotherapy regimens in combination with chemotherapy

Altered fractionated radiotherapy with concurrent chemotherapy has been also evaluated. In a phase II study at a single institution conducted by Prades et al. (Prades et al., 2002), there were no statistically significant differences observed in overall and disease-free survival between patients with pyriform sinus cancer treated with accelerated radiotherapy alone and those treated with intensified concurrent chemoradiotherapy. In a single institution phase II trial exploring organ preservation using split hyperfractionated accelerated radiation therapy and concomitant cisplatin in patients with advanced cancer of the larynx and hypopharynx, De la Vega et al. (De la Vega et al., 2003) found organ preservation possible in 44% of patients. The encouraging results of RTOG phase II trial 99-14 conducted to evaluate the accelerated radiotherapy using concomitant boost combined with two cycles of concurrent cisplatin in patients with stage III and IV squamous cell carcinoma of the oral cavity, oropharynx, hypopharynx, or larynx (Ang et al., 2005) suggesting that intensified radiotherapy regimens could be combined safely with chemotherapy motivated a phase III trial (RTOG H0129) predicted to determine whether accelerated fractionation using concomitant boost plus cisplatin can lead to better results compared with conventionally fractionated radiotherapy in combination with concurrent use of cisplatin.

Several randomised trials exploring intensified radiotherapy regimens in combination with chemotherapy in advanced head and neck cancer included patients with hypopharyngeal cancer (Brizel et al., 1998; Budach et al., 2005; Huguenin et al., 2004; 2004; Jeremic et al., 2000; Staar et al., 2001; Wendt et al., 1998) (Table 3). In a single institution study reported by Brizel et al. (Brizel et al., 1998) better locoregional control was achieved by concurrent chemoradiotherapy without any improvement in overall survival (Table 3). Wendt et al. (Wendt et al. 1998) reporting the results of a regimen consisting of split-course altered fractionation plus chemotherapy concluded that concurrent chemoradiotherapy offered significantly improved 3-year locoregional control and overall survival rate with acute reactions more pronounced in the concurrent chemoradiotherapy arm (Table 3). In a study of hyperfractionation, Jeremic et al. (Jeremic et al., 2000) reported a significant improvement in 3-year locoregional control, overall survival and distant-metastases-free survival with hyperfractionated radiotherapy and concurrent low-dose daily cisplatin as compared with hyperfractionation alone (Table 3). The reported frequency of acute mucositis and late complications were similar in both arms. The improvement of therapeutic index of hyperfractionated radiotherapy by concomitant cisplatin has been also confirmed in the randomised trial conducted by Huguenin et al. (Huguenin et al., 2004). In the multicentric randomised German trial conducted by German Cooperative Group (Staar et al., 2001), a concomitant boost accelerated fractionation alone was compared with the same radiotherapy regimen plus carboplatin and 5-fluorouracil (Table 3). The authors concluded that the efficiency of intensified concurrent chemoradiotherapy was less then expected when compared to radiotherapy alone. Updated results of this trial have shown no improvement in locoregional failure-free survival and overall survival among patients with hypopharyngeal cancer treated with intensified regimen (Semrau et al., 2006). Reporting final results of a prospective randomised study in locally advanced head and neck cancer comparing concurrent 5-fluorouracil and mitomycin chemotherapy and hyperfractionated accelerated radiotherapy to hyperfractionated accelerated radiotherapy alone, Budach et al. (Budach et al., 2005) have shown a locoregional control and survival benefit when altered fractionation in combination with chemotherapy was used without any efficacy benefit revealed in patients with advanced hypopharyngeal cancer (Table 3). It must be emphasized that in patients with advanced cancer of the hypopharynx intensified radiotherapy regimens in combination with chemotherapy currently do not represent a routinely recommended treatment.

6.3.4 Adjuvant neck dissection following concurrent chemoradiotherapy

General consensus exists that adjuvant neck dissection is not necessary for patients with N1 disease who have complete response to concurrent chemoradiotherapy in the neck. Although it has been shown that concurrent chemoradiotherapy provided good regional control even in patients with advanced N-stage disease, there was an increased risk of residual disease observed with the increased stage of nodal disease (Boyd et al., 1998) with residual tumour found in approximately one third of the surgical specimens when treatment included planned neck dissection following chemoradiotherapy (Haraf et al., 1991; Sanguineti et al., 1999). Randomised studies addressing the question of best approach for patients who achieved a clinical complete response after concurrent chemoradiotherapy for initial N2 or N3 disease are lacking. Although regional control remained higher with adjuvant neck dissection following hyperfractionated or accelerated radiotherapy regimens (Mendenhall et al., 2002) the role of adjuvant neck dissection following concurrent chemoradiotherapy for patients with N2 or N3 disease is controversial (Brizel et al., 2004; Grabenbauer et al., 2003). Current recommendations range from planned neck dissection for all patients with pretreatment N2 or N3 disease to neck dissection only in patients with radiographic or clinical evidence of residual disease. Adjuvant neck dissection should be performed 6 to 10 weeks after completion of concurrent chemoradiotherapy. The avoidance of expected increased treatment related morbidity should be obtained by performing modified or selective dissections with removal of nodes only from levels II-IV.

6.3.5 Induction chemotherapy

Several studies were performed to evaluate the role of induction chemotherapy followed by definitive radiotherapy in obtaining functional organ preservation in advanced resectable hypopharyngeal cancer. The general approach was that patients were given two to three cycles of induction chemotherapy followed by definitive radiotherapy, with surgery reserved for nonresponse to induction chemotherapy, persistent disease after radiation, or relapse. Results of retrospective studies on patients with resectable, locally advanced hypopharyngeal cancers requiring total laryngectomy treated with one to three cycles of induction cisplatin-based chemotherapy followed by definitive radiotherapy in the presence of complete or partial response to chemotherapy at the primary site have shown a rate of larynx preservation ranging between 32% and 52% (Kim et al., 1998; Kraus et al., 1994; Zelefsky et al., 1996). Comparing results regarding locoregional control, disease-free survival, and overall survival achieved with this treatment approach with results obtained with surgery and postoperative radiotherapy in patients with similarly staged disease, it has been suggested that induction chemotherapy followed by definitive radiotherapy could be considered an effective strategy to achieve organ preservation without compromising survival in patients with advanced cancer of the hypopharynx (Kim et al., 1998).

There were few randomised phase III studies conducted on patients with hypopharyngeal cancers eligible only for total laryngectomy with partial pharyngectomy, comparing surgery and postoperative radiotherapy with two or three cycles of induction cisplatin/5-fluorouracil chemotherapy followed by radiotherapy in clinically complete responders, or total laryngectomy for those who had not a complete response (Lefebvre et al., 1996), or induction chemotherapy plus radiotherapy with induction chemotherapy plus surgery plus radiotherapy (Beauvillain et al., 1997), or induction chemotherapy followed by radiotherapy with concurrent chemoradiotherapy (Prades et al., 2010). In the randomised phase III study 24891 conducted by EORTC, survival did not differ between treatment groups and functional larynx was retained in 50% of the survivors in the chemoradiotherapy group (Lefebvre et al., 1996). The results from this trial were confirmed by its long term evaluation

(Lefebvre et al., 2004). In the French randomised trial conducted by Beauvillian et al. (Beauvillain et al., 1997), statistically improved 5-year local control and overall survival was found in patients treated with induction chemotherapy followed by total laryngopharyngectomy and postoperative radiotherapy. Larynx preservation was obtained in 38% of patients treated with induction chemotherapy followed by definitive radiotherapy. Nevertheless, several meta-analyses have failed to demonstrate any significant improvement in survival after induction chemotherapy followed by radiotherapy (Browman, 1994; El-Sayed & Nelson, 1996; Pignon et al., 2000). The largest and most detailed of these, the meta-analysis of the MACH-NC Collaborative Group, analysed data from 31 trials of induction chemotherapy with more than 5,200 patients enrolled, and reported 2% 5-year improvement in overall survival being statistically nonsignificant ($p = 0.38$) (Pignon et al., 2000).

The renewed interest in induction chemotherapy arisen from data showing treatment failure due to the development of distant metastases in 1 of 5 patients with stage III-IV head and neck cancer treated with multimodality approaches including concurrent chemoradiotherapy (Bernier & Bentzen, 2003) led to the evaluation of the use of both induction chemotherapy and concurrent chemoradiotherapy in a sequential approach supposed to provide optimal benefit for this patients category. In the light of emerged need to improve overall treatment outcome in patients with locoregionally advanced head and neck cancer, the results of sequential therapy could be considered especially important for patients with advanced cancers of the hypopharynx because this primary site has been found to be an independent predictor for distant metastases development (Adelstein et al., 2006a). Both randomised phase III studies performed to evaluate sequential therapy with induction chemotherapy, the TAX 324 study (Posner et al., 2007) and the study conducted by the investigators in Madrid (Hitt et al., 2005) confirmed the benefit of induction chemotherapy using a triplet combination including taxane followed by concurrent chemoradiotherapy. However, there would be no level 1 of evidence data showing the superiority of induction chemotherapy followed by concurrent chemoradiotherapy over concurrent chemoradiotherapy until ongoing randomised, phase III trials comparing sequential therapy versus concurrent chemoradiotherapy complete (Adelstein et al., 2006b; Posner, 2005).

6.3.6 Targeted therapy with cetuximab

Based upon the evidence of increased levels of Epidermal Growth Factor Receptor (EGFR) expression in the majority of head and neck cancer, and the associated poor outcome with its presence (Chung et al., 2006), the addition of molecular targeted therapies in head and neck cancer was assumed as another potential method offering further improve outcome. A large international multicenter randomised phase III clinical study was performed in which radiotherapy alone was compared with radiotherapy plus weekly cetuximab at an initial dose of 400 mg/m^2 followed by 250 mg/m^2 weekly for the duration of radiotherapy in patients with stage III-IV cancer of the oropharynx, larynx or hypopharynx (Bonner et al., 2006). In this study, radiotherapy was delivered either with conventional fractionation or with altered fractionation (hyperfractionation or concomitant boost accelerated radiotherapy). The median survival, and the observed rates of locoregional control and overall survival at 3 years were significantly higher in patients treated with radiotherapy plus cetuximab than those in patients treated with radiotherapy alone. However, the median duration of overall survival for patients with hypopharyngeal cancer was equal in both treatment groups. Reporting the 5-year survival data from this study, Bonner et al. (Bonner et al., 2010) showed significantly improved overall survival at 5 years for patients treated with cetuximab and radiotherapy compared with that achieved in the radiotherapy-alone group. The results from this prospective randomised trial support the superiority of concurrent targeted antibody enhanced radiotherapy over radiotherapy alone for advanced disease (NCI level of evidence Iii A for a single phase III trial, level 2 for recommendation). It has been suggested that it is reasonable to consider this regimen of radiotherapy plus cetuximab in patients with coexisting medical conditions and poor performance status who are not good candidates for concurrent chemoradiotherapy or surgery (Garden et al., 2004b; Seiwert & Cohen, 2005).

6.4 Unresectable M0 disease

The published guidelines by the National Comprehensive Cancer Network (NCCN) for technical unresectability criteria including evidence for direct invasion of cervical vertebrae or brachial plexus and direct involvement of deep muscles of the neck or carotid artery, provided a general framework to clearly define tumours being unresectable if anatomic considerations make it unlikely that all gross tumour can be removed or that local control can be achieved after resection even with the addition of postoperative radiotherapy (Forastiere et al., 2005). Patients presenting with unresectable hypopharyngeal cancer without evidence of distant metastases may be considered appropriate for localised and systemic treatment. However, historically speaking, conventionally fractionated radiotherapy offering low probability of cure was considered palliative when used as a single treatment modality in patients with unresectable disease. In order to improve locoregional control and to influence on prolongation of survival, the integration of chemotherapy with radiotherapy has been used as multimodality treatment approach for unresectable disease (Vokes & Weichselbaum, 1990). Induction chemotherapy with rare exception has not been shown to improve survival in patients with unresectable disease. A benefit from induction chemotherapy in term of overall survival has been suggested in the subset analysis of inoperable patients in the large study by Paccagnella et al. (Paccagnella et al., 1994). The subset analysis of the updated results for overall survival after a minimum follow-up of 10 years reported by Zorat et al. (Zorat et al., 2004) showed that among inoperable patients, there was a statistically significant better survival observed in the induction chemotherapy group compared to patients who did not receive induction chemotherapy. The EORTC 24971/TAX 323, a phase III study of 358 patients with unresectable locoregionally advanced head and neck cancer showed that the addition of docetaxel to cisplatin and 5-fluorouracil for induction and given before radiotherapy improved both progression-free and overall survival with less toxicity compared to cisplatin and 5-fluorouracil induction chemotherapy (Vermorken et al., 2007). Analysing the results of EORTC 24971/TAX 323 study in terms of symptom control and quality of life, Van Herpen et al. (Van Herpen et al., 2010) revealed that induction chemotherapy with docetaxel, cisplatin and 5-fluorouracil followed by definitive radiotherapy not only improved survival and reduced toxicity compared with cisplatin plus 5-fluorouracil based induction chemotherapy, but also had a substantial impact on improvement of quality of life in patients with unresectable locoregionally advanced disease. Randomised phase II studies comparing concurrent cisplatin-based chemoradiotherapy and induction chemotherapy followed by definitive radiotherapy in patients with unresectable head and neck cancer did not reveal any statistically significant difference in the overall survival between treatment groups, but taking into account the similar activity of two treatment schedules and the better compliance associated with the concurrent treatment, authors suggested that concurrent chemoradiotherapy might be considered an option in this patients category (Pinnaro et al., 1994; Taylor et al., 1994). In the Intergroup phase III study of Southwest Oncology Group (SWOG) and Eastern Cooperative Oncology Group (ECOG) for locally advanced and unresectable head and neck cancer, statistically significant difference in favour of concurrent chemoradiotherapy was observed only between cisplatin plus radiotherapy and radiotherapy alone (Adelstein et al., 2003). However, although randomised phase III trials comparing radiotherapy alone to concurrent chemoradiotherapy in advanced head and neck cancer were not specific for unresectable disease and hypopharyngeal primaries, the consistent improvement in locoregional control and survival obtained with concurrent chemoradiotherapy as well as the small, but consistent statistically significant benefit of this treatment modality revealed in the meta-analyses (Bourhis et al., 2004; Pignon et al., 2000) led to recommendation supporting radiotherapy and concurrent cisplatin-based chemoradiotherapy as standard treatment for patients with unresectable hypopharyngeal cancers. Recently reported definitive results of a phase III prospective multicenter randomised study conducted in Italy in which 164 patients with unresectable head and neck cancer were randomised to receive radiotherapy alone or combined with daily low-dose carboplatin showed statistically significant improvement in 3, 5 and 10-year overall survival rates in the group treated with concurrent chemoradiotherapy (Ruo Redda et al., 2010). In the absence of conclusive arguments supporting exact schedule of cisplatin administration, a nonrandomised study was conducted to compare two courses cisplatin or two courses of cisplatin plus 5-fluorouracil in 128 patients with locally advanced unresectable head and neck cancer. The results showed that two courses of fractionated cisplatin were accompanied with less acute toxicity whereas similar outcome and incidence of late toxicities were observed with both chemotherapy schedules (Tribius et al., 2009). The use of altered fractionation regimes in the management of unresectable, locoregionally advanced head and neck cancer have also been a part of an intensive clinical research focused on the improvement of locoregional control and overall survival. Based on the results of a large non-site-specific randomised RTOG 90-03 trial demonstrating an improvement in local control with accelerated fractionation using concomitant boost and hyperfractionated radiotherapy compared with conventional fractionation (Fu et al., 2000), and in accordance with the assessment of MARCH Collaborative Group (Bourhis et al., 2006) showing statistically significant improvement in locoregional control and an improvement in overall survival achieved with the use of accelerated radiotherapy, and especially with hyperfractionated radiotherapy, altered fractionation has been recommended as an alternative to concurrent chemoradiotherapy in patients with unresectable head and neck cancer. Nevertheless, both concurrent chemoradiotherapy and altered fractionation are accompanied with increased rates of acute and late toxicity. Intensified radiotherapy regimens in combination with chemotherapy are not routinely recommended in patients with unresectable head and neck cancer. A TAX 324 randomised phase III trial (Posner et al., 2007) demonstrated significant advantage of cisplatin/5-

fluorouracil/docetaxel induction chemotherapy followed by concurrent platinum based chemoradiotherapy in patients with advanced or unresectable head and neck disease including patients with hypopharyngeal cancer. However, despite the encouraging results observed with sequential therapy incorporating taxane in the induction chemotherapy setting, because of the lack of published data from phase III trials comparing induction chemotherapy followed by concurrent chemoradiotherapy with the standard treatment of concurrent chemoradiotherapy alone, this treatment approach in patients with unresectable hypopharyngeal cancer remains investigational. Besides induction chemotherapy followed by concurrent chemoradiotherapy, targeted therapy with cetuximab, tyrosine kinase inhibitor drugs, and the association of cetuximab with cisplatin-based concurrent chemoradiotherapy, also represent treatment approaches whose role in the management of unresectable hypopharyngeal cancer is yet to be established.

6.5 Radiation techniques

6.5.1 Two-dimensional (2D) radiotherapy

In conventional 2D radiotherapy, treatment setup is customized using conventional simulator and the placement of the radiation fields and their shapes are based on the bony anatomy acquired by the simulator diagnostic-quality films. A shrinking field technique initiating with opposed pair of lateral fields and a low anterior field covering the postoperative bed in patients treated with postoperative radiotherapy, or the primary tumour and clinically positive neck nodes in patients treated with definitive radiotherapy, and subclinical disease in the neck nodes including node levels in accordance with the nodal status and the subsite and the extension of the primary tumour is used (see section 6.1.3).

6.5.2 Three-dimensional (3D) conformal radiotherapy

In 3D conformal radiotherapy, treatment planning CT scans are required to define and delineate gross tumour volumes (GTVs), and clinical target volumes (CTVs). Determination of postoperative treatment volumes (CTVs) is based on preoperative staging results, pathologic review of surgical specimens, operative findings, and postoperative clinical assessment (see section 6.1.3). In definitive radiotherapy, the GTV of the primary tumour and the metastatic lymph nodes is defined as any visible tumour and the gross nodal disease revealed on imaging studies and/or physical examination. The CTV encompasses the GTV plus a margin around the tumour for the potential microscopic extension of the disease according to anatomical barriers, and also includes node levels in the neck according to the nodal status as well as the subsite of the primary tumour (see section 6.1.3). The planning target volumes (PTVs) are obtained by adding a margin of 0.5 cm around the adequate CTVs. The definition of contoured volumes and organs of risk is as recommended by International Commission on Radiation Units and Measurements (ICRU) Report 62 (International Commission on Radiation Units and Measurements [ICRU] Report 62, 1999). Delineation of the neck lymph node levels should be realised according to DAHANCA, EORTC, GORTEC, NCIC, RTOG consensus guidelines (Gregoire et al., 2003) and proposals for the delineation of the nodal clinical target volume in the node positive and the postoperative neck (Gregoire et al., 2006) (Fig. 1 a-b).

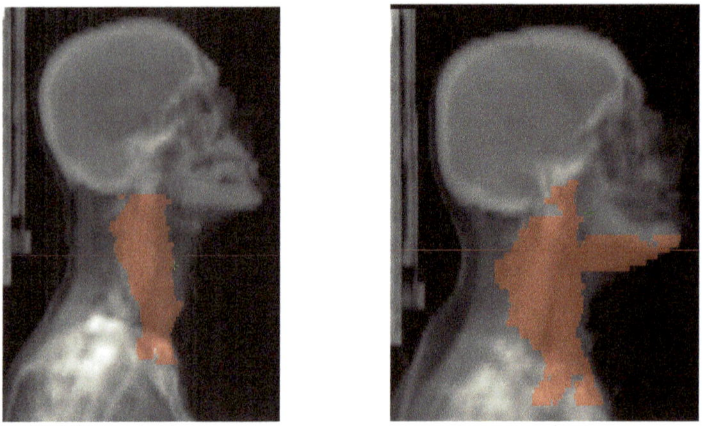

a b

Fig. 1. a-b. Sagital view of contoured clinical target volumes for elective neck nodal irradiation. a. Clinical target volume encompassing levels II, III, IV, and IV in patient with hypopharyngeal cancer arising from pyriform sinus apex with clinically negative neck. b. Clinical target volume encompassing levels I, II, III, IV, V, IV, retropharyngeal nodes and retrostyloid space in patient with hypopharyngeal cancer with esophageal extension and positive neck nodes in level II determined in the surgical specimen following neck dissection.

6.5.3 Intensity modulated radiotherapy (IMRT)

Clinical data evaluating the efficacy of IMRT for cancers of the hypopharynx are scarce, and the suggestions for satisfactory disease control come from small single-institution series with relatively short follow-up (Daly et al., 2011; Studer et al., 2006; Studer et al., 2010). Although prospective studies evaluating the efficacy and toxicity profile of IMRT to the hypopharynx are needed, IMRT techniques can be used to cover equivalent volumes of concern for hypopharyngeal cancers that involve the posterior pharyngeal wall, and for those primary tumours or metastatic lymphadenopathy that extending posterolaterally would overlie the spinal cord. The GTV is defined as all known gross disease determined from CT, MRI, clinical information, and endoscopic findings including abnormal lymph nodes identified on CT. The CTV1 is defined as the GTV with a 0.5-2 cm margin on primary and or nodal GTV (depending on the presence or absence of anatomic boundaries to microscopic spread). The CTV2 refers on the elective neck irradiation and includes the uninvolved neck lymph nodes. Final treatment target volumes include a PTV (GTV plus a margin of 0.3 to 0.5 cm margin), a PTV1 (CTV1 plus a margin of 0.3 to 0.5 cm margin), and a PTV2 (CTV2 plus a margin of 0.3 to 0.5 cm margin). Details about levels proposed for elective irradiation in dependence of the subsite of the primary tumour as well as with the nodal status are given in section 6.1.3.

6.5.4 Dose prescriptions

For small lesions (T1N0-1 and small T2N0), conventionally fractionated radiotherapy should be realised with a fraction size of 2 Gy to a total dose of 66 to 70 Gy.

For locally-regionally advanced lesions treated with concurrent chemoradiotherapy, conventional fractionation should be used with a total dose of 70 Gy in 7 weeks with a daily fraction of 2 Gy.

For locally-regionally advanced lesions treated with definitive radiotherapy using altered fractionation regimens following options can be offered: hyperfractionated radiotherapy with 79.2 Gy in 66 fractions over 6.5 weeks using 1.2 Gy per fraction twice a day, or accelerated fractionation with concomitant boost delivering a total dose of 72 Gy in 6 weeks, (1.8 Gy per fraction a day for the large field and 1.5 Gy boost as second daily fraction during the last 12 treatment days).

For lesions treated with postoperative radiotherapy or postoperative concurrent chemoradiotherapy, conventional fractionation with a total dose of 60 to 66 Gy at 2Gy per fraction to the postoperative bed and high-risk areas should be used.

Elective neck irradiation to uninvolved nodal regions should be realised with a total dose of 50 Gy using 2 Gy per fraction.

If simultaneous integrated boost IMRT technique in 33 fractions is used, the recommended dose to the planning target volume PTV (i.e., GTV with a margin) is ~ 70 Gy at 2.12 Gy per fraction. The PTV1 will receive 59.4 Gy at 1.8 Gy per fraction, and PTV2 will receive 54 Gy at 1.64 Gy per fraction.

If simultaneous integrated boost IMRT technique in 35 fractions is used, the PTV (i.e., GTV with a margin) will receive 70 Gy at 2 Gy per fraction, the PTV1 will receive 63 Gy at 1.8 Gy per fraction, and PTV2 will receive 56 Gy at 1.6 Gy per fraction.

If sequential IMRT technique is used, two to three different separate dose plans are used with initial lower dose phase (weeks 1-5) followed by high-dose boost volume phase (weeks 6 and 7).

If IMRT with concomitant boost schedule is used, the dose to subclinical targets is delivered once daily for 6 weeks, and a separate boost plan as second daily treatment is used for the last 12 treatment days.

6.5.5 Dose limitations

The maximum dose delivered to the spinal cord should range between 45 and 50 Gy. The maximum dose given to the brain stem is limited at 54 Gy. Mandible maximum dose is equal or less than 70 Gy. The mean dose to each parotid gland should be less than 26 Gy, and if possible, the dose to 50% of the volume of each parotid gland should be kept equal to or less than 20 Gy. The brachial plexus dose should be less than 60 Gy, and the dose to the tracheotomies is limited to 50 Gy. It should be also recognised that dose of 70 Gy carries 5% risk for laryngeal cartilage necrosis.

7. Treatment of recurrent and metastatic hypopharyngeal cancer

Surgery is the optimal therapy for patients with local and/or regional recurrence who were previously treated with radiotherapy alone or in combination with chemotherapy. The reported successful salvage rate for local recurrence in hypopharyngeal cancer in the retrospective study of Taki et al. (Taki et al., 2010) was 17%. In the randomised controlled trial conducted at the Princess Margaret Hospital in Toronto, the overall survival rate at 3 years after surgery salvage for patients with recurrent laryngopharyngeal cancer treated with primary radiotherapy was 22% (Davidson et al., 1997). Unfortunately, the vast majority of recurrent hypopharyngeal tumours appear to be unsuitable for surgical intervention because of their unresectibility mostly due to the presence of direct extension into the neck including encasement of the carotid artery. Additionally, there is also a proportion of recurrences that are technically resectable but could not be resected because of patient comorbidities or patient refusal.

Radiotherapy with or without chemotherapy is the treatment of choice for patients initially treated with surgery alone. Reirradiation as an approach appearing to be a treatment with the most potential for cure in selected patients who previously underwent radiotherapy or chemoradiotherapy remains to be investigational. The reported local control rates following reirradiation for patients with recurrent head and neck cancer range between 13% and 42%, and 5-year survival rates range from 13% in unselected to 93% in highly selected series (Goldstein et al., 2008). However, the efficacy of reirradiation for hypopharyngeal cancer is difficult to be evaluated because most of the data are coming from series of highly heterogeneous patients.

The addition of concurrent chemotherapy to reirradiation in the management of recurrences of head and neck cancer was a reasonable effort made to improve the results of treatment by improving the efficacy of radiotherapy through the radiosensitising effects of chemotherapy. Rates of overall survival at two years in multi-institutional trials of concurrent reirradiation and chemotherapy conducted by RTOG ranged between 17% and 25% (Horwitz et al., 2005; Spencer et al., 2001). Reirradiation alone and especially when combined with concurrent chemotherapy is associated with potentially severe and life-threatening treatment-related toxicities that occur in 9% to 32% of patients (Creak et al., 2005). Therefore, physicians, making a decision for the management of recurrent unresectable hypopharyngeal cancer, must be aware of the insufficient data confirming reirradiation as advocated standard of care and must balance the potential risk of severe complications and quality-of-life issues associated with reirradiation with only a small possibility for long-term survival.

For patients with recurrent, hypopharyngeal cancer who are not candidates for salvage surgery or radiation treatment as well as for patients presenting with metastatic disease and therefore not eligible for multimodality potentially curative treatment, chemotherapy, being the historical palliative option, often represents the treatment of last resort. Generally aimed at prolonging survival, and also at improving the quality of life by controlling existing symptoms, and preventing of new cancer-related symptoms, chemotherapy, despite the use of more aggressive combinations and the achievement of higher response rates, has not been convincingly demonstrated to improve survival (Colevas, 2006). Further, despite the palliative intent of chemotherapy in this patients category, there is infrequent assessment of the correlation between tumour shrinkage and benefit such as symptom reduction, and there are also no generated data to support a positive impact of chemotherapy on patients' quality of life. Clinical studies focused on the evaluation of the role of chemotherapy in patients with incurable locoregionally recurrent or metastatic head and neck cancer are not site specific. The best studied single agents are methotrexate, cisplatin, 5-fluorouracil and the taxanes (paclitaxel and docetaxel). In general, the response rate of single-agent and combination chemotherapy ranges between 10% and 40% (Colevas, 2006; Vokes & Choong, 2008). Various combinations of cytotoxic agents were compared in randomised clinical trials. The review analysis of these trials confirming the demonstrated statistically significant response superiority of combination versus monotherapy approaches has also shown that cisplatin and 5-fluorouracil was the only combination with superior response rate over single-agent chemotherapy without associated trend to a lower median survival (Browman & Cronin, 1994). Treatment results achieved in randomised studies exploring the role of different chemotherapy regimens in the treatment of recurrent or metastatic head and neck cancer are summarised in Table 4. The utility of paclitaxel plus cisplatin in patients with recurrent or metastatic head and neck cancer was defined in two randomised trials conducted by the ECOG (Forastiere et al., 2001b; Gibson et al., 2005) (Table 4). In the randomised study of Vermorken et al. (Vermorken et al., 2008) conducted to investigate the efficacy of cetuximab plus platinum-based chemotherapy as first-line treatment in patients with recurrent or metastatic head and neck cancer, the combination of platinum agent (either cisplatin or carboplatin), 5-fluorouracil, and cetuximab has been shown to significantly improve the median overall survival and progression-free survival as compared with chemotherapy alone consisting of platinum agent and 5-fluorouracil (Table 4). Although there are many options for palliative chemotherapy in patients with recurrent or metastatic head and neck cancer, treatment commencement should not ultimately follow the documentation of recurrent disease or presence of distant metastases. However, patients' selection focused on relation between possible benefits of palliation and the risks of treatment induced toxicity should represent more important procedure than the selection of particular cytotoxic agents. Regimens in wide clinical use are: methotrexate given at 40 to 60 mg/m^2 intravenously weekly; paclitaxel 80-100 mg/m^2 given as 1-hour weekly infusion; docetaxel given intravenously at 75-100 mg/m^2 over 1 hour every 21 days; cisplatin-5-fluorouracil combination with cisplatin 100 mg/m^2 given intravenously on day 1 and 5-fluorouracil 1,000 mg/m^2 every day given as continuous infusion over days 1 to 4, repeated every 21 to 28 days; cisplatin-paclitaxel combination with cisplatin 75 mg/m^2 given intravenously and paclitaxel 175 mg/m^2 given intravenously over 3 hours, both on day 1, repeated every 21 days; cisplatin-docetaxel combination with cisplatin 75 mg/m^2 given intravenously and docetaxel 75 mg/m^2 given intravenously over 1 hour, both on day 1 and repeated every 21 days; carboplatin-paclitaxel combination with carboplatin given at Area Under the Curve (AUC) 6 and paclitaxel 200 mg/m^2 given intravenously over 3 hours, both on day 1, every 21 days, or carboplatin given at AUC 2 and paclitaxel 80 mg/m^2 given intravenously over 1 hour, both on day 1 administered on a weekly basis.

8. Complications of treatment

Poor general health, chronic malnutrition, alcoholism, and advanced age of the patient, or the use of preoperative radiotherapy, represent factors influencing the increased risk for surgical complications. Hemorrhage and damage to cranial nerves are most frequently observed intraoperative complications. The most common complication after laryngopharyngectomy is pharyngocutaneous fistula as a result from a leakage at the site of the pharyngeal closure that might be a consequence of tight closure or presence of tumour at

Authors	*Therapy regimens*	*Response rate % (CR %)*	*Median survival (months)*
Taylor et al. (Taylor et al., 1984)	MTX 1,500 mg/m^2 given as continuous infusion over 24 hours with leucovorin vs. 40 mg/m^2 given i.m.	32 vs. 22; p=0.52	4.2 for both treatments
Vogl et al. (Vogl et al., 1985)	MTX 40 mg/m^2 i.v. weekly, with escalation to 60 mg/m^2 on day 8 and subsequently in the absence of toxicity vs. MTX 40 mg/m^2 i.m. on days 1 and 15, bleomycin 10 U i.m. on day 1, 8 and 15, and cisplatin 50 mg/m^2 i.v. on day 4, repeated every 21 days	35 vs. 48; p=0.04 (8 vs. 16; p=0.04)	5.6 for both treatments
Williams et al. (Williams et al., 1986)	MTX 45 mg/m^2 given as weekly i.v. bolus with escalation to 60 mg/m^2 in the absence of toxicity v.s. four-week courses of cisplatin 60 mg/m^2 on day 1 plus vinblastine 0.1 mg/kg on days 1 and 15 i.v. plus bleomycin 15 U i.v. weekly	16 vs. 24; n.s.	7.8 vs. 7.2; n.s.
Eisenberger et al. (Eisenberger et al., 1989)	MTX 40 mg/m^2 given i.v. weekly vs. carboplatin 400 mg/m^2 given i.v. monthly in combination with MTX given at the same dose/schedule	25 vs. 25; n.s.	2 vs. 3; n.s.
Forastiere et al. (Forastiere et al., 1992)	MTX 40 mg/m^2 given i.v. weekly (MTX) vs. cisplatin 100 mg/m^2 given i.v. on day 1 and 5-FU 1,000 mg/m^2 per day for a 96-hour continuous infusion, repeated every 21 days (CP + 5FU) vs. carboplatin 300 mg/m^2 given i.v. on day 1 and 5-FU 1,000 mg/m^2 per day for a 96-hour continuous infusion, repeated every 28 days (CB + 5-FU)	10 vs. 32 vs. 21; CP + 5-FU superior to MTX with p<0.001	5.6 vs. 6.6 vs. 5.0; n.s.
Jacobs et al. (Jacobs et al., 1992)	Cisplatin 100 mg/m^2 given i.v. on day 1 and 5-FU 1,000 mg/m^2 per day for a 96-hour continuous infusion, repeated every 21 days (CP + 5-FU) vs. cisplatin 100 mg/m^2 given i.v. on day 1 and repeated every 21 days (CP) v.s 5-FU 1,000 mg/m^2 per day for a 96-hour continuous infusion, repeated every 21 days (5-FU)	32 vs. 17 vs. 13; CP + 5-FU superior to CP and to 5-FU with p=0.035	5.7 for all treatments
Clavel et al. (Clavel et al., 1994)	MTX 40 mg/m^2 given i.v. on days 1 and 15, weekly, bleomycin 10 mg and vincristine 2 mg given on days 1, 8 and 15, CP 50 mg/m^2 given on day 4, repeated every 21 days (CABO) vs. cisplatin 100 mg/m^2 given i.v. on day 1 and 5-FU 1,000 mg/m^2 per day for a 96-hour continuous infusion, repeated every 21 days (CF) vs. cisplatin 50 mg/m^2 given on days 1 and 8, repeated every 28 days (C)	34 vs. 31 vs. 15; CABO and CF superior to C with p<0.001, p=0.003, respectively (9.5 vs. 1.7 vs. 2.5; CABO superior to CF with p=0.01 and superior to C with p=0.02)	7.3 for all treatments

Authors	*Therapy regimens*	*Response rate % (CR %)*	*Median survival (months)*
Schrijvers et al. (Schrijvers et al., 1998)	Cisplatin 100 mg/m² given i.v. on day 1 and 5-FU 1,000 mg/m² per day for a 96-hour continuous infusion, repeated every 21 days vs. same schedule with interferon alfa-2b given s.c. 3 x 10^6 U/day on days 1 to 5, repeated every 21 days	47 vs. 48; p<0.70 (10.7 vs. 6.8; p<0.50)	6.3 vs. 6; p=0.49
Forastiere et al. (Forastiere et al., 2001b)	Paclitaxel 200 mg/m² for a 24-hour continuous infusion plus cisplatin 75 mg/m² + granulocyte colony-stimulating factor, repeated every 21 days vs. paclitaxel 135 mg/m² for a 24-hour continuous infusion plus cisplatin 75 mg/m², repeated every 21 days	35 vs. 36; n.s. (4 vs. 12; p=0.038)	7.6 vs. 6.8; p=0.759
Gibson et al. (Gibson et al., 2005)	Cisplatin 100 mg/m² given i.v. on day 1 and 5-FU 1,000 mg/m² per day for a 96-hour continuous infusion, repeated every 21 days vs. cisplatin 75 mg/m² given i.v. on day 1 and paclitaxel 175 mg/m² given over 3 hours on day 1, repeated every 21 days	27 vs. 26; n.s. (6.7 vs. 7.0; n.s.)	8.7 vs. 8.1; n.s.
Burtness et al. (Burtness et al., 2005)	Cetuximab 200 mL/m² given i.v. on day 1 over 2 hours for cycle 1, and in subsequent cycles cetuximab 125 mL/m² given i.v. weekly over 1-hour plus cisplatin 100 mg/m² given i.v. on day 1 every 4 weeks vs. placebo plus cisplatin 100 mg/m² given i.v. on day 1 every 4 weeks	26 vs. 10; p=0.03	8.0 vs. 9.2; p=0.21
Vermorken et al. (Vermorken et al., 2008)	Cisplatin 100 mg/m² given i.v. on day 1 or carboplatin 5 mg per milliliter per minute at an AUC given on day 1 as a 1-hour infusion plus 5-FU 1,000 mg/m² per day for a 96-hour continuous infusion, repeated every 21 days vs. the same chemotherapy regimen plus cetuximab 400 mg/m² given initially as intravenous infusion over 2-hours, then 250 mg/m² given weekly as a 1-hour intravenous infusion	20 vs. 36; p<0.001	7.4 vs. 10; p=0.04

CR: complete response; MTX: methotrexate; i.m.: intramuscularly; i.v.: intravenously; U: units; 5-FU: 5-fluorouracil; s.c.: subcutaneously; AUC: area under the curve

Table 4. Randomised studies of chemotherapy in recurrent/metastatic head and neck cancer

the margins of resection. Aspiration pneumonia after partial laryngectomy is postoperative complication occasionally requiring total laryngectomy. Pharyngeal stenosis is commonly manifested following a jejunal free flap reconstruction of a total laryngopharyngectomy. Late complications include pharyngoesophageal stenosis and stricture, chronic pharyngocutaneous fistula and functional deficits in swallowing.

Acute ccomplications of radiotherapy include development of mucositis, dermatitis, xerostomia, and dysgeusia. Acute mucositis as the most frequently observed radiation-induced morbidity is related to the intensity of the treatment regimen with a greater incidence of grade 3-4 reactions associated with accelerated fractionation and concurrent chemoradiotherapy. The occurrence of arytenoid edema being well known consequence of radiotherapy lead to tracheotomy in less than 10% of patients. Late complications of radiotherapy include fibrosis of the soft tissues in the neck, fibrosis of the esophagus, which may develop into an esophageal stricture or tracheoesophageal fistula, and radiation-induced hypothyroidism requiring thyroid-replacement therapy. Rarely seen, but potentially serious late complications are carotid rupture, pharyngocutaneous fistula, laryngeal chondronecrosis or soft tissue necrosis of the posterior pharyngeal wall, laryngeal strictures, brachial plexus injury, and the possibility of spinal cord injury. When keeping the dose to the spinal cord under 50 Gy, myelitis is rarely occurred complication (Emami et al., 1991; Marcus & Million, 1990). However, L'Hermitte sign can occur 2 to 3 months after treatment and last several weeks to months.

Chemotherapy complications include adverse effects in dependence of the specific cytotoxic agents used. Cisplatin-based regimens induce nausea and vomiting, and cumulative toxicities from cisplatin such as ototoxicity, peripheral neuropathy, nephrotoxicity, or myelosuppression. The use of 5-fluorouracil can cause myelosuppression in addition to mucositis, diarrhoea, and vascular irritation. Common adverse effects of taxanes are peripheral neuropathy, myelosuppression, alopecia, and potential hypersensitivity reactions.

9. Follow-up

Post treatment follow-up is required to evaluate treatment response, and is also intended to detect early recurrence, and identify second primary cancers. The majority of local recurrences occur within the first 2 years of treatment (Fu et al., 2000; Ho et al., 1993). Independent second malignancies in the upper aerodigestive tract have an annual incidence of approximately 3% (Cooper et al., 1989; Spector et al., 2001), and the risk for their development is not time limited.

Patients should be followed up every 1-3 months over the first year after treatment, every 2-4 months in the second year after treatment, every 4-6 months in the third through the fifth years after treatment, and every 6-12 months thereafter (National Comprehensive Cancer Network [NCCN], 2011).

Each follow-up examination should include history, physical examination, and fiberoptic endoscopy, or indirect mirror exam. Diagnostic imaging of the neck should be performed for the assessment of response to treatment and must be also performed in any patient with new signs and symptoms suggesting recurrence development. If PET-CT scan is used for follow-up, the first scan should be performed at not less than 3 months after treatment to reduce false-positive scans that can result from active inflammation following treatment (Robson, 2002). Biopsy is mandatory if there is clinical suspicion of residual or recurrent disease. Annual chest is primarily recommended for detection of second primary tumours. In patients who received surgery or radiation to a substantial proportion of the thyroid gland, monitoring of thyroid-stimulating hormone (TSH) levels is recommended every 6 to 12 months.

10. Conclusion

Patients with early-stage hypopharyngeal cancers including T1N0-1 and small T2N0 lesions achieve satisfactory rates of local control when treated with either conservation surgery or radiotherapy as a single treatment modality. Patients with locally-regionally advanced resectable hypopharyngeal cancers could be treated with radical surgery followed by postoperative radiotherapy or postoperative concurrent chemoradiotherapy. In patients with advanced resectable hypopharyngeal cancers requiring laryngopharyngectomy for the surgical approach, concurrent chemoradiotherapy or altered fractionation radiotherapy are treatment modalities allowing anatomic and functional organ preservation while demonstrating equivalent results in terms of survival with those obtained with immediate surgery. For patients presenting with unresectable hypopharyngeal cancer without evidence of distant metastases, radiotherapy and concurrent cisplatin-based chemotherapy should be considered standard treatment approach. The adoption of IMRT, considering its more conformal dose distribution with steep gradients between planning target volumes and critical structures, should be advocated in the routine clinical practice as radiotherapy technique in the treatment of hypopharyngeal cancer.

However, patients with early stage disease are relatively rare, and for those with advanced disease being most frequently present, the results in the achievement of long-term control and survival with the advancement made using aggressive therapeutic approaches remain quite unsatisfactory. Sequential therapy (induction chemotherapy followed by concurrent chemoradiotherapy), intensified radiotherapy regimens in combination with chemotherapy, and the incorporation of molecular targeted therapies in combination with traditional chemotherapy and radiotherapy are strategies currently investigated in an effort to improve outcomes in patients with advanced hypopharyngeal cancer.

11. References

Adelstein, D.J. & LeBlanc, M. (2006b). Does Induction Chemotherapy Have a Role in the Management of Locoregionally Advanced Squamous Cell Head and Neck Cancer? *J Clin Oncol,* Vo.24, No.17, (June 2006), pp. 2624-2628, ISSN 0732-183X

Adelstein, D.J.; Lavertu, P.; Saxton, J.P.; Secic, M.; Wood, B.G.; et al. (2000). Mature Results of a Phase III Randomized Trial Comparing Chemoradiotherapy With Radiation Therapy Alone in Patients With Stage III and IV Squamous Cell Carcinoma of the Head and Neck. *Cancer,* Vol.88, No.4, (February 2000), pp. 876-883, ISSN 0008-543X

Adelstein, D.J.; Li, Y.; Adams, G.L.; Wagner, H.; Kish, J.A.; et al. (2003). An Intergroup Phase III Comparison of Standard Radiation and Two Schedules of Concurrent Chemoradiotherapy in Patients With Unresectable Squamous Cell Head and Neck Cancer. *J Clin Oncol,* Vol.21, No.1, (January 2003), pp. 92-98, ISSN 0732-183X

Adelstein, D.J.; Saxton, J.P.; Lavertu, P.; Tuason, L.; Wood, B.G.; et al. (1997). A Phase III Randomized Trial Comparing Concurrent Chemotherapy and Radiotherapy With Radiotherapy Alone in Resectable Stage III and IV Squamous Cell Head and Neck

Cancer: Preliminary Results. *Head Neck,* Vol.19, No.7, (October 1997), pp. 567-575, ISSN 1043-3074

Adelstein, D.J.; Saxton, J.P.; Rybicki, L.A.; Esclamado, R.M.; Wood, B.G.; et al. (2006a). Multiagent Concurrent Chemoradiotherapy for Locoregionally Advanced Squamous Cell Head and Neck Cancer: Mature Results from a Single Institution. *J Clin Oncol,* Vol.24, No.7, (March 2006), pp. 1064-1071, ISSN 0732-183X

Akimoto, T.; Mitsuhashi, N.; Sakurai, H.; Takahashi, T.; Yamakawa, M.; et al. (1996). Results of Radiation Therapy for Hypopharyngeal Carcinoma: Impact of Accelerated Hyperfractionation on Prognosis. *Japanese Journal of Clinical Oncology,* Vol.26, No.3, (June 1996), pp. 169-174, ISSN 0368-2811

Allal, A.S. (1997). Cancer of the Pyriform Sinus: Trends Towards Conservative Treatment. *Bulletin du Cancer,* Vol.84, No.7, (July 1997), pp. 757-762, ISSN 1769-6917

Aluffi, P.; Pisani, P.; Policarpo, M. & Pia F. (2006). Contralateral Cervical Lymph Node Metastases in Pyriform Sinus Carcinoma. *Otolaryngol Head Neck Surg,* Vol.134, No.4, (April 2006), pp. 650-653, ISSN 0194-5998

Amatsu, M.; Mohri, M. & Kinishi M. (2001). Significance of Retropharyngeal Node Dissection at Radical Surgery for Carcinoma of the Hypopharynx and Cervical Esophagus. *Laryngoscope,* Vol.111, No.6, (June 2001), pp. 1099-1103, ISSN 0023-852X

Ambrosch, P.; Kron, M.; Pradier, O. & Steiner W. (2001). Efficacy of Selective Neck Dissection: A Review of 503 Cases of Elective and Therapeutic Treatment of the Neck in Squamous Cell Carcinoma of the Upper Aerodigestive Tract. *Otolaryngol Head Neck Surg,* Vol.124, No.2, (February 2001), pp. 180-187, ISSN 0194-5998

Amdur, R.J.; Mendenhall, W.M.; Stringer, S.P.; Villaret, D.B. & Cassisi N.J. (2001). Organ Preservation With Radiotherapy for T1-T2 Carcinoma of the Pyriform Sinus. *Head Neck,* Vol.23, No.5, (May 2001), pp. 353-362, ISSN 1043-3074

Ang, K.K.; Harris, J.; Garden, A.S.; Trotti, A.; Jones, C.U.; et al. (2005). Concomitant Boost Radiation Plus Concurrent Cisplatin for Advanced Head and Neck Carcinomas: Radiation Therapy Oncology Group Phase II Trial 99-14. *J Clin Oncol,* Vol.23, No.13, (May 2005), pp. 3008-3015, ISSN 0732-183X

Ang, K.K.; Trotti, A.; Brown, B.W.; Garden, A.S.; Foote, R.L.; et al. (2001). Randomized Trial Addressing Risk Features and Time Factors of Surgery plus Radiotherapy in Advanced Head and Neck Cancer. *Int J Radiat Oncol Biol Phys,* Vol.51, No.3, (November 2001), pp. 571-578, ISSN 0360-3016

Antognoni, P.; Bossi, A.; Cerizza, L.; Esposito, E.; Molteni, M.; et al. (1991). Exclusive Radiotherapy of Carcinoma of the Hypopharynx. Retrospective Study of a Series of 100 Patients. *La Radiologia Medica,* Vol.82, No.3, (September 1991), pp. 328-333, ISSN 0033-8362

Arriagada, R.; Eschwege, F.; Cachin, Y. & Richard J.M. (1983). The Value of Combining Radiotherapy With Surgery in the Treatment of Hypopharyngeal and Laryngeal Cancers. *Cancer,* Vol.51, No.10, (May 1983), pp. 1819-1825, ISSN 0008-543X

Awwad, H.K.; Lotayef, M.; Shouman, T.; Begg, A.C.; Wilson, G.; et al. (2002). Accelerated Hyperfractionation (AHF) Compared to Conventional Fractionation (CF) in the Postoperative Radiotherapy of Locally Advanced Head and Neck Cancer: Influence of Proliferation. *Br J Cancer,* Vol.86, No.4, (February 2002), pp. 517-523, ISSN 0007-0920

Axon, P.R.; Woolford, T.J.; Hargreaves, P.; Yates, P.; Birzgalis, E.R.; et al. (1997). A Comparison of Surgery and Radiotherapy in the Management of Post-Cricoid Carcinoma. *Clinical Otolaryngology and Allied Sciences,* Vol.22, No.4, (August 1997), pp. 370-374, ISSN 0307-7772

Barton, R.T. (1973). Surgical Treatment of Carcinoma of the Pyriform Sinus. *Arch Otolaryngol,* Vol.97, No.4, (April 1973), pp. 337-339, ISSN 0003-9977

Barzan, L.; Veronesi, A.; Caruso, G.; Serraino, D.; Magri, D.; et al. (1990). Head and Neck Cancer and Ageing: A Retrospective Study in 438 Patients. *Journal of Laryngology and Otology,* Vol.104, No.8, (August 1990), pp. 634-640, ISSN 0022-2151

Bataini, J.P. (1993). Radiotherapy in N0 Head and Neck Cancer Patients. *European Archives of Oto-Rhino-Laryngology,* Vol.250, No.8, (February 1993), pp. 442-445, ISSN 0937-4477

Bataini, J.P.; Bernier, J.; Jaulerry, C.; Brunin, F. & Pontvert D. (1990). Impact of Cervical Disease and Its Definitive Radiotherapeutic Management on Survival: Experience in 2013 Patients With Squamous Cell Carcinomas of Oropharynx and Pharyngolarynx. *Laryngoscope,* Vol.100, No.7, (July 1990), pp. 716-723, ISSN 0023-852X

Bataini, P.; Brugere, J.; Bernier, J.; Jaulerry, C.H.; Picot, C. & Ghossein N.A. (1982). Results of Radical Radiotherapeutic Treatment of Carcinoma of the Pyriform Sinus: Experience of the Institut Curie. *Int J Radiat Oncol Biol Phys,* Vol.8, No.8, (August 1982), pp. 1277-1286, ISSN 0360-3016

Beauvillain, C.; Mahe, M.; Bourdin, S.; Peuvrel, P.; Bergerot, P.; et al. (1997). Final Results of a Randomized Trial Comparing Chemotherapy plus Radiotherapy With Chemotherapy plus Surgery plus Radiotherapy in Locally Advanced Resectable Hypopharyngeal Carcinomas. *Laryngoscope,* Vol.107, No.5, (May 1997), pp. 648-653, ISSN 0023-852X

Bernier, J. & Bentzen, S.M. (2003). Altered Fractionation and Combined Radio-Chemotherapy Approaches: Pioneering New Opportunities in Head and Neck Oncology. *Eur J Cancer,* Vol.39, No.5, (March 2003), pp. 560-571, ISSN 0014-2964

Bernier, J. & Cooper J.S. (2005). Chemoradiation After Surgery for High-Risk Head and Neck Patients: How Strong is the Evidence? *Oncologist,* Vol.10, No.3, (March 2005), pp. 215-224, ISSN 1083-7159

Bernier, J.; Domenge, C.; Ozsahin, M.; Matuszewska, K.; Levebvre, J.L.; et al. (2004). Postoperative Irradiation With or Without Concomitant Chemotherapy for Locally Advanced Head and Neck Cancer. *N Engl J Med,* Vol.350, No.19, (May 2004), pp. 1945-1952, ISSN 0028-4793

Bonner, J.A.; Harari, P.M.; Giralt, J. ; Cohen, R.B.; Jones, C.U.; et al. (2010). Radiotherapy plus Cetuximab for Locoregionally Advanced Head and Neck Cancer: 5-Year Survival Data from a Phase 3 Randomised Trial, and Relation Between Cetuximab-Induced Rash and Survival. *Lancet Oncol,* Vol.11, No.1, (January 2010), pp. 21-28, ISSN 1470-2045

Bonner, J.A.; Harari, P.M.; Giralt, J.; Azarnia, N.; Shin, D.M.; et al. (2006). Radiotherapy plus Cetuximab for Squamous-Cell Carcinoma of the Head and Neck. *N Engl J Med*, Vol.354, No.6, (February 2006), pp. 567–578, ISSN 0028-4793

Bourhis, J.; Amand, C.; Pignon, J.P.; MACH-NC Collaborative Group. (2004). Update of MACH-NC (Meta-Analysis of Chemotherapy in Head & Neck Cancer) Database Focused on Concomitant Chemotherapy. *J Clin Oncol, 2004 ASCO Annual Meeting Proceedings (Post-Meeting Edition)*, Vol.22, Suppl.14, (July 2004), 5505, ISSN 0732-183X

Bourhis, J.; Overgaard, J.; Audry, H.; Ang, K.K.; Saunders, M.; Bernier, J.; et al. (2006). Hyperfractionated or Accelerated Radiotherapy in Head and Neck Cancer: A Meta-Analysis. *Lancet*, Vol.368, No.9538, (September 2006), pp. 843-854, ISSN 0023-7507

Bova, R.; Goh, R.; Poulson, M. & Coman, W.B. (2005). Total Pharyngolaryngectomy for Squamous Cell Carcinoma of the Hypopharynx: A Review. *Laryngoscope*, Vol.115, No.5, (May 2005), pp. 864-69, ISSN 0023-852X

Boyd, T.S.; Harari, P.M.; Tannehill, S.P.; Voytovich, M.C.; Hartig, G.K.; et al. (1998). Planned Postradiotherapy Neck Dissection in Patients With Advanced Head and Neck Cancer. *Head Neck*, Vol.20, No.2, (March 1998), pp. 132-137, ISSN 1043-3074

Brennan, J.A.; Boyle, J.O.; Koch, W.M.; Goodman, S.N.; Hruban, R.H.; et al. (1995). Association Between Cigarette Smoking and Mutation of the P53 Gene in Squamous-Cell Carcinoma of the Head and Neck. *N Engl J Med*, Vol.332, No.11, (March 1995), pp. 712–717, ISSN 0028-4793

Brizel, D.M.; Albers, M.E.; Fisher, S.R.; Scher, R.L.; Richtsmeier, W.J.; et al. (1998). Hyperfractionated Irradiation With or Without Concurrent Chemotherapy for Locally Advanced Head and Neck Cancer. *N Engl J Med*, Vol.338, No.25, (June 1998), pp. 1798-1804, ISSN 0028-4793

Brizel, D.M.; Prosnitz, R.G.; Hunter, S.; Fisher, S.R.; Clough, R.L.; et al. (2004). Necessity for Adjuvant Neck Dissection in Setting of Concurrent Chemoradiation for Advanced Head-And-Neck Cancer. *Int J Radiat Oncol Biol Phys*, Vol.58, No.5, (April 2004), pp. 1418-1423, ISSN 0360-3016

Browman, G.P. & Cronin, L. (1994). Standard Chemotherapy in Squamous Cell Head and Neck Cancer: What We Have Learned from Randomized Trials. *Seminars in Oncology*, Vol.21, No.3, (June 1994), pp. 311-319, ISSN 0093-7754

Browman, G.P. (1994). Evidence-Based Recommendations Against Neoadjuvant Chemotherapy for Routine Management of Patients With Squamous Cell Head and Neck Cancer. *Cancer Investigation*, Vol.12, No.6, (January 1994), pp. 662-670, ISSN 0735-7907

Browman, G.P.; Hodson, D.I.; Mackenzie, R.J.; Bestic, N.; Zuraw, L.; Cancer Care Ontario Practice Guideline Initiative Head and Neck Cancer Disease Site Group. (2001). Choosing a Concomitant Chemotherapy and Radiotherapy Regimen for Squamous Cell Head and Neck Cancer: A Systematic Review of the Published Literature With Subgroup Analysis. *Head Neck*, Vol.23, No.7, (July 2001), pp. 579-589, ISSN 1043-3074

Buckley, J.G. & MacLennan K. (2000). Cervical Node Metastases in Laryngeal and Hypopharyngeal Cancer: A Prospective Analysis of Prevalence and Distribution. *Head Neck*, Vol.22, No.4, (July 2000), pp. 380-385, ISSN 1043-3074

Budach, V.; Stuschke, M.; Budach, W.; Baumann, M.; Geismar, D.; et al. (2005). Hyperfractionated Accelerated Chemoradiation With Concurrent Fluorouracil-Mitomycin is More Effective than Dose-Escalated Hyperfractionated Accelerated Radiation Therapy Alone in Locally Advanced Head and Neck Cancer: Final Results of the Radiotherapy Cooperative Clinical Trials Group of the German Cancer Society 95-06 Prospective Randomized Trial. *J Clin Oncol*, Vol.23, No.6, (February 2005), pp. 1125–1135, ISSN 0732–183X

Budach, W.; Hehr, T.; Budach, V.; Belka, C. & Dietz K. (2006). A Meta-Analysis of Hyperfractionated and Accelerated Radiotherapy and Combined Chemotherapy and Radiotherapy Regimens in Unresected Locally Advanced Squamous Cell Carcinoma of the Head and Neck. *BMC Cancer*, Vol.6, (January 2006), p. 28, ISSN 1471-2407

Burtness, B.; Goldwasser, M.A.; Flood, W.; Mattar, B.; Forastiere, A.A. (2005). Phase III Randomized Trial of Cisplatin Plus Placebo Compared With Cisplatin Plus Cetuximab in Metastatic/Recurrent Head and Neck Cancer: An Eastern Cooperative Oncology Group Study. *J Clin Oncol*, Vol.23, No.34, (December 2005), pp. 8646-8654, ISSN 0732–183X

Byers, R.M.; Wolf, P.F. & Ballantyne, A.J. (1988). Rationale for Elective Modified Neck Dissection. *Head Neck Surg*, Vol.10, No.3, (January-February 1988), pp. 160-7, ISSN 0148-6403

Carpenter, R.J. 3rd. & DeSanto, L.W. (1977). Cancer of the Hypopharynx. *Surgical Clinics of North America*, Vol.57, No.4, (August 1997), pp. 723–735, ISSN 0960-7404

Chen, S.W.; Yang, S.N.; Liang, J.A.; Lin, F.J. & Tsai, M.H. (2009). Prognostic Impact of Tumor Volume in Patients With Stage III-IVA Hypopharyngeal Cancer Without Bulky Lymph Nodes Treated With Definitive Concurrent Chemoradiotherapy. *Head Neck*, Vol.31, No.6, (June 2009), pp. 709-716, ISSN 1043-3074

Chevalier, D.; Watelet, J.B.; Darras, J.A. & Piquet J.J. (1997). Supraglottic Hemilaryngopharyngectomy plus Radiation for the Treatment of Early Lateral Margin and Pyriform Sinus Carcinoma. *Head Neck*, Vol.19, No.1, (January 1997), pp. 1-5, ISSN 1043-3074

Chu, P.Y.; Li, W.Y. & Chang, S.Y. (2008). Clinical and Pathologic Predictors of Survival in Patients With Squamous Cell Carcinoma of Hypopharynx After Surgical Treatment. *Annals of Otology, Rhinology and Laryngology*, Vol.117, No.3, (March 2008), pp. 201-06, ISSN 0003-4894

Chung, C.H.; Ely, K.; McGavran, L.; Varella-Garcia, M.; Parker. J.; et al. (2006). Increased Epidermal Growth Factor Receptor Gene Copy Number is Associated With Poor Prognosis in Head and Neck Squamous Cell Carcinomas. *J Clin Oncol*, Vol.24, No.25, (September 2006), pp. 4170-4176, ISSN 0732–183X

Clavel, M.; Vermorken, J.B.; Cognetti, F.; Cappelaere, P.; de Mulder, P.H.; et al. (1994). Randomized Comparison of Cisplatin, Methotrexate, Belomycin and Vincristine (CABO) Versus Cisplatin and 5-Fluorouracil (CF) Versus Cisplatin (C) in Recurrent or Metastatic Squamous Cell Carcinoma of the Head and Neck. A Phase III Study of the EORTC Head and Neck Cancer Cooperative Group. *Annals of Oncology*, Vol.5, No.6, (July 1994), pp. 521-526, ISSN 0923-7534

Clayman, G.L. & Frank, D.K. (1998). Selective Neck Dissection of Anatomically Appropriate Levels is as Efficacious as Modified Radical Neck Dissection for Elective Treatment of the Clinically Negative Neck in Patients With Squamous Cell Carcinoma of the Upper Respiratory and Digestive Tracts. *Archives of Otolaryngology – Head & Neck Surgery*, Vol.124, No.3, (March 1998), pp. 348-352, ISSN: 0886-4470

Clayman, G.L. & Weber, R.S. (1996). Cancer of the Hypopharynx and Cervical Esophagus, In: *Cancer of the Head and Neck*, E. Myers & J.Y. Suen, (Eds.), 423-438, W.B. Saunders, ISBN 978-0721655505, New York

Colevas, A.D. (2006). Chemotherapy Options for Patients With Metastatic or Recurrent Squamous Cell Carcinoma of the Head and Neck. *J Clin Oncol*, Vol.24, No.17, (June 2006), pp. 2644-2652, ISSN 0732–183X

Cooper, J.S.; Pajak, T.F.; Forastiere, A.; Jacobs, J.; Fu, K.K.; et al. (1998). Precisely Defining High-Risk Operable Head and Neck Tumors Based on RTOG #85-03 and #88-24: Targets for Postoperative Radiochemotherapy? *Head Neck*, Vol.20, No.7, (October 1998), pp. 588–594, ISSN 1043-3074

Cooper, J.S.; Pajak, T.F.; Rubin, P.; Tupchong, L.; Brady, L.W.; et al. (1989). Second Malignancies in Patients who Have Head and Neck Cancer: Incidence, Effect on Survival and Implications Based on RTOG Experience. *Int J Radiat Oncol Biol Phys*, Vol.17, No.3, (September 1989), pp. 449-456, ISSN 0360-3016

Cooper, J.S.; Pajak, T.H.; Forastiere, A.A.; Jacobs, J.; Campbell, B.H.; et al. (2004). Postoperative Concurrent Radiotherapy and Chemotherapy for High-Risk Squamous-Cell Carcinoma of the Head and Neck. *N Engl J Med*, Vol.350, No.19, (May 2004), pp. 1937-1944, ISSN 0028-4793

Cooper, J.S.; Porter, K.; Mallin, K.; Hoffman, H.T.; Weber, R.S.; et al. (2009). National Cancer Database Report on Cancer of the Head and Neck: 10-Year Update. *Head Neck*, Vol.31, No.6, (June 2009), pp. 748-758, ISSN 1043-30742009

Corvo, R. (2007). Evidence-Based Radiation Oncology in Head and Neck Squamous Cell Carcinoma. *Radiother Oncol*, Vol.85, No.1, (October 2007), pp. 156-170, ISSN 0167-8140

Creak, A.L.; Harrington, K. & Nutting, C. (2005). Treatment of Recurrent Head and Neck Cancer: Re-Irradiation or Chemotherapy? *Clinical Oncology (Royal College of Radiologists)*, Vol.17, No.3, (May 2005), pp. 138-147, ISSN 0936-6555

Daly, M.E.; Le, Q.T.; Jain, A.K.; Maxim, P.G.; Hsu, A.; et al. (2011). Intensity-Modulated Radiotherapy for Locally Advanced Cancers of the Larynx and Hypopharynx. *Head Neck*, Vol.33, No.1, (January 2011), pp. 103-111, ISSN 1043-3074

Davidge-Pitts, K.J. & Mannel A. (1983). Pharyngolaryngectomy With Extrathoracic Esophagectomy. *Head Neck Surg*, Vol.6, No.1, (September-October 1983), pp. 571–574 ISSN 0148-6403

Davidson, J.; Keane, T.; Brown, D.; Freeman, J.; Gullane, P.; et al. (1997). Surgical Salvage After Radiotherapy for Advanced Laryngopharyngeal Carcinoma. *Archives of*

Otolaryngology – Head & Neck Surgery, Vol.123, No.4, (April 1997), pp. 420-424, ISSN 0886-4470

De Bree, R.; Leemans, C.R.; Silver, C.E.; Robbins, K.T.; Rodrigo, J.P.; et al. (2011). Paratracheal Lymph Node Dissection in Cancer of the Larynx, Hypopharynx, and Cervical Esophagus: The Need for Guidelines. *Head Neck*, Vol.33, No.6, (June 2011), pp. 912-916, ISSN 1043-3074

De la Vega, F.A.; Garcia, R.V.; Dominguez, D.; Iturre, E.V.; Lopez, E.M.; et al. (2003). Hyperfractionated Radiotherapy and Concomitant Cisplatin for Locally Advanced Laryngeal and Hypopharyngeal Carcinomas: Final Results of a Single Institutional Program. *Am J Clin Oncol*, Vol.26, No.6, (December 2003), pp. 550-557, ISSN 0277-3732

Dinshaw, K.A.; Agarwal, J.P.; Laskar, S.G.; Gupta, T.; Shrivastava, S.K.; et al. (2005). Head and Neck Squamous Cell Carcinoma: The Role of Post-Operative Adjuvant Radiotherapy. *J Surg Oncol*, Vol.91, No.1, (July 2005), pp. 48-55, ISSN 0022-4790

Edge, S.B.; Byrd, D.R.; Compton, C.C.; Fritz, A.G.; Greene, F.L. & Trotti, A. (Eds). (2009). *AJCC Cancer Staging Manual*, Springer, ISBN 978-0-387-88440-0, New York

Eisenberger, M.; Krasnow, S.; Ellenberg, S.; Silva, H.; Abrams, J.; et al. (1989). A Comparison of Carboplatin Plus Methotrexate Versus Methotrexate Alone in Patients With Recurrent and Metastatic Head and Neck Cancer. *J Clin Oncol*, Vol.7, No.9, (September 1989), pp. 1341-1345, ISSN 0732-183X

El Badawi, S.A.; Goepfert, H.; Fletcher, G.H.; Herson, J. & Oswald, M.J. (1982). Squamous Cell Carcinoma of the Pyriform Sinus. *Laryngoscope*, Vol.92, No.4, (April 1982), pp. 357-364, ISSN 0023-852X

Elias, M.M.; Hilgers, F.J.M.; Keus, R.B.; Gregor, R.T.; Hart, A.A.M.; et al. (1995). Carcinoma of the Pyriform Sinus: A Retrospective Analysis of Treatment Results Over a 20-Year Period. *Clinical Otolaryngology and Allied Sciences*, Vol.20, No.3, (June 1995), pp. 249-53, ISSN 0307-7772

El-Sayed, S. & Nelson, N. (1996). Adjuvant and Adjunctive Chemotherapy in the Management of Squamous Cell Carcinoma of the Head and Neck Region. A Meta-Analysis of Prospective and Randomized Trials. *J Clin Oncol*, Vol.14, No.3, (March 1996), pp. 838-847, ISSN 0732-183X

Emami, B.; Lyman, J.; Brown, A.; Coia, L.; Goitein, M.; et al. (1991). Tolerance of Normal Tissue to Therapeutic Irradiation. *Int J Radiat Oncol Biol Phys*, Vol.21, No.1, (May 1991), pp. 109-122, ISSN 0360-3016

Ernoux-Neufcoeur, P.; Arafa, M.; Decaestecker, C.; Duray, A.; Remmelink, M.; et al. (2001). Combined Analysis of HPV DNA, P16, P21 and P53 to Predict Prognosis in Patients With Stage IV Hypopharyngeal Carcinoma. *Journal of Cancer Research and Clinical Oncology*, Vol.137, No.1, (January 2011), pp. 173-181, ISSN 0171-5216

Fakhry, C. & Gillison, M. (2006). Clinical Implications of Human Papillomavirus in Head and Neck Cancers. *J Clin Oncol*, Vol.24, No.17, (June 2006), pp. 2606-2611, ISSN 0732-183X

Farrington, W.T.; Weighill, J.S. & Jones P.H. (1986). Post-Cricoid Carcinoma (Ten-Year Retrospective Study). *Journal of Laryngology and Otology*, Vol.100, No.1, (January 1986), pp. 79-84, ISSN 0022-2151

Fein, D.A.; Mendenhall, W.M.; Parsons, J.T.; Stringer, S.P.; Cassisi, N.J.; et al. (1993). Pharyngeal Wall Carcinoma Treated With Radiotherapy: Impact of Treatment Technique and Fractionation. *Int J Radiat Oncol Phys*, Vol.26, No.5, (August 1993), pp. 751-757, ISSN 0360-3016

Flanders, W.D. & Rothman, K.J. (1982). Interaction of Alcohol and Tobacco in Laryngeal Cancer. *Am J Epidemiol*, Vol.115, No.3, (March 1982), pp. 371–379, ISSN 0002-9262

Forastiere, A.A.; Ang, K.; Brizel, D.; Brockstein, B.E.; Dunphy, F.; et al. (2005). Head and Neck Cancers. *Journal of the National Comprehensive Cancer Network*, Vol.3, No.3, (May 2005), pp. 316-391, ISSN 1540-1405

Forastiere, A.A.; Berkey, B.; Maor, M.; Weber, R.; Goephert, H.; et al. (2001a). Phase III Trial to Preserve the Larynx: Induction Chemotherapy and Radiotherapy Versus Concomitant Chemoradiotherapy Versus Radiotherapy Alone, Intergroup Trial R91-11, *Proceedings of the American Society of Clinical Oncology 2001 37th ASCO Annual Meeting*, 20(abstr. 4), ISSN 0732-183X, San Francisco, California, USA, May 12-15, 2001

Forastiere, A.A.; Leong, T.; Rowinsky, E.; Murphy, B.A.; Vlock, D.R.; et al. (2001b). Phase III Comparison of High-Dose Paclitaxel + Cisplatin + Granulocyte Colonystimulating Factor Versus Low-Dose Paclitaxel + Cisplatin in Advanced Head and Neck Cancer: Eastern Cooperative Oncology Group Study E1393. *J Clin Oncol*, Vol.19, No.4, (February 2001), pp. 1088-1095, ISSN 0732–183X

Forastiere, A.A.; Metch, B.; Schuller, D.E.; Ensley, J.F.; Hutchins, L.F.; et al. (1992). Randomized Comparison of Cisplatin Plus Fluorouracil and Carboplatin Plus Fluorouracil Versus Methotrexate in Advanced Squamous-Cell Carcinoma of the Head and Neck: A Southwest Oncology Group Study. *J Clin Oncol*, Vol.10, No.8, (August 1992), pp. 1245-1251, ISSN 0732–183X

Foucher, M.; Poissonnet, G.; Rame, J.P.; Toussaint, B.; Vedrine, P.O.; et al. (2009). T1-T2 N0 Hypopharyngeal Cancers Treated With Surgery Alone. A GETTEC Study (French Neck Study Group). *Annales d'Oto-Laryngologie et de Chirurgie Cervico- Faciale*, Vol.126, No.4, (September 2009), pp. 203-207, ISSN 0003-438X

Franceschi, S.; Munoz, N.; Bosch, X.F.; Snijders, P.J. & Walboomers, J.M. (1996). Human Papillomavirus and Cancers of the Upper Aerodigestive Tract: A Review of Epidemiological and Experimental Evidence. *Cancer Epidemiology, Biomarkers & Prevention*, Vol.5, No.7, (July 1996), pp. 567-575, ISSN 1055-9965

Frank, J.L.; Garb, J.L.; Kay, S.; McClish, D.K.; Bethke, K.P.; et al. (1994). Postoperative Radiotherapy Improves Survival in Squamous Cell Carcinoma of the Hypopharynx. *Am J Surg*, Vol.168, No.5, (November 1994), pp. 476–480, ISSN 0899-7403

Freeman, R.B.; Marks, J.E. & Ogura J.H. (1979). Voice Preservation in Treatment of Carcinoma of the Pyriform Sinus. *Laryngoscope*, Vol.89, No.11, (November 1979), pp. 1855–1863, ISSN 0023-852X

Fu, K.K.; Pajak, T.F, Trotti, A.; Jones, C.U.; Spencer, S.A.; et al. (2000). A Radiation Therapy Oncology Group (RTOG) Phase III Randomized Study to Compare Hyperfractionation and Two Variants of Accelerated Fractionation to Standard Fractionation Radiotherapy for Head and Neck Squamous Cell Carcinoma: First

Report of RTOG 9003. *Int J Radiat Oncol Biol Phys,* Vol.48, No.1, (August 2000), pp. 7-16, ISSN 0360-3016

Gale, N.; Cardesa, A. & Zidar N. (2006). Larynx and Hypopharynx, In: *Pathology of the Head and Neck,* A. Cardesa & P.J. Slootweg, (Eds), 198-226, Springer-Verlag, ISBN-10 3-540-30628-5, Berlin Heidelberg

Garden, A.S.; Asper, J.A.; Morrison, W.H.; Schechter, N.R.; Glisson, B.S.; et al. (2004b). Is Concurrent Chemoradiation the Treatment of Choice for All Patients With Stage III or IV Head and Neck Carcinoma? *Cancer,* Vol.100, No.6, (March 2004), pp. 1171-1178, ISSN 0008-543X

Garden, A.S.; Harris, J.; Vokes, E.E.; Forastiere, A.A.; Ridge, J.A.; et al. (2004a). Preliminary Results of Radiation Therapy Oncology Group 97-03: A Randomized Phase II Trial of Concurrent Radiation and Chemotherapy for Advanced Squamous Cell Carcinomas of the Head and Neck. *J Clin Oncol,* Vol.22, No.14, (July 2004), pp. 2856-2864, ISSN 0732-183X

Garden, A.S.; Morrison, W.H.; Ang, K.K. & Peters, L.J. (1995). Hyperfractionated Radiation in the Treatment of Squamous Cell Carcinomas of the Head and Neck: A Comparison of Two Fractionation Schedules. *Int J Radiat Oncol Biol Phys,* Vol.31, No.3, (February 1995), pp. 493–502, ISSN 0360-3016

Garden, A.S.; Morrison, W.H.; Clayman, G.L.; Ang, K.K. & Peters, L.J. (1996). Early Squamous Cell Carcinoma of the Hypopharynx: Outcomes of Treatment With Radiation Alone of the Primary Disease. *Head Neck,* Vol.18, No.4, (July-August 1996), pp. 317-322, ISSN 1043-3074

Gibson, M.K.; Li, Y.; Murphy, B.; Hussain, M.H.A.; DeConti, R.C.; et al. (2005). Randomized Phase III Evaluation of Cisplatin plus Fluorouracil Versus Cisplatin plus Paclitaxel in Advanced Head and Neck Cancer (E1395): An Intergroup Trial of the Eastern Cooperative Oncology Group. *J Clin Oncol,* Vol.23, No.15, (May 2005), pp. 3562-3567, ISSN 0732-183X

Glanz, H. (1999). Pathomorphological Aspects of Transoral Resection of Hypopharyngeal Carcinoma With Preservation of the Larynx. Patient Selection, Treatment Results. *Laryngorhinootologie,* Vol.78, No.12, (December 1999), pp. 654-662, ISSN 0935-8943

Goldstein, D.P.; Clark, J.; Gullane P.J.; Dawson, L.A.; Siu, L.L.; et al. (2008). Carcinoma of the Hypopharynx. In: *Head and Neck Cancer: An Evidence-based Team Approach,* E.M. Genden & M.A. Varvares, (Eds.), 44-69, Thieme Medical Publishers, Inc, ISBN 978-1-58890-636-6, New York

Grabenbauer, G.G.; Rodel, C.; Ernst-Stecken, A.; Brunner, T.; Hornung, J.; et al. (2003). Neck Dissection Following Radiochemotherapy of Advanced Head and Neck Cancer-for Selected Cases Only? *Radiother Oncol,* Vol.66, No.1, (January 2003), pp. 57-63, ISSN 0167-8140

Gregoire, V.; Coche, E.; Cosnard, G.; Hamoir, M. & Reychler H. (2000). Selection and Delineation of Lymph Node Target Volumes in Head and Neck Conformal Radiotherapy. Proposal for Standardizing Terminology and Procedure Based on Surgical Experience. *Radiother Oncol,* Vol.56, No.2, (August 2000), pp. 135-150, ISSN 0167-8140

Gregoire, V.; Eisbruch, A.; Hamoir, M. & Levendag P. (2006). Proposal for the Delineation of the Nodal CTV in the Node-Positive and Post-Operative Neck. *Radiother Oncol,* Vol.79, No.1, (April 2006), pp. 15-20, ISSN 0167-8140

Gregoire, V.; Levendag, P.; Ang, K.K.; Bernier, J.; Braaksma, M.; et al. (2003). CT-Based Delineation of Lymph Node Levels Related CTVs in the Node Negative Neck: DAHANCA, EORTC, GORTEC, NCIC, RTOG Consensus Guidelines. *Radiother Oncol,* Vol.69, No.3, (December 2003), pp. 227-236, ISSN 0167-8140

Gupta, T.; Agarwal, J.P.; Ghosh-Laskar, S.; Parikh, P.M.; D'Cruz, A.K.; et al. (2009b). Radical Radiotherapy With Concurrent Weekly Cisplatin in Locoregionally Advanced Squamous Cell Carcinoma of the Head and Neck: A Single-Institution Experience. *Head and Neck Oncology,* Vol.1, (June 2009), p. 17, ISSN1758-3284

Gupta, T.; Chopra, S.; Agarwal, J.P.; Ghosh-Laskar, S.; D'Cruz, A.; et al. (2010). Postoperative Radiotherapy in Hypopharyngeal Cancer: Single-Institution Outcome Analysis. *International Journal of Head and Neck Surgery,* Vol.1, No.1, (January-April 2010), pp. 1-8, ISSN 0975-7899

Gupta, T.; Chopra, S.; Agarwal, J.P.; Laskar, S.G.; D'Cruz, A.K.; et al. (2009a). Squamous Cell Carcinoma of the Hypopharynx: Single-Institution Outcome Analysis of a Large Cohort of Patients Treated With Primary Non-Surgical Approaches. *Acta Oncol,* Vol.48, No.4, (January 2009), pp. 541-548, ISSN 0284-186X

Gustavsson, P.; Jakobsson, R.; Johansson, H.; Lewin, F.; Norell, S.; et al. (1998). Occupational Exposures and Squamous Cell Carcinoma of the Oral Cavity, Pharynx, Larynx, and Oesophagus: A Case-Control Study in Sweden. *Occupational and Environmental Medicine,* Vol.55, No.6, (June 1998), pp. 393–400, ISSN 1351-0711

Hall, S.F.; Groome, P.A.; Irish, J. & O'Sullivan, B. (2009). Towards Further Understanding of Prognostic Factors for Head and Neck Cancer Patients: The Example of Hypopharyngeal Cancer. *Laryngoscope,* Vol.119, No.4, (April 2009), pp. 696-702, ISSN 0023-852X

Haraf, D.J.; Vokes, E.E.; Panje, W.R. & Weichselbaum R.R. (1991). Survival and Analysis of Failure Following Hydroxyurea, 5-Flourouracil and Concomitant Radiation Therapy in Poor Prognosis Head and Neck Cancer. *Am J Clin Oncol,* Vol.14, No.5, (October 1991), pp. 419-422, ISSN 0277-3732

Hasegawa, Y. & Matsuura, H. (1994). Retropharyngeal Node Dissection in Cancer of the Oropharynx and Hypopharynx. *Head Neck,* Vol.16, No.2, (March-April 1994), pp. 173-180, ISSN 1043-3074

Hirano, S.; Tateya, I.; Kitamura, M.; Kada, S.; Ishikawa, S.; et al. (2010). Ten Years Single Institutional Experience of Treatment for Advanced Hypopharyngeal Cancer in Kyoto University. *Acta Oto-Laryngologica.Supplementum,* Vol.563, (November 2010), pp. 56-61, ISSN 0365-5237

Hitt, R.; Lopez-Pousa, A.; Martinez-Trufero, J.; Escrig, V.; Carles, J.; et al. (2005). Phase III Study Comparing Cisplatin plus Fluorouracil to Paclitaxel, Cisplatin, and Fluorouracil Induction Chemotherapy Followed by Chemoradiotherapy in Locally Advanced Head and Neck Cancer. *J Clin Oncol,* Vol.23, No.34, (December 2005), pp. 8636-8645, ISSN 0732–183X

Ho, C.M.; Lam, K.H.; Wei, W.I.; Yuen, P.W. & Lam L.K. (1993). Squamous Cell Carcinoma of the Hypopharynx-Analysis of Treatment Results. *Head Neck,* Vol.15, No.5, (September-October 1993), pp. 405-412, ISSN 1043-3074

Hoffman, H.T.; Karnell, L.H.; Funk, G.F.; Robinson, R.A. & Menck, H.R. (1998). The National Cancer Data Base Report on Cancer of the Head and Neck. *Archives of Otolaryngology - Head & Neck Surgery,* Vol.124, No.9, (September 1998), pp. 951-962, ISSN 0886-4470

Hoffman, H.T.; Karnell, L.H.; Shah, J.P.; Ariyan, S.; Brown, G.S.; et al. (1997). Hypopharyngeal Cancer Patient Care Evaluation. *Laryngoscope,* Vol.107, No.8, (August 1997), pp. 1005-1017, ISSN 0023-852X

Hong, T.S.; Tome, W.A.; Chappell, R.J.; Chinnaiyan, P.; Mehta, M.P.; et al. (2005). The Impact of Daily Setup Variations on Head-And-Neck Intensity Modulated Radiation Therapy. *Int J Radiat Oncol Biol Phys,* Vol.61, No.3, (March 2005), pp. 779-788, ISSN 0360-3016

Horwitz, E.M.; Harris, J.; Langer, C.J.; Nicolaou, N.; Kies, M.; et al. (2005). Concurrent Split Course Hyperfractionated Radiotherapy (Hfx RT), Cisplatin (DDP) and Paclitaxel (P) in Patients With Recurrent, Previously Irradiated Squamous Cell Carcinoma of the Head and Neck (SCCHN): Update of RTOG 9911. *J Clin Oncol, 2005 ASCO Annual Meeting Proceedings,* Vol.23, Suppl.16, Part I of II, (June 2005), 5577, ISSN 0732-183X

Hsu, L.P. & Chen, P.R. (2005). Distant Metastases of Head and Neck Squamous Cell Carcinomas-Experience from Eastern Taiwan. *Tzu Chi Medical Journal,* Vol.17, No.2, pp. 99-104, ISSN 1016-3190

Huguenin, P.; Beer, K.T.; Allal, A.; Rufibach, K.; Friedli, C.; et al. (2004). Concomitant Cisplatin Significantly Improves Locoregional Control in Advanced Head and Neck Cancers Treated With Hyperfractionated Radiotherapy. *J Clin Oncol,* Vol.22, No.23, (December 2004), pp. 4665-4673, ISSN 0732-183X

International Commission on Radiation Units and Measurements (ICRU) Report 62. (1999). Prescribing, Recording, and Reporting Photon Beam Therapy (Supplement to ICRU Report 50), ICRU, pp. ix 52, ISBN 0-913394-61-0, Bethesda

Jacobs, C.; Lyman, G.; Velez-Garcia, E.; Sridhar, K.S.; Knight, W.; et al. (1992). A Phase III Randomized Study Comparing Cisplatin and Fluorouracil as Single Agents and in Combination for Advanced Squamous Cell Carcinoma of the Head and Neck. *J Clin Oncol,* Vol.10, No.2, (February 1992), pp. 257-263, ISSN 0732-183X

Jayant, K.; Balakrishnan, V.; Sanghvi, L.D. & Jussawalla, D.J. (1977). Quantification of the Role of Smoking and Chewing Tobacco in Oral, Pharyngeal and Oesophageal Cancers. *Br J Cancer,* Vol.35, No.2, (February 1977), pp. 232-235, ISSN 0007-0920

Jeremic, B.; Shibamoto, Y.; Milicic, B.; Nikolic, N.; Dagovic, A.; Aleksandrovic, J.; et al. (2000). Hyperfractionated Radiation Therapy With or Without Concurrent Low-Dose Daily Cisplatin in Locally Advanced Squamous Cell Carcinoma of the Head and Neck: A Prospective Randomized Trial. *J Clin Oncol,* Vol.18, No.7, (April 2000), pp. 1458-1464, ISSN 0732-183X

Jeremic, B.; Shibamoto, Y.; Stanisavljevic, B.; Milojevic, L.; Milicic, B. & Nikolic, N. (1997). Radiation Therapy Alone or With Concurrent Low-Dose Daily Either Cisplatin or

Carboplatin in Locally Advanced Unresectable Squamous Cell Carcinoma of the Head and Neck: A Prospective Randomized Trial. *Radiother Oncol*, Vol.43, No.1, (April 1997), pp. 29-37, ISSN 0167-81401997

Johansen, L.V.; Grau, C. & Overgaard, J. (2000). Hypopharyngeal Squamous Cell Carcinoma: Treatment Results in 138 Consecutively Admitted Patients. *Acta Oncol*, Vol.39, No.4, (January 2000), pp. 529-536, ISSN 0284-186X

Jol, J.K. ; Quak, J.J.; de Bree, R. & Leemans, C.R. (2003). Larynx Preservation Surgery for Advanced Posterior Pharyngeal Wall Carcinoma With Free Flap Reconstruction: A Critical Appraisal. *Oral Oncology*, Vol.39, No.6, (September 2003), pp. 552-558, ISSN 1368-8375

Jones, A.S. & Stell, P.M. (1991). Squamous Cell Carcinoma of the Posterior Pharyngeal Wall. *Clinical Otolaryngology and Allied Sciences*, Vol.16, No.5, (October 1991), pp. 462–465, ISSN 0307-7772

Jones, A.S.; McRae, R.D.; Phillips, D.E.; Hamilton, J.; Field, J.K.; et al. (1995). The Treatment of Node Negative Squamous Cell Carcinoma of the Postcriciod Region. *Journal of Laryngology and Otology*, Vol.109, No.2, (February 1995), pp. 114–119, ISSN 0022-2151

Jones, A.S.; Wilde, A.; McRae, R.D.; Phillips, D.E.; Field, J.K.; et al. (1994). The Treatment of Early Squamous Cell Carcinoma of the Piriform Fossa. *Clinical Otolaryngology and Allied Sciences*, Vol.19, No.6, (December 1994), pp. 485-490, ISSN 0307-7772

Joo, Y.H.; Sun, D.I.; Cho, K.J.; Cho, J.H. & Kim, M.S. (2010). The Impact of Paratracheal Lymph Node Metastasis in Squamous Cell Carcinoma of the Hypopharynx. *European Archives of Oto-Rhino-Laryngology*, Vol.267, No.6, (January 2010), pp. 945-950 ISSN 0937-4477

Kajanti, M. & Mantyla, M. (1990). Carcinoma of the Hypopharynx. *Acta Oncol*, Vol.29, No.7, (January 1990), pp. 903–907, ISSN 0284-186X

Kamiyama, R.; Saikawa, M. & Kishimoto, S. (2009). Significance of Retropharyngeal Lymph Node Dissection in Hypopharyngeal Cancer. *Japanese Journal of Clinical Oncology*, Vol.39, No.10, (October 2009), pp. 632-637, ISSN 0368-2811

Keane, T.J. (1982). Carcinoma of the Hypopharynx. *Journal of Otolaryngology*, Vol.11, No.4, (August 1982), pp. 227-231, ISSN 0381-6605

Keane, T.J.; Hawkins, N.V.; Beale, F.A.; Cummings, B.J.; Harwood, A.R.; et al. (1983). Carcinoma of the Hypopharynx-Results of Primary Radical Radiation Therapy. *Int J Radiol Oncol Biol Phys*, Vol.9, No.5, (May 1983), pp. 659-664, ISSN 0360-3016

Kim, K.H.; Sung, M.W.; Rhee, C.S.; Koo, J.W.; Koh, T.Y.; Lee, D.W.; et al. (1998). Neoadjuvant Chemotherapy and Radiotherapy for the Treatment of Advanced Hypopharyngeal Carcinoma. *American Journal of Otolaryngology*, Vol.19, No.1, (January-February 1998), pp. 40–44, ISSN 0196-0709

Kim, S.; Wu, H.G.; Heo, D.S.; Kim, K.H.; Sung, M.W.; et al. (2001). Advanced Hypopharyngeal Carcinoma Treatment Results According to Treatment Modalities. *Head Neck*, Vol.23, No.9, (September 2001), pp. 713–717, ISSN 1043-3074

Kim, W.T.; Ki, Y.K.; Nam, J.H.; Kim, D.W.; Lee, B.J.; et al. (2004). The Results of Postoperative Radiotherapy for Hypopharyngeal Carcinoma. *The Korean Society of*

Therapeutic Radiology and Oncology, Vol.22, No.4, (December 2004), pp254-264, ISSN 0368-2811

Kirchner, J.A. (1975). Pyriform Sinus Cancer: A Clinical and Laboratory Study. *Annals of Otology, Rhinology and Laryngology,* Vol.84, No.6, (November-December 1975), pp. 793–803, ISSN 0003-4894

Koch, W.M.; Lango, M.; Sewell, D.; Zahurak, M. & Sidransky, D. (1999). Head and Neck Cancer in Nonsmokers: A Distinct Clinical and Molecular Entity. *Laryngoscope,* Vol.109, No.10, (October 1999), pp. 1544–1551, ISSN 0023-852X

Koch, W.M.; Lee, D.J.; Eisele, D.W.; Miller, D.; Poole, M.; Cummings, C.W.; et al. (1995). Chemoradiotherapy for Organ Preservation in Oral and Pharyngeal Carcinoma. *Archives of Otolaryngology - Head & Neck Surgery,* Vol.121, No.9, (September 1995), pp. 974–980, ISSN 0886-4470

Koo, B.S.; Lim, Y.C.; Lee, J.S.; Kim, Y.H.; Kim, S.H.; et al. (2006). Management of Contralateral N0 Neck in Pyriform Sinus Carcinoma. *Laryngoscope,* Vol.116, No.7, (July 2006), pp. 1268-1272 ISSN 0023-852X

Kraus, D.H.; Pfister, D.G.; Harrison, L.B.; Shah, J.P.; Spiro, R.H.; et al. (1994). Larynx Preservation With Combined Chemotherapy and Radiation Therapy in Advanced Hypopharynx Cancer. *Otolaryngol Head Neck Surg,* Vol.111, No.1, (July 1994), pp. 31-37, ISSN 0194-5998

Kraus, D.H.; Zelefsky, M.J.; Brock, H.A.; Huo, J.; Harrison, L.B.; et al. (1997). Combined Surgery and Radiation Therapy for Squamous Cell Carcinoma of the Hypopharynx. *Otolaryngol Nead Neck Surg,* Vol.116, No.6, Pt.1, (June 1997), pp. 637-641, ISSN 0194-5998

Laccourreye, H.; Lacau St Guily, J.; Brasnu, D.; Fabre, A. & Menard, M. (1987). Supracricoid Hemilaryngopharyngectomy. Analysis of 240 Cases. *Annals of Otology, Rhinology and Laryngology,* Vol.96, No.2, Pt.1, (March-April 1987), pp. 217–221, ISSN 0003-4894

Laccourreye, O.; Merite-Drancy, A.; Brasnu, D.; Chabardes, E.; Cauchois, R.; et al. (1993). Supracricoid Hemilaryngopharyngectomy in Selected Pyriform Sinus Carcinoma Staged as T2. *Laryngoscope,* Vol.103, No.12, (December 1993), pp. 1373-1379, ISSN 0023-852X

Lajtmam, Z. & Manestar, D. (2001). A Comparison of Surgery and Radiotherapy in the Management of Advanced Pyriform Fossa Carcinoma. *Clin Otolaryngol,* Vol.26, No.1, (January 2001), pp. 59–61, ISSN 1749-4478

Layland, M.K. & Sessions, D.G. (2005). The Influence of Lymph Node Metastasis in the Treatment of Squamous Cell Carcinoma of the Oral Cavity, Oropharynx, Larynx and Hypopharynx: N0 Versus N+. *Laryngoscope,* Vol.115, No.4, (April 2005), pp. 629-639, ISSN 0023-852X

Lederman M. (1962). Carcinoma of Laryngopharynx. Results of Radiotherapy. *Journal of Laryngology and Otology,* Vol.76, No.5, (May 1962), pp. 317–334, ISSN 0022-2151

Lee, M.S.; Ho, H.C.; Hsiao, S.H.; Hwang, J.H.; Lee, C.C.; et al. (2008). Treatment Results and Prognostic Factors in Locally Advanced Hypopharyngeal Cancer. *Acta Otolaryngol,* Vol.128, No.1, (January 2008), pp. 103-109, ISSN 0001-6489

Lee, W.R.; Berkey, B.; Marcial, V.; Fu, K.K.; Cooper, J.S.; et al. (1998). Anemia is Associated With Decreased Survival and Increased Locoregional Failure in Patients With

Locally Advanced Head and Neck Carcinoma: A Secondary Analysis of RTOG 85-27. *Int J Radiat Oncol Biol Phys*, Vol.42, No.5, (December 1998), pp.1069-1075, ISSN 0360-3016

Lefebvre, J. & Chevalier, D. (2004). Cancer De l'Hypopharynx, *EMC - Oto-rhino-laryngologie,* Vol.1, No.4, (November 2004), pp. 274-289, ISSN 1762-5688

Lefebvre, J.L.; Castelain, B.; La De Torre, J.C.; Delobelle-Deroide, A. & Vankemmel, B. (1987). Lymph Node Invasion in Hypopharynx and Lateral Epilarynx: A Prognostic Factor. *Head Neck Surg,* Vol.10, No.1, (September-October 1987), pp 14–18 ISSN 0148-6403

Lefebvre, J.L.; Chevalier, D.; Luboinski, B.; Kirkpatrick, A.; Collette, L.; et al. (1996). Larynx Preservation in Pyriform Sinus Cancer: Preliminary Results of a European Organization for Research and Treatment of Cancer Phase III Trial. EORTC Head and Neck Cancer Cooperative Group. *The Journal of the National Cancer Institute,* Vol.88, No.13, (July 1996), pp. 890–899, ISSN 0027-8874

Lefebvre, J.L.; Chevalier, D.; Luboinski, B.; Traissac, L.; Andry, G.; et al. (2004). Is Laryngeal Preservation (LP) With Induction Chemotherapy (ICT) Safe in the Treatment of Hypopharyngeal SCC? Final Results of the Phase III EORTC 24891 Trial. *J ClinOncol, 2004 ASCO Annual Meeting Proceedings (Post-Meeting Edition),* Vol.22, Suppl.14, (July 2004), 5505, ISSN 0732–183X

Levebvre, J.L. & Lartigau, E. (2003). Preservation of Form and Function during Management of Cancer of the Larynx and Hypopharynx. *World Journal of Surgery,* Vol.27, No.7, (July 2003), pp. 811-816, ISSN 0364-2313

Levebvre, J.L. (2000). What is the Role of Primary Surgery in the Treatment of Laryngeal and Hypopharyngeal Cancer? Hayes Martin Lecture. *Archives of Otolaryngology – Head & Neck Surgery,* Vol.126, No.3, (March 2000), pp. 285-288, ISSN 0886-4470

Llatas, M.C.; Molla, C.L.; Garcia, R.B.; Ramirez, M.J.F.; Domenech, F.G.; et al. (2009). Hypopharyngeal Cancer: Analysis of Evolution and Treatment Results. *Acta Otorrinolaringologica Espanola,* Vol.60, No.1, (January-February 2009), pp. 3-8, ISSN 0001-6519

Lou, H.F.; Xiao, S.F.; Zhao, E.M.; Guo, M.; Wang, Q.G.; et al. (2008). Selective Neck Dissection on the Treatment of Neck Metastases in 63 Patients With Squamous Cell Carcinoma of Hypopharynx. *Zhonghua Er Bi Yan Hou Tou Jing Wai Ke Za Zhi,* Vol.43, pp. 202-207, ISSN 1673-0860

Lundahl, R.E.; Foote, R.L.; Bonner, J.A.; Suman, V.J.; Lewis, J.E.; et al. (1998). Combined Neck Dissection and Postoperative Radiation Therapy in the Management of High-Risk Neck: A Matched-Pair Analysis. *Int J Radiat Oncol Biol Phys,* Vol.40, No.3, (February 1998), pp. 529-534, ISSN 0360-3016

Makeieff, M.; Mercante, G.; Jouzdani, E.; Garrel, R.; Crampette, L.; et al. (2004). Supraglottic Hemipharyngolaryngectomy for the Treatment of T1 and T2 Carcinomas of Laryngeal Margin and Piriform Sinus. *Head Neck,* Vol.26, No.8, (August 2004), pp. 701-705, ISSN 1043-3074

Marchand, J.L.; Luce, D.; Leclerc, A.; Goldberg, P.; Orlowski, E.; et al. (2000). Laryngeal and Hypopharyngeal Cancer and Occupational Exposure to Asbestos and Man-Made

Vitreous Fibers: Results of a Case-Control Study. *American Journal of Industrial Medicine,* Vol.37, No.6, (June 2000), pp. 581-589, ISSN 0271-3586

Marcus, R.B. Jr. & Million, R.R. (1990). The Incidence of Myelitis After Irradiation of the Cervical Spinal Cord. *Int J Radiat Oncol Biol Phys,* Vol.19, No.1, (July 1990), pp. 3-8, ISSN 0360-3016

Marks, J.E.; Kurnik, B.; Powers, W.E. & Ogura, J.H. (1978). Carcinoma of the Pyriform Sinus. An Analysis of Treatment Results and Patterns of Failure. *Cancer,* Vol.41, No.3, (March 1978), pp. 1008-1015, ISSN 0008-543X

McKaig, R.G.; Baric, R.S. & Olshan, A.F. (1998). Human Papillomavirus and Head and Neck Cancer: Epidemiology and Molecular Biology. *Head Neck,* Vol.20, No.3, (May 1998), pp. 250-65, ISSN 1043-3074

Mendenhall, W.M.; Million, R.R. & Bova, F.I. (1984). Analysis of Time-Dose Factors in Clinically Positive Neck Nodes Treated With Irradiation Alone in Squamous Cell Carcinoma of the Head and Neck. *Int J Radiat Oncol Biol Phys,* Vol.10, No.5, (April 1984), pp. 639-643, ISSN 0360-3016

Mendenhall, W.M.; Parsons, J.T.; Cassisi, N.J. & Million, R.R. (1987a). Squamous Cell Carcinoma of the Pyriform Sinus Treated With Radical Radiation Therapy. *Radiother Oncol,* Vol.9, No.3, (July 1987), pp. 201–208, ISSN 0167-8140

Mendenhall, W.M.; Parsons, J.T.; Devine, J.W.; Cassisi, N.J. & Million, R.R. (1987b). Squamous Cell Carcinoma of the Pyriform Sinus Treated With Surgery and/or Radiotherapy. *Head Neck Surg,* Vol.10, No.2, (November-December 1987), pp. 88-92, ISSN 0148-6403

Mendenhall, W.M.; Villaret, D.B.; Amdur, R.J.; Hinerman, R.W. & Mancuso, A.A. (2002). Planned Neck Dissection After Definitive Radiotherapy for Squamous Cell Carcinoma of the Head and Neck. *Head Neck,* Vol.24, No.11, (November 2002), pp. 1012-1018, ISSN 1043-3074

Menvielle, G.; Luce, D.; Goldberg, P.; Bugel, I. & Leclerc, A. (2004). Smoking, Alcohol Drinking and Cancer Risk for Various Sites of the Larynx and Hypopharynx. A Case-Control Study in France. *European Journal of Cancer Prevention,* Vol.13, No.3, (June 2004), pp. 165-172, ISSN: 0959-8278

Meoz-Mendez, R.T.; Fletcher, G.H.; Guillamondegui, O.M. & Peters, L.J. (1978). Analysis of the Results of Irradiation in the Treatment of Squamous Cell Carcinomas of the Pharyngeal Walls. *Int J Radiat Oncol Biol Phys,* Vol.4, No.7, (July 1978), pp. 579–585, ISSN 0360-3016

Million, R.R. & Cassisi, N.J. (1981). Radical Irradiation for Carcinoma of the Pyriform Sinus. *Laryngoscope,* Vol.91, No.3, (March 1981), pp. 439–450, ISSN 0023-852X

Mineta, H.; Ogino, T.; Amano, H.M.; Ohkawa, Y.; Araki, K.; et al. (1998). Human Papilloma Virus (HPV) Type 1 and 18 Detected in Head and Neck Squamous Cell Carcinoma. *Anticancer Research,* Vol.18, No.6B, (November-December 1998), pp. 4765-4768, ISSN 0250-7005

Mirimanoff, R.O.; Wang, C.C. & Doppke, K.P. (1985). Combined Surgery and Postoperative Radiation Therapy for Advanced Laryngeal and Hypopharyngeal Carcinomas. *Int JRadiat Oncol Biol Phys,* Vol.11, No.3, (March 1985), pp. 499-504, ISSN 0360-3016

Mochiki, M.; Sugawasa, M.; Nibu, K.; Asai, M.; Nakao, K.; et al. (2007). Prognostic Factors for Hypopharyngeal Cancer: A Univariate and Multivariate Study of 142 Cases. *Acta Oto-Laryngologica. Supplementum,* Vol.559, (December 2007), pp. 136-144, ISSN 0365-5237

Moore, K.L.; Agur, A.M.R & Dalley, A.F. (Eds). (2010). *Essential Clinical Anatomy,* Lippincott Williams & Wilkins, ISBN 978-0-7817-9915-7, Baltimore

Muller, D.; Millon, R.; Velten, M.; Bronner, G.; Jung, G.; et al. (1997). Amplification of 11q13 DNA Markers in Head and Neck Squamous Cell Carcinomas: Correlation With Clinical Outcome. *Eur J Cancer,* Vol.33, No.13, (November 1997), pp. 2203-2210, ISSN 0014-2964

Munro, A.J. (1995). An Overview of Randomized Controlled Trials of Adjuvant Chemotherapy in Head and Neck Cancer. *Br J Cancer,* Vol.71, No.1, (January 1995), pp. 83-91, ISSN 0007-0920

Nakamura, K.; Shioyama, Y.; Kawashima, M.; Saito, Y.; Nakamura, N.; et al. (2006). Multi-Institutional Analysis of Early Squamous Cell Carcinoma of the Hypopharynx Treated With Radical Radiotherapy. *Int J Radiat Oncol Biol Phys,* Vol.65, No.4, (July 2006), pp. 1045-1050, ISSN 0360-3016

National Comprehensive Cancer Network (NCCN) Clinical Practice Guidelines in Oncology: Head and Neck Cancers - V.2.2011, 30.04.2011, Available from http://www.nccn.org/professionals/physicians_gls/PDF/head-and-neck.pdf

Niibe, Y.; Karasawa, K.; Mitsuhashi, T. & Tanaka, Y. (2003). Hyperfractionated Radiation Therapy for Hypopharyngeal Carcinoma Compared With Conventional Radiation Therapy: Local Control, Laryngeal Preservation and Overall Survival. *Japanese Journal of Clinical Oncology,* Vol.33, No.9, (September 2003), pp. 450–455, ISSN 0368-2811

Nishimaki, T.; Kanda, T.; Nakagawa, S.; Kosuqi, S.; Tanabe, T.; et al. (2002). Outcomes and Prognostic Factors After Surgical Resection of Hypopharyngeal and Cervical Esophageal Carcinomas. *International Surgery,* Vol.87, No.1, (January-March 2002), pp. 38-44, ISSN: 0020-8868

Paccagnella, A.; Orlando, A.; Marchiori, C.; Zorat, P.L.; Cavaniglia, O.; et al. (1994). Phase III Trial of Initial Chemotherapy in Stage III or IV Head and Neck Cancers: A Study by the Gruppo di Studio sui Tumori della Testa e del Collo. *The Journal of the National Cancer Institute,* Vol.86, No.4, (February 1994), pp. 265-272, ISSN 0027-8874

Pameijer, F.A.; Mancuso, A.A.; Mendenhall, W.M.; Parsons, J.T.; Mukherji, S.K.; et al. (1998). Evaluation of Pretreatment Computed Tomography as a Predictor of Local Control in T1/T2 Pyriform Sinus Carcinoma Treated With Definitive Radiotherapy. *Head Neck,* Vol.20, No.2, (March 1998), pp. 159–168, ISSN 1043-3074

Park, Y.M.; Kim, W.S.; Byeon, H.K.; De Virgilio, A.; Jung, J.S.; et al. (2010). Feasibility of Transoral Robotic Hypopharyngectomy for Early-Stage Hypopharyngeal Carcinoma. *Oral Oncology,* Vol.46, No.8, (August 2010), pp. 597-602, ISSN 1368-8375

Parsons, J.T.; Cassisi, N.J. & Million, R.R. (1984). Results of Twice-a-Day Irradiation of Squamous Cell Carcinomas of the Head and Neck. *Int J Radiat Oncol Biol Phys,* Vol.10, No.11, (November 1984), pp. 2041–2051, ISSN 0360-3016

Parsons, J.T.; Mendenhall, W.M.; Stringer, S.P.; Cassisi, N.J. & Million, R.R. (1993). Twice-a-Day Radiotherapy for Squamous Cell Carcinoma of the Head and Neck: The University of Florida Experience. *Head Neck,* Vol.15, No.2, (April 1993), pp. 87–96, ISSN 1043-3074

Pene, F.; Avedian, V.; Eschwege, F.; Barrett, A.; Schwaab, G.; et al. (1978). A Retrospective Study of 131 Cases of Carcinoma of the Posterior Pharyngeal Wall. *Cancer,* Vol.42, No.5, (November 1978), pp. 2490–2493, ISSN 0008-543X

Pfister, D.G.; Hu, K.S. & Levebvre, J.L. (2009). Cancer of the Hypopharynx and Cervical Esophagus. Part A: General Principles and Management. In: *Head and Neck Cancer: A Multidisciplinary Approach,* L.B. Harrison, R.B. Session & W.K. Hong, (Eds.), 398-436, Lippincott Williams & Wilkins, ISBN 978-0-7817-7136-8, Philadelphia

Pignon, J.P.; Baujat, B. & Bourhis, J. (2005). Individual Patient Data Meta-Analyses in Head and Neck Carcinoma: What Have We Learnt? *Cancer Radiotherapie,* Vol.9, No.1, (February 2005), pp. 31-36, ISSN 1278-3218

Pignon, J.P.; Bourhis, J.; Domenge, C. & Designe, L. (2000). Chemotherapy Added to Locoregional Treatment for Head and Neck Squamous-Cell Carcinoma: Three Meta-Analyses of Updated Individual Data. MACH-NC Collaborative Group. Meta-Analysis of Chemotherapy on Head and Neck Cancer. *Lancet,* Vol.355, No.9208, (March 2000), pp. 949–955, ISSN 0023-7507

Pignon, J.P.; le Maitre, A.; Maillard, E. & Bourhis, J. (2009). Meta-Analysis of Chemotherapy in Head and Neck Cancer (MACH-NC): An Update on 93 Randomized Trials and 17,346 Patients. *Radiother Oncol,* Vol.92, No.1, (July 2009), pp. 4-14, ISSN 0167-8140

Pillsbury, H.C. & Clark, M. (1997). A Rationale for Therapy of the N0 Neck. *Laryngoscope,* Vol.107, No.10, (October 1997), pp. 1294-1315, ISSN 0023-852X

Pingree, T.F.; Davis, R.K.; Reichman, O. & Derrick, L. (1987). Treatment of Hypopharyngeal Carcinoma: A 10-Year Review of 1,362 Cases. *Laryngoscope,* Vol.97, No.8, Pt.1, (August 1987), pp. 901–904, ISSN 0023-852X

Pinnaro, P.; Cercato, C.; Giannarelli, D.; Carlini, P.; Del Vecchio, M.R.; et al. (1994). A Randomized Phase II Study Comparing Sequential Versus Simultaneous Chemo-Radiotherapy in Patients With Unresectable Locally Advanced Squamous Cell Cancer of the Head and Neck. *Annals of Oncology,* Vol.5, No.6, (July 1994), pp. 513-519, ISSN 0923-7534

Pivot, X.; Felip, E.; ESMO Guidelines Working Group. (2008). Squamous Cell Carcinoma of the Head and Neck: ESMO Clinical Recommendations for Diagnosis, Treatment and Follow-Up. *Annals of Oncology,* Vol.19, Suppl.2, (May 2008), ii79-ii80, ISSN 0923-7534

Pivot, X.; Magne, N.; Guadiola, E.; Poissonnet, G.; Dassonville, O. ; et al. (2005). Prognostic Impact of the Epidermal Growth Factor Receptor Levels for Patients With Larynx and Hypopharynx Cancer. *Oral Oncology,* Vol.41, No.3, (March 2005), pp. 320-327, ISSN 1368-8375

Plataniotis, G.A.; Theofanopoulou, M.E.; Kalogera-Fountzila, A.; Haritanti, A.; Ciuleanou, E.; et al. (2004). Prognostic Impact of Tumor Volumetry in Patients With Locally Advanced Head and Neck Carcinoma (Non-Nasopharyngeal) Treated by

Radiotherapy Alone or Combined Radiochemotherapy in a Randomized Trial. *Int J Radiat Oncol Biol Phys*, Vol.59, No.4, (July 2004), pp. 1018-1026, ISSN 0360-3016

Popescu, C.R.; Bertesteanu, S.V.G.; Mirea, D.; Grigore, R.; Ionescu, D.; et al. (2010). The Epidemiology of Hypopharynx and Cervical Esophagus Cancer. *Journal of Medicine and Life*, Vol.3, No.4, (November 2010), pp. 396-401, ISSN 1844-122x

Posner, M.R. (2005). Paradigm Shift in the Treatment of Head and Neck Cancer: The Role of Neoadjuvant Chemotherapy. *Oncologist*, Vol.10, Suppl3, (October 2005), pp. 11-19, ISSN 1083-7159

Posner, M.R.; Hershock, D.M.; Blajman, C.R.; Mickiewicz, E.; Winquist, E.; et al. (2007). Cisplatin and Fluorouracil Alone or With Docetaxel in Head and Neck Cancer. *N Engl J Med*, Vol.357, No.17, (October 2007), pp. 1705-1715, ISSN 0028-4793

Prades, J.M.; Lallemant, B.; Garrel, R.; Reyt, E.; Righini, C.; et al. (2010). Randomized Phase III Trial Comparing Induction Chemotherapy Followed by Radiotherapy to Concomitant Chemoradiotherapy for Laryngeal Preservation in T3M0 Pyriform Sinus Carcinoma. *Acta Otolaryngol*, Vol.130, No.1, (May 2010), pp. 150-155, ISSN 0001-6489

Prades, J.M.; Schmitt, T.M.; Timoshenko, A.P.; Simon, P.G.; de Cornulier, J.; et al. (2002). Concomitant Chemoradiotherapy in Pyriform Sinus Carcinoma. *Archives of Otolaryngology – Head & Neck Surgery*, Vol.128, No.4, (April 2002), pp. 384-388, ISSN 0886-4470

Prosnitz, R.G.; Yao, B.; Farell, C.L.; Clough. R. & Brizel, D.M. (2005). Pretreatment Anemia is Correlated With the Reduced Effectiveness of Radiation and Concurrent Chemotherapy in Advanced Head and Neck Cancer. *Int J Radiat Oncol Biol Phys*, Vol.61, No.4, (March 2005), pp. 1087-95, ISSN 0360-3016

Rapoport, A. & Franco, E.L. (1993). Prognostic Factors and Relative Risk in Hypopharyngeal Cancer-Related Parameters Concerning Stage, Therapeutics and Evolution. *Revista Paulista de Medicina*, Vol.111, No.2, (March-April 1993), pp. 337-343, ISSN, 0035-0362

Richards, B.L. & Spiro, J.D. (2000). Controlling Advanced Neck Disease: Efficacy of Neck Dissection and Radiotherapy. *Laryngoscope*, Vol.110, No.7, (July 2000), pp. 1124-1127, ISSN 0023-852X

Robbins, K.T.; Shaha, A.R.; Medina, J.E.; Califano, J.A.; Wolf, G.T.; et al. (2008). Consensus Statement on the Classification and Terminology of Neck Dissection. *Archives of Otolaryngology – Head & Neck Surgery*, Vol.134, No.5, (May 2008), pp. 536-538, ISSN 0886-4470

Robson, A. (2002). Evidence-Based Management of Hypopharyngeal Cancer. *Clinical Otolaryngology and Allied Sciences*, Vol.27, No.5, (October 2002), pp. 413-420, ISSN 0307-7772

Rosenthal, D.I. & Ang, K.K. (2004). Altered Radiation Therapy Fractionation, Chemoradiation, and Patient Selection for the Treatment of Head and Neck Squamous Carcinoma. *Seminars in Radiation Oncology*, Vol.14, No.2, (April 2004), pp. 153-166, ISSN 1053-4296

Rudert, H.H. & Hoft, S. (2003). Transoral Carbon-Dioxide Laser Resection of Hypopharyngeal Carcinoma. *European Archives of Oto-Rhino-Laryngology,* Vol.260, No.4, (April 2003), pp. 198-206, ISSN 0937-4477

Ruo Redda, M.G.; Ragona, R.; Ricardi, U.; Beltramo, G.; Rampino, M.; et al. (2010). Radiotherapy Alone or With Concomitant Daily Low-Dose Carboplatin in Locally Advanced, Unresectable Head and Neck Cancer: Definitive Results of a Phase III Study With a Follow-Up Period of up to Ten Years. *Tumori,* Vol.96, No.2, (March-April 2010), pp. 246-253, ISSN 0300-8916

Sakata, K.; Aoki, Y.; Karasawa, K.; Nakagawa, K.; Hasezawa, K.; et al. (1998). Analysis of Treatment Results of Hypopharyngeal Cancer. *Radiation Medicine,* Vol.16, No.1, (January-February 1998), pp. 31-36, ISSN 0288-2043

Samant, S.; Kumar, P.; Wan, J.; Hanchett, C.; Vieira, F.; et al. (1999). Concomitant Radiation Therapy and Targeted Cisplatin Chemotherapy for the Treatment of Advanced Pyriform Sinus Carcinoma: Disease Control and Preservation of Organ Function. *Head Neck,* Vol.21, No.7, (October 1999), pp. 595-601, ISSN 1043-3074

Sanchiz, F.; Milla, A.; Torner, J.; Bonet, F.; Artola, N.; et al. (1990). Single Fraction per Day Versus Two Fractions per Day Versus Radiochemotherapy in the Treatment of Head and Neck Cancer. *Int J Radiat Oncol Biol Phys,* Vol.19, No.6, (December 1990), pp. 1347-1350, ISSN 0360-3016

Sanguineti, G.; Corvo, R.; Benasso, M.; Margarino, G.; Sormani, M.; et al. (1999). Management of the Neck After Alternating Chemoradiotherapy for Advanced Head and Neck. *Head Neck,* Vol.21, No.3, (May 1999), pp. 223-228, ISSN 1043-3074

Sanguineti, G.; Richetti, A.; Bignardi, M.; Corvo, R.; Gabriele, P.; et al. (2005). Accelerated Versus Conventional Fractionated Postoperative Radiotherapy for Advanced Head and Neck Cancer: Results of a Multicenter Phase III Study. *Int J Radiat Oncol Biol Phys,* Vol.61, No.3, (March 2005), pp. 762-771, ISSN 0360-3016

Schrijvers, D.; Johnson, J.; Jiminez, U.; Gore, M.; Kosmidis, P.; et al. (1998). Phase III Trial of Modulation of Cisplatin/Fluorouracil Chemotherapy by Interferon Alfa-2b in Patients With Recurrent or Metastatic Head and Neck Cancer. *J Clin Oncol,* Vol.16, No.3, (March 1998), pp. 1054-1059, ISSN 0732–183X

Schwager, K.; Hoppe, F.; Hagen, R. & Brunner, F.X. (1999). Free-Flap Reconstruction for Laryngeal Preservation After Partial Laryngectomy in Patients With Extended Tumors of the Oropharynx and Hypopharynx. *European Archives of Oto-Rhino-Laryngology,* Vol.256, No.6, (July 1999), pp. 280-282, ISSN 0937-4477

Seiwert, T.Y. & Cohen, E.E.W. (2005). State-of-the-Art Management of Locally Advanced Head and Neck Cancer. *Br J Cancer,* Vol.92, No.8, (April 2005), pp. 1341–1348, ISSN 0007-0920

Semrau, R.; Mueller, R.P.; Stuetzer, H.; Staar, S.; Schroeder, U.; et al. (2006). Efficacy of Intensified Hyperfractionated and Accelerated Radiotherapy and Concurrent Chemotherapy With Carboplatin and 5-Flurouracil: Updated Results of a Randomized Multicentric Trial in Advanced Head-and-Neck Cancer. *Int J Radiat Oncol Biol Phys,* Vol.64, No.5 (April 2006), pp. 1308–1316, ISSN 0360-30162001

Sewnaik, A.; Hoorweg, J.J.; Knegt, P.P.; Wieringa, M.H.; van der Beek, J.M.H.; et al. (2005). Treatment of Hypopharyngeal Carcinoma: Analysis of Nationwide Study in the

Netherlands Over a 10-Year Period. *Clin Otolaryngol*, Vol.30, No.1, (February 2005), pp. 52-57, ISSN 1749-4478

Shah, H.K.; Khuntia, D.; Hoffman, H.T. & Harari, P.M. (2008). Hypopharyngeal Cancer, In: *Perez and Brady's Principles and Practice of Radiation Oncology*, E.C. Halperin, C.A. Perez, L.W. Brady LW, (Eds.), 958-974, Lippincot Williams & Wilkins, a Wolters Kluwer business, ISBN 078176369X, Philadelphia

Shangina, O.; Brennan, P.; Szeszenia-Dabrowska, N.; Mates, D.; Fabianova, E.; et al. (2006). Occupational Exposure and Laryngeal and Hypopharyngeal Cancer Risk in Central and Eastern Europe. *American Journal of Epidemiology*, Vol.164, No.4, (August 2006), pp. 367-375, ISSN 0002-9262

Siddiqui, F.; Sarin, R.; Agarwal, J.P.; Thotathil, Z.; Mistry, R.; et al. (2003). Squamous Carcinoma of the Larynx and Hypopharynx in Children: A Distinct Clinical Entity? *Medical and Pediatric Oncology*, Vol.40, No.5, (May 2003), pp. 322-324, ISSN 0098-1532

Slaughter, D.P.; Southwick, H.W. & Smejkal, W. (1953). Field Cancerization in Oral Stratified Squamous Epithelium; Clinical Implications of Multicentric Origin. *Cancer*, Vol.6, No.5, (September 1952), pp. 963–968, ISSN 0008-543X

Smeele, L.E.; Leemans, C.R.; Langendijk, J.A.; Tiwari, R.; Slotman, B.J.; et al. (2000). Positive Surgical Margins in Neck Dissection Specimens in Patients With Head and Neck Squamous Cell Carcinoma and the Effect of Radiotherapy. *Head Neck*, Vol.22, No.6, (September 2000), pp. 559-563, ISSN 1043-3074

Somers, K.D.; Merrick, M.A.; Lopez, M.E.; Incognito, L.S.; Schechter, G.L.; et al. (1992). Frequent P53 Mutations in Head and Neck Cancer. *Cancer Research*, Vol.52, No.21, (November 1992), pp. 5997–6000, ISSN 0008-5472

Sorensen, D.M.; Lewark, T.M.; Haney, J.L.; Meyers, A.D.; Krause, G.; et al. (1997). Absence of P53 Mutations in Squamous Carcinomas of the Tongue in Nonsmoking and Nondrinking Patients Younger than 40 Years. *Archives of Otolaryngology – Head & Neck Surgery*, Vol.123, No.5, (May 1997), pp. 503–506, ISSN 0886-4470

Spector, G.J. (2001). Distant Metastases from Laryngeal and Hypopharyngeal Cancer. *Journal for Oto-Rhino-Laryngology and Its Related Specialties*, Vol.63, No.4, (July-August 2001), pp. 224-228, ISSN 0301-1569

Spector, G.J.; Sessions, D.G.; Emami, B.; Simpson, J.; Haughey, B.; et al. (1995). Squamous Cell Carcinoma of the Pyriform Sinus: A Nonrandomized Comparison of Therapeutic Modalities and Long Term Results. *Laryngoscope*, Vol.105, No.4, (April 1995), pp. 397-406, ISSN 0023-852X

Spector, G.J.; Sessions, D.G.; Haughey, B.H.; Chao, K.S.C.; Simpson, J.; et al. (2001). Delayed Regional Metastases, Distant Metastases, and Second Primary Malignancies in Squamous Cell Carcinomas of the Larynx and Hypopharynx. *Laryngoscope*, Vol.111, No.6, (June 2001), pp. 1079-1087, ISSN 0023-852X

Spencer, S.A.; Harris, J.; Wheeler, R.H.; Machtay, M.; Schultz, C.; et al. (2001). RTOG 96-10: Reirradiation With Concurrent Hydroxyurea and 5-Fluorouracil in Patients With Squamous Cell Cancer of the Head and Neck. *Int J Radiat Oncol Biol Phys*, Vol.51, No.5, (December 2001), pp. 1299-1304, ISSN 0360-3016

Staar, S.; Rudat, V.; Stuetzer, H.; Dietz, A.; Volling, P.; et al. (2001). Intensified Hyperfractionated Accelerated Radiotherapy Limits the Additional Benefit of Simultaneous Chemotherapy-Results of a Multicentric Randomized German Trial in Advanced Head-and-Neck Cancer. *Int J Radiat Oncol Biol Phys,* Vol.50, No.5, (August 2001), pp. 1161-1171, ISSN 0360-30162001

Standring, S. (Ed). (2004). *Gray's Anatomy: The Anatomical Basis of Clinical Practice,* Churchill Livingstone, ISBN 0-443-07168-3, Philadelphia

Steiner, W.; Ambrosch, P.; Hess, C.F. & Kron, M. (2001). Organ Preservation by Transoral Laser Microsurgery in Piriform Sinus Carcinoma. *Otolaryngology-Head and Neck Surgery,* Vol.124, No.1, (January 2001), pp. 58-67, ISSN 0194-5998

Stell, P.M.; Carden, E.A.; Hibbert. J. & Dalby, J.E. (1978). Post Cricoid Carcinoma. *Clin Oncol,* Vol.4, No.3, (September 1978), pp. 215-226, ISSN 0305-7399

Stell, P.M; Ramadan, M.F.; Dalby, J.E.; Hibbert, J.; Raab, G.M.; et al. (1982). Management of Postcricoid Carcinoma. *Clinical Otolaryngology and Allied Sciences,* Vol.7, No.3, (June 1982), pp. 145-152, ISSN 0307-7772

Studer, G.; Lutolf, U.M.; Davis, J.B. & Glanzmann, C. (2006). IMRT in Hypopharyngeal Tumors. *Strahlenther Onkol,* Vol.182, No.6, (June 2006), pp. 331-335, ISSN 0179-7158

Studer, G.; Peponi, E.; Kloeck, S.; Dossenbach, T.; Huber, G.; et al. (2010). Surviving Hypopharynx-Larynx Carcinoma in the Era of IMRT. *Int J Radiat Oncol Biol Phys,* Vol.77, No.5, (August 2010), pp. 1391-1396, ISSN 0360-3016

Tai, S.K.; Yang, M.H.; Wang, L.W.; Tsai, T.L.; Chu, P.Y.; et al. (2008). Chemoradiotherapy Laryngeal Preservation for Advanced Hypopharyngeal Cancer. *Japanese Journal of Clinical Oncology,* Vol.38, No.8, (August 2008), pp. 521-527, ISSN 0368-2811

Taki, S.; Homma, A.; Oridate, N.; Suzuki, S.; Suzuki, F.; et al. (2010). Salvage Surgery for Local Recurrence After Chemoradiotherapy or Radiotherapy in Hypopharyngeal Cancer Patients. *European Archives of Oto-Rhino-Laryngology,* Vol.267, No.11, (November 2010), pp. 1765-1769, ISSN 0937-4477

Talton, B.M.; Elkon, D.; Kim, J.A.; Fitz-Hugh, G.S. & Constable, W. (1981). Cancer of the Posterior Hypopharyngeal Wall. *Int J Radiat Oncol Biol Phys,* Vol. 7, No.5, (May 1981), pp. 597-599, ISSN 0360-3016

Tandon, D.A.; Bahadur, S.; Chatterji, T.K. & Rath, G.K. (1991). Carcinoma of the Hypopharynx: Results of Combined Therapy. *Indian Journal of Cancer,* Vol.28, No.3, (September 1991), pp. 131-138, ISSN 0019-509X

Tani, M. & Amatsu, M. (1987). Discrepancies Between Clinical and Histopathologic Diagnoses in T3 Pyriform Sinus Cancer. *Laryngoscope,* Vol.97, No.1, (January 1987), pp. 93-96, ISSN 0023-852X

Taylor, J.M.; Mendenhall, W.M. & Lavey, R.S. (1991). Time-Dose Factors in Positive Neck Nodes Treated With Irradiation Only. *Radiother Oncol,* Vol.22, No.3, (November 1991), pp. 167-173, ISSN 0167-8140

Taylor, S.G. 4th; McGuire, W.P.; Hauck, W.W.; Showel, J.L. & Lad T.E. (1984). A Randomized Comparison of High-Dose Infusion Methotrexate Versus Standard-Dose Weekly Therapy in Head and Neck Squamous Cancer. *J Clin Oncol,* Vol.2, No.9, (September 1984), pp. 1006-1010, ISSN 0732-183X

Taylor, S.G. 4th; Murthy, A.K.; Vannetzel, J.M.; Colin, P.; Dray, M.; et al. (1994). Randomized Comparison of Neoadjuvant Cisplatin and Fluorouracil Infusion Followed by Radiation Versus Concomitant Treatment in Advanced Head and Neck Cancer. *J Clin Oncol*, Vol.12, No.2, (February 1994), pp. 385-395, ISSN 0732–183X

Teshima, T.; Chatani, M.; Inoue, T.; Miyahara, H. & Sato, T. (1988). Radiation Therapy for the Carcinoma of the Hypopharynx With Special Reference to Nodal Control. *Laryngoscope*, Vol.98, No.5, (May 1988), pp. 564-567, ISSN 0023-852X

Timon, C.V.; Toner, M. & Conlon, B.J. (2003). Paratracheal Lymph Node Involvement in Advanced Cancer of the Larynx, Hypopharynx and Cervical Oesophagus. *Laryngoscope*, Vol.113, No.9, (September 2003), pp. 1595-1599, ISSN 0023-852X

Toita, T.; Nakano, M.; Ogawa, K.; Koja, S.; Maeshiro, N.; et al. (1996). Prognostic Factors for Local Control in Hypopharyngeal Cancer Treated With Radical Irradiation. *Strahlenther Onkol*, Vol.172, No.1, (January 1996), pp. 30-33, ISSN 0179-7158

Tribius, S.; Kronemann, S.; Kilic, Y.; Schroeder, U.; Hakim, S.; et al. (2009). Radiochemotherapy Including Cisplatin Alone Versus Cisplatin + 5-Fluorouracil for Locally Advanced Unresectable Stage IV Squamous Cell Carcinoma of the Head and Neck. *Strahlenther Onkol*, Vol.185, No.10, (October 2009), pp. 675-681, ISSN 0179-7158

Tsikoudas, A.; Ghuman, N. & Riad, M.A. (2007). Globus Sensation as Early Presentation of Hypopharyngeal Cancer. *Clin Otolaryngol*, Vol.32, No.6, (December 2007), pp. 452-456, ISSN 1749-4478

Tsou, Y.A.; Hua, J.H.; Lin, M.H. & Tsai, M.H. (2006). Analysis of Prognostic Factors of Chemoradiation Therapy for Advanced Hypopharyngeal Cancer-Does Tumor Volume Correlate With Central Necrosis and Tumor Pathology? *Journal for Oto-Rhino-Laryngology and Its Related Specialties*, Vol.68, No.4, (February 2006), pp. 206-212, ISSN: 0301-1569

Tuyns, A.J.; Esteve, J.; Raymond, L.; Berrino, F.; Benhamou, E.; et al. (1988). Cancer of the Larynx/Hypopharynx, Tobacco and Alcohol: IARC International Case-Control Study in Turin and Varese (Italy), Zaragoza and Navarra (Spain), Geneva (Switzerland) and Calvados (France). *International Journal of Cancer*, Vol.41, No.4, (April 1988), pp. 483-491, ISSN 0020-7136

Uzcudun, A.E.; Bravo Fernández, P.; Sánchez, J.J.; Garcia Grane, A.; Rabanal Retolaza, I.; et al. (2001). Clinical Features of Pharyngeal Cancer: A Retrospective Study of 258 Consecutive Patients. *Journal of Laryngology and Otology*, Vol.115, No.2, (February 2001), pp. 112-118 ISSN 0022-2151

Van der Riet, P.; Nawroz, H.; Hruban, R.H.; Corio, R.; Tokino, K.; et al. (1994). Frequent Loss of Chromosome 9p21-22 Early in Head and Neck Cancer Progression. *Cancer Research*, Vol.54, No.5, (March 1994), pp. 1156–1158, ISSN 0008-5472

Van Herpen, C.M.; Mauer, M.E.; Mesia, R.; Degardin, M.; Lelic, S.; et al. (2010). Short-Term Health-Related Quality of Life and Symptom Control With Docetaxel, Cisplatin, 5-Fluorouracil and Cisplatin (TPF), 5-Fluorouracil (PF) for Induction in Unresectable Locoregionally Advanced Head and Neck Cancer Patients (EORTC 24971/TAX 323). *Br J Cancer*, Vol.103, No.8, (October 2010), pp. 1173-1181, ISSN 0007-0920

Van Mierlo, I.J.; Levendag, P.C.; Eijkenboom, W.M.; Jansen, P.P.; Meeuwis, C.A.; et al. (1995). Radiation Therapy for Cancer of the Piriform Sinus. A Failure Analysis. *Am J Clin Oncol*, Vol.18, No.6, (December 1995), pp. 502-509, ISSN 0277-3732

Van Oijen, M.G.C.T. & Slootweg P.J. (2000). Oral Field Cancerization: Carcinogen-Induced Independent Events or Micrometastatic Deposits? *Cancer Epidemiology, Biomarkers & Prevention*, Vol. 9, No.3, (March 2000), pp. 249–256, ISSN 1055-9965

Vandenbrouck, C.; Eschwege, F.; De La Rochefordiere, A.; Sicot, H.; Mamelle, G.; et al. (1987). Squamous Cell Carcinoma of the Pyriform Sinus: A Retrospective Study of 351 Cases Treated at the Institut Gustave-Roussy. *Head Neck Surg*, Vol.10, No.1, (September-October 1987), pp. 4–13, ISSN 0148-6403

Vermorken, J.B.; Mesia, R.; Rivera, F.; Remenar, E., Kawecki, A.; et al. (2008). Platinum-Based Chemotherapy Plus Cetuximab in Head and Neck Cancer. *N Engl J Med*, Vol.359, No.11, (September 2008), pp. 1116-1127, ISSN 0028-4793

Vermorken, J.B.; Remenar, E.; van Herpen, C.; Gorlia, T.; Mesia, R.; et al. (2007). Cisplatin, Fluorouracil, and Docetaxel in Unresectable Head and Neck Cancer. *N Engl J Med*, Vol.357, No.17, (October 2007), pp. 1695-1704, ISSN 0028-4793

Vilaseca, I.; Blanch, J.L.; Bernal-Sprekelsen, M. & Moragas, M. (2004). CO2 Laser Surgery: A Larynx Preservation Alternative for Selected Hypopharyngeal Carcinomas. *Head Neck*, Vol.26, No.11, (November 2004), pp. 953-959, ISSN 1043-3074

Vogl, S.E.; Schoenfeld, D.A.; Kaplan, B.H.; Lerner, H.J.; Engstrom, P.F.; et al. (1985). A Randomized Prospective Comparison of Methotrexate With a Combination of Methotrexate, Bleomycin, and Cisplatin in Head and Neck Cancer. *Cancer*, Vol.56, No.3, (August 1985), pp. 432-442, ISSN 0008-543X

Vokes, E.E. & Choong, N. (2008). Chemotherapy of Head and Neck Cancer. In: *The Chemotherapy Source Book*, M.C. Perry, (Ed.), 324-340, Lippincott Williams & Wilkins, ISBN 978-0-7817-7328-7, Philadelphia.

Vokes, E.E. & Weichselbaum, R.R. (1990). Concomitant Chemoradiotherapy: Rationale and Clinical Experience in Patients With Solid Tumors. *J Clin Oncol*, Vol.8, No.5, (May 1990), pp. 911–934, ISSN 0732–183X

Wang, C.C.; Blitzner, P.H. & Suit, H.D. (1985). Twice-a-Day Radiation Therapy for Cancer of the Head and Neck. *Cancer*, Vol.55, Suppl.9, (May 1985), pp. 2100–2104, ISSN 0008-543X

Weber, R.S.; Marvel, J.; Smith, P.; Hankins, P.; Wolf, P. & Goepfert, H. (1993). Paratracheal Lymph Node Dissection for Carcinoma of the Larynx, Hypopharynx, and Cervical Esophagus. *Otolaryngol Head Neck Surg*, Vol.108, No.1, (January 1993), pp. 11–17, ISSN 0194-5998

Wendt, T.G.; Grabenbauer, G.G.; Rodel, C.M.; Thiel, H.J.; Aydin, H.; et al. (1998). Simultaneous Radiochemotherapy Versus Radiotherapy Alone in Advanced Head and Neck Cancer: A Randomized Multicenter Study. *J Clin Oncol*, Vol.16, No.4, (April 1998), pp. 1318-1324, ISSN 0732–183X

Williams, M.E.; Gaffey, M.J.; Weiss, L.M.; Wilczynski, S.P.; Schuuring, E.; et al. (1993). Chromosome 11Q13 Amplification in Head and Neck Squamous Cell Carcinoma. *Archives of Otolaryngology – Head & Neck Surgery*, Vol.119, No.11, (November 1993), pp. 1238-1243 ISSN: 0886-4470

Williams, S.D.; Velez-Garcia, E.; Essessee, I.; Ratkin, G.; Birch, R.; et al. (1986). Chemotherapy for Head and Neck Cancer. Comparison of Cisplatin + Vinblastine + Bleomycin Versus Methotrexate. *Cancer,* Vol.57, No.1, (January 1986), pp. 18-23, ISSN 0008-543X

Wygoda, A.; Skladowski, K.; Tarnawski, R.; Sasiadek, W.; Mucha, A.; et al. (2000). Prognostic Factors in Radiotherapy for Hypopharyngeal Cancer. *Otolaryngologia Polska,* Vol. 54, Suppl.31, (January 2000), pp. 33-36, ISSN 0030-6657

Yates, A. & Crumley, R.L. (1984). Surgical Treatment of Pyriform Sinus Cancer: A Retrospective Study. *Laryngoscope,* Vol.94, No.12, Pt.1, (December 1984), pp. 1586–1590, ISSN 0023-852X

Zackrisson, B.; Nilsson, P.; Kjellen, E.; Johansson, K.A.; Modig, H.; et al. (2011). Two-Year Results from a Swedish Study on Conventional Versus Accelerated Radiotherapy in Head and Neck Squamous Cell Carcinoma - The ARTSCAN Study. *Radiother Oncol,* (2011), doi:10.1016/j.radonc.2010.12.010

Zelefsky, M.J.; Kraus, D.H.; Pfister, D.G.; Raben, A.; Shah, J.P.; et al. (1996). Combined Chemotherapy and Radiotherapy Versus Surgery and Postoperative Radiotherapy for Advanced Hypopharyngeal Cancer. *Head Neck,* Vol.18, No.5, (September-October 1996), pp. 405–411, ISSN 1043-3074

Zorat, P.L.; Paccagnella, A.; Cavaniglia, G.; Loreggian, L.; Gava, A.; et al. (2004). Randomized Phase III Trial of Neoadjuvant Chemotherapy in Head and Neck Cancer: 10-Year Follow-Up. *The Journal of the National Cancer Institute,* Vol.96, No.22, (November 2004), pp. 1714-1717, ISSN 0027-8874

2

Laryngeal Cancers in Sub-Saharan Africa

Mala Bukar Sandabe,
Hamman Garandawa and Abdullahi Isa
Department of ENT University of Maiduguri Teaching Hospital Nigeria

1. Introduction

Laryngeal cancers are not common[1]. Squamous cell carcinomas of the larynx are the commonest head and neck tumour in the western world. It represents approximately 1% of all malignancy in males [1]. It's about five times common in men than in women. The cause is unknown but tobacco smoking and alcohol acting synergistically increases the risk, radiation, asbestos and a number of occupational factors are implicated. Patients usually present with progressive hoarseness and difficulty in breathing, pain is an uncommon symptom whereas dysphagia, neck swelling, cachexia and fetor indicate advance disease. All patients in our series are black Africans and unfortunately they presents late. The cancer is confirmed by biopsy of the tumour through direct laryngoscopy under general anaesthesia. And tentative treatment depends on the stage of the tumour.

2. Research methodology

This would be 10 years retrospective studies of black African patients with laryngeal carcinomas carried out in University of Maiduguri Teaching Hospital Maiduguri, Federal Medical Centre Nguru, Federal Medical Centre, Yola. These hospitals are located in the North Eastern region of Nigeria, Sub-Saharan Africa. These centers also receive patients from neighboring countries of Niger, Chad and Cameroon. Clinical records of all patients with histologically confirmed laryngeal carcinoma from January 2001 - December 2010 were reviewed, data extracted from the records includes biodata, presenting complaints (the main complaints for which the patient sought medical advice), and associated complaints (complaints regarded as unimportant by the patient), duration of presenting complaints, duration of symptoms on first presentation, Social habit, physical examination findings, X-ray of soft tissue neck, CT-Scan/MRI of the Larynx findings, the site of the lesion in the larynx, histopathological types, treatment offered and symptom free period after treatment (last entry in the case note) . Data was analyzed using Statistical Package for Social Sciences (SPSS) - version 15 software. Descriptive analysis done for all data; Chi square test, and correlation studies were applied where appropriate. Results was presented in tables and graphs. P - Value < 0.05 was considered significant.

3. Literature review

Grossly the larynx extends from the superior border of the epiglottis to the inferior border of the cricoid cartilage. Anteriorly, it is related to the lingual epiglottis, the thyrohyoid membrane, the anterior commissure, thyroid cartilage, cricothyroid membrane and the anterior arch of the cricoid cartilage. The posterior relations are the posterior commissure the arytenoids, and the interarytenoid Space. [1.] Squamous cell carcinoma of the larynx is the commonest head and neck cancer in the Western world. In the UK it represents approximately 1% of all malignancies in men. (Powell and Robin, 1983). It is about five times commoner in males than in females. The incidence increases with age, but the peak age of presentation is in the seventh decade. The cause of cancer of the larynx is not known, but there is an indisputable relationship between tobacco smoking and alcohol consumption, (US surgeon general, 1979; Hinds, Thomas and O'Reilly, 1979). Verrucous carcinoma is a distinct variant of well differentiated Squamous cell carcinoma. (Ackerman's tumour). Other malignant tumour types include adenocarcinoma, adenoid cystic carcinoma, fibrosarcoma, Chondrosarcoma and lymphomas. Spread and growth depends on the site of origin of the primary tumour. Anatomical barriers are important factors in determining the direction and extend of tumour growth.

1. **Supraglottis**. This comprises the larynx superior to the apex of the ventricle. Exophytic supraglottic cancers do not often extends to the glottic region and seldom involve the thyroid cartilage, Ulcerative lesions may extend down below the anterior commissure, Cranially supraglottic cancers extend to the vallecular and base of the tonque, arytenoids cartilage and pyriform sinus is reach by deep invasion.[1,2.]
2. **Glottis.** This comprises the vocal cords and the anterior and posterior commissures. Most of the tumours originates in the free margins of the vocal cords which are covered by squamous epithelium. Tumour may extend along the cord to the anterior commissure and to the muscles of the vocal cord. Fixation of the vocal cords indicate deep invasion
3. **Subglottis.** This extends from the inferior border of the glottis to the lower border of the cricoids cartilage, tumours are rare, grow circumferentially, usually extensive before symptoms appear which is mainly inspiratory sridor.[1,2.]

4. Clinical features

Hoarseness is the main symptoms; [1, 2, 3.] Dyspnoea and stridor are late symptoms and usually indicate an advanced tumour. Pain in the throat is an uncommon symptom. Dysphagia indicates pharyngeal invasion Neck swelling indicate extra laryngeal extension or lymph nodes involvement. Symptoms of anorexia, cachexia and fetor imply advanced disease. Indirect laryngoscopy should reveal the site and size of the lesions however because of difficulty in examining the subglottic and the laryngeal surface of the epiglottis. Flexible Fibre optic laryngoscopy helps in visualizing all part of the larynx. The neck should be palpated for the presence of enlarged lymph nodes. Laryngeal tumours usually metastasize to the upper deep cervical lymph nodes, but supraglottic tumours may cause bilateral nodes, and some subglottic tumours may spread to the upper mediastinal nodes.

Palpable lymph nodes are important in determining prognosis, about one-third of patients with no palpable lymph nodes have histologically positive nodes, and a similar number of palpable nodes are histologically negative.

5. Investigations of patients with laryngeal cancer

The main stay of investigation in our center was radiography. Plain X-rays soft tissue neck was done by the entire patient studied. Although plain X-rays soft tissue neck has no role in the current management of patients with carcinoma of the larynx, prevertebral soft tissue thickness, the epiglottis can be visualized; it is also affordable in the developing countries. Cost about 8USD. Computerized tomography scan(CT-Scan) which include contrast enhanced helical CT scanning has a high sensitivity 91% and high negative predictive values of 95% in detecting cartilage invasion of CA larynx[7]. In our survey only 15(16.1%) of our patients had CT scanning done. This is due to the high cost of CT scan per session. It cost about 300USD and most of the patients live on less than a Dollar a day. Magnetic resonance imaging(MRI) which has several advantages over CT-scan especially in pre- surgical planning can only be done by 6(6.5%) of our patients due to the cost per session of 400USD. The multiplanner capabilities of MRI are superior to the reformations available with the traditional CT-scan. MRI has been found to have a sensitivity of 89-94%, specificity 74-88% and a negative predictive value of 94-96% for the detection of neoplastic invasion[7]. Positron emission tomography (PET) which is critical in detection of metastasis and for follow-up of treated patients, but sadly such services is nonexistent in most developing nations.

6. Treatment options 1, 2, 3, 5, 6

The standard treatment of laryngeal carcinoma is surgery and radiotherapy in varying combinations. Surgery involves partial or total removal of the larynx to achieve cure, radiotherapy have been found to be effective in early laryngeal cancers (T1 and T2) with local control ranging from 70-100%. In advance laryngeal cancers (T3 and T4) post operative chemoradiation can achieve loco-regional control.[4].

	frequency	Percentage (%)
Partial laryngectomy and radiotherapy	6	6.5
Total laryngectomy and radiotherapy	18	19.3
Radiotherapy alone	32	34.4
Chemotherapy and radiotherapy	37	39.7

Table 1.

	1-2 years	3-4years	5-6 years	7-8 years	9-10 years	Total
Male	30	17	6	0	3	78
Female	6	3	0	3	0	15
Total	36	20	6	3	3	93

Table 2. Symptom free period

	<1year	1-2years	3-4years	5-6years	7-8years	9-10years	Total
supraglottic	9	12	5	3	3	3	35
glottic	0	0	6	3	0	0	9
subglottic	3	0	6	0	0	0	9
transglottic	13	24	3	0	0	0	40
total	25	36	20	6	3	3	93

Table 3. Symptom free period

Most patients in our series where offered synchronous therapy of chemoradiation because of late presentation 54(58%) and 27(29%) presented in stage III and stage IV respectively, however the survival rate barely 1-2years and because of late presentation in our series most glottis tumour have progress to transglottic on presentation with average symptom free period of 3years after treatment. Overall 6(6.5%) had partial laryngectomy and post-operative radiotherapy, 18(19.3%) had total laryngectomy and post-operative radiotherapy, 32(34.4%) had radiotherapy alone and 37(39.7%) had chemotherapy and radiotherapy. The common agents used in our series include cisplatin, 5-florouracil, docetaxel and Adriamycin in varying combinations and administered either as neoadjuvant, adjuvant or concomitant chemotherapy.

7. Discussion

Laryngeal cancer is the most common cancer of the aerodigestive track, it accounts for 20% of all head and neck cancers. The incidence of these tumours is closely correlated with smoking cigarettes, as head and neck tumours occur 6(six) times more often among cigarettes smokers then among non smokers.

Cancer of the larynx has been found to be commoner in males, it occurs in increasing age with the peak incidence being in the 5th decade.

In our study, 93 patients were surveyed with carcinoma of the larynx, 78 (83.9%) male and females constituted 15 (16.1%) mean age of 56 years (+ 6- 8yrs), M: F=5.2:1.

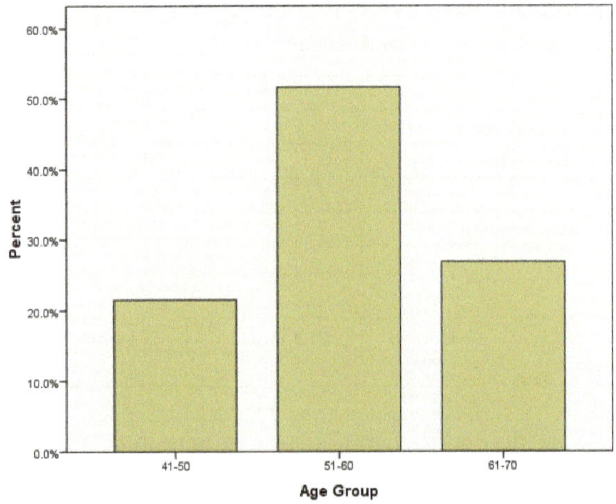

Fig. 1. Age distribution

The estimated incidence of carcinoma of the larynx in the United States is about 12,000 per annum while in Nigeria the incidence is estimated at 783 per annum. Squamous cell carcinoma is the commonest histological type; in our series it constituted 90.3% other were verrucous Carcinoma, 32% and Adenocarcinoma 6.5%. Studies conducted elsewhere in the country by Amusa et al also showed the histological type to be predominantly squamous cell. [8]

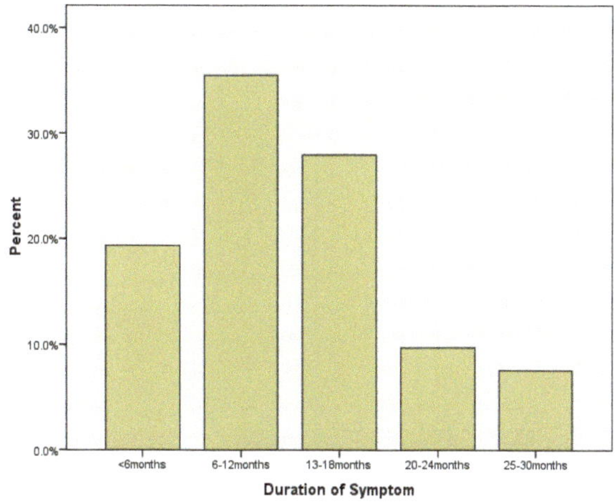

Fig. 2. Duration of symtoms

	frequency	Percentage (%)
Squamous cell carcinoma	84	90.3
Verrucous carcinoma	3	3.2
Adenocarcinoma	6	6.5
Total	93	100.0

Table 4. Histological types

Transglottic carcinoma was found to be the commonest with 40 (43.0%), supraglottic, 35 (37.6%): table V. This is in contrast to other studies in which most laryngeal cancers arise from the glottis,[9] this could be due to the late presentation in most of the patients with loco-regional involvement, (images 1, 2 and 3)

Site	N (%)
Transglottic	40(43.0)
Supraglottic	35(37.6)
Glottic	9(9.7)
Subglottic	9(9.7)
Total	93(100.0)

Table 5.

Most of the patient presented with stage - III tumours, this is in agreement with most head and neck tumour presentation in developing countries.

	Supraglottic	Glottic	Subglottic	Transglottic	Total
Male	29	9	6	34	78
Female	6	0	3	6	15
TOTAL	35	9	9	40	93

Table 6. Site of lesion

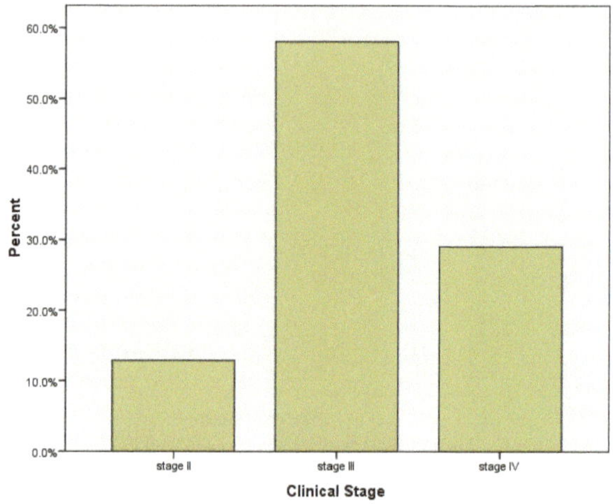

Fig. 3. Clinical stage at presentation

There was a significant correlation between the clinical stage of the tumour at presentation and the site of the lesion, most patient present with stages III &IV transglottic or supraglottic tumour. P<0.05 (0.000).

	Stage II	Stage III	Stage IV	Total
Supraglottc	3	20	12	35
Glottic	9	0	0	9
Subglottic	0	9	0	9
Transglottic	0	25	15	40
Total	12	54	27	93

Table 7. Correlation between clinical stage of patient and site of lesion

Correlation also exist between the site of the lesion and the social habit of the patients, with those who smoke cigarettes and drink alcohol presenting more with glottis tumours P< 0.05(0.00) This could be due to the synergistic effect of cigarette smoking and alcohol on head and neck tumours.

	Supraglottic	Glottic	Subglottic	Transglottic	Total
smoke	12	0	0	15	27
alcohol	0	0	0	3	3
Smoke and alcohol	3	6	3	3	15
None	20	3	6	19	48
Total	35	9	9	40	93

P<0.05(0.000)

Table 8. Correlation between social habit of patients and site of lesion

Site of lesion	Stage II	Stage III	Stage IV	Total
Supraglottic	3	20	12	35
Glottic	9	0	0	9
Subglottic	0	9	0	9
Transglottic	0	25	15	40
Total	12	54	27	93

And the site of lesion $P<0.05$ (0.000)

Table 9. Correlation between the clinical stages of the tumour

8. Conclusion

In conclusion black African patients in our study typically present late which accounts for the higher number of transglottic and supraglottic cancers. Among some of the reasons for late presentations are lack of affordability and accessibility by most patients to tertiary health facility in developing countries like Nigeria. The national health insurance scheme covers less than 10% of the population of 150million Nigerians thus living the majority to pay an exorbitant fee for health care services. Another reason is the absence of radiotherapy centers in most tertiary health facility in developing countries such that patient have to travel a long distance with their relatives to access such services further increasing the cost of treatment and delay before presentation.

Finally there is a need to educate the general public and especially health care providers to promptly refer patients with hoarseness of more than 2 weeks duration for direct laryngoscopy and biopsy by an otolaryngologist.

Most countries in sub-Saharan Africa are now emerging democracies, and thus the challenges of infrastructural development and health care reforms are central to effective governance.

In Nigeria for instance in the last ten years about 20 tertiary health centers are established by the governments and the existing teaching hospitals are completely overhauled to improve service delivery particularly in the area of cancer management, new radiotherapy centers are established to complement the old existing ones, which are also upgraded. Also most states in Nigeria have upgraded some of their secondary health centers to specialist tertiary health care centers while the existing secondary health centers are renovated and equipped with modern facilities. Personnel are also trained to reduce the doctor to patient's ratio and also to manage the new and modern equipments, for example a decade ago there are about 30 trained ENT surgeons practicing in Nigeria but with better facilities and more training centers there are now about 350 ENT surgeons in Nigeria. Patients are now seeking prompt medical consultations to find solutions to their health problems, this is partly made possible by continuous health education through both electronic and prints media. However there are some problems militating against improved health care services particularly in cancer management, these are, paucity of clinical pathologist, lack of regular maintenance of medical hardware's partly because of lack of spare parts and the technical knowhow in sub-Saharan Africa.

The future direction in head and neck cancer management in Africa is promising because both governments and non-governmental organizations are establishing various cancer treatment centers to complement the existing centers. Through the non-governmental organizations doctors and other health care workers all over the world are visiting and assisting African patients from all field of medical specialty.

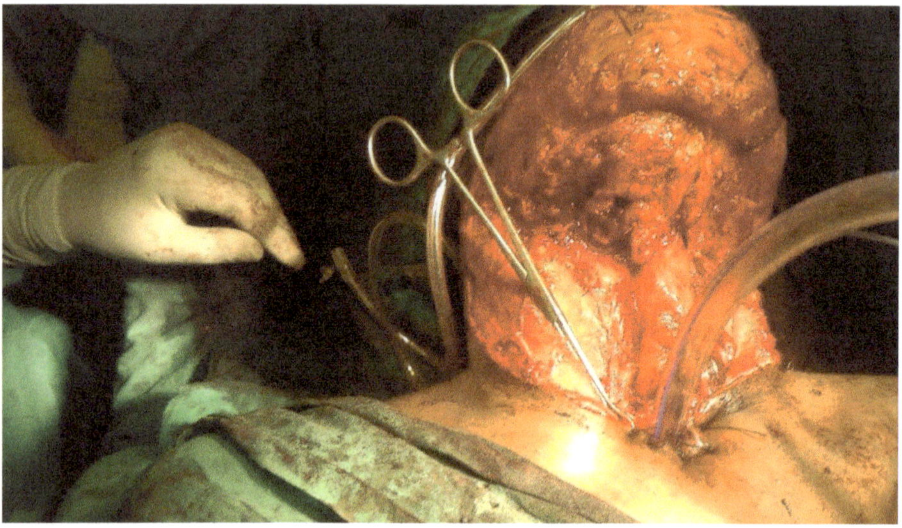

Picture 1. Gluck Sorenson incision and flap Secured to the chin, with tracheostomy Pre-operatively done to relieve airway obstruction.

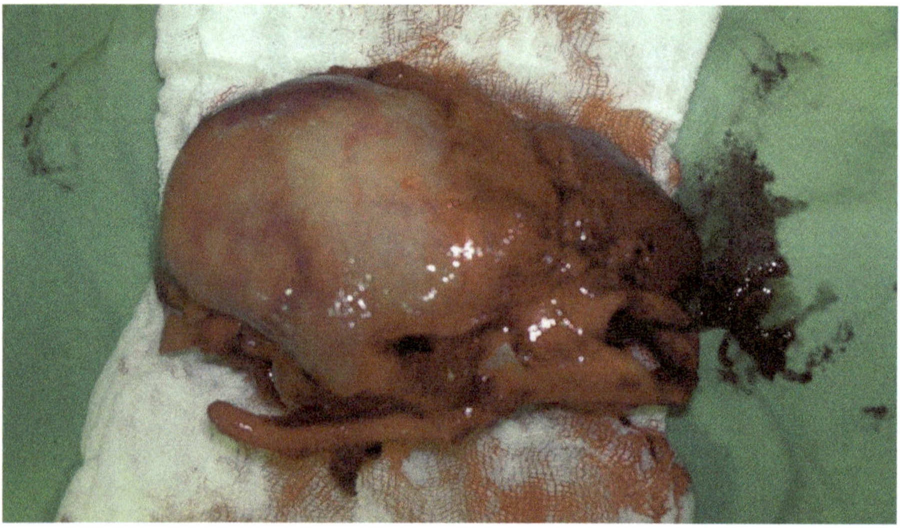

Picture 2. A complete surgical specimen of the larynx with hyoid bone.

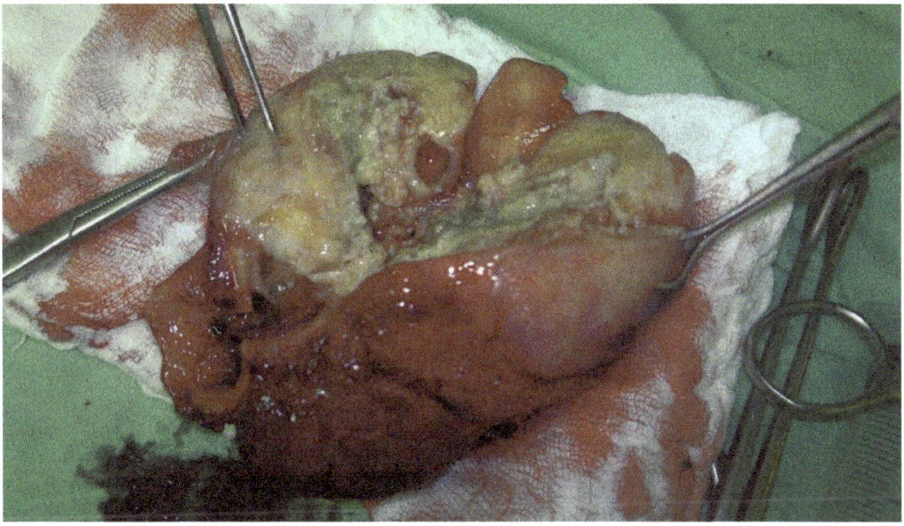

Picture 3. A Longitudinal cut through laryngeal specimen showing the Transglottic spread of the tumour

9. References

[1] P.E.Robin and Jan Olofsson; Scott-Brown's otolaryngology and head and neck surgery, vol 5, 6th ed. 1997.

[2] NJ Roland, RDR McRae, AW McCombe; Key Topics in otolaryngology and head and neck surgery,2nd ed.2001.

[3] Iseh KR, Abdullahi M, Aliyu D; Laryngeal tumours: Clinical pattern in Sokoto, Northwestern, Nigeria, Nig journal of medicine, vol. 20, No.1.2011.

[4] Babagana M. Ahmad; Laryngeal carcinoma-current treatment options, Nig journal of medicine, vol. 8, No. 1.1999.

[5] Otoh EC, Johnson NW, Danfillo IS, Adeleke OA, Olasoji HA. Primary head and neck cancers in Northeastern Nigeria. West Afr J. Med. 2004, oct-dec; 23(4): 305-13.

[6] Bhatia PL. Head and neck cancers in plateau state of Nigeria. West Afr J of Med.1990, oct-dec; 9(4): 304-10.

[7] Becker M, Burkhardt K, Dulgnerov P, et al. imaging of the larynx and hypopharynx. Eur J Radiol, Jun 2008, 66(3):460-79.

[8] YB Amusa, A Balmus, JK Olabanji, EO Oyebanjo. Laryngeal carcinoma: Experience in Ile-ife, Nigeria, Nigerian Journal of clinical practice 2011, 14 (1):74- 78.

[9] Samuel W.B., Marshall M., Roy R.C. Laryngeal cancer, www.health.am/cr/laryngeal-cancer.

[10] Nasir Iqbal, James S, Simon L, Arthur J.F, Harold E.K, Michelle L.M, Ayeesha W, Sameer R. K. Laryngeal carcinoma imaging, www.emedicine/ medscape.com/article/383230. May 27, 2011

[11] Incidence (Annual) of larynx cancer,www.health24.com/medical/condition_centres.

[12] Devleena M. A., Soumita P., Anondiya C. Comparison of vindrelbine with cisplatin in concomitant chemoradiotherapy in head and neck cancer; Ind. J Med. Peadtr Onco 2010 31 (1): 4-7

Part 2

Biology of Head and Neck Cancer

3

Molecular Genetics and Biology of Head and Neck Squamous Cell Carcinoma: Implications for Diagnosis, Prognosis and Treatment

Federica Ganci, Andrea Sacconi, Valentina Manciocco, Renato Covello, Giuseppe Spriano, Giulia Fontemaggi and Giovanni Blandino
Regina Elena Cancer Institute
Italy

1. Introduction

Head and neck cancers are different types of tumours found in the upper aero-digestive tract. The vast majority of them (more than 90%) are squamous cell carcinomas (HNSCC) that originate in the epithelium lining of the oral cavity, pharynx and larynx. There is a higher incidence rate in males compared to females (Ragin et al, 2007). The median age of patients with HNSCC is about 60 years (Ragin et al, 2007). Young patients make up 1-8% (Llewellyn et al, 2004). HNSCC comprise 5.5% of all incidence cancers (Mitra et al, 2007) and is the sixth leading cancer worldwide with approximately 600,000 cases reported annually (Leemans et al, 2011). Local recurrence affects about 60% of patients and metastases develop in 15-20% of cases (Choi & Chen, 2005). About 40-50% of patients with HNSCC survive for 5 years (Leemans et al, 2011). About one third of patients are diagnosed with early-stage disease, whereas the majority are diagnosed with advanced stage cancer with lymph node metastases. Early stage tumours are treated by surgery or radiotherapy ensuing more favourable prognosis. Surgery is the main source of treating advanced tumors combined with post-operative chemo- and radio-therapy. Over the past two decades, the quality of life of patients with HNSCC has increased due to the ample use of more advanced surgical and radiotheraupeutic techniques, as well as organ preservation protocols. Despite these improvements, survival has not markedly improved because patients still frequently develop local-regional recurrences, distant metastases and second primary tumors. The TNM staging system, that is most often used to classify patients with HNSCC, is based on the clinical, radiological and pathological examination of tumor specimens. This system does not adequately address the molecular heterogeneity of HNSCC and the ability of staging to predict prognosis in HNSCC is limited because patients with tumours with the same clinicopathologic stage do not have the same disease progression, response to therapy, rate of disease recurrence and survival (Leemans et al, 2011; Choi & Chen, 2005). Ongoing molecular studies show that these HNSCC may not be considered as homogenous as previously supposed (Pai & Westra, 2009). Recognition of distinct molecular and genetic profiles could permit finer resolution of HNSCC into distinct subtypes that differ with regard to risk factors, pathogenesis and clinical behavior. A more detailed molecular characterization ultimately is likely to improve the development of new therapeutic strategies, potentially relevant to diagnosis and prognosis of this poorly defined subset of head and neck cancers.

2. Risk factors

The main risk factor for HNSCC is tobacco smoking. This risk is strongly correlated with the time and rate who person smokes. In fact, when a person stops smoking it reduces the risk of developing cancer (Schlecht et al, 1999). Besides environmental exposure to tobacco smoke, passive smoking appears to increase the risk of developing HNSCC, even for individuals who have never actively smoked (Zhang et al, 2000). This increased risk is mostly attributable to the genotoxic effects of carcinogens in tobacco smoke, including nitrosamines and polycyclic hydrocarbons. Tobacco smoking has showed to have site specific differences in the anatomical sub-regions, with an increase in sensitivity from the oral cavity down to the larynx (Werbrouck et al, 2008). Tobacco has also proven to be a significant prognostic marker (Ragin et al, 2007; Leemans et al, 2011). Identifying the molecular targets of cigarette smoking in order to discern a specific profile of tobacco-induced mutations is still currently being studied. *TP*53 mutations and overexpression in HNSCC, for example, occur more frequently in patients who smoke than in patients who do not smoke (Field et al, 1991; Ronchetti et al, 2004). Much attention has been focused on genetic polymorphisms in those enzymes that activate pro-carcinogens and detoxify carcinogens; however no clear-cut association has been established yet. Heavy use of alcohol has also been recognized as an independent risk factor for HNSCC, particularly for cancer of the hypopharynx (Sturgis et al, 2004). However, alcohol consumption is mainly relevant for its ability in magnifying its effects with tobacco smoke in a synergistic manner (Talamini et al, 2002). Its ability in enhancing the effects of smoking most likely resides in its nature as a chemical solvent, increasing and prolonging mucosal exposure to the carcinogens present in tobacco (Pai & Westra, 2009). In addition, although alcohol itself is not a direct carcinogen, its metabolites and acetaldehyde form DNA adducts that interfere with DNA synthesis and repair. Polymorphisms in the enzymes that metabolize alcohol to acetaldehyde have not been conclusively associated with modifying cancer risk. A subgroup of HNSCC, particularly those of the oropharynx and oral cavity, is also caused by high risk infection types of human papillomavirus (especially HPV-16 and 18) (Chung & Gillison, 2009; Leemans et al, 2011). HPV has been established as a causative agent in about 70% of oral cavity and oropharyngeal cancers. The vast majority of HPV-positive HNSCC localizes to the tonsillar crypts of the lingual and palate tonsils. Its structural features render them particularly vulnerable to HPV attack (Pai & Westra, 2009). The traditional risk factors, tobacco and alcohol use, do not appear to play a contributing role in HPV-related cancers (D'Souza et al, 2007). Certain sexual practices that facilitate repeated viral exposure are strongly associated with HPV oral infection (Smith et al, 2004). Although the risk factors for HPV viral infection are well recognized, those associated with subsequent HPV-induced tumorigenesis are now only coming into focus. However, it is known that HPV-positive and negative tumours represent different clinical pathological and molecular entities (Table 1) and that HPV-related tumours, which constitute about 20% of all HNSCC subtypes, are associated with a more favorable outcome (Chung & Gillison, 2009, Leemans et al, 2011).

	HPV positive	HPV negative
Risk factors	High-risk sexual behavior	Smoking and alcohol use
Predilection site	Oropharynx and oral cavity especially lingual and palatine tonsil	None
Main molecular genetic alterations	Infrequent p53 mutations, degradation of p53-Rb pathway by HPV E6/E7 protein	High frequency of p53 mutations, 17p and 9p loh, loss of p16 expression
Prognosis	Better	Worse

Table 1. Main characteristics of HPV+ and HPV- HNSCC

3. Genetic alterations

It is well known that HNSCC is the result of a multistep process characterized by the accumulation of genetic and epigenetic alterations (Ha et al, 2009). The genetic alterations associated with HNSCC are numerous and include a variety of different pathways (Table 2). The accumulation and selection of these aberrant pathways may sometimes be due to random chance, but more commonly, they are attributable to a lifetime of environmental exposure to tobacco, alcohol and HPV infection. Therefore, the chance of DNA damage is high and often there is an accumulation of genetic events that lead to the development of HNSCC (Ha et al, 2009). Genetic alterations, including copy number variations (CNV), gains or losses of heterozigosity (LOH) may cause the inactivation of tumor suppressor genes and the activation of oncogenes, which in turn lead to uncontrolled cell growth and metastasis (Chen & Chen, 2009). In order to identify the genetic alterations, such as chromosomal deletions and/or amplifications, the presence of Single Nucleotide Polymorphisms SNPs or mutations in oncogenes/tumour suppressor genes or other genes, different techniques can be adopted from various low throughput and high throughput methods (Ha et la, 2009). The low throughput resolution methods are brought about by a study of CNV/LOH using polymerase chain reaction (PCR) -related methods and fluorescence in situ hybridization (FISH). The high throughput resolution methods are the array-related methods, such as Comparative Genomic Hybridization (CGH) array, to identify genome wide CNV/LOH events. The arrays have the ability to finely map regions of chromosomal gain or loss, much more accurately than the conventional molecular techniques. Regions of chromosomal loss commonly reported are at 1p, 3p, 4p, 5q, 8p, 10p, 11q, 13q and 18q, while those that are frequently gained are at 1q, 3q, 5p, 7q, 8q, 9q, 11q, 12p, 14q and 15q (Ha et al, 2009; Wreesmann & Singh, 2005). Most possibly, the presence of CNV/LOH has the potential to

Locus or gene	Frequency in HNSCC
LOH 3p	60-70%
LOH 9p	70-80%
LOH 11q	30%
LOH 13q	30%
LOH 17p	50-70%
p16 inactivation	80%
Cyclin D1 amplification	30%
FHIT, RASSF1A inactivation	50-80%
*TP*53 mutations	60-80%

Table 2. Frequent molecular abnormalities in HNSCC (Perez-Ordonez et al, 2006)

serve as a prognostic indicator, alone or in combination with other markers, to identify HNSCC patients at high risk of recurrence and death (Chen & Chen, 2008).

3.1 The molecular biology of field cancerization of HNSCC

In 1953, the term "field cancerization" was introduced to explain two phenomena: (1) the high tendency to develop local recurrences after treatment of HNSCC and, (2) the high likelihood that multiple independent tumours would develop in the head neck mucosa (Ha & Califano, 2003). According to this concept, molecular genetic approaches have recently shown that when a primary HNSCC is compared with a second tumour elsewhere in the respiratory tract, the paired tumours often harbor some identical patterns of genetic alterations (Pai & Westra, 2009). In all probability, a critical genetic alteration may be a single cell providing a growth advantage over its neighboring cells. These cells can migrate to populate continuous tracts of mucosa, accumulate other alterations, acquire additional growth advantage and ultimately transform into aggressive subclones separated by time and space (Califano et al, 2000). It is important to note that, the epithelium of the upper respiratory tract may be populated by these genetically damaged clones and may lack hystopathological evidence of dysplasia. Thus, the presence of morphologically intact but genetically damaged cells may perhaps explain the mechanism underlying cancerization as well as certain distress patterns of tumour behavior, such as local recurrences following seemingly to complete surgical resection. A current model of HNSCC progression associates the loss of chromosomal arms 3p, 9p and 17p with conversion from normal to dysplastic epithelium. Subsequent loss of 11q, 13q and 14q is associated with progression to carcinoma in situ, with the loss of 6p, 8p, 8q and 4q seen in more advanced stages with invasive property (Califano et al, 1996; Choi & Chen, 2005; Perez-Ordonez et al, 2006) (fig.1).

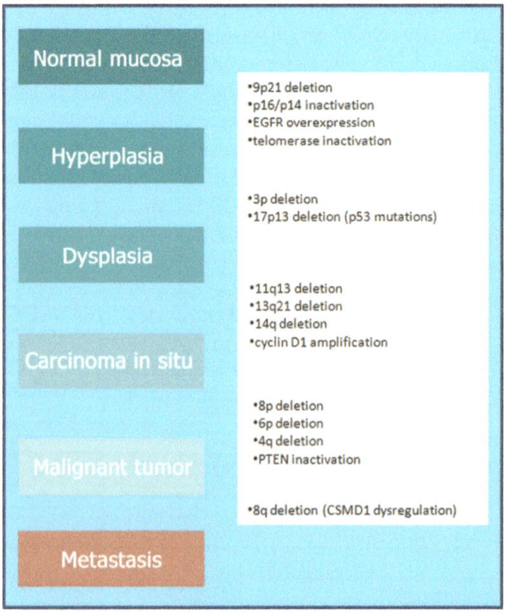

Fig. 1. HNSCC carcinogenesis model, modified from Califano et al. (1996)

3.2 Molecular genetics of premalignant oral lesions

HNSCC develops from normal aereodigestive mucosa progressing through a series of histological identifiable pre-malignant stages. In particular, oral squamous cell carcinomas (OSCC) may be preceded by the appearance of lesions, which have the potential to develop into cancer in the oral cavity. The development of OSCC is generally expected upon the development of multiple, clonal, genetic alterations, which lend a clonal population of cells a growth advantage over others. The distinction between benign and potentially malignant oral lesions is currently based upon the histological examination of biopsy specimens. In the absence of a carcinoma or dysplasia, the ability to quantify the risk associated with malignant transformation is limited. It is for this reason that a molecular and genetic characterization of premalignant lesions may be very important in predicting their malignant potential. There are several histologically distinct lesions of the oral cavity that have malignant potential. These are leukoplakia, erythroplakia, lichen planus and submucous fibrosis, together with a spectrum of chromosomal, genetic and molecular alterations. The degree of similarity to OSCC found in premalignant lesions is dependent upon the presence of atypia. However, individual lesions may present molecular genetic alterations similar to OSCC, even in the absence of histologically defied dysplasia (Mithani et al, 2007).

Leukoplakia, defined as a predominantly white lesion of oral mucosa that cannot be characterized by any other definable lesion, is the most commonly diagnosed premalignant lesions in the oral cavity (Mithani et al, 2007). It is also strongly associated with the development of OSCC. Patients with oral leokoplakia have up to 36% incidence of subsequent OSCC development, only if the lesion demonstrates dysplastic features. In the absence of dysplasia, these lesions still possess a 15% incidence of cancer development (Mithani et al, 2007). In particular, increased LOH was correlated to the histopathological progression in the upper aereodigestive tract (Califano et al, 1996). 50% of leukoplastic lesions contain allelic loss of either the 3p or 9p chromosome arms, which are associated with higher risk of malignant transformation. This risk increases further in the presence of additional LOH at the 4q, 8p, 11q, 13q and 17p loci (Rosin et al, 2000). Insertions or deletions of base pairs at microsatellites, termed microsatellite instability (MSI), are another cytogenetic feature shared between premalignant lesions and OSCC. The MSI is present in 55% of leukoplakia and there is a trend towards increasing MSI prevalence associated with histological progression of premalignant lesions (Mithani et al, 2007). In addition, many studies have demonstrated a trend in increasing polysomy at several loci, such as chromosomes 7 and 17, in the progression of the aeredigestive tract. For example, lesions with a >3% proportion of cells with trisomy 9 have a significantly higher likelihood of progression in cancer (Lee et al, 2000; Mithani et al, 2007). It is also demonstrated that telomerase activity is correlated with the degree of atypia and dysplastic changes (Mithani et al, 2007). Finally, mitochondrial genomic mutations, which occur in response to oxidative damage and stress, may have a role in the development of cancer, including HNSCC (Sanchez-Cespedes et al, 2001). The mechanism by which these mutations contribute to carcinogenesis has not yet been demonstrated. It has been postulated to occur because of mitochondrial dysfunction in apoptosis or through reactive oxygen species generation (Gottlieb & Tomlinson, 2005). Epigenetic changes are also important. An aberrant methylation of CpG-rich regions of the promoters prevents gene transcription by altering the structure of histone complex. Promoter hypermetilation is a mechanism by which tumour suppressor genes are transcriptionally inactivated (Ha & Califano, 2006). There are few studies on the aberrant methylation occurring in leukoplakia, where the hypermetylation of RAR-b2 (Youssef et al, 2004), p16 and MGMT (Lopez et al, 2003) has been shown. These genes are metylated also in OSCC.

3.3 Association between genetic alterations and poor outcome of HNSCC patients

Various studies indicate that many of the LOH events in certain chromosomal regions are associated with shorter survival of HNSCC patients. The most commonly reported CNV and LOH associated with survival pertain to chromosomal regions 11q, 3q, 7p and 22q (for CNV) and in 3p, 8p and 9p, 13q (for LOH) (Chen & Chen, 2008). For example, many studies identified a consistent amplification in the head and neck tumours at region 11q13. Possibly the amplification of this region plays an important role in HNSCC survival, given the many known oncogenes, such as bcl-1, Int-2, hst-1, EMS1, CCND1 and PRAD1, in turn are correlated with clinical outcomes, that reside in this region (Chen & Chen, 2008). As far as recurrence is concerned, the most commonly reported CNV/LOH events associated with recurrence involved CNV at 11q and LOH at 9p and 17p (Chen & Chen, 2008). Only few papers focus on the combination of histopathological and clinical characteristics, such as tumour size, lymph node status and metastasis (TNM) staging or treatment condition and the data results from CNV and/or LOH to predict survival. For example, the association between 3p LOH and poor outcome in HNSCC patients with early stage I and II tumours was shown (Partridge et al, 1996). Other research has also shown that patients who received radiotherapy, 6q LOH was associated with reduced survival (Jamieson et al, 2003).

3.3.1 Genetic polymorphism and their association with outcomes in HNSCC

Single nucleotides polymorphisms (SNPs) are a DNA sequence variation occurring when a single nucleotide in the genome differs between members of a biological species or paired chromosomes in an individual. This variation in DNA sequences may not lead to an amino acid alteration and do not seem to have any adverse effects in "normal" individuals. It is possible to perform the analysis of SNPs using PCR-related methods, such as direct sequencing, or using SNP arrays. These SNPs may be markers for disease predisposition, or may be used to genetically identify patients, as they tend to cluster with ethnic background. Recent results from case-control studies of several phenotypic and genotypic assays support the hypothesis that genetic susceptibility or predisposition plays an important role in HNSCC aetiology (Negri et al, 2009; Garavello et al, 2008; Ingelman-Sundberg, 2001). It has been hypothesized that susceptibility to disease development is based on inherited differences in the efficiency of carcinogen metabolism, DNA repair and cell cycle control, or a combination of these. SNPs located in DNA repair genes can modulate DNA repair capacity and, consequently, alter cancer risk. In particular, it was shown that, among all DNA repair pathways, the sequence variations in the base excision repair (BER) pathway may contribute to HNSCC susceptibility. For example, a significantly decreased risk of HNSCC was associated with the adenosine diphosphate ribosyl transferase (ADPRT) 762Ala/Ala genotype and the combined ADPRT Val/Ala and ADPRT Ala/Ala genotypes, compared with the ADPRT Val/Val genotype (Li et al, 2007). An association between the presence of cytocrome P450 (CYP) and GSTs allelic variants, which are families of enzymes involved in the metabolism of many environmental agents, including tobacco and alcohol, and increased risk of HNSCC was also demonstrated. In particular, it was observed that the CYP1A2*1D variant allele confers an increased risk of HNSCC, while the CYP1A2*1C polymorphism was associated with tumour recurrence (Olivieri et al, 2009). Finally, CYP2E1*5B and GSTM1 null alleles were associated with advanced clinical stages (Olivieri, 2009). In conclusion, it is clear that genetic polymorphisms may act as predictors of risk and are also associated with tumour recurrence, since they are important for determining the parameters associated with tumour progression and poor outcomes in HNSCC. For these reasons, the identification of individuals presenting polymorphic variations would have an impact on primary prevention and early detection strategies.

3.3.2 Genetic polymorphism and their association to tobacco and alcohol use

Smoking and the consumption of alcohol are the main risk factors for head/neck cancer. Although the chance of developing HNSCC increases with the level of tobacco smoking and alcohol use, it is obvious that not every (heavy) smoker and/or drinker develops HNSCC. The risk for an individual to develop HNSCC after exposure to tobacco carcinogens, may therefore also depend on sequence variation in the genes (genetic polymorphisms) coding for the enzymes involved in the detoxification of tobacco smoke carcinogens, such as microsomal epoxide hydrolase (mHE), gluthatione-S-transferase (GSTs) and uridine 5'-diphosphate (UDP)-glucuronosyltransferase (UGTs). Genetic polymorphisms in these genes may alter their activity and may thus modulate the risk of HNSCC. For example, the presence of null polymorphism in GSTM1 or GSTT1 was associated with an increased risk for HNSCC in smokers (Lacko et al, 2009). For the UGTs, both the variants UGT1A7 and UGT1A10 were associated with an altered risk of developing cancer (Lacko et al, 2009). Tobacco smoke is associated with the increased formation of DNA lesions, which can be repaired also by BER pathway. Therefore, also an individual variation in BER, is one of the host factors that may influence tobacco smoking-related HNSCC risk. The Rad1 c.3429 G>C polymorphism has a more evident association with cancer risk in the group of heavy smokers (Werbrouck et al, 2008). Detoxification of tobacco smoke carcinogens, together with DNA repair and apoptotic pathways, is probably the most important rescue pathways in preventing the development of tobacco-induced HNSCC. In fact, the activity of such enzymes may differ between individuals and this is one of the possible explanations for the differences in inter-individual susceptibility for the development of HNSCC.

3.4 Epigenetic alterations

HNSCC is a result of multiple genetic and epigenetic alterations. Epigenetic is defined as the stable inheritance of information based on gene expression levels without changing the underlying genetic code (Esteller et al, 2002). These heritable modifications of the DNA molecule itself occur through several pathways including alterations in DNA methylation and histone modifications mediated by: DNA methyltransferases (DNMT), methyl-CpG-binding domain proteins, histoneacethyltranferases (HAT), histone deacetylases (HDAC), histone methyltransferases (HMT) and histone demethylases (Glazer et al, 2009). Epigenetic changes have been associated with cancer specific expression differences in human malignancies, including HNSCC (Herman et al, 2003). These alterations are known to occur early in tumoriginesis and are associated with distinctive cancer types. The main epigenetic modification found in humans is the methylation of the 5′ carbon of the cytosine ring within cytosine-guanine dinucleotides (CpGs) by the enzyme class methyltransferases. CpG methylation occurs in patterns both species and tissue specific, serving to block transcription and recruit histone and modifying tightly packed heterochromatin and gene silencing. DNMTs are responsible for maintaining the methylation status of a gene in the cell's progeny. In addition, histone modification has also been shown to play an active role in regulating gene expression. Histone modifications and DNA methylations play a significant role in the organization of nuclear structure, ultimately influencing gene expression. The epigenetic inactivation of tumor suppressor genes is an important event in HNSCC (Steinmann et al, 2009; Glazer et al, 2009). In recent years, new assays, such as sodium bisolfite treatment of DNA, which converts the non-methylated cytosines to uracyl, and methylation sensitive quantitative PCR, have further advanced the ability to evaluate the methylation status of tissue samples. In HNSCC, the promoter hypermethylation of p16 is a frequent event (Reed et al, 1996; Glazer et al, 2009; Steinmann et al, 2009). Studies on promoter methylation have uncovered many other genes in HNSCC, such as DIM-6, ATM, p15, TIMP-3, MGMT, RARB-2, DAP-K, E-cadherin, Cyclin A1, RASSF1A, CDKN2A, CDH1 and DCC (Steinmann et al, 2009). These genes are involved in pathways that control cell cycle progression, apoptosis, cell-cell adhesion, DNA repair and tumour invasion. A trend toward an increased methylation of these genes in more advanced tumour stages and less differentiated HNSCC was observed. In particular, p16 methylation was significantly high in poorly differentiated HNSCC and RASSF5 methylation occurred preferentially in advanced tumour stages, while methylation of RASSF4 was higher in patients with recurrence (Steinmann et al, 2009). A relationship between methylation profiling, tumour stage and age of patients was also shown (Marsit et al, 2009). A borderline significant association between tumour site and methylation pattern was also observed (Marsit et al, 2009). These data reveal that patterns of epigenetic alteration may hold a relevant role in identifying the process through which carcinogens act epigenetically to drive tumourigenesis as well as in providing useful tools with diagnostic value.

3.4.1 Epigenetic alterations and correlation with aetiologic agents and clinical parameters

DNA methylation-associated epigenetic silencing of tumor suppressor genes is an aberrant marker of cancer with considerable specificity. An association among HPV, tobacco smoking and alcohol exposure and methylation of specific genes has been identified. In particular, using a whole genome profiling approach, not only was there a correlation between methylation and tobacco and alcohol use, but also in considering smoking intensity (packs per day) and lifetime average drinks per week (Marsit et al, 2009). Tumour HPV16 DNA status also demonstrated to have an association with methylation, showing that HPV+ and HPV- HNSCC patients do not only have a different pattern of methylation, but have a more pronounced hypomethylation in HPV-negative tumours than in HPV-positive tumours (Richards et al, 2009). In addition, genomic instability, as measured by genome-wide loss of heterozogosity (LOH) and single nucleotide polymorphism (SNP) analysis, is greater in HNSCC samples with more pronounced hypomethylation. For example, epigenetic inactivation of the SFRP genes is associated with drinking, smoking and HPV. Promoter methylation of SFRP1 occurred more often in both heavy and light drinkers compared to non drinkers. SFRP4 promoter methylation, on the other hand, occurred at a higher prevalence in never smokers and former smokers than in current smokers, and also was independently associated with HPV16 viral DNA (Marsit et al, 2006).

4. Potential molecular prognosis markers in HNSCC

HNSCC has long been a challenge in regards to treatment because of the high rate of recurrences and advanced diseases at the time of diagnosis. Molecular identification of tissue biomarkers in diagnostic biopsy specimens may not only identify patients at risk for developing HNSCC but also select patients that may benefit from more aggressive treatment methods. In addition, they may potentially offer new methods for early diagnosis, monitoring and treatment alternatives for HNSCC patients. Some emerging molecular markers include *TP53*, epidermal growth factor receptor (EGFR), cyclin D1, transforming growth factor alpha (TGF-alfa), p16^{INK4A}, cyclooxigenase-2 (*Cox-2*), vascular endothelial growth factor (VEGF) and matrix metallo proteinases (MMPs) (Table 3).

Molecule name	Genomic localization	Function	From literature	References
TP53	17p13	A tumor-suppressor regulating cell cycle progression, apoptosis and cell survival	➢ 60-80% of HNSCC shows *TP53* somatic mutations causing mostly p53 protein overexpression. ➢ Predictive and prognostic value for survival, recurrence, treatments response and lymph node status	- Bradford et al, 2003 - Cabanillas et al, 2007 - Cabelguenne et al, 2000 - Gasco and Crook, 2003 - Graveland et al, 2011 - Lassaletta et al, 1999 - Leemans et al, 2011 - Nees et al,1993 - Nogueria et al, 1998 - Nylander et al, 2000 - Perrone et al, 2010 - Poeta et al, 2007 - Quon et al, 2001 - Temam et al, 2000 - Thomas et al, 2005
p16^{INK4A} (CDKN2A)	9p21	A tumor-suppressor regulating senescence and cell-cycle progression by acting as an inhibitor of cyclin dependent kinase 4 and 6-cyclin D complexes	➢ 50-80% of HNSCC shows loss of p16 expression, mostly by promoter hypermethylation or homozygous deletion. ➢ Prognostic value for survival and development of distant metastases ➢ High p16 expression in combination with persistent HPV16-18 infection predicts a better prognosis	- Ambrosch et al, 2001 - Bazan et al, 2002 - Broek et al, 2009 - Thomas et al, 2005 - Namazie et al, 2002 - Thomas et al, 2005 - Yuen et al, 2002

Molecule name	Genomic localization	Function	From literature	References
PTEN	10q23	A tumor suppressor gene regulating signaling pathways controlling cell proliferation and apoptosis	➢ 30% of HNSCC shows loss of PTEN ➢ Potential prognostic value in relation to poor outcome. ➢ Association between PTEN overexpression and increase of radioresistance	- Mriouah et al, 2010 - Pai and Westra, 2009 - Pattje et al, 2010 - Pedrero et al, 2005
Cyclin D1	11q13	Proto-oncogene regulating cell cycle progression	➢ 17-79% of HNSCC shows amplification and overexpression of cyclin D1 ➢ Prognostic value in relation to more advanced, aggressive disease, lymph node metastasis and reduced survival	- Akervall et al, 1997 - Capaccio et al, 2000 - Holley et al, 2005 - Kumar et al, 2003 - Leemans et al, 2011 - Marsit et al, 2008 - Michalides et al, 1997 - Namazie et el, 2002 - Nimeus et al, 2004 - Okami et al, 1999 - Pyeon et al, 2007 - Thomas et al, 2005 - Volavsek et al, 2003
EGFR	7p11	Trans membrane TK acting as a central transducer in multiple pathways that mediate cell cycle progression, angiogenesis, inhibition of apoptosis, tumor invasion and metastasis	➢ 34-90% of HNSCC shows overexpression of EGFR ➢ Prognostic value in relation to disease free survival and overall survival; association with a shorter overall survival and poor outcomes. ➢ From 2006 use of therapy based on EGFR inhibitors	- Carracedo et al, 2008 - Chang et Califano, 2008 - Hama et al, 2009 - Kalyankrishna and Grandis, 2006 - Quon et al, 2001 - Smilek et al, 2006 - Uribe & Gonzalez, 2011
VEGFs		Ligands of trans membrane TK promoting cell proliferation, migration and survival of endothelial cells during tumor growth	➢ 90% of HNSCC shows overexpression of VEGFs (especially A and C forms), ➢ They are important pro-angiogenic factors, which promote neovascularization in cancer. ➢ They are associated with tumor growth, metastasis, treatment failure and shorter overall survival	- Kyzas et al, 2004 - Kyzas et al, 2005 - Lentsch et al, 2006 - Mineta et al, 2000 - Moryama et al, 1997 - Neuchrist et al, 2001 - Neuchrist et al, 2003 - Petruzzelli et al, 1997

Molecule name	Genomic localization	Function	From literature	References
Cox2	1q25.2–25.3	Catalytic enzyme decreasing apoptosis, increasing inflammation and important for tumor progression	➢ Presence of Cox 2 up regulation in tumor (150 folds) and adjacent tissues (50 folds) compared to nomal epithelium. ➢ It seem to be an early event in HNSCC carcinogenesis ➢ Prognostic value for survival; Cox 2 overexpression in combination with PEG2 is associated with a shorter overall survival ➢ Prognostic marker in premalignant lesions. ➢ Low levels of Cox 2 are associated with poorer overall survival in larynx cancer ➢ Independent predictor of disease-free survival. ➢ Ongoing preclinical studies with therapy based on Cox-2 inhibitors in combination with EGFR inhibitors	- Gallo et al, 2002 - Itoh et al, 2003 - Ranelletti et al, 2001 - Sudbo et al, 2003 - Thomas et al, 2005
TGF alfa	2p13	Growth factor inducing epithelial development and primary ligand of the EGFR	➢ Association between TGFA overexpression and poor outcome and response to anti-EGFR therapy	- Logullo et al, 2003 - Quon et al, 2001 - White et al, 2010
MMPs		Family of Zn-dependent proteolytic enzymes that degrade the basement membrane and other components of the extracellular matrix	➢ Overexpression in HNSCC of various MMPs, including MMP2, MMP8, MMP13 ➢ Association with poor outcome, cisplatin resistance, lymph node metastasis and early recurrence. ➢ Evidences about association between the EGFR signaling and MMPs activation	- Kusukawa et al, 1996 - O-Charoenrat et al, 2000 - Patel et al, 2005 - Sinpitaksakul et al, 2008 - Thomas et al, 2005

Table 3. Biomarkers in head and neck cancers

4.1 *TP53*

TP53 is a tumour suppressor gene located on chromosome 17p13 and consists of 11 exons that encode protein p53, and functions in carcinogenesis by initiating G1 arrest in response to certain DNA damage and apoptosis. Studies suggest that after mutation in one *TP53* allele, the remaining wild type (w.t.) allele is often deleted and therefore the mutant phenotype is expressed (Yin et al, 1993; Kiuru et al, 1997). The prevalence of *TP53* mutations is 20-70% in HNSCC (Blons et al, 2003). The reported frequency of the mutations varies among different studies. This is related, at least in part, to techniques used for detecting mutations, the regions of the *TP53* gene analyzed, and the anatomic site of the analyzed sample tumours. Exons 5 to 8 (encoding the "core" domain) of *TP53* are the most analyzed because they represent the major site of *TP53* mutations. However, other studies report that a considerable amount of HNSCC carries *TP53* mutations outside the core domain of p53 (Balz et al, 2003; Saunders et al, 1999).

4.1.1 Tobacco and *TP53*

An explanation for the heterogeneity of *TP53* mutation frequency could be the different levels of exposure to risk factors in the population studied. In fact, the frequency of *TP53* mutation in patients with invasive HNSCC was related to the level of exposure to cigarette smoke and alcohol (Blons et al, 2003; Ronchetti et al, 2004; Hussain et al, 1999). The frequency of somatic *TP53* mutation in smoking HNSCC patients was at least double compared to non-smoking HNSCC patients (Field et al, 1991). DNA can be damaged by numerous tobacco carcinogens and environmental chemicals that can be activated or degraded by specific enzymes termed xenobiotic-matabolizing enzymes (XMEs). The existence of XMEs variants may explain individual susceptibility to *TP53* mutations. An XME genotype that results in increased DNA damage as a consequence of altered carcinogen metabolism could increase the incidence of *TP53* mutations (Blons et al, 2003). For example, a strong association between *TP53* mutation and CYP1B1 genotypes was found in smokers (Ko et al, 2001; Thier et al, 2002). Finally, an increased sensitivity to mutagens as a result of low DNA repair capacity increases the frequency or modify the pattern of *TP53* mutations (Casse et al, 2003; Wong et al, 2002). As expected from experimental tobacco carcinogenesis, the most prevalent mutations in HNSCC are G:C>A:T transitions and G:C>T:A tranversions. It is also interesting to note that frameshift mutations, which are more frequent in patients exposed to both alcohol and tobacco, occur more frequently in HNSCC than in other tobacco-independent cancer types (Blons et al, 2003).

4.1.2 Is *TP53* mutation an early or a late event?

The expression of the p53 protein has been detected also in oral premalignant lesions (such as leukoplakia), where it may indicate an impending malignancy. Specifically, suprabasal expression has been highly predictive of malignant development (Cruz et al, 1998). In addition, when surgical margins of primary HNSCC are examined for mutational changes, there is an increased risk of local recurrence when positive margins demonstrating clonal alterations in *TP53* are observed (Graveland et al, 2011). However, there have been conflicting conclusions concerning the stage at which *TP53* mutations occur during HNSCC carcinogenesis. Early studies performed by immunocytochemistry suggested that *TP53* alterations are an early event in the carcinogenesis of HNSCC. In contrast, subsequent studies have found that *TP53* mutations represent a late event and are associated with an invasive phenotype (Shahnavaz et al, 2000; Shin et al, 2000). Whether this is due to different methods in the evaluation of *TP53* mutations or whether they define new subgroups in the HNSCC is still an open question. As described, *TP53* mutations are frequently detected by immunohistochemical analysis. This simple analysis is based on the finding that mutant p53 protein, adopting an altered conformation, becomes very stable, facilitating its detection and allowing its use as a marker for gene mutation. However, not all types of mutations are detected by this method, because some of them do not lead to protein stabilization. It is possible that some *TP53* mutations result in negative immunostaining or wild type *TP53* gene may be associated with p53 protein overexpression (Strano et al, 2007). Consequently, direct sequencing of the *TP53* gene is probably the most important component for any *TP53* evaluation at present.

4.1.3 Clinical evaluation of *TP53* status

When the mutational analysis of *TP53* and the clinical outcome in patients with HNSCC as a whole are correlated, studies have reported contradictory results even when using the same molecular techniques. The correlation between p53 expression and clinical outcome in patients with HNSCC, however, has been questioned (Thomas et al, 2005) (Table 3). A number of studies have shown that *TP53* gene mutations are associated with an increased risk for locoregional recurrence and poor outcome (Thomas et al, 2005). Furthermore, a significant correlation between p53 expression and clinical outcome appears to be strongest in the subgroup of patients with laryngeal SCC (Narayana et al, 1998; Nylander et al, 2000). Although there are many studies correlating mutations or overexpression of p53 with poor outcomes, others have shown that *TP53* mutations or overexpression do not independently predict clinical outcomes in patients with HNSCC (Thomas et al, 2005). Possible explanations for incongruity between these studies may be due to a failure of immunohistochemical techniques to detect actual *TP53* mutations, differences between races, variation in tissue handling and analysis techniques and variation in the definition of overexpression (Strano et al, 2007(b); Thomas et al, 2005). In addition, differences observed in the impact of *TP53* alterations on prognosis may be due to different treatment methods. In fact, a predictive role of *TP53* mutations on treatment responses, in particular in radiotherapy and chemotherapy, was demonstrated (Blons et al, 2003). Furthermore, in the *TP53* mutations located in the DNA binding domain, the chance of a major response to chemotherapy treatments were inferior. Finally, the accumulation of mutant p53 protein leads to the production of anti-p53 antibodies. Their presence is significantly correlated with increased risks of recurrence and death (Blons et al, 2003).

4.1.4 Therapy by reactivation or elimination of mutant p53 protein

HNSCC has been one of the first tumour localities to benefit from gene transfer therapy. The transfection of wild type *TP53* into cell lines induced growth arrest and reduced tumourigenicity in nude mice. This suggested that restoring p53 function in HNSCC could inhibit cell growth (Strano et al, 2007(b)). Therapeutic strategies based on p53 tumour suppressor function were initiated. One of these approaches is based on the functional correction of mutant p53 protein using short synthetic peptides derived from the C-terminus of wt-p53. In particular, these peptides can increase the DNA binding ability of wt-p53 and restore the transcriptional activity of some gain of function mutants. This application is severely restricted by the complexity of the synthesis, stability limitations, restricted uptake and intracellular processing. Stabilizing the native form of p53 protein (correctly folded) by shifting the equilibrium from its denatured form was another idea. As a consequence of the re-acquired native folding, some p53 mutants are able to activate wt-p53 target genes and promote apoptosis (Strano et al, 2007(b)). Finally, the last therapeutic strategy is based on the elimination of mutant p53. The efficient replication of adenovirus requires the neutralization of p53 function through E1B viral protein. ONYX-015 is an engineered adenovirus that does not express E1B protein and consequently is unable to inactivate p53. The infection of tumour cells carrying *TP53* mutations with ONYX-15 provokes apoptosis. Clinical trials are underway in HNSCC patients. While the treatment with ONYX-15 alone gave only marginal effects, its combination with cisplatin and 5-fluorouracil had a more profound impact on the response of patients (Strano et al, 2007(b)); Perrone et al, 2010).

4.1.5 Oncogenic properties: Gain of function of mutant p53

Mutant p53 proteins are unable to transcriptionally regulate wt-p53 target genes and to exert its antitumoral effects such as apoptosis, growth arrest, differentiation and senescence. On the other hand, countless evidence has demonstrated that at least certain mutant forms of the p53 protein may possess gain of function activity, thereby positively contributing to the development, maintenance and spreading of many types of tumours, including HNSCC (Gasco & Crook, 2003; Strano et al, 2007(a)). A great amount of in vitro and in vivo evidence have firmly established an oncogenic role of certain missense *TP53* mutations (such as p53R175H), located especially in the DNA binding domain (Strano et al, 2007). The resulting protein is a full-length protein, with a single aminoacid change that is sufficient to make them unable to recognize the wt-*TP53*-DNA consensus on target gene promoters. In addition, the half-life of mutant p53 protein is extremely prolonged compared to that of w.t.-p53. It has been hypothesized that mutant p53 proteins could serve as oncogenic transcription factors. By genome-wide expression profile techniques it has been shown that p53 mutant proteins can modulate sets of genes involved in oncogenic activities (Strano et al, 2007). Furthermore, the semiquantitative SnaPshot analysis in HNSCC *TP53* mutant patients shows a higher expression of missense mutant allele compared to w.t. These data demonstrate that *TP53* missense and nonsense mutations have a dissimilar allelic expression imbalance (AEI) behavior in HNSCC, mostly likely independent from the LOH *TP53* status. The positive AEI in favour of *TP53* missense mutations could be due to the inactivation of w.t. allele, as well as to the higher expression or mRNA stability of mutant allele (Ganci et al, 2011). Comparatively, the low expression of the nonsense mutations compared to the w.t. allele in HNSCC tissue may be due to the nonsense mediated decay (MND) surveillance pathway, which ensures the rapid degradation of the mRNAs containing premature translation termination codons (Behm-Ansmant et al, 2007).

4.1.6 p53 as a marker for the clonal heterogeneity identification of tumor cells

The most striking features of HNSCC are its histopatological heterogeneity and the disparity between biological behavior, which is extremely variable, and morphological classification. It is well recognized that patients with similar stages of head and neck cancer may have a diverse clinical course and response to similar treatment (Kearsley et al, 1990). Considerable intratumor heterogeneity for genetic alterations has been demonstrated, as shown in the genetic analysis by LOH and MSI on chromosomes 17p13 (p53) and 9p21 (RPS6) (Wang et al, 2006). They examined the differential genetic composition of the histological high-grade and low-grade areas showing an increase of aberration proportions for both loci in the poorly differentiated region of the tumour. Similar results were obtained by the immunohistochemistry (IHC) analysis of mutant p53 staining from hematoxylin and eosin HNSCC sections (Ganci et al, 2011; Wang et al, 2006; Boyle et al, 1993). A higher number of p53 positive cells were observed in poorly differentiated regions than in moderately or well differentiated ones (fig.2). Furthermore, data from cloning and sequencing p53 cDNA in tumours carrying double and triple p53 mutations showed that different p53 mutated alleles were present (Ganci et al, 2011). On the other hand, HNSCC tissues carrying double/triple p53 mutations on different alleles showed a positive, but not homogenous p53 staining, independently from the state of tumour cell differentiation, probably relying on the presence of clonal populations carrying different *TP*53 mutations in the same tumour (Ganci et al, 2011) (fig.2). The intratumour heterogeneity, which was also demonstrated for the methylation status (Varley et al, 2009), could be due to multiple different processes of carcinogenesis, where clonal populations arising within tumours may undergo separate individual genetic changes conferring different aggressiveness capacity.

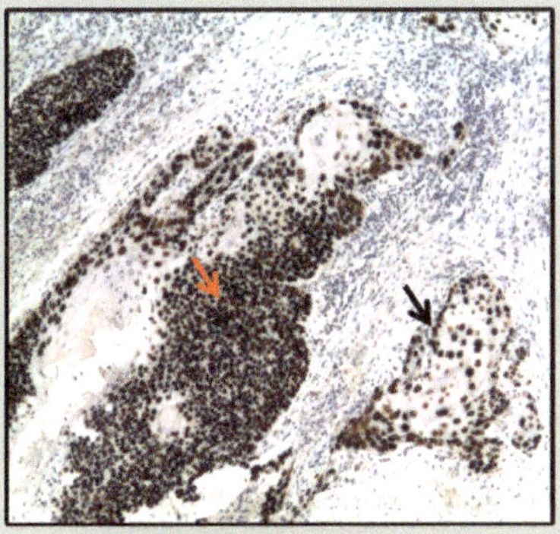

(a)

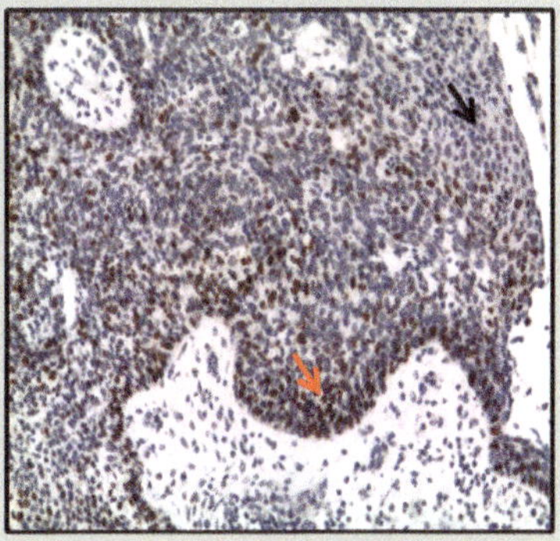

(b)

(a) p53 Y234C protein shows positive staining by IHC. A higher number of p53 positive cells was observed in poorly differentiated (red arrow) tissue areas than in moderately or well differentiated ones (black arrow). (b) The tissue carrying the two *TP*53 mutations C242Y and Del.T155-M169 (deletion of 40bp) on separate alleles shows overexpression of p53 protein. A positive, but not homogeneous, p53 staining was observed by IHC independently from the tumor cell differentiation state, probably relying on the presence of clonal populations carrying different *TP*53 mutations in this tumor. Red and black arrows indicate regions with positive and negative p53 staining, respectively, in a poorly differentiated tumor area.

Fig. 2. p53 as a marker for the clonal heterogeneity in HNSCC

4.1.7 HPV infection and correlation with p53 status

Similar to tobacco and alcohol use, oral human papilloma virus (HPV) infection, plays a role in the pathogenesis of HNSCC. The transforming potential of high-risk, oncogenic types (as

HPV-16, 18), is largely a result of the function of two viral proteins, E6 and E7, which functionally inactivate two human tumour suppressor proteins, p53 and pRB, respectively. Expression of high-risk HPV E6 and E7 results in cellular proliferation, loss of cell cycle regulation, impaired cellular differentiation, increased frequency of spontaneous and mutagen-induced mutations and chromosomal instability (Chung & Gillison, 2009) (fig. 3). HPV was detected in about 20% of HNSCC cases especially in oropharynx and oral cancer (Leemans et al, 2011; Rosenquist et al, 2007). The possible involvement of *TP53* status and HPV infection was suggested by several studies in which HPV DNA was detected and almost all positive cases were w.t. for *TP53* (fig. 4) (Smith et al, 2010; Mitra et al, 2007). HPV positive cancer was also associated with a significantly better prognosis than HPV negative cases, which have a higher frequency of *TP53* mutations. Altogether, these data support the evidence that HPV positive HNSCC is a distinct pathobiological and clinical disease component (Leemans et al, 2011).

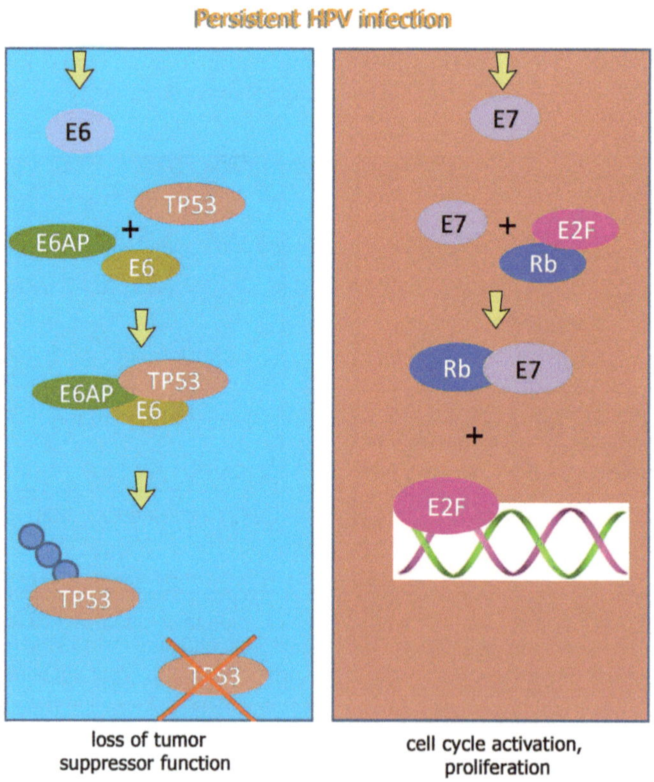

The human papillomavirus (HPV) genome contains various early and late open reading frames and encodes two viral oncoproteins: E6 and E7. The E6 protein binds p53 and targets the protein for degradation (by ubiquitination), whereas the E7 protein binds and inactivates the Rb pocket proteins. The molecular consequence of the expression of these viral oncoproteins is cell cycle entry and inhibition of p53-mediated apoptosis, which allows the virus to replicate E6AP=E6 adaptor protein.

Fig. 3. HPV infection affects cell cycle.

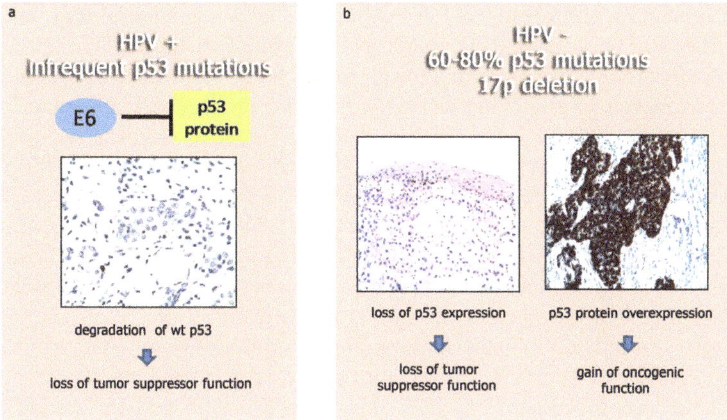

a) b)

a) In HPV + HNSCC the oncoprotein HPV E6 promotes p53 degradation. Consequently p53 protein expression is not detected in the tumor by IHC. p53 inactivation by HPV causes loss of its tumor suppressor function.
b) In HPV- HNSCC, p53 tumor suppressor function is mainly inactivated by 17p13 deletion and/or *TP*53 mutations. A subset of *TP*53 mutations, mainly missense mutations, show not only loss of tumor suppressor properties, but also gain of oncogenic functions. These mutations are often associated with p53 protein overexpression by IHC.

Fig. 4. Correlation of *TP53* status and HPV infection in HNSCC

4.1.8 P72R *TP*53 polymorphism

A common polymorphism exists in exon 4 of the *TP*53 gene resulting in the expression of either arginine (R) or proline (P) at codon 72 (Matlashewski et al, 1987). This sites is within the apoptosis-signalling domain of the protein. The R form of w.t. p53 is more leading to the hypothesis that individuals homozygous for R in the germ-line are at higher risk of HPV associated cancers than carriers of other genotypes (Storey et al, 1998). Several studies have addressed this possibility in HNSCC, but none have identified an increased frequency of any codon 72 genotype. Despite the apparent absence in the association between codon 72 genotype and risk of HNSCC, there is evidence demonstrating that the clinico-pathological characteristics of cancers may be affected by polymorphism (Gasco & Crook, 2003). Loss of the 72P allele has been reported in several studies. In a small series of HNSCC from northern Europe and Japan, there was a clear bias for *TP*53 mutants to target the 72R allele and for LOH to involve the 72P. 72R mutants more potently inhibit p73, a protein belonging to the p53 family, than equivalent 72P mutants. It is a persuasive possibility that preferential retention of 72R mutants in HNSCC is a reflection of this activity (Gasco & Crook, 2003). The study of the effect of this polymorphism on clinical outcomes of HNSCC will be of great interest.

4.2 Other potential molecular prognostic markers

EGFR is a transmembrane tyrosine kinase capable of promoting neoplastic transformation. Binding to the extracellular domain of EGFR causes the activation of a number of downstream effectors including the activation of tyrosine kinase and activation of intracellular Ras, Raf and mitogen-activated protein kinase cascades. They are involved in malignant transformation and tumour growth through the inhibition of apoptosis, cellular proliferation, promotion of angiogenesis and metastasis. The EGFR family includes EGFR, c-erbB2, c-erbB3 and c-erbB4, which have the ability to form receptor heterodimers and crosstalk between them. Both EGF and the transforming growth factor (TGF)-alpha are ligands that bind to EGFR (Thomas et al, 2005; Kalyanrshna & Grandis, 2006). EGFR expression has been extensively studied in HNSCC and its overexpression reported in 34-80% of HNSCC using IHC (Beckhardt et al, 1995; Grandis et al, 1993). However, EGFR expression may occur in two stages, the over-expression in normal and well-differentiated epithelia adjacent to the tumour and the upregulation from dysplasia to HNSCC that may result from gene amplification. This marker has been significantly associated with short disease-free survival, overall survival and poor prognosis in HNSCC patients (Table 3). Data showing an increased expression of EGFR in well and moderately differentiated tumour cells and in dysplastic tissue compared with poorly differentiated tissue, suggest that EGFR upregulation may be an early event during HNSCC carcinogenesis. Co-expression of Her2 and Her3, which do not have intrinsic tyrosine kinase activity, is reported to increase transforming activity, and their expression has been strongly associated with shortened patient survival (Thomas et al, 2005). EGFR over-expression has been shown to be an independent prognostic factor for neck node relapse in primary specimens of patients with laryngeal cancer (Almadori et al, 1999). Increased tumour resistance to cytotoxic agents, including radiotherapy has been associated with EGFR over-expression in HNSCC, in addition to its association with more aggressive tumour behavior (Thomas et al, 2005). This suggests that the evaluation of EGFR status at the time of diagnosis may help identify subsets of patients, who are at increased risk of neck node metastasis, may have an unfavorable radiotherapy treatment outcome and may therefore benefit from more aggressive treatments. Several studies, however, have found no association between EGFR and clinical stage, including lymph node status, extracapsular invasion, recurrence or survival in specimens from HNSCC patients using IHC, Western or Southern blot techniques (Thomas et al, 2005; Glazer et al, 2009). Qualitative and quantitative differences in techniques for determining EGFR positivity and cut-off levels may be significant factors contributing to the disagreement between studies. Nonetheless, the prognostic significance of EGFR in HNSCC in a great number of studies has compelled the development of therapeutic strategies to block EGFR signal transduction system and, theoretically, downregulate tumour growth. The use of antibodies against EGFR or inhibitors of tyrosine kinase in combination with chemotherapy or radiotherapy are underway in various cancer systems including HNSCC (Glazer et al, 2009; Chang & Califano, 2008; Uribe & Gonzalez; 2011).

Cyclin D1 (CCND1) is a proto-oncogene located on chromosome 11q13 involved in the regulation of cell cycle transitions. Overexpression of *CCND1* has been shown to shorten the G1 phase of the cell cycle (Motokura & Arnold, 1993). Abnormalities in cyclin D1 may result from genomic inversion, transloction or gene amplification (Leemans et al, 2011). However, overexpression may occur in the absence of gene amplification through a not well-characterized mechanism, which may precede gene amplification. Early dysregulation of *CCND1* expression may occur during head and neck tumourigenesis (Izzo et al, 1998). Amplification and/or over-expression of *CCND1* have been demonstrated in 17-79% of tumour specimens from HNSCC patients by IHC, FISH or RT-PCR. *CCND1* shows a higher incidence in hypopharyngeal and laryngeal carcinomas between 41% and 64% and a rare incidence (8%) in tonsillar carcinomas. Gene amplification is the most commonly reported alteration of *CCND1.* Its amplification and/or overexpression have been shown to correlate significantly with tumour extension, regional lymph node metastases and advanced clinical stage of HNSCC (Thomas et al, 2005; Quon et al, 2001). In addition, many studies show convincing data of *CCND1* aberration as a prognostic marker for disease-free survival and overall survival in patients with this disease (Table 3). In particular, its overexpression was associated with an adverse disease free survival, independent of T and N (Quon et al, 2001). In contrast, other data found no significant associations between levels of *CCND1* and survival of patients with HNSCC (Vielba et al, 2003). As most of the studies on *CCND1* utilize IHC in paraffin-embedded tissue from patients with HNSCC to examine the expression of *CCND1*, reasons for the differences between these studies are not clearly evident. However, differences in parameters for grading immunohistochemical staining may account for some of these discrepancies. In addition, the retrospective selection of patients for analysis may influence the outcome of these studies. Several studies documented the independent value of cyclin D1 overexpression, particularly when combined with the loss p16 expression. In fact, significant correlation with poor clinical outcome measures of recurrence, metastasis and survival was seen when both of these genetic aberrations occur together than either alone (Thomas et al, 2005).

p16 protein, which is encoded by the *CDKN2A* tumour suppressor gene on chromosome 9p21, inactivates the function of cdk4-cdk6-cyclin D complexes (Leemans et al, 2011). Loss of heterozygosity of the short arm of chromosome 9 (9p21-22) has been reported with high frequency in dysplasia, carcinoma in situ and HNSCC, suggesting that this genetic alteration may be involved in the early developmental stages of this disease (Thomas et al, 2005). Loss of p16 expression, mostly homozygous deletions and methylations is present in 52–82% of tumours from HNSCC patients using various detection techniques such as IHC and RT-PCR (Thomas et al, 2005). Using fluorescence in situ hybridization (FISH), p16 deletion was significantly associated with development of distant metastases (Table 3) (Namazie et al, 2002). In addition, using PCR-based techniques, a prospective study of locally advanced laryngeal SCC identified p16 mutation as an independent predictive factor for disease relapse and death (Bazan et al, 2002). In addition, downregulation of p16 was associated with a more locally advanced tumour (Thomas et al, 2005). HPV infection has an important role in understanding p16 role as a prognostic marker in HNSCC. It is well established that in HNSCC detected with HPV oncoproteins, p16 overexpression or *TP*53 wild type have a better prognosis (Leemans et al, 2011; Smith et al; 2010). In particular, HPV infection has been demonstrated to play a role in the molecular pathways through its viral oncoproteins, E6 and E7 (Chung & Gillison, 2009). They increase degradation of p53 and interfere with pRB function leading to upregulation of p16 by loss of negative feedback control. It was shown that recurrence free-survival were highest in the HNSCC patients positive for HPV infection, having p53 wild type and overexpressing p16 (Leemans et al, 2011).

Cyclooxygenase (COX) is an enzyme that is responsible for the formation of prostanoids (prostaglandins, prostacyclins, and thromboxanes) which are involved in the inflammatory response. Two isoforms of Cox, Cox-1 and Cox-2, have been described. Although Cox-1 is constitutively expressed in various tissues, Cox-2 expression is undetectable in most tissues and may play an important role in carcinogenesis and in the pathophysiologic progression of HNSCC (Thomas et al, 2005; Lin et al, 2002). Overexpression of Cox-2 in premalignant lesions such as oral Leukoplakia and HNSCC by the techniques of quantitative RT-PCR, IHC or immunoblotting has detected (Thomas et al, 2005). Cox-2 expression can be induced by various stimuli including a variety of cytokines, hormones and tumour promoters such as benzopyrene, a carcinogenic agent involved in head and neck tumorigenesis. Cox-2 enzyme contributes to carcinogenesis by catalysing the synthesis of mutagens decreasing programmed cell death or apoptosis, increasing inflammation and immunosuppression, increasing new blood vessel formation or angiogenesis and increasing potential for invasion and metastasis (Eling et al, 1990; Tsujii & DuBois, 1995; Gallo et al, 2001; Thomas et al, 2005). Cytoplasmic expression of Cox-2 has been demonstrated in 70–88% of specimens from HNSCC patients with HNSCC using IHC and in 87% of tumour specimens using RT-PCR. In addition, expression of Cox-2 is significantly higher in tumour specimens with confirmed cervical lymph node metastasis and in advanced and poorly differentiated tumours of HNSCC (Table 3) (Thomas et al, 2005). Expression of Cox-2 was also found to be a significant prognostic marker in patients with premalignant lesions (Sudbo et al, 2003), and is an independent predictor of disease-free survival (Itoh et al, 2003), but not overall survival in patients with OSCC. Interestingly, one study suggested that patients with Cox-2-negative tumours, measured using IHC and Western blot analysis, had a worse clinical outcome as compared to patients bearing a Cox-2-positive laryngeal SCC (Ranelletti et al, 2001). Furthermore, COX-2 expression was noted in all laryngeal cancer specimens using IHC, and again, a lack of correlation between Cox-2 expression and clinicopathologic variables such as primary tumour size, stage, survival, recurrence or metastases was reported for these patients (Thomas et al, 2005). Despite these results, numerous studies in various cancer systems suggest that Cox-2 activity is important in the progression of epithelial cancers.

Vascular endothelial growth factor-A (VEGF-A) is one of the key angiogenic factors promoting neovascularization in cancer, including HNSCC (Lim, 2005). It induces proliferation, migration and survival of endothelial cells during tumour growth by binding to specific tyrosine receptor kinases. Six members of the VEGF family have been identified: VEGF-A/ vascularpermeability factor (four isoforms), VEGF-B/VEGF-related factor, VEGF-C/VEGF-related protein, VEGF-D/c-fos-induced growth factor, VEGF-E and placenta growth factor, and abnormal regulation of angiogenic factors have been implicated in the pathogenesis of cancer. In particular, VEGF-A has been described as an important prognostic factor in many types of human cancer (Thomas et al, 2005). Several retrospective studies in HNSCC have demonstrated that VEGF-A (Teknos et al, 2002) and VEGF-C (Tanigaki et al, 2004) expression is associated with clinicopathological factors and/or poor patient's outcome, suggesting that they could serve as a prognostic marker also in HNSCC (Table 3). Many studies have shown that VEGF-A, as well as VEGF-C, are upregulated in head and neck cancers, thus stimulating proliferation of vascular and lymphatic endothelial cells, and increasing vessel permeability (Thomas et al, 2005). The enhanced angiogenic activity could sustain growth of the primary tumour, potentiate dissemination and also support the establishment of micrometastases (Onesto et al, 2006). This is consistent with the strong association observed in different studies between VEGF-A expression and distant recurrence. It was also demonstrated that VEGF-A protein levels are closely associated to overall survival (Onesto et al, 2006). Subsequently, multivariate analysis showed that VEGF-

A expression is an independent prognostic factor for overall survival. However, the status of VEGF-A remains unclear since other HNSCC retrospective studies have shown no correlation between VEGF-A expression and prognosis (Onesto et al, 2006; Thomas et al, 2005). These conflicting results may be due partly to the method of detection of VEGF-A expression (i.e.IHC), used in most of the previous reports, and which is a semiquantitative method. A contributing factor for these discrepant studies may be related to the lack of a direct technique to measure angiogenic activity in tissue specimens. By using a semiquantitative method (i.e. IHC) as well as a quantitative method (i.e. ELISA), it is shown that VEGF-A expression is significantly associated with the tumour differentiation stage, poorly differentiated tumours expressing higher VEGF-A levels than highly differentiated tumours in head and neck carcinomas (Onesto et al, 2006; Thomas et al, 2005). In conclusion, markers related to tumour neovascularization can also predict the outcome in head and neck cancer patients.

Transforming growth factor **alpha (TGF-α)** is upregulated in some human cancers, including HNSCC. It is produced in macrophages, brain cells, and keratinocytes, and induces epithelial development. It competes with EGF for EGFR binding, which also results in receptor activation and cellular proliferation. By using IHC analysis, it was demonstrated that TGF alfa is elevated in HNSCC and in the adjacent histologically normal mucosa compared to normal control mucosa. The prognostic significance of TGF alfa has not been as widely studied as that of EGFR, but there is suggestive evidence that its overexpression may predict an increased risk of recurrence and adverse survival in HNSCC patients (Table 3) (Quon et al, 2001; Leemans et al, 2011).

MMPs. The capacity of head and neck cancer to invade adjacent tissues and develop locoregional metastasis often presents serious problems in clinical management. Cancer cell invasion, metastasis and angiogenesis is a complex, multistep process, involving the cooperation of multiple proteolytic enzymes that are secreted by tumour and/or host cells and whose substrates include extracellular matrix (ECM) components. The matrix metalloproteinases (MMPs) are a family of zinc- and calcium-dependent endopeptidases that can collectively degrade virtually all protein components of the ECM. Degradation of collagen matrix is important for HNSCC to invade surrounding tissues and metastasize to regional and distant organs (Thomas et al, 2005; Lim, 2005) MMP-2 and MMP-9, believed to play a major role in tumour invasion and metastasis in HNSCC, degrade type IV collagen, the main component of basement membrane (Stetler-Stevenson et al, 1993). MMPs can be inactivated by naturally occurring tissue inhibitors of MMPs (TIMPs). Expression of TIMPs has also been associated with poor prognosis in HNSCC patients (Thomas et al, 2005). Various MMPs are over-expressed in HNSCC including MMP-2, MMP-8, MMP-9 and MMP-13 (Thomas et al, 2005; Ha et al, 2009). These have been detected mainly with the immunohistochemical analysis of paraffin-embedded primary tumours. MMP-9 is over-expressed in 60-92% of HNSCC and was positively correlated to the over-expression of proto-oncogene eIF4E (Nathan et al, 2002). Correlation of expression of MMP-9 with traditional clinicopathogic variables or with measures of clinical outcome in patients with HNSCC remains controversial (Table 3). Over-expression of MMP-9 has been significantly correlated with histologic grade, advanced tumour stage and lymph node metastases of HNSCC at diagnosis. Alternatively, the correlation between the expression of MMP-9 and traditional clinical prognostic factors such as tumour and lymph node stages has not been demonstrated in HNSCC patients (Thomas et al, 2005). Differences in the clinical stages of patients at presentations and differences in treatment modalities have been proposed as possible factors contributing to the discrepancies between these studies. The MMP-2 expression in HNSCC at the invasive front in advanced HNSCC was significantly correlated with overall survival, early recurrence in lymph node negative patients and lymph node metastasis (Table 3). In addition, studies from serum samples of HNSCC patients showed that high serum levels of soluble E-cadherine, MMP-9, active MMP-13, and presence of antibody anti-p53 were found to be significantly associated with poor survival and the presence of lymph node metastasis (Thomas et al, 2005). This demonstrates that the combined determination and evaluation of tumour markers may improve the diagnosis of lymph node metastasis in HNSCC. Finally, a recent study from a genome-wide transcriptional analysis of 25 HNSCC cell lines, having a different intrinsic cisplatin sensitivity, showed the possible use of MMP-7 and MMP-13, as novel predictive biomarkers for cisplatin resistance (Ansell et al, 2009).

FHIT, which is located at chromosome 3p14.2, is a tumour suppressor gene that is frequently deleted in human cancers, including HNSCC. Loss of Fhit protein expression has also been reported in some precancerous lesions of the oral cavity and esophagus (Tai et al, 2004). It has been found to be associated with exposure to environmental carcinogens, such as smoking and alcohol consumption. The loss or alterations of normal FHIT function in the context of cell growth or tumour suppression is still not known. The role of Fhit as a prognostic marker in patients with HNSCC has not yet been clearly ascertained (Table 3). Reduction or loss of Fhit expression can be found in 53–68% of tumour samples from patients with HNSCC (Thomas et al, 2005). Data obtained by using IHC, Western blot and RT-PCR methods, show that a low FHIT expression correlated with high expression of Ki-67, suggest that FHIT-altered tumour cells may have high proliferation potential (Mineta et al, 2003). However, only a few studies have found a significant correlation between Fhit expression and prognosis of patients with HNSCC. Patients whose tumours showed low or no expression of Fhit had significantly shorter disease-free survival (Lee et al, 2001; Tai et al, 2004). Interestingly, it has been shown that no reduction in Fhit expression by IHC predicted a significantly poorer outcome in patients with advanced oropharyngeal cancer (Otero-Garcia et al, 2004). In this study, tumours from all patients that subsequently developed distant metastases showed no reduction of expression of Fhit. The authors did not provide a rationale for the discrepancy between their and other studies. In other studies, authors showed that loss of Fhit expression by IHC predicted significantly poorer overall survival and an increased rate of distant metastases in patients with HNSCC (Tai et al, 2004). The results of these studies suggest that Fhit expression, as a potential new marker in HNSCC, is still in question. Further studies to elucidate the potential role of this gene in HNSCC carcinogenesis are needed.

Several other molecular factors may provide potential prognostic information for HNSCC patients. PTEN (Table 3), Ki67 and Bcl-2 are three of them. Ki67 is a marker reflecting cellular proliferation. Bcl-2 plays an important role in regulating apoptosis. The data on the prognostic role for Bcl-2 in HNSCC remain contradictory. Existing data show an association of Bcl-2 overexpression with recurrence and poor survival. On the other hand, there are also studies in which no correlations with clinical outcomes are reported (Ha et al, 2009; Quon et al, 2001).

5. Molecular study of HNSCC

HNSCC is a heterogeneous disease with complex molecular abnormalities. By using high throughput approaches generating gene expression and, more recently, microRNAs expression profiling, researchers may obtain a molecular classification and characterization of HNSCC, also in association with clinical parameters.

5.1 Gene expression

Gene expression signatures constitute an additional biological approach used to: identify screening and diagnostic molecular markers, improve tumour staging (cervical lymph node and distant metastasis prediction), differentiate lung metastasis of HNSCC from primary lung squamous cell carcinomas, predict tumour response to therapy, and provide outcome predictors (Lallemant et al, 2010). Two technologies are currently used: DNA microarrays, which extensively measures the expression of thousands of genes, and qRT-PCR, which provides a more accurate quantification of the expression of more limited number of transcripts. From a clinical point of view, gene expression profiling should provide more accurate information about the cancer consequently leading to a more personalized and improved treatment strategy (Choi & Chen, 2005). To date, more than 60 gene expression profiling studies from human clinical samples of HNSCC have been published, with variable objectives, methods and results. The most significant source of heterogeneity among DNA microarray profiling studies comes from the various methods of data generation and analysis. All microarray data analyses consist of two basic steps: 1) establishing a normalized hybridization signal for each transcript and 2) the subsequent statistical determination of the signal variations. Perhaps, the largest drawback of microarray-based examinations of HNSCC is the lack of a well-defined standard for their use, interpretation and validation. Variability in tissue procurement, tumour cell isolation, RNA extraction, choice of array platform can also explain the differences among several HNSCC gene expression studied. For instance, some authors included samples from different HNSCC locations, others focused on a specific site; some analyzed microdissected tumour epitheliums, others including the surrounding stroma (Choi & Chen, 2005). Furthermore, most studies relied on a very limited number of samples. Consequently, it is important to set a threshold percentage value of tumour cells content and the contribution of stromal cell contamination to genetic expression profiles. Another consideration in microarray experimental planning is choosing appropriate controls. It is possible to use matched or unmatched normal tissue samples as a control, in which matched tissue is taken from the same patient from whom the tumour sample was obtained, while unmatched sample is obtained from subjects without cancer. However, from the pooled gene expression data, it was possible to identify a group of genes reported by multiple studies to be significantly up-regulated and down-regulated in HNSCC (Choi & Chen, 2005; Lallemant et al, 2010). These genes were used to encode cytoskeletal and extracellular matrix proteins, inflammatory mediators, proteins involved in epidermal differentiation and cell adhesion molecules (Choi & Chen, 2005). Data suggested a global downregulation of genes that encode ribosomal proteins and enzymes in the cholesterol biosynthesis pathway, and an upregulation of genes that encode matrix metalloproteinases and genes involved in the inflammatory response (Choi & Chen, 2005).

5.1.1 Identification of HNSCC in body fluids: Blood and saliva

During carcinogenesis, some cancer cells may migrate into the blood stream or be eliminated into natural cavities like the bladder, mouth and intestines. Recovering transcriptional biomarkers representing genetic cancer alterations in the serum, plasma, urine, semen or saliva of patients, have already proven to be feasible and potentially useful, even if to date there are a few and preliminary results (Sidransky et al, 1997; Lallelmant et al, 2010). In a study, researchers compared a gene expression profile in the blood serum of HNSCC patients and control cases, aiming to identify a signature of 5 overexpressed genes and demonstrate the utility of serum in the HNSCC diagnosis. It is important to note that diagnostic biomarker detection in saliva of HNSCC patients is a promising field of research. To date, most studies have focused on DNA alterations (mutations or methylation) and only recently on mRNA detection. Among the genes correlated with the HNSCC diagnosis identified from the saliva, there are *IL1beta, OAZ1, SAT, IL8, SAT* and *H3F3A* (Li et al, 2006; Lallelmant et al, 2010).

5.1.2 Gene expression profile and local metastasis prediction

Metastatic spread is an extremely bad prognostic factor. It is responsible for the cause of death in 90% of all cancer patients (Mehlen & Puisieux, 2006). When cervical lymph node metastases are identified, more aggressive treatments are proposed either by surgery or radiotherapy. In presence of distant metastases, the disease is considered incurable and palliative treatments are indicated. Differences between metastatic and non-metastatic tumours may be detected. Data from fourteen studies demonstrated that specific differences in gene expression exist between N+ and N0 HNSCC (Lallemant et al, 2010).This difference can be used to predict the N status on initial diagnostic biopsy. On the contrary, a few studies have tried to find gene expression signatures that could predict the development of distant metastasis in HNSCC, but to date, poor results have been obtained (Choi & Chen, 2005). Insufficient samples number may in part explain the failure of these studies. In this aspect HNSCC differs from other tumour types, such as breast or prostate cancer, where a metastasis signature was identified. Cervical lymph nodes seem to work as a filter for metastatic cells and could be a prerequisite in hematologic spread. The acquisition by the primary tumour of a metastatic genetic profile is not inevitably associated with the occurrence of a distant metastasis because this cervical immunological fence can prevent or delay their appearance (Braakhuis et al, 2006).

One of the main difficulties during the diagnosis of HNSCC is detecting microscopic tumour clusters, known to be easily overlooked by conventional histopathological methods in lymph nodes and/or surgical margins (Lallemant et al, 2010). Micrometastases are responsible for cancer recurrence in the neck of patients classified as N0 and, who consequently did not receive a prophylactic treatment either by neck dissection or radiotherapy. Additional biomarkers may be of help to improve stratifying patients selected for sentinel node biopsy. As suggested by preliminary results, gene expression signatures may greatly facilitate the identification of micrometastases in N0 patients. In the same way, the development of high frequency recurrence may be due to the presence of microscopic cancer cells cluster in the resection margins disregarded by conventional microscopy (Lallemant et al, 2010). Among the molecular markers with proven predictive value for lymphatic disease are E-cadherin, podoplanin, p16, bmi-1 and LOX (Huber et al, 2011;

Lallemant et al, 2010). Until now, the published predictive factors for metastatic disease in early HNSCC are histomorphological parameters, like mode of invasion, depth of tumour infiltrations, grade of differentiation, lymphatic invasion and intratumoral lymphatic density (Huber et al, 2011). The combination of these identified molecular markers and the histopatological features could allow individual risk stratification with possible impact on treatment strategy.

5.1.3 Gene expression to distinguish HNSCC lung metastasis

In many cases, the most common site of a HNSCC distant metastasis is the lung tissue (Ferlito et al, 2001). Knowledge of whether this tumour is a lung primary cancer or an HNSCC metastasis is crucial in the patient's decision making process in choosing treatment. Unfortunately, in the presence of a single pulmonary nodule of squamous cell origin, the distinction between the primary lung tumour and HNSCC metastasis is impossible to discern (Lallemant et al, 2010). To date, only two studies have tried to address this issue by using gene expression approach. A signature of 10 genes correctly predicted and identified the origin of the tumour, thus suggesting the likelihood in identifying the origin of histologically similar malignant lesions based on expression profiling (Vachani et al, 2007).

5.1.4 Correlation between gene expression profiling and clinical outcomes

Gene expression profiling in relation to outcome prediction has been investigated to help clinicians to better stratify patients according to tumour aggressiveness, define prognosis, and subsequently modulate treatment intensity. The first study that reported the possible use of gene expression profiling for outcome prediction identified a 375 gene signature that divides the 17 patients of their cohort into two groups with slightly different survivals (Belbin et al, 2002). Data from different studies show a set of genes which identify HNSCC patients with high and low risk of recurrence and survival (Lallemant et al, 2010). For instance, it seems that high level of osteonectin may be a powerful, independent predictor for short-disease free survival interval and poor overall survival. A few studies also combined DNA microarray and CGH data to correlate the gene expression changes with chromosomal dosage and structure alterations (Lallemant et al, 2010). To date, the ability of gene expression profiling to provide effective outcome predictor remains questionable and extremely challenging.

In HNSCC, choosing the most efficient treatment for each patient is based on a TNM evaluation. However, a certain percentage of patients do not respond to treatment. Thus, the differences in gene expression profiles between responders and non responders may be identified. To date, only few studies have addressed this specific issue in relation to HNSCC (Lallemant et al, 2010). Among the identified potentially predictive genes for therapy response there are MDM2, erb2, H-ras, VCAM-1 (Ganly et al, 2007). However, although these studies provide support for the use of gene expression in predicting treatment response, their results are disappointing. Another confounding factor could be the combination of treatments used, consisting of two distinct biological mechanisms of action. Ongoing studies focusing on the development of a predictive response signature for radiotherapy alone or chemotherapy alone are more likely to be successful (Lallemant et al, 2010).

5.2 microRNAs expression profiling in HNSCC

A class of small non-coding RNAs termed microRNAs (miRNAs) has recently been indicated as biomarker of some types of cancers (Nana-Sinkam & Croce, 2010). miRNAs are endogenous, small, non-coding RNAs of 17-25 nucleotides that are thought to regulate approximately 30% of human genes. miRNAs modulate gene expression at post-transcriptional level, primarily through their partial complementarity with the coding region or 3′ untranslated region (UTR) of target mRNAs. This then leads to translational repression and/or degradation, therefore, the regulation of gene expression (Babu et al, 2011). In rare cases, they may also promote translation (Lin et al, 2011).They are involved in essential biological activities such as cellular differentiation, proliferation, development, apoptosis and cell cycle regulation (Shiiba et al, 2010). The roles of miRNAs in cancer have been extensively investigated in the past few years. The relevance of miRNAs in cancer was suggested by the observed changes in expression patterns and recurrent amplification as well as deletion of miRNA genes in cancer (Shiiba et al, 2010; Chen et al, 2010). It has been shown that there are two types of cancer-related miRNAs: oncogenic or tumour suppressor miRNAs (Table 4) (Babu et al, 2011). miRNAs expression profiling has been performed by microarray analysis or qRT-PCR methods. Some microRNAs show consistently altered expressions by different studies. For example, the upregulated expression of miR-21, -31, -18 and -221 has been reported in at least two different studies. Similarly, the expression of the miR-133a, -133b, -125a, -138, -139, -200c, -26b, -302b, -302c, -342, -371, and -373 is consistently reported to be down regulated in HNSCC (Shiiba et al, 2010). Except certain miRNAs, all published miRNAs profiling show little agreement. This may be due to various types of samples applied, to different qualities of material (FFPE or fresh tissue), different sampling locations/cell lines, methods for performing the assay and scope of the array. The sampling technique of the tumour tissue also influenced the proportion of tumor cells to non-tumor cells that may interfere with the sensitivity of real time PCR and microarray analysis.

5.2.1 Functional analysis of miRNAs in HNSCC

Potential tumour suppressor miRs: Several miRNAs are found to act as tumour suppressors in cancer and in HNSCC (Table 4). Reduced expression of almost all members of let-7 family has been observed in HNSCC by several studies (Babu et al, 2011). For example, it is shown that exogenous expression of let-7a promotes laryngeal cancer cells dysfunction by modulating proliferation, inhibiting metastasis and inducing apoptosis (Long et al, 2009). In addition, it was shown that let-7a affects RAS and c-Myc expression at protein level, thus leading to the modulation of apoptotic genes and oncogenes expression. Furthermore, reducing it into let-7d expression is associated with poor prognosis (Childs et al, 2009). Down regulation of miR-125a/b is also observed in HNSCC by independent studies. Functional data that involve introducing miR-125b into HNSCC cell lines result in a reduced cell proliferation. A possible molecular mechanism contributing to this effect might be ERBB2 targeting by miR-125a/b which has experimentally been demonstrated. In fact, a high level of ERBB2 expression was observed in HNSCC suggesting disruption of miRNA suppression of this gene (Babu et al, 2011). Down regulation of miR-133a/b was also reported. Knocking-in these miRs in HNSCC cells resulted in reduced cell proliferation or increased apoptosis (Wong et al, 2008 (a)). An increased levels of PKM2, the validated cellular target of miR-133a/b, has also been associated with cancer progression (Wong et al,

2008 (a)). Members of miR-200 family, such as miR-200a and miR-200b, are also down regulated in HNSCC. They target ZEB1/2, which act as transcriptional repressors of E-cadherin. In this way, the down modulation with the miR-200 family, concomitantly to the overexpression of miR-155, may promote epithelial mesenchymal transition (EMT) (Babu et al, 2011; Chen et al, 2010). In addition, the role of miR-138 in metastasis has also been demonstrated; miR-138 modulates migration and invasion through targeting RhoC and ROCK2. The inhibition of miR-138 enhanced cell migration as well as invasion (Liu et al, 2009). The expression of other miRs, such as miR-34c and miR-204, also correlates with invasion. Enhancing miR-204 expression directly leads to the reduction of proliferation, invasion and migration in HNSCC cell lines (Lee et al, 2010). Also microRNAs can be silenced by hypermethylation for the tumor suppressor genes. miR-137 and 193a are an example; they are downregulated in HNSCC (Kozaki et al, 2008). In addition, miR-137 promoter hypermethylation is significantly associated with poorer average survival in a study of 67 HNSCC patients (Langevin et al, 2010).

Potentional oncogenic miRs: Several miRNAs are found to act as oncogenic miRs in cancer and in HNSCC (Table 4). Overexpression of miR-106b-25 and 17-92 clusters was observed in cancer, including HNSCC, by independent studies (Babu et al, 2011; Shiiba et al, 2010). These clusters, targeting p21 mRNA, are linked with cell cycle dysfunction. In fact, knock-down of both clusters in HNSCC cells results in a reduced proliferation rate. miRNA-mediated deregulation of p21 is likely to play an important role in tobacco associated HNSCC carcinogenesis because it can negatively regulate p53-mediated DNA damage induced by carcinogens in tobacco smoke (Ivanovska et al, 2008). Another overexpressed putative oncogenic miR identified in HNSCC is miR-221, which is able to suppress the expression of cell cycle regulators p27 and p57 (Babu et al, 2011). Reduced expression of p27 has been well reported in HNSCC. It has even been suggested that it may act as a biomarker for cancer progression (Queiroz et al, 2010). In addition, a role of the miR-106b-25 and 17-92 clusters in controlling TGF-beta signaling pathway, which is deregulated in HNSCC, is emerging (Leemans et al, 2011). Another common deregulation in miRs expression in HNSCC is the upregulation of miR-21. Transfection of this miR into HNSCC cell lines results in significant increased growth rate whereas inhibitor-driven knock-down of miR-21 reduces cell proliferation. Furthermore, the inhibition of miR-21 was demonstrated to enhance cytocrome-c release, thereby promoting apoptosis (Babu et al, 2011). Finally, miR-155 shows an increased level of expression in several cancers including HNSCC and its possible role in the carcinogenesis has been investigated (Babu et al, 2011).

5.2.2 miRNAs as prognostic and diagnostic biomarkers associated with HNSCC: Correlation with clinical outcomes

Several investigators have empathized the role of miRs as biomarkers for HNSCC (Table 5). In a recent study focusing on identifying miRNAs expression signatures in association with progressive leukoplakia using sequentially progressive samples, researches built a multi-miR prognosis predictor (Cervigne et al, 2009; Babu et al, 2011). The predictors are composed of eight miRs. According to the proposed model of miR changes during the progression from leukoplakia to OSCC, the over-expression of a subset of miRs (miR-146b, miR-181b, miR-21, miR-345, mR-518b, miR-520g, miR-649 and miR-184) may be considered an early detectable event in oral tumour progression. This is because they were commonly

Oncogenic miRs	References
miR-106b-25 cluster	- Ivanovoska et al, 2008; - Petrocca et al, 2008.
miR-17-92 cluster	- Petrocca et al, 2008
miR-221	- Avissar et al, 2009 (a)
miR-21	- Cervigne et al, 2009; - Kimura et al, 2010.
miR-155	- Chang et al, 2008; - Hui et al, 2010; - Ramdas et al, 2009 .
miR-31	- Liu et al, 2010
miR-184	- Wong et al, 2008 (b); - Wong et al, 2009.
Tumor suppressor miRs	**- References**
Let-7 family	- Chang et al, 2008; - Hui et al, 2010; - Ramdas et al, 2009.
miR-125a/b	- Henson et al, 2009; - Park et al, 2009.
miR-133a/b	- Nohata et al, 2011
miR-200 family	- Park et al, 2009;
miR-1	- Nohata et al, 2011

Table 4. Altered microRNAs in HNSCC

deregulated in progressive and malignant lesions and were unchanged or under-expressed in non-progressive lesions. In particular, miR-345, miR-21 and miR-181b are strongly associated with increased lesion severity during the transition from histologically pre-malignant to malignant lesions. According to this model, the final stages of carcinogenesis may also involve changes in miR-196a and miR-206, which appear under-expressed in premalignant lesions and over-expressed in carcinomas. Interestingly, these miRs are predicted to target cancer-associated genes, e.g. *TNFRSF10B, ACAT1, NFIB, CCL1, MSH2, ACYP1 and PCBP2* (miR-21); *GRM1, MAP3K10, CCDC42, SNHG5* (miR-181b); *TSPO, RFXDC1, ZNF133, MORN3* (miR-345) (Cervigne et al, 2009). However, the usefulness of miRs as prognostic factors has only begun to be explored. Data from the study of miR-205 and Let-7d expression showed their association with locoregional occurrence and shorter survival (Childs et al, 2009). In addition, high expression of miR-205 can be used to detect positive lymph nodes, suggesting that this miR can be considered as a marker for metastatic HNSCC (Fletcher et al, 2008). Another similar study identified lower expression levels of miR-451 in HNSCC tumours as a strong predictor for recurrence (Hui et al, 2010). In a study that looked into identifying diagnostic miRs in the saliva, researchers reported significantly low levels of miR-125a and 200a in the saliva of OSCC patients compared to control subjects (Park et al, 2009). Another recent study reported high levels of miR-184 and miR-31 in plasma of OSCC (Wong et al, 2008 (b), 2009). The study also showed that miR-184 has antiapoptotic functions in HNSCC cell lines. In fact, the inhibition of its expression can reduce cell proliferation rates. Finally, an association with higher expression of miR-211 and most advanced nodal metastases, vascular invasion and poor prognosis was demonstrated in HNSCC (Chang et al, 2008).

Putative miR marker	Properties as marker	References
mir-205	➢ Prognostic value: ➢ low expression is associated with loco-regional recurrence. ➢ low expression of both miR-205 and let-7d is associated with poor survival ➢ role of miR-205 down-regulation in epithelial-mesenchymal transition of head and neck spindle cell carcinoma ➢ miR-205 expression as a marker for detection of metastatic HNSCC	- Childs et al, 2009; - Fletcher et al, 2008; - Kimura et al, 2010; - Zidar et al, 2011.
Let-7d	➢ Prognostic value: ➢ down-regulation of let-7d in combination with miR-205 low expression is associated with poor survival ➢ let-7d down-regulation promotes epithelial-mesenchymal transition (EMT) and have a role in chemoresistance	- Chang et al, 2011; - Childs et al, 2009.
miR-211	➢ Prognostic value: ➢ high miR-211 expression is associated with a worse survival rate	- Chang et al, 2008
miR-31	➢ Diagnostic marker: ➢ detection of high miR-31 expression in plasma from oral cancer patients ➢ miR-31 expression in plasma is remarkably reduced after tumor resection	- Liu et al, 2010.
miR-125a, 200a	➢ Diagnostic marker: ➢ detection of low miR-125a and miR-200a expression levels in the saliva of oral cavity cancers	- Park et al, 2009.
miR-184	➢ Diagnostic marker: ➢ detection of high mir-184 expression in plasma from oral cancer patients ➢ miR-184 expression in plasma is remarkably reduced after tumor resection	- Wang et al, 2009; - Wong et al, 2008 (b).
miR-137	➢ Prognostic marker: ➢ miR-137 promoter methylation is associated with poor overall survival ➢ miR-137 aberrant methylation is more evident in female gender	- Langevin et al, 2010.
miR-21	➢ Prognostic value: ➢ elevated miR-21 level was associated with worse survival outcome; ➢ high expression of miR-21, in combination with miR-181b and miR-345 is associated with increased severity during progression	- Avissar et al, 2009 (a); - Cervigne et al, 2009; - Fu et al, 2011; - Kimura et al, 2010.

Putative miR marker	Properties as marker	References
miR-210	➢ Marker of hypoxia and prognostic/predictive value: demonstrated functional role in tumor survival under hypoxia	- Gee et al, 2010
miR-451	➢ Strong predictor for relapse	- Hui et al, 2010
miR-221, miR-375	➢ Diagnostic marker: ➢ the expression ratio of miR-221 to miR-375 can distinguish the normal from tumor tissue	- Avissar et al, 2009 (a)

Table 5. microRNAs as putative biomarker in HNSCC

5.2.3 Aetiologic agents and correlation with miRNAs expression

Despite the relative recent discovery of microRNAs and their association with cancer, their correlation with the aetiologic agents of HNSCC is still ongoing. Until now, very few studies have focused on this area. Data from multivariate analyses showed that expression of miR-375 increases with alcohol consumption. Though expression of miR-375 is lower in tumours compared to normal tissues, fine-tuning of miRNA expression can occur at the level of the tumour microenvironment and can vary according to exposures and locations of the tumour (Avissar et al, 2009 (b)). In this case, alcohol consumption may contribute to the altered expression of miR-375 within HNSCC tumours. The regulation of miRNAs is complex and perturbations of the normal homeostatic mechanisms responsible for overall epigenetic stability could play a crucial role in potentially carcinogenic gene expression. Higher expression of miR-375 was also found in pharyngeal and laryngeal tumours compared with tumours of the oral cavity (Avissar et al, 2009 (b)). This observation is consistent with several findings indicating that miRNA profiles are tumour and cell-type specific which can even accurately differentiate tumour subtypes. Furthermore, the productivity for differential expression of miR-375 in tissues might reflect etiology. The significant association observed between drinking and miR-375 expression coupled with its tendency for higher expression in pharyngeal and laryngeal tumours may suggest that the deregulation of miRNA by exposures occurs preferentially in certain tissues (Avissar et al, 2009 (b)). Until now, there is no apparent evidence on the correlation of microRNAs expression and tobacco smoke in HNSCC. It is known that alcohol and tobacco use are predisposing factors for developing HNSCC, but HPV is also known to be associated with HNSCC, especially in the oral cavity and oropharynx cancer. HPV positive tumours have distinct clinical, molecular and prognostic features (Leemans et al, 2011). Until now, there is only one study on the microRNAs expression profiling analysis and HPV status information of HNSCC patients (Lajer et al, 2011). Researchers using a microarray approach have observed that HPV clearly has an influence on the miRNAs expression profile on a set of 49 oral cavity and oropharynx patients compared to 39 control subjects. In particular, miR-145, 125a, and 126 were reduced in HPV-positive HNSCC patients, while miR-363 expression was increased (Lajer et al, 2011).

5.4.4 An overview on therapy in HNSCC: Curcumin as a potential therapeutic agent

Standard treatment regimens for head and neck cancer depend on the stage of the disease. Early stage (stage I and II) tumours are treated primarily with surgery or radiotherapy, or with a combination of both modalities resulting in similar local control and survival rates. Radiation may also be used postoperatively when surgical margins are close or positive, or if a perineural or lymphovascular invasion by tumour is found. More advanced (stage III and IV) cancers often require a combination of therapies consisting of surgery, radiation and chemotherapy which can result in a very high morbidity (Wilken et al, 2011). Platinum-based agents form the backbone of the standard chemotherapeutic regimens for head and neck cancer. Cisplatin (cis diamminedichloroplatinum) is a widely used drug in the class of platinum-based chemotherapies. The efficacy of cisplatin in HNSCC is greatly increased when combined with other chemotherapeutic agents, such as taxanes (paclitaxel and docetaxel) and 5 fluorouracil (5-FU) (Adelstein et al, 2010). The potential adverse effects from the treatment for HNSCC are numerous (Wilken et al, 2011). Despite continuing research and advances in treatment, the clinical outcomes and overall survival rates for HNSCC have not improved significantly over the last several decades, with an overall 5-year survival rate as low as 50%. As a result, there has been continuing investigation into potential alternative and less toxic therapies for head and neck cancer, aiming to achieve a more favorable clinical outcome while reducing treatment morbidity. The class of molecularly targeted therapies against the epidermal growth factor receptor (EGFR) is one such example, as EGFR is overexpressed in a number of head and neck cancers (Chang & Califano, 2008). Cetuximab is an anti-EGFR monoclonal antibody that was approved by the Food and Drug Administration in 2004 for the treatment of advanced colon cancer. In 2006, Cetuximab was approved for use in head and neck squamous cell carcinoma both in combination with radiotherapy for advanced HNSCC as well as single-agent therapy for platinum-refractory head and neck cancer. Several studies of cetuximab as an adjuvant agent with radiotherapy have demonstrated improved locoregional control and statistically significant increases in both progression-free and overall survival (Wilken et al, 2011). The addition of cetuximab to standard platinum-based chemotherapy in platinum-resistant recurrent or metastatic head and neck cancer has also been studied and demonstrated increased treatment efficacy and improved overall survival without a significant increase in toxicity (Wilken et al, 2011). Multiple molecular pathways such as NF-kB activation, EGFR and PI3K/AKT/mTOR signaling, STAT3 expression, the MAP kinase cascade and VEGF mediated angiogenesis have been shown to be deregulated in HNSCC and represent potential therapeutic targets (Choi & Chen, 2005; Leemans et al, 2011). While some promising results from such targeted therapies have been obtained, the complexity of interaction between these signaling pathways may contribute to the limited clinical response seen with the use of single-agent biologic therapies. Curcumin (diferuloylmethane) is a polyphenol derived from the *Curcuma longa* plant, commonly known as turmeric. Curcumin has been used extensively in Ayurvedic medicine for centuries, as it is nontoxic and has a variety of therapeutic properties including anti-oxidant, analgesic, anti-inflammatory and antiseptic activity (Wilken et al, 2011). More recently curcumin has been found to possess anti-cancer activities, mostly via its effect on a variety of biological pathways involved in mutagenesis, oncogene expression, cell cycle regulation, apoptosis, tumorigenesis and metastasis (Wilken et al, 2011). Curcumin has shown an anti-proliferative effect in multiple cancers, and is an inhibitor of the transcription factor NF-kB and downstream gene products (including c-myc, Bcl-2, COX-2, NOS, Cyclin D1, TNF-alpha, interleukins and MMP-9). In addition, curcumin affects a variety of growth factor receptors and cell adhesion molecules involved in tumour growth, angiogenesis and metastasis (Wilken et al, 2011). As a natural product, curcumin is nontoxic. It has been studied in various in vitro and vivo models of head and neck squamous cell carcinoma with promising results. An overview of the current literature supports the spice's utility in the treatment of head and neck cancer and its effect as a chemopreventive agent (Wilken et al, 2011).

6. Conclusions

To date, the study of molecular prognostic factors has been an evolution motivated by the desire to define more homogenous groups of patients for treatment selection. Expression of these markers in diagnostic biopsy specimens may be an additional tool for selecting patients that may benefit from more aggressive treatment. Although these findings may help focus on selecting markers for further analysis for their value in the understanding and management of HNSCC, there are limitations to utilizing the list of molecules such as genes, microRNAs or proteins. Disagreement between studies may be due to the variety of tumour sites, sensitivity of the techniques used, quality of the specimens studied and the arbitrary cut-off values setted. More importantly, a lack of uniformed curative protocols throughout these studies may significantly affect their outcome, as the choice of a treatment method may have a great impact on long term survival of HNSCC patients. Although the pathobiology of many of the biomarkers in HNSCC provides sufficient rationale for clinical trials on single potential therapeutic agents, a multimarker strategy in addition to clinical parameters, is likely to add importance to the risk management of patients with or at risk of HNSCC. In this regard, microarray technology may provide a means for screening HNSCC samples for the presence or absence of a large number of genes or other molecules simultaneously. Many studies strongly suggest that miRNAs play a crucial role and may be a biomarker in HNSCC. There is a great deal of evidence demonstrating how altered expression of selected miRNAs may contribute to the deregulation of biological pathways involved in cancer such as cell cycle, apoptosis, epithelial-mesenchimal transition. Elucidation of the molecular mechanisms for miRNAs that are strong predictors of clinical outcomes can lead to a more complete picture of the role of miRNAs in HNSCC. Thus, detailed investigations of miRNAs, concerning intercommunication among miRNAs and between miRNAs and mRNAs, altered protein expression induced by miRNAs and site specific miRNAs expression profiling, are required accordingly before future clinical trials of therapeutic applications. For instance, antisense targeting of miRNAs for therapeutic purposes is emerging as a promising approach.

7. References

Adelstein, D. J., Moon, J., Hanna, E., Giri, P. G., Mills, G. M., Wolf, G. T., & Urba, S. G. (2010). Docetaxel, Cisplatin, and Fluorouracil Induction Chemotherapy Followed by Accelerated Fractionation/Concomitant Boost Radiation and Concurrent Cisplatin in Patients with Advanced Squamous Cell Head and Neck Cancer: A Southwest Oncology Group Phase II Trial (S0216). *Head Neck*, Vol. 32, No. 2, (Feb 2010), pp. 221-228, ISSN 1097-0347

Akervall, J. A., Michalides, R. J., Mineta, H., Balm, A., Borg, A., Dictor, M. R., Jin, Y., Loftus, B., Mertens, F., &Wennerberg, J. P. (1997). Amplification of Cyclin D1 in Squamous Cell Carcinoma of the Head and Neck and the Prognostic Value of Chromosomal

Abnormalities and Cyclin D1 Overexpression. *Cancer*, Vol. 79, No. 2, (Jan 1997), pp. 380-389, ISSN 0008-543X

Almadori, G., Cadoni, G., Galli, J., Ferrandina, G., Scambia, G., Exarchakos, G., Paludetti, G., & Ottaviani, F. (1999). Epidermal Growth Factor Receptor Expression in Primary Laryngeal Cancer: An Independent Prognostic Factor of Neck Node Relapse. *Int J Cancer*, Vol. 84, No. 2, (Apr 1999), pp. 188-191, ISSN 0020-7136

Ambrosch, P., Schlott, T., Hilmes, D., &Ruschenburg, I. (2001). P16 Alterations and Retinoblastoma Protein Expression in Squamous Cell Carcinoma and Neighboring Dysplasia from the Upper Aerodigestive Tract. *Virchows Arch*, Vol. 438, No. 4, (Apr 2001), pp. 343-349, ISSN 0945-6317

Ansell, A., Jerhammar, F., Ceder, R., Grafstrom, R., Grenman, R., &Roberg, K. (2009). Matrix Metalloproteinase-7 and -13 Expression Associate to Cisplatin Resistance in Head and Neck Cancer Cell Lines. *Oral Oncol*, Vol. 45, No. 10, (Oct 2009), pp. 866-871, ISSN 1368-8375

Avissar, M., Christensen, B. C., Kelsey, K. T., &Marsit, C. J. (2009). MicroRNA Expression Ratio Is Predictive of Head and Neck Squamous Cell Carcinoma. *Clin Cancer Res*, Vol. 15, No. 8, (Apr 15 2009), pp. 2850-2855, ISSN 1078-0432

Avissar, M., McClean, M. D., Kelsey, K. T., &Marsit, C. J. (2009). MicroRNA Expression in Head and Neck Cancer Associates with Alcohol Consumption and Survival. *Carcinogenesis*, Vol. 30, No. 12, (Dec 2009), pp. 2059-2063, ISSN 1460-2180

Babu, J. M., Prathibha, R., Jijith, V. S., Hariharan, R., &Pillai, M. R. (2011). A Mir-Centric View of Head and Neck Cancers. *Biochim Biophys Acta*, Vol. 1816, No. 1, (Aug 2011), pp. 67-72, ISSN 0006-3002

Baez, A. (2008). Genetic and Environmental Factors in Head and Neck Cancer Genesis. *J Environ Sci Health C Environ Carcinog Ecotoxicol Rev*, Vol. 26, No. 2, (Apr-Jun 2008), pp. 174-200, ISSN 1532-4095

Balz, V., Scheckenbach, K., Gotte, K., Bockmuhl, U., Petersen, I., & Bier, H. (2003). Is the P53 Inactivation Frequency in Squamous Cell Carcinomas of the Head and Neck Underestimated? Analysis of p53 Exons 2-11 and Human Papillomavirus 16/18 E6 Transcripts in 123 Unselected Tumor Specimens. *Cancer Res*, Vol. 63, No. 6, (Mar 2003), pp. 1188-1191, ISSN 0008-5472

Bazan, V., Zanna, I., Migliavacca, M., Sanz-Casla, M. T., Maestro, M. L., Corsale, S., Macaluso, M., Dardanoni, G., Restivo, S., Quintela, P. L., Bernaldez, R., Salerno, S., Morello, V., Tomasino, R. M., Gebbia, N., & Russo, A. (2002). Prognostic Significance of P16^{ink4a} Alterations and 9p21 Loss of Heterozygosity in Locally Advanced Laryngeal Squamous Cell Carcinoma. *J Cell Physiol*, Vol. 192, No. 3, (Sep 2002), pp. 286-293, ISSN 0021-9541

Beckhardt, R. N., Kiyokawa, N., Xi, L., Liu, T. J., Hung, M. C., el-Naggar, A. K., Zhang, H. Z., & Clayman, G. L. (1995). Her-2/Neu Oncogene Characterization in Head and Neck Squamous Cell Carcinoma. *Arch Otolaryngol Head Neck Surg*, Vol. 121, No. 11, (Nov 1995), pp. 1265-1270, ISSN 0886-4470

Behm-Ansmant, I., Kashima, I., Rehwinkel, J., Sauliere, J., Wittkopp, N., &Izaurralde, E. (2007). mRNA Quality Control: An Ancient Machinery Recognizes and Degrades mRNA with Nonsense Codons. *FEBS Lett*, Vol. 581, No. 15, (Jun 2007), pp. 2845-2853, ISSN 0014-5793

Belbin, T. J., Singh, B., Barber, I., Socci, N., Wenig, B., Smith, R., Prystowsky, M. B., & Childs, G. (2002). Molecular Classification of Head and Neck Squamous Cell Carcinoma Using cDNA Microarrays. *Cancer Res*, Vol. 62, No. 4, (Feb 2002), pp. 1184-1190, ISSN 0008-5472

Blons, H., & Laurent-Puig, P. (2003). TP53 and Head and Neck Neoplasms. *Hum Mutat*, Vol. 21, No. 3, (Mar 2003), pp. 252-257, ISSN 1098-1004

Boyle, J. O., Hakim, J., Koch, W., Van der Riet, P., Hruban, R. H., Roa, R. A., Correo, R., Eby, Y. J., Ruppert, J. M., & Sidransky, D. (1993). The Incidence of p53 Mutations Increases with Progression of Head and Neck Cancer. *Cancer Res*, Vol. 53, No. 19, (Oct 1993), pp. 4477-4480, ISSN 0008-5472

Braakhuis, B. J., Senft, A., de Bree, R., de Vries, J., Ylstra, B., Cloos, J., Kuik, D. J., Leemans, C. R., & Brakenhoff, R. H. (2006). Expression Profiling and Prediction of Distant Metastases in Head and Neck Squamous Cell Carcinoma. *J Clin Pathol*, Vol. 59, No. 12, (Dec 2006), pp. 1254-1260, ISSN 0021-9746

Braakhuis, B. J., Tabor, M. P., Kummer, J. A., Leemans, C. R., &Brakenhoff, R. H. (2003). A Genetic Explanation of Slaughter's Concept of Field Cancerization: Evidence and Clinical Implications. *Cancer Res*, Vol. 63, No. 8, (Apr 2003), pp. 1727-1730, ISSN 0008-5472

Bradford, C. R., Zhu, S., Ogawa, H., Ogawa, T., Ubell, M., Narayan, A., Johnson, G., Wolf, G. T., Fisher, S. G., & Carey, T. E. (2003). p53 Mutation Correlates with Cisplatin Sensitivity in Head and Neck Squamous Cell Carcinoma Lines. *Head Neck*, Vol. 25, No. 8, (Aug 2003), pp. 654-661, ISSN 1043-3074

Cabanillas, R., Rodrigo, J. P., Astudillo, A., Dominguez, F., Suarez, C., & Chiara, M. D. (2007). p53 Expression in Squamous Cell Carcinomas of the Supraglottic Larynx and Its Lymph Node Metastases: New Results for an Old Question. *Cancer*, Vol. 109, No. 9, (May 2007), pp. 1791-1798, ISSN 0008-543X

Cabelguenne, A., Blons, H., de Waziers, I., Carnot, F., Houllier, A. M., Soussi, T., Brasnu, D., Beaune, P., Laccourreye, O., & Laurent-Puig, P. (2000). p53 Alterations Predict Tumor Response to Neoadjuvant Chemotherapy in Head and Neck Squamous Cell Carcinoma: A Prospective Series. *J Clin Oncol*, Vol. 18, No. 7, (Apr 2000), pp. 1465-1473, ISSN 0732-183X

Califano, J., van der Riet, P., Westra, W., Nawroz, H., Clayman, G., Piantadosi, S., Corio, R., Lee, D., Greenberg, B., Koch, W., & Sidransky, D. (1996). Genetic Progression Model for Head and Neck Cancer: Implications for Field Cancerization. *Cancer Res*, Vol. 56, No. 11, (Jun 1996), pp. 2488-2492, ISSN 0008-5472

Califano, J., Westra, W. H., Meininger, G., Corio, R., Koch, W. M., & Sidransky, D. (2000). Genetic Progression and Clonal Relationship of Recurrent Premalignant Head and Neck Lesions. *Clin Cancer Res*, Vol. 6, No. 2, (Feb 2000), pp. 347-352, ISSN 1078-0432

Capaccio, P., Pruneri, G., Carboni, N., Pagliari, A. V., Quatela, M., Cesana, B. M., & Pignataro, L. (2000). Cyclin D1 Expression Is Predictive of Occult Metastases in Head and Neck Cancer Patients with Clinically Negative Cervical Lymph Nodes. *Head Neck*, Vol. 22, No. 3, (May 2000), pp. 234-240, ISSN 1043-3074

Carracedo, D. G., Astudillo, A., Rodrigo, J. P., Suarez, C., & Gonzalez, M. V. (2008). Skp2, P27kip1 and Egfr Assessment in Head and Neck Squamous Cell Carcinoma: Prognostic Implications. *Oncol Rep*, Vol. 20, No. 3, (Sep 2008), pp. 589-595, ISSN 1021-335X

Casse, C., Hu, Y. C., & Ahrendt, S. A. (2003). The Xrcc1 Codon 399 Gln Allele Is Associated with Adenine to Guanine p53 Mutations in Non-Small Cell Lung Cancer. *Mutat Res*, Vol. 528, No. 1-2, (Jul 2003), pp. 19-27, ISSN 0027-5107

Cervigne, N. K., Reis, P. P., Machado, J., Sadikovic, B., Bradley, G., Galloni, N. N., Pintilie, M., Jurisica, I., Perez-Ordonez, B., Gilbert, R., Gullane, P., Irish, J., & Kamel-Reid, S. (2009). Identification of a MicroRNA Signature Associated with Progression of Leukoplakia to Oral Carcinoma. *Hum Mol Genet*, Vol. 18, No. 24, (Dec 2009), pp. 4818-4829, ISSN 1460-2083

Chang, C. J., Hsu, C. C., Chang, C. H., Tsai, L. L., Chang, Y. C., Lu, S. W., Yu, C. H., Huang, H. S., Wang, J. J., Tsai, C. H., Chou, M. Y., Yu, C. C., & Hu, F. W. (2011). Let-7d Functions as Novel Regulator of Epithelial-Mesenchymal Transition and Chemoresistant Property in Oral Cancer. *Oncol Rep*, Vol. 26, No. 4, (Oct 2011), pp. 1003-1010, ISSN 1791-2431

Chang, K. W., Liu, C. J., Chu, T. H., Cheng, H. W., Hung, P. S., Hu, W. Y., & Lin, S. C. (2008). Association between High Mir-211 MicroRNA Expression and the Poor Prognosis of Oral Carcinoma. *J Dent Res*, Vol. 87, No. 11, (Nov 2008), pp. 1063-1068, ISSN 1544-0591

Chang, S. S., & Califano, J. (2008). Current Status of Biomarkers in Head and Neck Cancer. *J Surg Oncol*, Vol. 97, No. 8, (Jun 2008), pp. 640-643, ISSN 0022-4790

Chang, S. S., Jiang, W. W., Smith, I., Poeta, L. M., Begum, S., Glazer, C., Shan, S., Westra, W., Sidransky, D., & Califano, J. A. (2008). MicroRNA Alterations in Head and Neck Squamous Cell Carcinoma. *Int J Cancer*, Vol. 123, No. 12, (Dec 2008), pp. 2791-2797, ISSN 1097-0215

Chen, H. C., Chen, G. H., Chen, Y. H., Liao, W. L., Liu, C. Y., Chang, K. P., Chang, Y. S., & Chen, S. J. (2009). MicroRNA Deregulation and Pathway Alterations in Nasopharyngeal Carcinoma. *Br J Cancer*, Vol. 100, No. 6, (Mar 2009), pp. 1002-1011, ISSN 1532-1827

Chen, L. H., Tsai, K. L., Chen, Y. W., Yu, C. C., Chang, K. W., Chiou, S. H., Ku, H. H., Chu, P. Y., Tseng, L. M., Huang, P. I., & Lo, W. L. (2010). MicroRNA as a Novel Modulator in Head and Neck Squamous Carcinoma. *J Oncol*, Vol. 2010, No., (Feb 2010), pp. 135632, ISSN 1687-8469

Chen, Y., & Chen, C. (2008). DNA Copy Number Variation and Loss of Heterozygosity in Relation to Recurrence of and Survival from Head and Neck Squamous Cell Carcinoma: A Review. *Head Neck*, Vol. 30, No. 10, (Oct 2008), pp. 1361-1383, ISSN 1097-0347

Childs, G., Fazzari, M., Kung, G., Kawachi, N., Brandwein-Gensler, M., McLemore, M., Chen, Q., Burk, R. D., Smith, R. V., Prystowsky, M. B., Belbin, T. J., & Schlecht, N. F. (2009). Low-Level Expression of MicroRNAs Let-7d and Mir-205 Are Prognostic Markers of Head and Neck Squamous Cell Carcinoma. *Am J Pathol*, Vol. 174, No. 3, (Mar 2009), pp. 736-745, ISSN 1525-2191

Choi, P., & Chen, C. (2005). Genetic Expression Profiles and Biologic Pathway Alterations in Head and Neck Squamous Cell Carcinoma. *Cancer*, Vol. 104, No. 6, (Sep 2005), pp. 1113-1128, ISSN 0008-543X

Chung, C. H., & Gillison, M. L. (2009). Human Papillomavirus in Head and Neck Cancer: Its Role in Pathogenesis and Clinical Implications. *Clin Cancer Res*, Vol. 15, No. 22, (Nov 2009), pp. 6758-6762, ISSN 1078-0432

Chung, C. H., Parker, J. S., Karaca, G., Wu, J., Funkhouser, W. K., Moore, D., Butterfoss, D., Xiang, D., Zanation, A., Yin, X., Shockley, W. W., Weissler, M. C., Dressler, L. G., Shores, C. G., Yarbrough, W. G., & Perou, C. M. (2004). Molecular Classification of Head and Neck Squamous Cell Carcinomas Using Patterns of Gene Expression. *Cancer Cell*, Vol. 5, No. 5, (May 2004), pp. 489-500, ISSN 1535-6108

Cruz, I. B., Snijders, P. J., Meijer, C. J., Braakhuis, B. J., Snow, G. B., Walboomers, J. M., & van der Waal, I. (1998). P53 Expression above the Basal Cell Layer in Oral Mucosa Is an Early Event of Malignant Transformation and Has Predictive Value for Developing Oral Squamous Cell Carcinoma. *J Pathol*, Vol. 184, No. 4, (Apr 1998), pp. 360-368, ISSN 0022-3417

D'Souza, G., Kreimer, A. R., Viscidi, R., Pawlita, M., Fakhry, C., Koch, W. M., Westra, W. H., & Gillison, M. L. (2007). Case-Control Study of Human Papillomavirus and Oropharyngeal Cancer. *N Engl J Med*, Vol. 356, No. 19, (May 2007), pp. 1944-1956, ISSN 1533-4406

Eling, T. E., Thompson, D. C., Foureman, G. L., Curtis, J. F., & Hughes, M. F. (1990). Prostaglandin H Synthase and Xenobiotic Oxidation. *Annu Rev Pharmacol Toxicol*, Vol. 30, No., (Apr 1990), pp. 1-45, ISSN 0362-1642

Esteller, M., & Herman, J. G. (2002). Cancer as an Epigenetic Disease: DNA Methylation and Chromatin Alterations in Human Tumours. *J Pathol*, Vol. 196, No. 1, (Jan 2002), pp. 1-7, ISSN 0022-3417

Ferlito, A., Shaha, A. R., Silver, C. E., Rinaldo, A., & Mondin, V. (2001). Incidence and Sites of Distant Metastases from Head and Neck Cancer. *ORL J OtorhinolaryngolRelat Spec*, Vol. 63, No. 4, (Jul-Aug 2001), pp. 202-207, ISSN 0301-1569

Field, J. K., Spandidos, D. A., Malliri, A., Gosney, J. R., Yiagnisis, M., & Stell, P. M. (1991). Elevated p53 Expression Correlates with a History of Heavy Smoking in Squamous Cell Carcinoma of the Head and Neck. *Br J Cancer*, Vol. 64, No. 3, (Sep 1991), pp. 573-577, ISSN 0007-0920

Fletcher, A. M., Heaford, A. C., & Trask, D. K. (2008). Detection of Metastatic Head and Neck Squamous Cell Carcinoma Using the Relative Expression of Tissue-Specific Mir-205. *Transl Oncol*, Vol. 1, No. 4, (Dec 2008), pp. 202-208, ISSN 1936-5233

Fu, X., Han, Y., Wu, Y., Zhu, X., Lu, X., Mao, F., Wang, X., He, X., & Zhao, Y. (2011). Prognostic Role of MicroRNA-21 in Various Carcinomas: A Systematic Review and Meta-Analysis. *Eur J Clin Invest*, Vol., No., (Apr 2011), pp., ISSN 1365-2362

Gallo, O., Franchi, A., Magnelli, L., Sardi, I., Vannacci, A., Boddi, V., Chiarugi, V., & Masini, E. (2001). Cyclooxygenase-2 Pathway Correlates with Vegf Expression in Head and Neck Cancer. Implications for Tumor Angiogenesis and Metastasis. *Neoplasia*, Vol. 3, No. 1, (Jan-Feb 2001), pp. 53-61, ISSN 1522-8002

Gallo, O., Masini, E., Bianchi, B., Bruschini, L., Paglierani, M., & Franchi, A. (2002). Prognostic Significance of Cyclooxygenase-2 Pathway and Angiogenesis in Head and Neck Squamous Cell Carcinoma. *Hum Pathol*, Vol. 33, No. 7, (Jul 2002), pp. 708-714, ISSN 0046-8177

Ganci, F., Conti, S., Fontemaggi, G., Manciocco, V., Donzelli, S., Covello, R., Muti, P., Strano, S., Blandino, G., & Spriano, G. (2011). Allelic Expression Imbalance of TP53 Mutated and Polymorphic Alleles in Head and Neck Tumors. *OMICS*, Vol. 15, No. 6, (Jun 2011), pp. 375-381, ISSN 1557-8100

Ganly, I., Talbot, S., Carlson, D., Viale, A., Maghami, E., Osman, I., Sherman, E., Pfister, D., Chuai, S., Shaha, A. R., Kraus, D., Shah, J. P., Socci, N. D., & Singh, B. (2007). Identification of Angiogenesis/Metastases Genes Predicting Chemoradiotherapy Response in Patients with Laryngopharyngeal Carcinoma. *J Clin Oncol*, Vol. 25, No. 11, (Apr 2007), pp. 1369-1376, ISSN 1527-7755

Garavello, W., Foschi, R., Talamini, R., La Vecchia, C., Rossi, M., Dal Maso, L., Tavani, A., Levi, F., Barzan, L., Ramazzotti, V., Franceschi, S., & Negri, E. (2008). Family History and the Risk of Oral and Pharyngeal Cancer. *Int J Cancer*, Vol. 122, No. 8, (Apr 2008), pp. 1827-1831, ISSN 1097-0215

Gasco, M., & Crook, T. (2003). The p53 Network in Head and Neck Cancer. *Oral Oncol*, Vol. 39, No. 3, (Apr 2003), pp. 222-231, ISSN 1368-8375

Gee, H. E., Camps, C., Buffa, F. M., Patiar, S., Winter, S. C., Betts, G., Homer, J., Corbridge, R., Cox, G., West, C. M., Ragoussis, J., & Harris, A. L. (2010). Hsa-Mir-210 Is a Marker of Tumor Hypoxia and a Prognostic Factor in Head and Neck Cancer. *Cancer*, Vol. 116, No. 9, (May 2010), pp. 2148-2158, ISSN 0008-543X

Glazer, C. A., Chang, S. S., Ha, P. K., & Califano, J. A. (2009). Applying the Molecular Biology and Epigenetics of Head and Neck Cancer in Everyday Clinical Practice. *Oral Oncol*, Vol. 45, No. 4-5, (Apr-May 2009), pp. 440-446, ISSN 1368-8375

Gottlieb, E., & Tomlinson, I. P. (2005). Mitochondrial Tumour Suppressors: A Genetic and Biochemical Update. *Nat Rev Cancer*, Vol. 5, No. 11, (Nov 2005), pp. 857-866, ISSN 1474-175X

Grandis, J. R., & Tweardy, D. J. (1993). Elevated Levels of Transforming Growth Factor Alpha and Epidermal Growth Factor Receptor Messenger RNA Are Early Markers of Carcinogenesis in Head and Neck Cancer. *Cancer Res*, Vol. 53, No. 15, (Aug 1993), pp. 3579-3584, ISSN 0008-5472

Graveland, A. P., Golusinski, P. J., Buijze, M., Douma, R., Sons, N., Kuik, D. J., Bloemena, E., Leemans, C. R., Brakenhoff, R. H., & Braakhuis, B. J. (2011). Loss of Heterozygosity at 9p and p53 Immunopositivity in Surgical Margins Predict Local Relapse in Head and Neck Squamous Cell Carcinoma. *Int J Cancer*, Vol. 128, No. 8, (Apr 2011), pp. 1852-1859, ISSN 1097-0215

Ha, P. K., & Califano, J. A. (2003). The Molecular Biology of Mucosal Field Cancerization of the Head and Neck. *Crit Rev Oral Biol Med*, Vol. 14, No. 5, (Sep 2003), pp. 363-369, ISSN 1544-1113

Ha, P. K., & Califano, J. A. (2006). Promoter Methylation and Inactivation of Tumour-Suppressor Genes in Oral Squamous-Cell Carcinoma. *Lancet Oncol*, Vol. 7, No. 1, (Jan 2006), pp. 77-82, ISSN 1470-2045

Ha, P. K., Chang, S. S., Glazer, C. A., Califano, J. A., & Sidransky, D. (2009). Molecular Techniques and Genetic Alterations in Head and Neck Cancer. *Oral Oncol*, Vol. 45, No. 4-5, (Apr-May 2009), pp. 335-339, ISSN 1368-8375

Hama, T., Yuza, Y., Saito, Y., J, O. uchi, Kondo, S., Okabe, M., Yamada, H., Kato, T., Moriyama, H., Kurihara, S., & Urashima, M. (2009). Prognostic Significance of Epidermal Growth Factor Receptor Phosphorylation and Mutation in Head and Neck Squamous Cell Carcinoma. *Oncologist*, Vol. 14, No. 9, (Sep 2009), pp. 900-908, ISSN 1549-490X

Henson, B. J., Bhattacharjee, S., O'Dee, D. M., Feingold, E., & Gollin, S. M. (2009). Decreased Expression of Mir-125b and Mir-100 in Oral Cancer Cells Contributes to

Malignancy. *Genes Chromosomes Cancer*, Vol. 48, No. 7, (Jul 2009), pp. 569-582, ISSN 1098-2264

Herman, J. G., & Baylin, S. B. (2003). Gene Silencing in Cancer in Association with Promoter Hypermethylation. *N Engl J Med*, Vol. 349, No. 21, (Nov 2003), pp. 2042-2054, ISSN 1533-4406

Holley, S. L., Matthias, C., Jahnke, V., Fryer, A. A., Strange, R. C., & Hoban, P. R. (2005). Association of Cyclin D1 Polymorphism with Increased Susceptibility to Oral Squamous Cell Carcinoma. *Oral Oncol*, Vol. 41, No. 2, (Feb 2005), pp. 156-160, ISSN 1368-8375

Huber, G. F., Fritzsche, F. R., Zullig, L., Storz, M., Graf, N., S, K. Haerle, Jochum, W., Stoeckli, S. J., & Moch, H. (2011). Podoplanin Expression Correlates with Sentinel Lymph Node Metastasis in Early Squamous Cell Carcinomas of the Oral Cavity and Oropharynx. *Int J Cancer*, Vol. 129, No. 6, (Sep 2011), pp. 1404-1409, ISSN 1097-0215

Huber, G. F., Zullig, L., Soltermann, A., Roessle, M., Graf, N., Haerle, S. K., Studer, G., Jochum, W., Moch, H., &Stoeckli, S. J. (2011). Down Regulation of E-Cadherin (Ecad) - a Predictor for Occult Metastatic Disease in Sentinel Node Biopsy of Early Squamous Cell Carcinomas of the Oral Cavity and Oropharynx. *BMC Cancer*, Vol. 11, No.,(June 2011), pp. 217, ISSN 1471-2407

Hui, A. B., Lenarduzzi, M., Krushel, T., Waldron, L., Pintilie, M., Shi, W., Perez-Ordonez, B., Jurisica, I., O'Sullivan, B., Waldron, J., Gullane, P., Cummings, B., & Liu, F. F. (2010). Comprehensive MicroRNA Profiling for Head and Neck Squamous Cell Carcinomas. *Clin Cancer Res*, Vol. 16, No. 4, (Feb 2010), pp. 1129-1139, ISSN 1078-0432

Hussain, S. P., & Harris, C. C. (1999). p53 Mutation Spectrum and Load: The Generation of Hypotheses Linking the Exposure of Endogenous or Exogenous Carcinogens to Human Cancer. *Mutat Res*, Vol. 428, No. 1-2, (Jul 1999), pp. 23-32, ISSN 0027-5107

Ingelman-Sundberg, M. (2001). Genetic Variability in Susceptibility and Response to Toxicants. *Toxicol Lett*, Vol. 120, No. 1-3, (Mar 2001), pp. 259-268, ISSN 0378-4274

Itoh, S., Matsui, K., Furuta, I., & Takano, Y. (2003). Immunohistochemical Study on Overexpression of Cyclooxygenase-2 in Squamous Cell Carcinoma of the Oral Cavity: Its Importance as a Prognostic Predictor. *Oral Oncol*, Vol. 39, No. 8, (Dec 2003), pp. 829-835, ISSN 1368-8375

Ivanovska, I., Ball, A. S., Diaz, R. L., Magnus, J. F., Kibukawa, M., Schelter, J. M., Kobayashi, S. V., Lim, L., Burchard, J., Jackson, A. L., Linsley, P. S., & Cleary, M. A. (2008). MicroRNAs in the Mir-106b Family Regulate P21/Cdkn1a and Promote Cell Cycle Progression. *Mol Cell Biol*, Vol. 28, No. 7, (Apr 2008), pp. 2167-2174, ISSN 1098-5549

Izzo, J. G., Papadimitrakopoulou, V. A., Li, X. Q., Ibarguen, H., Lee, J. S., Ro, J. Y., El-Naggar, A., Hong, W. K., & Hittelman, W. N. (1998). Dysregulated Cyclin D1 Expression Early in Head and Neck Tumorigenesis: In Vivo Evidence for an Association with Subsequent Gene Amplification. *Oncogene*, Vol. 17, No. 18, (Nov 1998), pp. 2313-2322, ISSN 0950-9232

Jamieson, T. A., Brizel, D. M., Killian, J. K., Oka, Y., Jang, H. S., Fu, X., Clough, R. W., Vollmer, R. T., Anscher, M. S., &Jirtle, R. L. (2003). M6p/Igf2r Loss of Heterozygosity in Head and Neck Cancer Associated with Poor Patient Prognosis. *BMC Cancer*, Vol. 3, No., (Feb 2003), pp. 4, ISSN 1471-2407

Kalyankrishna, S., & Grandis, J. R. (2006). Epidermal Growth Factor Receptor Biology in Head and Neck Cancer. *J Clin Oncol*, Vol. 24, No. 17, (Jun 2006), pp. 2666-2672, ISSN 1527-7755

Kearsley, J. H., Furlong, K. L., Cooke, R. A., & Waters, M. J. (1990). An Immunohistochemical Assessment of Cellular Proliferation Markers in Head and Neck Squamous Cell Cancers. *Br J Cancer*, Vol. 61, No. 6, (Jun 1990), pp. 821-827, ISSN 0007-0920

Kimura, S., Naganuma, S., Susuki, D., Hirono, Y., Yamaguchi, A., Fujieda, S., Sano, K., & Itoh, H. (2010). Expression of MicroRNAs in Squamous Cell Carcinoma of Human Head and Neck and the Esophagus: Mir-205 and Mir-21 Are Specific Markers for HNSCC and Escc. *Oncol Rep*, Vol. 23, No. 6, (Jun 2010), pp. 1625-1633, ISSN 1791-2431

Kiuru, A., Servomaa, K., Grenman, R., Pulkkinen, J., & Rytomaa, T. (1997). p53 Mutations in Human Head and Neck Cancer Cell Lines. *Acta Otolaryngol Suppl*, Vol. 529, No., (1997), pp. 237-240, ISSN 0365-5237

Ko, Y., Abel, J., Harth, V., Brode, P., Antony, C., Donat, S., Fischer, H. P., Ortiz-Pallardo, M. E., Thier, R., Sachinidis, A., Vetter, H., Bolt, H. M., Herberhold, C., & Bruning, T. (2001). Association of Cyp1b1 Codon 432 Mutant Allele in Head and Neck Squamous Cell Cancer Is Reflected by Somatic Mutations of p53 in Tumor Tissue. *Cancer Res*, Vol. 61, No. 11, (Jun 2001), pp. 4398-4404, ISSN 0008-5472

Kojima, M., Morisaki, T., Uchiyama, A., Doi, F., Mibu, R., Katano, M., & Tanaka, M. (2001). Association of Enhanced Cyclooxygenase-2 Expression with Possible Local Immunosuppression in Human Colorectal Carcinomas. *Ann Surg Oncol*, Vol. 8, No. 5, (Jun 2001), pp. 458-465, ISSN 1068-9265

Kozaki, K., Imoto, I., Mogi, S., Omura, K., & Inazawa, J. (2008). Exploration of Tumor-Suppressive MicroRNAs Silenced by DNA Hypermethylation in Oral Cancer. *Cancer Res*, Vol. 68, No. 7, (Apr 2008), pp. 2094-2105, ISSN 1538-7445

Kumar, R. V., Kadkol, S. S., Daniel, R., Shenoy, A. M., & Shah, K. V. (2003). Human Papillomavirus, p53 and Cyclin D1 Expression in Oropharyngeal Carcinoma. *Int J Oral MaxillofacSurg*, Vol. 32, No. 5, (Oct 2003), pp. 539-543, ISSN 0901-5027

Kusukawa, J., Harada, H., Shima, I., Sasaguri, Y., Kameyama, T., & Morimatsu, M. (1996). The Significance of Epidermal Growth Factor Receptor and Matrix Metalloproteinase-3 in Squamous Cell Carcinoma of the Oral Cavity. *Eur J Cancer B Oral Oncol*, Vol. 32B, No. 4, (Jul 1996), pp. 217-221, ISSN 0964-1955

Kyzas, P. A., Cunha, I. W., & Ioannidis, J. P. (2005). Prognostic Significance of Vascular Endothelial Growth Factor Immunohistochemical Expression in Head and Neck Squamous Cell Carcinoma: A Meta-Analysis. *Clin Cancer Res*, Vol. 11, No. 4, (Feb 2005), pp. 1434-1440, ISSN 1078-0432

Kyzas, P. A., Stefanou, D., & Agnantis, N. J. (2004). Immunohistochemical Expression of Vascular Endothelial Growth Factor Correlates with Positive Surgical Margins and Recurrence in T1 and T2 Squamous Cell Carcinoma (Scc) of the Lower Lip. *Oral Oncol*, Vol. 40, No. 9, (Oct 2004), pp. 941-947, ISSN 1368-8375

Lacko, M., Oude Ophuis, M. B., Peters, W. H., & Manni, J. J. (2009). Genetic Polymorphisms of Smoking-Related Carcinogen Detoxifying Enzymes and Head and Neck Cancer Susceptibility. *Anticancer Res*, Vol. 29, No. 2, (Feb 2009), pp. 753-761, ISSN 0250-7005

Lajer, C. B., Nielsen, F. C., Friis-Hansen, L., Norrild, B., Borup, R., Garnaes, E., Rossing, M., Specht, L., Therkildsen, M. H., Nauntofte, B., Dabelsteen, S., & von Buchwald, C. (2011). Different MirRNA Signatures of Oral and Pharyngeal Squamous Cell Carcinomas: A Prospective Translational Study. *Br J Cancer*, Vol. 104, No. 5, (Mar 2011), pp. 830-840, ISSN 1532-1827

Lallemant, B., Evrard, A., Chambon, G., Sabra, O., Kacha, S., Lallemant, J. G., Lumbroso, S., & Brouillet, J. P. (2010). Gene Expression Profiling in Head and Neck Squamous Cell Carcinoma: Clinical Perspectives. *Head Neck*, Vol. 32, No. 12, (Dec 2010), pp. 1712-1719, ISSN 1097-0347

Langevin, S. M., Stone, R. A., Bunker, C. H., Grandis, J. R., Sobol, R. W., &Taioli, E. (2010). MicroRNA-137 Promoter Methylation in Oral Rinses from Patients with Squamous Cell Carcinoma of the Head and Neck Is Associated with Gender and Body Mass Index. *Carcinogenesis*, Vol. 31, No. 5, (May 2010), pp. 864-870, ISSN 1460-2180

Langevin, S. M., Stone, R. A., Bunker, C. H., Lyons-Weiler, M. A., Laframboise, W. A., Kelly, L., Seethala, R. R., Grandis, J. R., Sobol, R. W., &Taioli, E. (2010). MicroRNA-137 Promoter MethylationIs Associated with Poorer Overall Survival in Patients with Squamous Cell Carcinoma of the Head and Neck. *Cancer*, Vol., No., (Nov 2010), pp., ISSN 0008-543X

Lassaletta, L., Brandariz, J. A., Benito, A., de la Cruz, J., Gomez, C., Ballestin, C., Hitt, R., Colomer, R., & Alvarez-Vicent, J. J. (1999). p53 Expression in Locally Advanced Pharyngeal Squamous Cell Carcinoma. *Arch Otolaryngol Head Neck Surg*, Vol. 125, No. 12, (Dec 1999), pp. 1356-1359, ISSN 0886-4470

Lee, J. I., Soria, J. C., Hassan, K., Liu, D., Tang, X., El-Naggar, A., Hong, W. K., & Mao, L. (2001). Loss of Fhit Expression Is a Predictor of Poor Outcome in Tongue Cancer. *Cancer Res*, Vol. 61, No. 3, (Feb 2001), pp. 837-841, ISSN 0008-5472

Lee, J. J., Hong, W. K., Hittelman, W. N., Mao, L., Lotan, R., Shin, D. M., Benner, S. E., Xu, X. C., Lee, J. S., Papadimitrakopoulou, V. M., Geyer, C., Perez, C., Martin, J. W., El-Naggar, A. K., &Lippman, S. M. (2000). Predicting Cancer Development in Oral Leukoplakia: Ten Years of Translational Research. *Clin Cancer Res*, Vol. 6, No. 5, (May 2000), pp. 1702-1710, ISSN 1078-0432

Lee, Y., Yang, X., Huang, Y., Fan, H., Zhang, Q., Wu, Y., Li, J., Hasina, R., Cheng, C., Lingen, M. W., Gerstein, M. B., Weichselbaum, R. R., Xing, H. R., &Lussier, Y. A. (2010). Network Modeling Identifies Molecular Functions Targeted by Mir-204 to Suppress Head and Neck Tumor Metastasis. *PLoS Comput Biol*, Vol. 6, No. 4, (Apr 2010), pp. e1000730, ISSN 1553-7358

Leemans, C. R., Braakhuis, B. J., & Brakenhoff, R. H. (2011). The Molecular Biology of Head and Neck Cancer. *Nat Rev Cancer*, Vol. 11, No. 1, (Jan 2011), pp. 9-22, ISSN 1474-1768

Lentsch, E. J., Goudy, S., Sosnowski, J., Major, S., &Bumpous, J. M. (2006). Microvessel Density in Head and Neck Squamous Cell Carcinoma Primary Tumors and Its Correlation with Clinical Staging Parameters. *Laryngoscope*, Vol. 116, No. 3, (Mar 2006), pp. 397-400, ISSN 0023-852X

Li, C., Hu, Z., Lu, J., Liu, Z., Wang, L. E., El-Naggar, A. K., Sturgis, E. M., Spitz, M. R., & Wei, Q. (2007). Genetic Polymorphisms in DNA Base-Excision Repair Genes Adprt, Xrcc1, and Ape1 and the Risk of Squamous Cell Carcinoma of the Head and Neck. *Cancer*, Vol. 110, No. 4, (Aug 2007), pp. 867-875, ISSN 0008-543X

Li, Y., Elashoff, D., Oh, M., Sinha, U., St John, M. A., Zhou, X., Abemayor, E., & Wong, D. T. (2006). Serum Circulating Human Mrna Profiling and Its Utility for Oral Cancer Detection. *J Clin Oncol*, Vol. 24, No. 11, (Apr 2006), pp. 1754-1760, ISSN 1527-7755

Li, Z., Guan, W., Li, M. X., Zhong, Z. Y., Qian, C. Y., Yang, X. Q., Liao, L., Li, Z. P., & Wang, D. (2011). Genetic Polymorphism of DNA Base-Excision Repair Genes (Ape1, Ogg1 and Xrcc1) and Their Correlation with Risk of Lung Cancer in a Chinese Population. *Arch Med Res*, Vol. 42, No. 3, (Apr 2011), pp. 226-234, ISSN 1873-5487

Lim, S. C. (2005). Expression of C-Erbb Receptors, Mmps and Vegf in Head and Neck Squamous Cell Carcinoma. *Biomed Pharmacother*, Vol. 59 Suppl 2, No., (Oct 2005), pp. S366-369, ISSN 0753-3322

Lin, C. C., Liu, L. Z., Addison, J. B., Wonderlin, W. F., Ivanov, A. V., &Ruppert, J. M. (2011). A Klf4-Mirna-206 Autoregulatory Feedback Loop Can Promote or Inhibit Protein Translation Depending Upon Cell Context. *Mol Cell Biol*, Vol. 31, No. 12, (Jun 2011), pp. 2513-2527, ISSN 1098-5549

Lin, D. T., Subbaramaiah, K., Shah, J. P., Dannenberg, A. J., & Boyle, J. O. (2002). Cyclooxygenase-2: A Novel Molecular Target for the Prevention and Treatment of Head and Neck Cancer. *Head Neck*, Vol. 24, No. 8, (Aug 2002), pp. 792-799, ISSN 1043-3074

Liu, C. J., Kao, S. Y., Tu, H. F., Tsai, M. M., Chang, K. W., & Lin, S. C. (2010). Increase of MicroRNA Mir-31 Level in Plasma Could Be a Potential Marker of Oral Cancer. *Oral Dis*, Vol. 16, No. 4, (May 2010), pp. 360-364, ISSN 1601-0825

Liu, C. J., Tsai, M. M., Hung, P. S., Kao, S. Y., Liu, T. Y., Wu, K. J., Chiou, S. H., Lin, S. C., & Chang, K. W. (2010). Mir-31 Ablates Expression of the Hif Regulatory Factor Fih to Activate the Hif Pathway in Head and Neck Carcinoma. *Cancer Res*, Vol. 70, No. 4, (Feb 2010), pp. 1635-1644, ISSN 1538-7445

Liu, X., Jiang, L., Wang, A., Yu, J., Shi, F., & Zhou, X. (2009). MicroRNA-138 Suppresses Invasion and Promotes Apoptosis in Head and Neck Squamous Cell Carcinoma Cell Lines. *Cancer Lett*, Vol. 286, No. 2, (Dec 2009), pp. 217-222, ISSN 1872-7980

Llewellyn, C. D., Johnson, N. W., & Warnakulasuriya, S. (2004). Factors Associated with Delay in Presentation among Younger Patients with Oral Cancer. *Oral Surg Oral Med Oral Pathol Oral Radiol Endod*, Vol. 97, No. 6, (Jun 2004), pp. 707-713, ISSN 1079-2104

Llewellyn, C. D., Linklater, K., Bell, J., Johnson, N. W., & Warnakulasuriya, S. (2004). An Analysis of Risk Factors for Oral Cancer in Young People: A Case-Control Study. *Oral Oncol*, Vol. 40, No. 3, (Mar 2004), pp. 304-313, ISSN 1368-8375

Logullo, A. F., Nonogaki, S., Miguel, R. E., Kowalski, L. P., Nishimoto, I. N., Pasini, F. S., Federico, M. H., Brentani, R. R., & Brentani, M. M. (2003). Transforming Growth Factor Beta1 (Tgfbeta1) Expression in Head and Neck Squamous Cell Carcinoma Patients as Related to Prognosis. *J Oral Pathol Med*, Vol. 32, No. 3, (Mar 2003), pp. 139-145, ISSN 0904-2512

Long, X. B., Sun, G. B., Hu, S., Liang, G. T., Wang, N., Zhang, X. H., Cao, P. P., Zhen, H. T., Cui, Y. H., & Liu, Z. (2009). Let-7a MicroRNA Functions as a Potential Tumor Suppressor in Human Laryngeal Cancer. *Oncol Rep*, Vol. 22, No. 5, (Nov 2009), pp. 1189-1195, ISSN 1021-335X

Lopez, M., Aguirre, J. M., Cuevas, N., Anzola, M., Videgain, J., Aguirregaviria, J., & Martinez de Pancorbo, M. (2003). Gene Promoter Hypermethylation in Oral Rinses of Leukoplakia Patients-a Diagnostic and/or Prognostic Tool? *Eur J Cancer*, Vol. 39, No. 16, (Nov 2003), pp. 2306-2309, ISSN 0959-8049

Marsit, C. J., Black, C. C., Posner, M. R., & Kelsey, K. T. (2008). A Genotype-Phenotype Examination of Cyclin D1 on Risk and Outcome of Squamous Cell Carcinoma of the Head and Neck. *Clin Cancer Res*, Vol. 14, No. 8, (Apr 2008), pp. 2371-2377, ISSN 1078-0432

Marsit, C. J., Christensen, B. C., Houseman, E. A., Karagas, M. R., Wrensch, M. R., Yeh, R. F., Nelson, H. H., Wiemels, J. L., Zheng, S., Posner, M. R., McClean, M. D., Wiencke, J. K., & Kelsey, K. T. (2009). Epigenetic Profiling Reveals Etiologically Distinct Patterns of DNA Methylation in Head and Neck Squamous Cell Carcinoma. *Carcinogenesis*, Vol. 30, No. 3, (Mar 2009), pp. 416-422, ISSN 1460-2180

Marsit, C. J., McClean, M. D., Furniss, C. S., & Kelsey, K. T. (2006). Epigenetic Inactivation of the Sfrp Genes Is Associated with Drinking, Smoking and Hpv in Head and Neck Squamous Cell Carcinoma. *Int J Cancer*, Vol. 119, No. 8, (Oct 2006), pp. 1761-1766, ISSN 0020-7136

Matlashewski, G. J., Tuck, S., Pim, D., Lamb, P., Schneider, J., & Crawford, L. V. (1987). Primary Structure Polymorphism at Amino Acid Residue 72 of Human p53. *Mol Cell Biol*, Vol. 7, No. 2, (Feb 1987), pp. 961-963, ISSN 0270-7306

Mehlen, P., & Puisieux, A. (2006). Metastasis: A Question of Life or Death. *Nat Rev Cancer*, Vol. 6, No. 6, (Jun 2006), pp. 449-458, ISSN 1474-175X

Michalides, R. J., van Veelen, N. M., Kristel, P. M., Hart, A. A., Loftus, B. M., Hilgers, F. J., & Balm, A. J. (1997). Overexpression of Cyclin D1 Indicates a Poor Prognosis in Squamous Cell Carcinoma of the Head and Neck. *Arch Otolaryngol Head Neck Surg*, Vol. 123, No. 5, (May 1997), pp. 497-502, ISSN 0886-4470

Mineta, H., Miura, K., Ogino, T., Takebayashi, S., Misawa, K., Ueda, Y., Suzuki, I., Dictor, M., Borg, A., & Wennerberg, J. (2000). Prognostic Value of Vascular Endothelial Growth Factor (Vegf) in Head and Neck Squamous Cell Carcinomas. *Br J Cancer*, Vol. 83, No. 6, (Sep 2000), pp. 775-781, ISSN 0007-0920

Mineta, H., Miura, K., Takebayashi, S., Misawa, K., Ueda, Y., Suzuki, I., Ito, M., & Wennerberg, J. (2003). Low Expression of Fragile Histidine Triad Gene Correlates with High Proliferation in Head and Neck Squamous Cell Carcinoma. *Oral Oncol*, Vol. 39, No. 1, (Jan 2003), pp. 56-63, ISSN 1368-8375

Mithani, S. K., Mydlarz, W. K., Grumbine, F. L., Smith, I. M., & Califano, J. A. (2007). Molecular Genetics of Premalignant Oral Lesions. *Oral Dis*, Vol. 13, No. 2, (Mar 2007), pp. 126-133, ISSN 1354-523X

Mitra, S., Banerjee, S., Misra, C., Singh, R. K., Roy, A., Sengupta, A., Panda, C. K., & Roychoudhury, S. (2007). Interplay between Human Papilloma Virus Infection and p53 Gene Alterations in Head and Neck Squamous Cell Carcinoma of an Indian Patient Population. *J Clin Pathol*, Vol. 60, No. 9, (Sep 2007), pp. 1040-1047, ISSN 0021-9746

Moriyama, M., Kumagai, S., Kawashiri, S., Kojima, K., Kakihara, K., & Yamamoto, E. (1997). Immunohistochemical Study of Tumour Angiogenesis in Oral Squamous Cell Carcinoma. *Oral Oncol*, Vol. 33, No. 5, (Sep 1997), pp. 369-374, ISSN 1368-8375

Motokura, T., & Arnold, A. (1993). Cyclin D and Oncogenesis. *Curr Opin Genet Dev*, Vol. 3, No. 1, (Feb 1993), pp. 5-10, ISSN 0959-437X

Mriouah, J., Boura, C., Pinel, S., Chretien, A. S., Fifre, A., Merlin, J. L., & Faivre, B. (2010). Cellular Response to Cetuximab in PTEN-Silenced Head and Neck Squamous Cell Carcinoma Cell Line. *Int J Oncol*, Vol. 37, No. 6, (Dec 2010), pp. 1555-1563, ISSN 1791-2423

Namazie, A., Alavi, S., Olopade, O. I., Pauletti, G., Aghamohammadi, N., Aghamohammadi, M., Gornbein, J. A., Calcaterra, T. C., Slamon, D. J., Wang, M. B., & Srivatsan, E. S. (2002). Cyclin D1 Amplification and P16(Mts1/Cdk4i) Deletion Correlate with Poor Prognosis in Head and Neck Tumors. *Laryngoscope*, Vol. 112, No. 3, (Mar 2002), pp. 472-481, ISSN 0023-852X

Nana-Sinkam, S. P., & Croce, C. M. (2010). MicroRNA Dysregulation in Cancer: Opportunities for the Development of MicroRNA-Based Drugs. *IDrugs*, Vol. 13, No. 12, (Dec 2010), pp. 843-846, ISSN 2040-3410

Narayana, A., Vaughan, A. T., Gunaratne, S., Kathuria, S., Walter, S. A., & Reddy, S. P. (1998). Is p53 an Independent Prognostic Factor in Patients with Laryngeal Carcinoma? *Cancer*, Vol. 82, No. 2, (Jan 1998), pp. 286-291, ISSN 0008-543X

Nathan, C. O., Amirghahri, N., Rice, C., Abreo, F. W., Shi, R., &Stucker, F. J. (2002). Molecular Analysis of Surgical Margins in Head and Neck Squamous Cell Carcinoma Patients. *Laryngoscope*, Vol. 112, No. 12, (Dec 2002), pp. 2129-2140, ISSN 0023-852X

Nees, M., Homann, N., Discher, H., Andl, T., Enders, C., Herold-Mende, C., Schuhmann, A., & Bosch, F. X. (1993). Expression of Mutated p53 Occurs in Tumor-Distant Epithelia of Head and Neck Cancer Patients: A Possible Molecular Basis for the Development of Multiple Tumors. *Cancer Res*, Vol. 53, No. 18, (Sep 1993), pp. 4189-4196, ISSN 0008-5472

Negri, E., Boffetta, P., Berthiller, J., Castellsague, X., Curado, M. P., Dal Maso, L., Daudt, A. W., Fabianova, E., Fernandez, L., Wunsch-Filho, V., Franceschi, S., Hayes, R. B., Herrero, R., Koifman, S., Lazarus, P., Lence, J. J., Levi, F., Mates, D., Matos, E., Menezes, A., Muscat, J., Eluf-Neto, J., Olshan, A. F., Rudnai, P., Shangina, O., Sturgis, E. M., Szeszenia-Dabrowska, N., Talamini, R., Wei, Q., Winn, D. M., Zaridze, D., Lissowska, J., Zhang, Z. F., Ferro, G., Brennan, P., La Vecchia, C., & Hashibe, M. (2009). Family History of Cancer: Pooled Analysis in the International Head and Neck Cancer Epidemiology Consortium. *Int J Cancer*, Vol. 124, No. 2, (Jan 2009), pp. 394-401, ISSN 1097-0215

Neuchrist, C., Erovic, B. M., Handisurya, A., Fischer, M. B., Steiner, G. E., Hollemann, D., Gedlicka, C., Saaristo, A., & Burian, M. (2003). Vascular Endothelial Growth Factor C and Vascular Endothelial Growth Factor Receptor 3 Expression in Squamous Cell Carcinomas of the Head and Neck. *Head Neck*, Vol. 25, No. 6, (Jun 2003), pp. 464-474, ISSN 1043-3074

Neuchrist, C., Erovic, B. M., Handisurya, A., Steiner, G. E., Rockwell, P., Gedlicka, C., & Burian, M. (2001). Vascular Endothelial Growth Factor Receptor 2 (Vegfr2) Expression in Squamous Cell Carcinomas of the Head and Neck. *Laryngoscope*, Vol. 111, No. 10, (Oct 2001), pp. 1834-1841, ISSN 0023-852X

Nimeus, E., Baldetorp, B., Bendahl, P. O., Rennstam, K., Wennerberg, J., Akervall, J., & Ferno, M. (2004). Amplification of the Cyclin D1 Gene Is Associated with Tumour Subsite, DNA Non-Diploidy and High S-Phase Fraction in Squamous Cell

Carcinoma of the Head and Neck. *Oral Oncol*, Vol. 40, No. 6, (Jul 2004), pp. 624-629, ISSN 1368-8375

Nogueira, C. P., Dolan, R. W., Gooey, J., Byahatti, S., Vaughan, C. W., Fuleihan, N. S., Grillone, G., Baker, E., & Domanowski, G. (1998). Inactivation of p53 and Amplification of Cyclin D1 Correlate with Clinical Outcome in Head and Neck Cancer. *Laryngoscope*, Vol. 108, No. 3, (Mar 1998), pp. 345-350, ISSN 0023-852X

Nohata, N., Hanazawa, T., Kikkawa, N., Mutallip, M., Fujimura, L., Yoshino, H., Kawakami, K., Chiyomaru, T., Enokida, H., Nakagawa, M., Okamoto, Y., & Seki, N. (2011). Caveolin-1 Mediates Tumor Cell Migration and Invasion and Its Regulation by Mir-133a in Head and Neck Squamous Cell Carcinoma. *Int J Oncol*, Vol. 38, No. 1, (Jan 2011), pp. 209-217, ISSN 1791-2423

Nylander, K., Dabelsteen, E., & Hall, P. A. (2000). The p53 Molecule and Its Prognostic Role in Squamous Cell Carcinomas of the Head and Neck. *J Oral Pathol Med*, Vol. 29, No. 9, (Oct 2000), pp. 413-425, ISSN 0904-2512

Okami, K., Reed, A. L., Cairns, P., Koch, W. M., Westra, W. H., Wehage, S., Jen, J., & Sidransky, D. (1999). Cyclin D1 AmplificationIs Independent of P16 Inactivation in Head and Neck Squamous Cell Carcinoma. *Oncogene*, Vol. 18, No. 23, (Jun 1999), pp. 3541-3545, ISSN 0950-9232

Olivieri, E. H., da Silva, S. D., Mendonca, F. F., Urata, Y. N., Vidal, D. O., Faria Mde, A., Nishimoto, I. N., Rainho, C. A., Kowalski, L. P., & Rogatto, S. R. (2009). Cyp1a2*1c, Cyp2e1*5b, and Gstm1 Polymorphisms Are Predictors of Risk and Poor Outcome in Head and Neck Squamous Cell Carcinoma Patients. *Oral Oncol*, Vol. 45, No. 9, (Sep 2009), pp. e73-79, ISSN 1368-8375

Onesto, C., Hannoun-Levi, J. M., Chamorey, E., Formento, J. L., Ramaioli, A., & Pages, G. (2006). Vascular Endothelial Growth Factor-a and Poly(a) Binding Protein-Interacting Protein 2 Expression in Human Head and Neck Carcinomas: Correlation and Prognostic Significance. *Br J Cancer*, Vol. 94, No. 10, (May 2006), pp. 1516-1523, ISSN 0007-

Otero-Garcia, J. E., Youssef, E., Enamorado, II, Du, W., Yoo, G. H., Merati, K., Kewson, D., Lonardo, F., Jacobs, J. R., & Kim, H. (2004). Prognostic Significance of p53 and Fhit in Advanced Oropharyngeal Carcinoma. *Am J Otolaryngol*, Vol. 25, No. 4, (Jul-Aug 2004), pp. 231-239, ISSN 0196-0709

P, O. charoenrat, Modjtahedi, H., Rhys-Evans, P., Court, W. J., Box, G. M., &Eccles, S. A. (2000). Epidermal Growth Factor-Like Ligands Differentially up-Regulate Matrix Metalloproteinase 9 in Head and Neck Squamous Carcinoma Cells. *Cancer Res*, Vol. 60, No. 4, (Feb 2000), pp. 1121-1128, ISSN 0008-5472

Pai, S. I., & Westra, W. H. (2009). Molecular Pathology of Head and Neck Cancer: Implications for Diagnosis, Prognosis, and Treatment. *Annu Rev Pathol*, Vol. 4, No., (Aug 2009), pp. 49-70, ISSN 1553-4014

Park, N. J., Zhou, H., Elashoff, D., Henson, B. S., Kastratovic, D. A., Abemayor, E., & Wong, D. T. (2009). Salivary MicroRNA: Discovery, Characterization, and Clinical Utility for Oral Cancer Detection. *Clin Cancer Res*, Vol. 15, No. 17, (Sep 2009), pp. 5473-5477, ISSN 1078-0432

Partridge, M., Emilion, G., & Langdon, J. D. (1996). Loh at 3p Correlates with a Poor Survival in Oral Squamous Cell Carcinoma. *Br J Cancer*, Vol. 73, No. 3, (Feb 1996), pp. 366-371, ISSN 0007-0920

Patel, B. P., Shah, P. M., Rawal, U. M., Desai, A. A., Shah, S. V., Rawal, R. M., & Patel, P. S. (2005). Activation of Mmp-2 and Mmp-9 in Patients with Oral Squamous Cell Carcinoma. *J Surg Oncol*, Vol. 90, No. 2, (May 2005), pp. 81-88, ISSN 0022-4790

Pattje, W. J., Schuuring, E., Mastik, M. F., Slagter-Menkema, L., Schrijvers, M. L., Alessi, S., van der Laan, B. F., Roodenburg, J. L., Langendijk, J. A., & van der Wal, J. E. (2010). The Phosphatase and Tensin Homologue Deleted on Chromosome 10 Mediates Radiosensitivity in Head and Neck Cancer. *Br J Cancer*, Vol. 102, No. 12, (Jun 2010), pp. 1778-1785, ISSN 1532-1827

Pedrero, J. M., Carracedo, D. G., Pinto, C. M., Zapatero, A. H., Rodrigo, J. P., Nieto, C. S., & Gonzalez, M. V. (2005). Frequent Genetic and Biochemical Alterations of the Pi 3-K/Akt/Pten Pathway in Head and Neck Squamous Cell Carcinoma. *Int J Cancer*, Vol. 114, No. 2, (Mar 2005), pp. 242-248, ISSN 0020-7136

Perez-Ordonez, B., Beauchemin, M., & Jordan, R. C. (2006). Molecular Biology of Squamous Cell Carcinoma of the Head and Neck. *J Clin Pathol*, Vol. 59, No. 5, (May 2006), pp. 445-453, ISSN 0021-9746

Perrone, F., Bossi, P., Cortelazzi, B., Locati, L., Quattrone, P., Pierotti, M. A., Pilotti, S., & Licitra, L. (2010). TP53 Mutations and Pathologic Complete Response to Neoadjuvant Cisplatin and Fluorouracil Chemotherapy in Resected Oral Cavity Squamous Cell Carcinoma. *J Clin Oncol*, Vol. 28, No. 5, (Feb 2010), pp. 761-766, ISSN 1527-7755

Petrocca, F., Vecchione, A., & Croce, C. M. (2008). Emerging Role of Mir-106b-25/Mir-17-92 Clusters in the Control of Transforming Growth Factor Beta Signaling. *Cancer Res*, Vol. 68, No. 20, (Oct 2008), pp. 8191-8194, ISSN 1538-7445

Petruzzelli, G. J., Benefield, J., Taitz, A. D., Fowler, S., Kalkanis, J., Scobercea, S., West, D., & Young, M. R. (1997). Heparin-Binding Growth Factor(S) Derived from Head and Neck Squamous Cell Carcinomas Induce Endothelial Cell Proliferations. *Head Neck*, Vol. 19, No. 7, (Oct 1997), pp. 576-582, ISSN 1043-3074

Poeta, M. L., Manola, J., Goldwasser, M. A., Forastiere, A., Benoit, N., Califano, J. A., Ridge, J. A., Goodwin, J., Kenady, D., Saunders, J., Westra, W., Sidransky, D., & Koch, W. M. (2007). TP53 Mutations and Survival in Squamous-Cell Carcinoma of the Head and Neck. *N Engl J Med*, Vol. 357, No. 25, (Dec 2007), pp. 2552-2561, ISSN 1533-4406

Pyeon, D., Newton, M. A., Lambert, P. F., den Boon, J. A., Sengupta, S., Marsit, C. J., Woodworth, C. D., Connor, J. P., Haugen, T. H., Smith, E. M., Kelsey, K. T., Turek, L. P., & Ahlquist, P. (2007). Fundamental Differences in Cell Cycle Deregulation in Human Papillomavirus-Positive and Human Papillomavirus-Negative Head/Neck and Cervical Cancers. *Cancer Res*, Vol. 67, No. 10, (May 2007), pp. 4605-4619, ISSN 0008-5472

Queiroz, A. B., Focchi, G., Dobo, C., Gomes, T. S., Ribeiro, D. A., & Oshima, C. T. (2010). Expression of P27, P21(Waf/Cip1), and P16(Ink4a) in Normal Oral Epithelium, Oral Squamous Papilloma, and Oral Squamous Cell Carcinoma. *Anticancer Res*, Vol. 30, No. 7, (Jul 2010), pp. 2799-2803, ISSN 1791-7530

Quon, H., Liu, F. F., & Cummings, B. J. (2001). Potential Molecular Prognostic Markers in Head and Neck Squamous Cell Carcinomas. *Head Neck*, Vol. 23, No. 2, (Feb 2001), pp. 147-159, ISSN 1043-3074

Ragin, C. C., Modugno, F., & Gollin, S. M. (2007). The Epidemiology and Risk Factors of Head and Neck Cancer: A Focus on Human Papillomavirus. *J Dent Res*, Vol. 86, No. 2, (Feb 2007), pp. 104-114, ISSN 0022-0345

Ramdas, L., Giri, U., Ashorn, C. L., Coombes, K. R., El-Naggar, A., Ang, K. K., & Story, M. D. (2009). MiRNA ExpressionProfiles in Head and Neck Squamous Cell Carcinoma and Adjacent Normal Tissue. *Head Neck*, Vol. 31, No. 5, (May 2009), pp. 642-654, ISSN 1097-0347

Ranelletti, F. O., Almadori, G., Rocca, B., Ferrandina, G., Ciabattoni, G., Habib, A., Galli, J., Maggiano, N., Gessi, M., & Lauriola, L. (2001). Prognostic Significance of Cyclooxygenase-2 in Laryngeal Squamous Cell Carcinoma. *Int J Cancer*, Vol. 95, No. 6, (Nov 2001), pp. 343-349, ISSN 0020-7136

Reed, A. L., Califano, J., Cairns, P., Westra, W. H., Jones, R. M., Koch, W., Ahrendt, S., Eby, Y., Sewell, D., Nawroz, H., Bartek, J., & Sidransky, D. (1996). High Frequency of P16 (Cdkn2/Mts-1/Ink4a) Inactivation in Head and Neck Squamous Cell Carcinoma. *Cancer Res*, Vol. 56, No. 16, (Aug 1996), pp. 3630-3633, ISSN 0008-5472

Richards, K. L., Zhang, B., Baggerly, K. A., Colella, S., Lang, J. C., Schuller, D. E., & Krahe, R. (2009). Genome-Wide Hypomethylation in Head and Neck Cancer Is More Pronounced in Hpv-Negative Tumors and Is Associated with Genomic Instability. *PLoS One*, Vol. 4, No. 3, (Mar 2009), pp. e4941, ISSN 1932-6203

Ronchetti, D., Neglia, C. B., Cesana, B. M., Carboni, N., Neri, A., Pruneri, G., & Pignataro, L. (2004). Association between p53 Gene Mutations and Tobacco and Alcohol Exposure in Laryngeal Squamous Cell Carcinoma. *Arch Otolaryngol Head Neck Surg*, Vol. 130, No. 3, (Mar 2004), pp. 303-306, ISSN 0886-4470

Rosenquist, K., Wennerberg, J., Annertz, K., Schildt, E. B., Hansson, B. G., Bladstrom, A., & Andersson, G. (2007). Recurrence in Patients with Oral and Oropharyngeal Squamous Cell Carcinoma: Human Papillomavirus and Other Risk Factors. *Acta Otolaryngol*, Vol. 127, No. 9, (Sep 2007), pp. 980-987, ISSN 0001-6489

Rosin, M. P., Cheng, X., Poh, C., Lam, W. L., Huang, Y., Lovas, J., Berean, K., Epstein, J. B., Priddy, R., Le, N. D., & Zhang, L. (2000). Use of Allelic Loss to Predict Malignant Risk for Low-Grade Oral Epithelial Dysplasia. *Clin Cancer Res*, Vol. 6, No. 2, (Feb 2000), pp. 357-362, ISSN 1078-

Rubin Grandis, J., Tweardy, D. J., & Melhem, M. F. (1998). Asynchronous Modulation of Transforming Growth Factor Alpha and Epidermal Growth Factor Receptor Protein Expression in Progression of Premalignant Lesions to Head and Neck Squamous Cell Carcinoma. *Clin Cancer Res*, Vol. 4, No. 1, (Jan 1998), pp. 13-20, ISSN 1078-0432

Sanchez-Cespedes, M., Parrella, P., Nomoto, S., Cohen, D., Xiao, Y., Esteller, M., Jeronimo, C., Jordan, R. C., Nicol, T., Koch, W. M., Schoenberg, M., Mazzarelli, P., Fazio, V. M., & Sidransky, D. (2001). Identification of a Mononucleotide Repeat as a Major Target for Mitochondrial DNA Alterations in Human Tumors. *Cancer Res*, Vol. 61, No. 19, (Oct 2001), pp. 7015-7019, ISSN 0008-5472

Saunders, M. E., MacKenzie, R., Shipman, R., Fransen, E., Gilbert, R., & Jordan, R. C. (1999). Patterns of p53 Gene Mutations in Head and Neck Cancer: Full-Length Gene Sequencing and Results of Primary Radiotherapy. *Clin Cancer Res*, Vol. 5, No. 9, (Sep 1999), pp. 2455-2463, ISSN 1078-0432

Schlecht, N. F., Franco, E. L., Pintos, J., & Kowalski, L. P. (1999). Effect of Smoking Cessation and Tobacco Type on the Risk of Cancers of the Upper Aero-Digestive Tract in Brazil. *Epidemiology*, Vol. 10, No. 4, (Jul 1999), pp. 412-418, ISSN 1044-3983

Shahnavaz, S. A., Regezi, J. A., Bradley, G., Dube, I. D., & Jordan, R. C. (2000). p53 Gene Mutations in Sequential Oral Epithelial Dysplasias and Squamous Cell Carcinomas. *J Pathol*, Vol. 190, No. 4, (Mar 2000), pp. 417-422, ISSN 0022-3417

Shiiba, M., Uzawa, K., & Tanzawa, H. (2010). MicroRNAs in Head and Neck Squamous Cell Carcinoma (HNSCC) and Oral Squamous Cell Carcinoma (OSCC). *Cancers*, Vol. 2 , No. 2, (Apr 2010), pp. 653-669, ISSN 2072-6694

Shin, D. M., Mao, L., Papadimitrakopoulou, V. M., Clayman, G., El-Naggar, A., Shin, H. J., Lee, J. J., Lee, J. S., Gillenwater, A., Myers, J., Lippman, S. M., Hittelman, W. N., & Hong, W. K. (2000). Biochemo preventive Therapy for Patients with Premalignant Lesions of the Head and Neck and p53 Gene Expression. *J Natl Cancer Inst*, Vol. 92, No. 1, (Jan 2000), pp. 69-73, ISSN 0027-8874

Sidransky, D. (1997). Nucleic Acid-Based Methods for the Detection of Cancer. *Science*, Vol. 278, No. 5340, (Nov 1997), pp. 1054-1059, ISSN 0036-8075

Sinpitaksakul, S. N., Pimkhaokham, A., Sanchavanakit, N., & Pavasant, P. (2008). Tgf-Beta1 Induced Mmp-9 Expression in HNSCC Cell Lines Via Smad/Mlck Pathway. *Biochem Biophys Res Commun*, Vol. 371, No. 4, (Jul 2008), pp. 713-718, ISSN 1090-2104

Smilek, P., Dusek, L., Vesely, K., Rottenberg, J., & Kostrica, R. (2006). Correlation of Expression of Ki-67, Egfr, C-Erbb-2, Mmp-9, p53, Bcl-2, Cd34 and Cell Cycle Analysis with Survival in Head and Neck Squamous Cell Cancer. *J ExpClin Cancer Res*, Vol. 25, No. 4, (Dec 2006), pp. 549-555, ISSN 0392-9078

Smith, E. M., Ritchie, J. M., Summersgill, K. F., Klussmann, J. P., Lee, J. H., Wang, D., Haugen, T. H., & Turek, L. P. (2004). Age, Sexual Behavior and Human Papillomavirus Infection in Oral Cavity and Oropharyngeal Cancers. *Int J Cancer*, Vol. 108, No. 5, (Feb 2004), pp. 766-772, ISSN 0020-7136

Smith, E. M., Rubenstein, L. M., Hoffman, H., Haugen, T. H., & Turek, L. P. (2010). Human Papillomavirus, P16 and p53 Expression Associated with Survival of Head and Neck Cancer. *Infect Agent Cancer*, Vol. 5, No., (Feb 2010), pp. 4-13, ISSN 1750-9378

Snyder, M. B., Stacey, A. J., Davis, R., Cawson, R. A., & Binnie, W. H. (1977). The Advantages of Xeroradiography for Panoramic Examination of the Jaws and Teeth. *J Periodontol*, Vol. 48, No. 8, (Aug 1977), pp. 467-472, ISSN 0022-3492

Steinmann, K., Sandner, A., Schagdarsurengin, U., & Dammann, R. H. (2009). Frequent Promoter Hypermethylation of Tumor-Related Genes in Head and Neck Squamous Cell Carcinoma. *Oncol Rep*, Vol. 22, No. 6, (Dec 2009), pp. 1519-1526, ISSN 1791-2431

Stetler-Stevenson, W. G., Liotta, L. A., & Kleiner, D. E., Jr. (1993). Extracellular Matrix 6: Role of Matrix Metalloproteinases in Tumor Invasion and Metastasis. *FASEB J*, Vol. 7, No. 15, (Dec 1993), pp. 1434-1441, ISSN 0892-6638

Storey, A., Thomas, M., Kalita, A., Harwood, C., Gardiol, D., Mantovani, F., Breuer, J., Leigh, I. M., Matlashewski, G., & Banks, L. (1998). Role of a p53 Polymorphism in the Development of Human Papillomavirus-Associated Cancer. *Nature*, Vol. 393, No. 6682, (May 1998), pp. 229-234, ISSN 0028-0836

Strano, S., Dell'Orso, S., Di Agostino, S., Fontemaggi, G., Sacchi, A., & Blandino, G. (2007). Mutant p53: An Oncogenic Transcription Factor. *Oncogene*, Vol. 26, No. 15, (Apr 2007), pp. 2212-2219, ISSN 0950-9232

Strano, S., Dell'Orso, S., Mongiovi, A. M., Monti, O., Lapi, E., Di Agostino, S., Fontemaggi, G., & Blandino, G. (2007). Mutant p53 Proteins: Between Loss and Gain of Function. *Head Neck*, Vol. 29, No. 5, (May 2007), pp. 488-496, ISSN 1043-3074

Sturgis, E. M., Sacks, P. G., Masui, H., Mendelsohn, J., & Schantz, S. P. (1994). Effects of Antiepidermal Growth Factor Receptor Antibody 528 on the Proliferation and Differentiation of Head and Neck Cancer. *Otolaryngol Head Neck Surg*, Vol. 111, No. 5, (Nov 1994), pp. 633-643, ISSN 0194-5998

Sturgis, E. M., Wei, Q., & Spitz, M. R. (2004). Descriptive Epidemiology and Risk Factors for Head and Neck Cancer. *Semin Oncol*, Vol. 31, No. 6, (Dec 2004), pp. 726-733, ISSN 0093-7754

Sudbo, J., Ristimaki, A., Sondresen, J. E., Kildal, W., Boysen, M., Koppang, H. S., Reith, A., Risberg, B., Nesland, J. M., &Bryne, M. (2003). Cyclooxygenase-2 (Cox-2) Expression in High-Risk Premalignant Oral Lesions. *Oral Oncol*, Vol. 39, No. 5, (Jul 2003), pp. 497-505, ISSN 1368-8375

Tai, S. K., Lee, J. I., Ang, K. K., El-Naggar, A. K., Hassan, K. A., Liu, D., Lee, J. J., Ren, H., Hong, W. K., & Mao, L. (2004). Loss of Fhit Expression in Head and Neck Squamous Cell Carcinoma and Its Potential Clinical Implication. *Clin Cancer Res*, Vol. 10, No. 16, (Aug 2004), pp. 5554-5557, ISSN 1078-0432

Talamini, R., Bosetti, C., La Vecchia, C., Dal Maso, L., Levi, F., Bidoli, E., Negri, E., Pasche, C., Vaccarella, S., Barzan, L., & Franceschi, S. (2002). Combined Effect of Tobacco and Alcohol on Laryngeal Cancer Risk: A Case-Control Study. *Cancer Causes Control*, Vol. 13, No. 10, (Dec 2002), pp. 957-964, ISSN 0957-5243

Tanigaki, Y., Nagashima, Y., Kitamura, Y., Matsuda, H., Mikami, Y., & Tsukuda, M. (2004). The Expression of Vascular Endothelial Growth Factor-a and -C, and Receptors 1 and 3: Correlation with Lymph Node Metastasis and Prognosis in Tongue Squamous Cell Carcinoma. *Int J Mol Med*, Vol. 14, No. 3, (Sep 2004), pp. 389-395, ISSN 1107-3756

Teknos, T. N., Cox, C., Yoo, S., Chepeha, D. B., Wolf, G. T., Bradford, C. R., Carey, T. E., & Fisher, S. G. (2002). Elevated Serum Vascular Endothelial Growth Factor and Decreased Survival in Advanced Laryngeal Carcinoma. *Head Neck*, Vol. 24, No. 11, (Nov 2002), pp. 1004-1011, ISSN 1043-3074

Temam, S., Flahault, A., Perie, S., Monceaux, G., Coulet, F., Callard, P., Bernaudin, J. F., St Guily, J. L., & Fouret, P. (2000). p53 Gene Status as a Predictor of Tumor Response to Induction Chemotherapy of Patients with Locoregionally Advanced Squamous Cell Carcinomas of the Head and Neck. *J Clin Oncol*, Vol. 18, No. 2, (Jan 2000), pp. 385-394, ISSN 0732-183X

Thier, R., Bruning, T., Roos, P. H., & Bolt, H. M. (2002). Cytochrome P450 1b1, a New Keystone in Gene-Environment Interactions Related to Human Head and Neck Cancer? *Arch Toxicol*, Vol. 76, No. 5-6, (Jun 2002), pp. 249-256, ISSN 0340-5761

Thomas, G. R., Nadiminti, H., & Regalado, J. (2005). Molecular Predictors of Clinical Outcome in Patients with Head and Neck Squamous Cell Carcinoma. *Int J Exp Pathol*, Vol. 86, No. 6, (Dec 2005), pp. 347-363, ISSN 0959-9673

Tran, N., McLean, T., Zhang, X., Zhao, C. J., Thomson, J. M., O'Brien, C., & Rose, B. (2007). MicroRNA Expression Profiles in Head and Neck Cancer Cell Lines. *Biochem Biophys Res Commun*, Vol. 358, No. 1, (Jun 2007), pp. 12-17, ISSN 0006-291X

Tsujii, M., & DuBois, R. N. (1995). Alterations in Cellular Adhesion and Apoptosis in Epithelial Cells Overexpressing Prostaglandin Endoperoxide Synthase 2. *Cell*, Vol. 83, No. 3, (Nov 1995), pp. 493-501, ISSN 0092-8674

Uribe, P., & Gonzalez, S. (2011). Epidermal Growth Factor Receptor (Egfr) and Squamous Cell Carcinoma of the Skin: Molecular Bases for Egfr-Targeted Therapy. *Pathol Res Pract*, Vol. 207, No. 6, (Jun 15 2011), pp. 337-342, ISSN 1618-0631

Vachani, A., Nebozhyn, M., Singhal, S., Alila, L., Wakeam, E., Muschel, R., Powell, C. A., Gaffney, P., Singh, B., Brose, M. S., Litzky, L. A., Kucharczuk, J., Kaiser, L. R., Marron, J. S., Showe, M. K., Albelda, S. M., & Showe, L. C. (2007). A 10-Gene Classifier for Distinguishing Head and Neck Squamous Cell Carcinoma and Lung Squamous Cell Carcinoma. *Clin Cancer Res*, Vol. 13, No. 10, (May 2007), pp. 2905-2915, ISSN 1078-0432

Van Den Broek, G. B., Wildeman, M., Rasch, C. R., Armstrong, N., Schuuring, E., Begg, A. C., Looijenga, L. H., Scheper, R., van der Wal, J. E., Menkema, L., van Diest, P. J., Balm, A. J., van Velthuysen, M. L., & Van den Brekel, M. W. (2009). Molecular Markers Predict Outcome in Squamous Cell Carcinoma of the Head and Neck after Concomitant Cisplatin-Based Chemoradiation. *Int J Cancer*, Vol. 124, No. 11, (Jun 2009), pp. 2643-2650, ISSN 1097-0215

Varley, K. E., Mutch, D. G., Edmonston, T. B., Goodfellow, P. J., & Mitra, R. D. (2009). Intra-Tumor Heterogeneity of Mlh1 Promoter Methylation Revealed by Deep Single Molecule Bisulfite Sequencing. *Nucleic Acids Res*, Vol. 37, No. 14, (Aug 2009), pp. 4603-4612, ISSN 1362-4962

Vielba, R., Bilbao, J., Ispizua, A., Zabalza, I., Alfaro, J., Rezola, R., Moreno, E., Elorriaga, J., Alonso, I., Baroja, A., & De La Hoz, C. (2003). p53 and Cyclin D1 as Prognostic Factors in Squamous Cell Carcinoma of the Larynx. *Laryngoscope*, Vol. 113, No. 1, (Jan 2003), pp. 167-172, ISSN 0023-852X

Volavsek, M., Bracko, M., & Gale, N. (2003). Distribution and Prognostic Significance of Cell Cycle Proteins in Squamous Carcinoma of the Larynx, Hypopharynx and Adjacent Epithelial Hyperplastic Lesions. *J Laryngol Otol*, Vol. 117, No. 4, (Apr 2003), pp. 286-293, ISSN 0022-2151

Wang, X., Fan, M., Chen, X., Wang, S., Alsharif, M. J., Wang, L., Liu, L., & Deng, H. (2006). Intratumor Genomic Heterogeneity Correlates with Histological Grade of Advanced Oral Squamous Cell Carcinoma. *Oral Oncol*, Vol. 42, No. 7, (Aug 2006), pp. 740-744, ISSN 1368-8375

Werbrouck, J., De Ruyck, K., Duprez, F., Van Eijkeren, M., Rietzschel, E., Bekaert, S., Vral, A., De Neve, W., & Thierens, H. (2008). Single-Nucleotide Polymorphisms in DNA Double-Strand Break Repair Genes: Association with Head and Neck Cancer and Interaction with Tobacco Use and Alcohol Consumption. *Mutat Res*, Vol. 656, No. 1-2, (Oct 2008), pp. 74-81, ISSN 0027-5107

White, R. A., Malkoski, S. P., & Wang, X. J. (2010). Tgf beta Signaling in Head and Neck Squamous Cell Carcinoma. *Oncogene*, Vol. 29, No. 40, (Oct 2010), pp. 5437-5446, ISSN 1476-5594

Wilken, R., Veena, M. S., Wang, M. B., & Srivatsan, E. S. (2011). Curcumin: A Review of Anti-Cancer Properties and Therapeutic Activity in Head and Neck Squamous Cell Carcinoma. *Mol Cancer*, Vol. 10, No., (Feb 2011), pp. 12-31, ISSN 1476-4598

Wong, R. H., Du, C. L., Wang, J. D., Chan, C. C., Luo, J. C., & Cheng, T. J. (2002). Xrcc1 and Cyp2e1 Polymorphisms as Susceptibility Factors of Plasma Mutant p53 Protein and Anti-P53 Antibody Expression in Vinyl Chloride Monomer-Exposed Polyvinyl Chloride Workers. *Cancer Epidemiol Biomarkers Prev*, Vol. 11, No. 5, (May 2002), pp. 475-482, ISSN 1055-9965

Wong, T. S., Ho, W. K., Chan, J. Y., Ng, R. W., & Wei, W. I. (2009). Mature Mir-184 and Squamous Cell Carcinoma of the Tongue. *Scientific World Journal*, Vol. 9, No., (Feb 2009), pp. 130-132, ISSN 1537-744X

Wong, T. S., Liu, X. B., Chung-Wai Ho, A., Po-Wing Yuen, A., Wai-Man Ng, R., & Ignace Wei, W. (2008). Identification of Pyruvate Kinase Type M2 as Potential Oncoprotein in Squamous Cell Carcinoma of Tongue through MicroRNA Profiling. *Int J Cancer*, Vol. 123, No. 2, (Jul 2008), pp. 251-257, ISSN 1097-0215

Wong, T. S., Liu, X. B., Wong, B. Y., Ng, R. W., Yuen, A. P., & Wei, W. I. (2008). Mature Mir-184 asPotential Oncogenic MicroRNA of Squamous Cell Carcinoma of Tongue. *Clin Cancer Res*, Vol. 14, No. 9, (May 2008), pp. 2588-2592, ISSN 1078-0432

Wreesmann, V. B., & Singh, B. (2005). Chromosomal Aberrations in Squamous Cell Carcinomas of the Upper Aerodigestive Tract: Biologic Insights and Clinical Opportunities. *J Oral Pathol Med*, Vol. 34, No. 8, (Sep 2005), pp. 449-459, ISSN 0904-2512

Yin, X. Y., Smith, M. L., Whiteside, T. L., Johnson, J. T., Herberman, R. B., & Locker, J. (1993). Abnormalities in the p53 Gene in Tumors and Cell Lines of Human Squamous-Cell Carcinomas of the Head and Neck. *Int J Cancer*, Vol. 54, No. 2, (May 1993), pp. 322-327, ISSN 0020-7136

Youssef, E. M., Lotan, D., Issa, J. P., Wakasa, K., Fan, Y. H., Mao, L., Hassan, K., Feng, L., Lee, J. J., Lippman, S. M., Hong, W. K., & Lotan, R. (2004). Hypermethylation of the Retinoic Acid Receptor-Beta(2) Gene in Head and Neck Carcinogenesis. *Clin Cancer Res*, Vol. 10, No. 5, (Mar 2004), pp. 1733-1742, ISSN 1078-0432

Yuen, P. W., Man, M., Lam, K. Y., & Kwong, Y. L. (2002). Clinicopathological Significance of P16 Gene Expression in the Surgical Treatment of Head and Neck Squamous Cell Carcinomas. *J Clin Pathol*, Vol. 55, No. 1, (Jan 2002), pp. 58-60, ISSN 0021-9746

Zhang, Z. F., Morgenstern, H., Spitz, M. R., Tashkin, D. P., Yu, G. P., Hsu, T. C., & Schantz, S. P. (2000). Environmental Tobacco Smoking, Mutagen Sensitivity, and Head and Neck Squamous Cell Carcinoma. *Cancer Epidemiol Biomarkers Prev*, Vol. 9, No. 10, (Oct 2000), pp. 1043-1049, ISSN 1055-9965

Zidar, N., Bostjancic, E., Gale, N., Kojc, N., Poljak, M., Glavac, D., & Cardesa, A. (2011). Down-Regulation of MicroRNAs of the Mir-200 Family and Mir-205, and an Altered Expression of Classic and Desmosomal Cadherins in Spindle Cell Carcinoma of the Head and Neck--Hallmark of Epithelial-Mesenchymal Transition. *Hum Pathol*, Vol. 42, No. 4, (Apr 2011), pp. 482-488, ISSN 1532-8392

4

Role of ING Family Genes in Head and Neck Cancer and Their Possible Applications in Cancer Diagnosis and Treatment

Esra Gunduz[1], Mehmet Gunduz[1,2,3,*], Levent Beder[3],
Ramazan Yigitoglu[4], Bunyamin Isik[5] and Noboru Yamanaka[3]
[1]Departments of Medical Genetics,
[2]Otolaryngology Head and Neck Surgery,
[3]Department of Otolaryngology Head and Neck Surgery,
Faculty of Medicine, Wakayama Medical University, Wakayama,
[4]Medical Biochemistry,
[5]Family Medicine, Faculty of Medicine, Fatih University, Ankara,
[1,2,4,5]Turkey
[3]Japan

1. Introduction

Cancer is one of the most common diseases, which treat human life. It produces huge psychological, economical and social burdens. Enormous preventive, diagnostic and therapeutic research efforts have been done to eradicate this deadly disease. Though some success have been obtained in terms of disease control for some of the neoplasms such as some of the lymphoma types, thyroid cancer and for some of the other solid tumors such as breast cancer in case of early detection, most still are left as a deadly disease. On the other hand current treatment modalities including surgery or/and chemoradiotherapy bring a huge hand local damage to the tissues and thus decrease the quality of life yet most shows recurrence and metastasis, which also questions the efficiency of these treatments.

Head and neck squamous cell carcinoma (HNSCC) is one of the most frequent cancers that lead to death, making it a major health problem in the world. HNSCC includes oral, oro/nasopharyngeal and laryngeal cancers and accounts for more than 644,000 new cases worldwide, with a mortality of 0.53 and a male predominance of 3:1 [1,2]. Despite advanced technology in the detection and treatment of HNSCC, it continues to pose a great threat for human life. Most patients suffering from this malignancy are at an advanced stage upon diagnosis in which 51% present regional metastasis and 10% with distant metastasis. The 5-year relative survival rate with regional metastasis is about 51% and with distant metastases is 28% [1,3].

Though much development has been obtained in surgical techniques, chemoradiation protocols, little progress was shown in terms of long-term survivals during several decades.

* Corresponding Author

Moreover, surgery now one of the main therapeutic options in these cancers gives rise to extensive local damage. Many patients lose partially or completely the organs in head and neck area, which have important functions such as speaking, eating, swallowing and respiration. Thus these patients finally fall into huge psychological and functional burden. On the other hand, last 2-3 decades provided great developments and progress in human genome technology, which warranted development novel diagnostic and therapeutic methods, which are finally supposed to be more effective and to preserve functional properties.

As for most cancer types, head and neck cancer is basically a genetic associated disease. Cumulative alterations of various genes are responsible for development of this cancer type. Environmental and personal factors such as smoking, drinking, dirty air, exposure to carcinogenic chemicals through working environment or foods finally influence on genes. These affected genes are altered either as genetically or epigenetically and mutated nonfunctional or deficient products then result in cancer development.

Our current knowledge on human genome showed that two major groups of tumor-associated genes, oncogenes and tumor suppressor genes (TSG) have been implicated in the carcinogenic process (**Figure 1**). In normal cell, a critical balance between TSG and oncogenes is necessary for physiological survival of the cell. In normal cell, product of oncogene is needed for its proliferation, survival and growth. On the other hand, TSG is necessary for balancing and suppressing excessive growth of the cell and entering into carcinogenic process. Most oncogenes are growth factors or their receptors, as well as various molecules of signaling pathways, proapoptotic genes, cell cycle proteins and transcription factors. These proteins finally induce cell cycle, proliferation and growth. As same for most genes, oncogenes have two alleles in nuclear genome. Role of oncogenes in human cancer is mediated through enforcement of protein function upon activated mutation of one of the alleles in its genomic location. The rest allele is usually not affected and final output is more cell proliferation, growth and cancer when other factors such inactivation of tumor suppressors, inability of immunological as well as apoptotic mechanisms are added.

On the other hand, tumor suppressors have been defined as genetic elements whose inactivation allows cell to display one or more phenotypes of neoplastic growth [4]. Products of TSG usually include inhibitors of cell cycle, chromatin remodeling factors, anti-apoptotic genes and some genes regulating gene expression at genetic and epigenetic levels. Similar to oncogenes, TSG also consist of two copies at their chromosomal loci. Inactivation of TSG leads to carcinogenic process. Until recently, Knudson two-hit hypothesis has been known as an explanation of inactivation of TSG during carcinogenesis [5]. According to this hypothesis, one of the alleles of a TSG is lost through carcinogenic effect, while the rest allele is usually inactivated through mutation of the gene (**Figure 2**). However, a novel class of TSG with haploid insufficiency, in which one allele is lost and the remaining allele is haplo-insufficient, has been described recently, and the patients with these hemizygous TSG in their genome are accepted as carriers for deficient allele of a TSG and they show a tumor-prone phenotype especially when challenged with carcinogens such as smoking, alcohol, x-ray, chemicals etc (Class II TSG) [6-10].

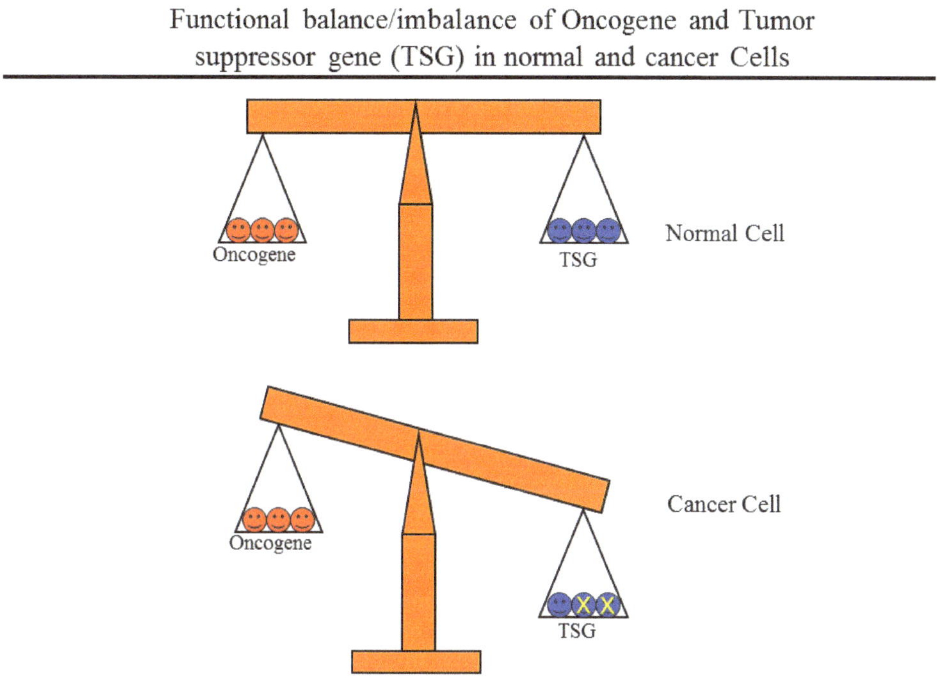

Fig. 1. Schematic representation of two major groups of genes on cell growth and cancer development.

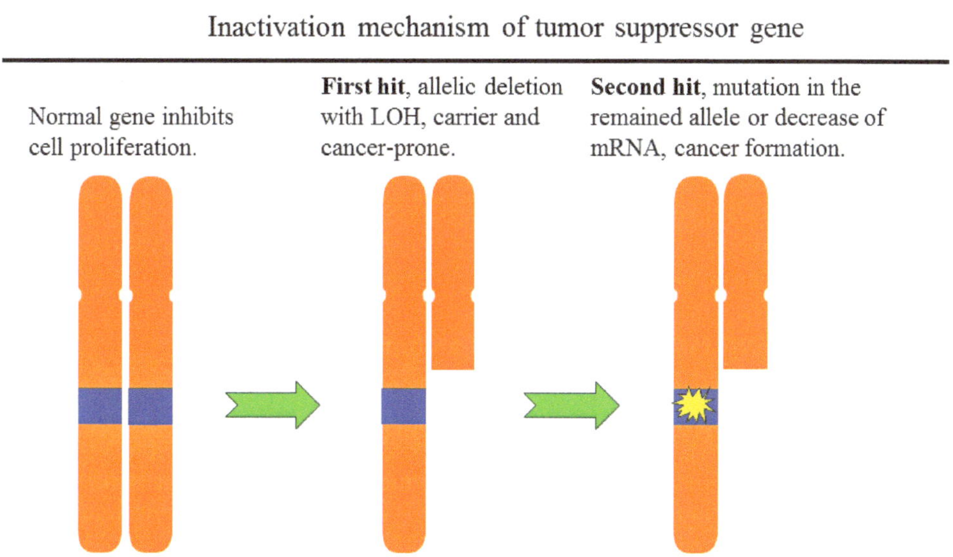

Fig. 2. Schematic representation of two-hit mechanism for inactivation of tumor suppressor gene

In the current review, we will focus on a recently identified TSG group, ING family tumor suppressors. Thus this review will mainly include alterations of ING family tumor suppressor in human cancer and their possible applications in molecular diagnosis and therapy of cancer. The five members of the ING family were recently identified by our group and other researchers in the field [11-17]. All proteins of ING family genes contain a highly conserved plant homeodomain (PHD) finger motif in the carboxy (C)-terminal end that is commonly detected in various chromatin remodeling proteins [18,19]. The N-terminal part of each ING protein seems to be unique, which determines the structure and different functions of various ING genes [11,12,16]. Although exact functions of ING family genes have not been clarified, the gene products have been reported to be involved in transcriptional regulation, apoptosis, cell cycle, angiogenesis and DNA repair through p53-dependent and -independent pathways. Moreover, ING family genes have also been known to constitute complexes with histone acetyltransferases (HAT) and histone deacetylases (HDAC) [11, 12, 16,20].

Within the members, ING1 is the founding member and thus most information about the family genes comes from the researches on ING1. ING1 was first isolated using subtractive hybridization between short segments of cDNAs from normal and a number of breast cancer cell lines [21]. These randomly fragmented cDNAs interfered with the activity of tumor suppressors by either blocking protein production through anti-sense sequences or abrogating function in a dominant-negative fashion through truncated sense fragments [21]. The other four members of ING gene family have been identified through sequence homologies with ING1, followed by functional in-vitro and then in-vivo cancer patient tissue analysis [11,12,19,22,23].

We characterized the genomic structure of ING1 gene and showed that ING1 gene produced at least 4 mRNA variants from 3 different promoters for the first time. Two of these variants, p33ING1b consisting of exons 1a and 2, and p24ING1c consisting of a truncated p47ING1a message including the first ATG codon in exon 2, are expressed majorly, while p47ING1a consisting exon 1b and exon 2, was not detected in head and neck tissues [13]. Our continuous efforts led to identification of ING3 [14]. Following these works, other groups and our group published investigations on other members of ING family including ING2, ING4 and ING5 [15,16,24-32]. Although almost all of the ING family members are known to be negative regulator of the cell growth, recent studies also demonstrated some of the members or splicing variants also functioning as oncogene, thus complicating the role of these genes in human carcinogenesis [31,32].

2. Disorders of ING family genes in human tumors

Rearrangement of ING1 gene locus was demonstrated in one neuroblastoma cell line and reduced expression in primary cancers and cell lines in early clinical studies at the time of ING1 cloning [11-17,21]. Following ING1 cDNA cloning, we identified the genomic structure of the human ING1 gene and showed its tumor suppressor character for the first time by finding its chromosomal deletion at the 13q34 locus and tumor-specific mutations in a number of head and neck squamous cell carcinoma (HNSCC) samples [13].

Regarding with the mRNA expression status of ING family genes, only a few studies exist in the literature. Toyama et al. detected 2–10-fold decreases in ING1 mRNA expression in 44%

of breast cancer and in all of 10 breast cancer cell lines examined [33]. Interestingly, the majority of breast cancers showing decreased ING1 expression had metastasized to regional lymph nodes, whereas only a small subset of cancers with elevated ING1 expression compared to adjacent normal tissues were metastatic. Another study also revealed reduced expression of breast cancer samples [34]. Down-regulation of ING1 mRNA has also been demonstrated in various other cancer types, including lymphoid malignancies, gastric tumors, brain tumors, lung cancer, ovarian cancer and esophagogastric carcinomas, though no comprehensive clinical correlation was performed [11,12,17,20,35-43]. Uncommon missense mutations and reduced protein expression of ING1 have also been detected in esophageal carcinomas [44], and colon cancer cell lines [36] while no mutation was detected in leukemia [37,45], oral cancers [46] and lymphoid malignancies [35].

For loss of ING gene and their protein functions, loss of heterozygosity (LOH), promoter CpG hypermetylation and nucleo-cytoplasmic protein mislocalization have been proposed [11,12,17,20]. Using methylation-specific PCR, the p33ING1b promoter was methylated and silenced in almost a quarter of all cases in primary ovarian tumors [42]. No differences or increased expression of ING1 were observed in recent studies of myeloid leukemia or melanoma [45,47].

Recently reduced expression of ING2 mRNA as well as protein was observed in hepatocellular carcinoma (HCC) [48]. Decreased ING2 expression (but not ING2 mutation) has been observed in lung cancer [49]. Decrease of nuclear ING2 protein was observed in melanoma [50]. On the other hand increased expression of ING2 mRNA was shown in colon cancer [51]. Moreover, ING2 may play a role in melanoma initiation, since reduction of nuclear ING2 has been reported in radial as well as vertical growth phases in metastatic melanoma as compared to dysplastic nevi [52]. On the other hand, reduced ING2 expression was associated with tumor progression and shortened survival time in HCC [48]. These epidemiological studies suggest that ING2 loss or reduction may be important for tumor initiation and/or progression [11,12,17,20].

As shown for ING2, decreased nuclear ING3 protein expression was associated with a poor survival rate. The survival rate was 93% for the patients with strong nuclear ING3 staining, whereas it declined to 44% for the patients with negative-to-moderate nuclear staining [52]. In a recent study, we also demonstrated frequent deletion of chromosomal locus of each of ING family member including ING3 in ameloblastomas [53].

ING4 mRNA was decreased in glioblastoma and associated with tumor progression [54]. Decreased ING4 has been associated with increased expression of IL-8 and osteopontin (OPN) in myeloma [11,55]. In both reports, decreased ING4 expression was associated with higher tumor grade and increased tumor angiogenesis. In myeloma, it was also associated with increased expression of interleukin-8 and osteopontin [11,55]. Expression of ING4 was decreased in malignant melanoma as compared to dysplastic nevi, and was found to be an independent poor prognostic factor for the patients [56]. ING4 was found to suppress the loss of contact inhibition and growth. Moreover some mutation and deletion were detected in cell lines derived from human cancers such as breast and lung [57].

Significant reduced expression of ING4 was detected in gliomas as compared with normal human brain tissue, and the extent of reduction correlated with the progression from lower to higher grades of tumours [54]. Klironomos et al. investigated immunohistochemically the expression pattern of ING4, NF-kappaB and the NF-kappaB downstream targets MMP-2, MMP-9 and u-PA in human astrocytomas from 101 patients. They found that ING-4 expression was significantly reduced in astrocytomas, and it was associated with tumor grade progression. Expression of a NF-kappaB subunit p65 was significantly higher in grade IV than in grade III and grade I/II tumors, and a statistical significant negative correlation between expression of ING4 and expression of nuclear p65 was noticed [58].

Recently Nagahama et al. reported up-regulation of ING4 in a human gastric carcinoma cell line (MKN-1) by promoting mitochondria-mediated apoptosis via the activation of p53 [59]. Both mRNA and protein of ING4 expression were down regulated in hepatocellular carcinoma tissues. ING4 expression level correlated with prognosis and metastatic potential of hepatocellular carcinoma [60]. In another recent study, ING4 mRNA and protein expression were examined in gastric adenocarcinoma tissues and human gastric adenocarcinoma cell lines by RT-PCR, real-time RT-PCR, tissue microarray immunohistochemistry, and western blot analysis [61]. Their data showed that ING4 mRNA and protein were dramatically reduced in stomach adenocarcinoma cell lines and tissues, and significantly less in female than in male patients. Decrease of ING4 mRNA expression was found to correlate with the stage of the tumour [61]. Wang et al. examined ING4 protein expression in 246 lung cancer samples and overall reduced ING4 expression and higher ING4 expression in cytoplasm than in nucleus of tumour cells were detected, suggesting its involvement in the initiation and progression of lung cancers [62].

Examination of ING4 protein expression levels in colorectal cancer samples from 97 patients showed that ING4 protein was down regulated in adenoma relative to normal mucosa and further reduced in colorectal cancer tissues. Decrease of ING4 protein expression was also related to the more advanced Dukes' stages and ING4 expression levels in patients with lymphatic metastasis were lower than those without metastasis, suggesting that ING4 play a role in colorectal carcinoma progression [63].

Xing et al. analyzed ING5 expression in gastric carcinoma tissues and cell lines (MKN28, MKN45, AGS, GT-3 TKB, and KATO-III) by Western blot and reverse transcriptase-polymerase chain reaction. An increased expression of ING5 messenger RNA was found in gastric carcinoma in comparison with paired mucosa and lower expression of nuclear ING5 protein and cytoplasmic translocation was detected in gastric dysplasia and carcinoma than that in nonneoplastic mucosa [64]. Nuclear ING5 expression was negatively correlated with tumor size, depth of invasion, lymph node metastasis, and clinicopathologic staging, whereas cytoplasmic ING5 was positively associated with depth of invasion, venous invasion, lymph node metastasis, and clinicopathologic staging in colorectal carcinomas [65].

3. Abnormalities of ING family genes in head and neck cancer

At the time of ING1 cloning, deletion of chromosome 13q34 was shown in head and neck cancer but ING1 gene was not known to be responsible for this deletion. Later in a comprehensive study, our group demonstrated tumor specific missense mutations in ING1 gene and frequent deletion at long arm of chromosome 13 for the first time in a human cancer [13]. Of 34 informative cases of head and neck squamous cell carcinoma, 68% of tumors showed loss of heterozygosity at chromosome 13q33-34, where the ING1 gene is located. By this study, ING1 has been recognized to be an important TSG at least in head and neck cancer. These mutations were found in the PHD zinc finger domain and putative nuclear localization signal, which may abrogate the normal function of ING1 protein (**Figure 3**). Following this study, our group led most of the researches for ING family genes in head and neck cancer.

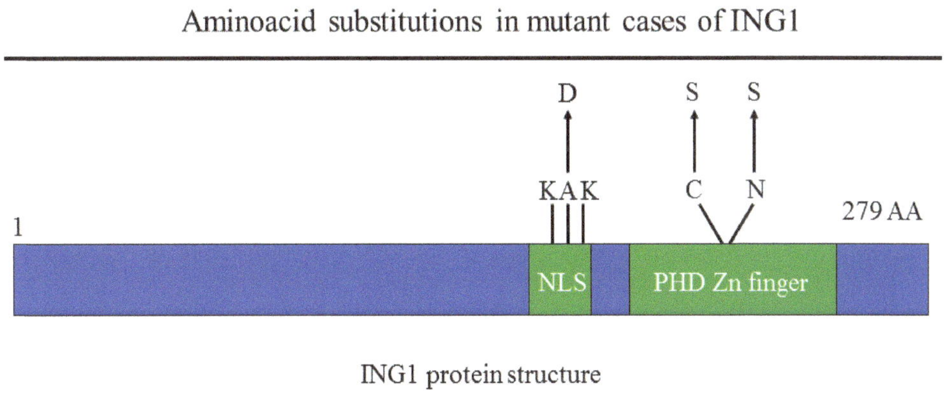

Fig. 3. Mutations detected at PHD zinc finger domain and nuclear localization signal (NLS) of ING1 protein, which may abrogate its function

On the other hand, examination of 71 indian oral cancer cases demonstrated only polymorphic changes but not somatic possible function effective alterations [66]. However, analysis of esophageal cancer, which display some similarities especially for hypopharyngeal cancer, also demonstrated somatic mutations in ING1, supporting our results [44].

We recently demonstrated that frequent deletion of ING2 locus at 4q35.1 associated with advanced tumor stage in HNSCC [67]. LOH was detected in about 55% of the informative samples and high LOH frequency was statistically associated with advanced T stage, suggesting that ING2 LOH might occur in late stages during HNSCC progression. On the other hand, positive node status (N) appeared to be the only independent prognostic factor for both overall and disease free survivals.

We showed frequent allelic loss of ING3 in HNSCC [14]. We analysed LOH at 7q31 region in 49 HNSCC by using six polymorphic microsatellite markers and found allelic deletion in 48% (22/46) of the informative cases. We detected two preferentially deleted regions, one is around D7S643 and the other around D7S486. When we redefined the map of 7q31 region according to the contiguous sequences, a recently identified gene, ING3, was found in the proximity of D7S643. But ING3 mutation was very rare in our study (a sole missense mutation of ING3 at codon 20). In another recent our study using a large study population, about half of the 71 tumor samples demonstrated downregulation of ING3 compared to their matched normal counterparts. We revealed that down-regulation of ING3 was more evident in late-stage tumors as compared with early stage patients, and patients with low ING3 mRNA expression demonstrated worse survival rates as compared to the patients with normal-high ING3 expression [68]. We also examined p53 mutation status and investigated its relationship with ING3, as well its clinicopathological characteristics. Although most clinicopathological variables were not significantly related to ING3 downregulation or p53 mutation status, a significant relationship was detected in terms of overall survival between the cases with low and normal to high ING3 expression. At 5 years follow up, approximately 60% of the patients with normal to high ING3 expression survived, whereas this was 35% in the patients with low ING3 expression. Multivariate analysis also showed downregulation of ING3 as an independent prognostic factor for poor overall survival. These results reveal that ING3 would function as a potential tumor suppressor molecule and that low levels of ING3 may indicate an aggressive nature of head and neck cancer.

We analyzed loss of heterozygosity at 12p12-13 region in 50 head and neck squamous cell carcinomas by using six highly polymorphic microsatellite markers and found allelic loss in 66% of the informative cases. To identify ING4 function, mutation analysis was performed. Though mutation of the ING4 gene was not found in head and neck cancers, the mRNA expression level examined by quantitative real-time RT-PCR analysis demonstrated decreased expression of ING4 mRNA in 76% of primary tumors as compared to matched normal samples. Since p53 dependent pathways of other ING family members have been shown, we examined p53 mutation status and compared with ING4 mRNA expression in tumor samples. However, no such direct relationship has been detected. In conclusion, frequent deletion and decreased mRNA expression of ING4 suggested it as a class two tumor suppressor gene and may play an important role in head and neck cancer [15].

In a recent study, nuclear expression of ING4 was found to gradually decrease from non-cancerous epithelium and dysplasia to HNSCC and was negatively correlated with a poorly-differentiated status, T staging, and TNM staging in HNSCC. On the other hand, cytoplasmic expression of ING4 was significantly enhanced in HNSCC and was significantly associated with lymph node metastasis and 14-3-3η expression. Moreover, nuclear expression of ING4 was positively correlated with p21 and p300 expression and with the apoptotic index. Their results suggested that the decreases in nuclear ING4 and cytoplasmic translocation of ING4 protein play important roles in tumorigenesis, progression and tumor differentiation in HNSCC [69].

Our group reported the first study linking ING5 chromosome locus to a human cancer. We demonstrated a high ratio of LOH in oral cancer using 16 microsatellite markers on the long arm of chromosome 2q21-37.3 [24]. ING5 appeared to be a strong candidate tumor suppressor in this study though several other candidate TSGs including ILKAP, HDAC4, PPP1R7, DTYMK, STK25, BOK are also localized at the area, where frequent deletion has been detected [11,12,24]. Moreover, our recent study revealed decreased expression of ING5 mRNA and mutations in oral cancer samples as compared to their corresponding normal controls, suggesting its tumor suppressive role in cancer [25]. Examination of 172 cases of HNSCC for ING5 protein by immunohistochemistry using tissue microarray, and in 3 oral SCC cell lines by immunohistochemistry and Western blot showed that a decrease in nuclear ING5 localization and cytoplasmic translocation were detected, supporting the previous studies and strong involvement of ING5 in tumorigenesis and tumor differentiation in HNSCC [70].

4. Possible applications of ING family genes in molecular diagnosis and therapy of cancer

So far most of the studies for possible applications of ING family genes in molecular diagnosis and therapy of cancer include cancer types other than head and neck cancer. However, ING family genes express ubiquitously and are involved in carcinogenesis of many cancer types especially in head and neck carcinogenesis. Thus the following section of the review is added as a model for possible application of ING family genes as diagnostic and therapeutic target.

4.1 Use of ING family genes for prediction of cancer behavior

4.1.1 Sub-cellular localization of ING proteins as a biomarker

Most tumor suppressors contain nuclear transport signals that facilitate their shuttling between the nucleus and the cytoplasm. This type of dynamic intracellular movement not only regulates protein localization, but also often impacts on function. Shuttling of tumor suppressor proteins between nucleus and cytoplasm has been reported to be involved in the regulation of cell cycle and proliferation. Deregulation of the nucleocytoplasmic cargo system results in the mislocalization of TSG proteins, which then alter function of TSG proteins [71]. The mistargeting of tumor suppressors can finally reveal direct cellular consequences and potentially lead to the initiation and progression of cancer. Abnormalities in nucleocytoplasmic cargo system leading the mislocalization of tumor suppressors were reported for p53, BRCA1, APC, VHL, BRG1 and ING1, and these abnormalities driven by genetic and epigenetic alterations in the tumor suppressor or their partners generally occur during the carcinogenic process [72-76]. For ING1, 2 of 3 different tumor specific somatic mutations that we detected in head and neck cancer were located at or near nuclear targeting domain, which could possibly abolish its functions through accumulation of the protein in the cytoplasm instead of in the nucleus [13].

In a recent study, Nouman et al. reported that translocation of p33ING1b from the nucleus into the cytoplasm of melanocytes may have an important role in the development and progression of melanomas [77]. Immunostaining with new monoclonal antibodies (MAb) of GN1 and GN2 showed that ING1b product, a nuclear protein, was accumulated in the cytoplasm and was closely associated with malignant melanoma development. The authors suggested that detection of this subcellular mobilization with MAb ING1b may be an early indicator and could be of value in diagnostic approach.

In another study of Nouman et al. nuclear expression of p33 (ING1b) was decreased in breast cancer cells, both in intensity and proportion of the cells stained. Reduction in nuclear expression of ING1 protein was associated with enhanced cytoplasmic p33 (ING1b) expression in a considerable number of cases. Those cases, which show p33 (ING1b) protein mislocalization, were also associated with more poorly differentiated tumors. Thus the authors suggested that p33 (ING1b) expression could be used as a marker of differentiation in invasive breast cancer. These results support the view that loss of p33 (ING1b) in the nucleus may be an important molecular event in the differentiation and pathogenesis of invasive breast cancer [78].

Similarly loss of nuclear expression of p33 (ING1b) was detected in 78% of cases of acute lymphoblastic leukemia (ALL). This loss in nuclear expression was associated with increased cytoplasmic expression of the protein. Kaplan Meier survival analysis demonstrated a trend towards a better prognosis for patients with tumors that had lost nuclear p33 (ING1b), suggesting that the loss of nuclear p33 (ING1b) expression may be an important molecular event in the pathogenesis of childhood ALL and can be used as a biomarker for prognosis [79].

In another similar study, Vieyra et al. demonstrated that sub-cellular mislocalization of p33ING1b is a commonly seen in gliomas and glioblastomas [80]. Overexpression and aberrant localization of ING1b into the cytoplasm were observed in all of the 29 brain tumors. p33 (ING1b) normally contains a nuclear targeting sequence [11,12,16]. It has been previously demonstrated that altered sub-cellular localization of p33 (ING1b) abrogates its proapoptotic functions [81]. Loss of targeting domains that ensure the proper intracellular localization of p33 (ING1b) or physical association of ING with p53 could account for the abnormal localization of p33 (ING1b) in cancer. Recent experimental observations, including post-translational stabilization of p53 by p33 (ING1b) [82], and the discovery of the p53 associated a parkin-like cytoplasmic-anchoring protein, PARC [83] and its p53-regulatory role support the possibility that association of ING proteins with p53 could account for the abnormal localization. Further studies in this field will clarify this point.

For a normal function of ING1, the protein should be in the nucleus. ING1b protein phosphorylated on serine residue at position 199 has been reported to bind 14-3-3 proteins and subsequently be exported from the nucleus [84]. It has recently been shown that ING1 also binds karyopherin proteins and that disruption of this interaction affects subcellular localization and activity of the ING as a transcriptional regulator [84].

For ING1, few studies exist regarding with its subcellular localization. However for other member of ING family proteins, it mostly remains unkown and only few studies exist for subcellular alterations during carcinogenesis. Similar to the study of Nouman et al. [77] nuclear ING3 expression was found to be remarkably reduced in malignant melanomas compared with dysplastic nevi, which was significantly correlated with the increased ING3 level in cytoplasm. Moreover the reduced nuclear ING3 expression was significantly correlated with a poorer disease-specific 5-year survival of the patients with primary melanoma, especially for the high-risk melanomas with the survival rate reducing from 93% for patients with strong nuclear ING3 staining in their tumor biopsies to 44% for those with negative-to-moderate nuclear ING3 staining. Interestingly, the multivariate Cox regression analysis revealed that reduced nuclear ING3 expression is an independent prognostic factor to predict patient outcome in primary melanomas [85].

By using tissue microarray technology and immunohistochemistry, ING2 expression in human nevi and melanoma biopsies was examined. The data showed that nuclear ING2 expression was significantly reduced in radial and vertical growth phases, and metastatic melanomas compared with dysplastic nevi. Reduced ING2 has been suggested as an important indicator in the initiation of melanoma development [86].

In a recent study, the subcellular localization of ING4 has been shown to be modulated by two wobble-splicing events at the exon 4-5 boundary, causing displacement from the nucleolus to the nucleus. The authors provided evidence that ING4 was degraded through the ubiquitin-proteasome pathway and that it is subjected to N-terminal ubiquitination. It has also been demonstrated that nucleolar accumulation of ING4 prolongs its half-life, but lack of nucleolar targeting potentially increases ING4 degradation. Taken together, data of this work suggested that the two wobble-splicing events at the exon 4-5 boundary influenced subnuclear localization and degradation of ING4 [87].

ING4 has been reported to interact with a novel binding partner, liprin alpha 1, which results in suppression of the cell spreading and migration [88]. Liprin α1/PPFIA1 (protein tyrosine phosphatase, receptor type f polypeptide) is known to be a cytoplasmic protein necessary for focal adhesion formation and axon guidance. Cytoplasmic ING4 may regulate cell migration through interacting with liprin α1, and with its known anti-angiogenic function, may prevent invasion and metastasis. This interaction could explain the specific property of ING4 from other ING proteins.

In summary, sub-cellular localization of ING proteins or their interaction partners could be detected with various molecular and immunohistopathological methods and may be used as a biomarker for the behavior of the tumor and prediction of the disease progress.

4.1.2 Genetic and epigenetic alterations of TSG as prognostic biomarker

Alterations in allelic status, expression of mRNA and/or protein of the ING family genes provide potential usage of these genes as biomarkers in human cancer. Regarding with relation between genetic alterations of various genes and clinical outcome has recently been investigated. Since only few studies regarding with ING family genes exist in the literature, we will first give examples, which has been reported for other genes and summarize those published for ING tumor suppressors. In such a research, FHIT gene methylation has been found as a prognostic marker for progressive disease of early lung cancer [89]. Methylation and LOH analysis of FHIT gene showed that loss or reduced FHIT expression was significantly associated with squamous cell carcinoma type and smokers. Also methylation in normally appearing lung mucosa was related with an increased risk for progression into lung cancer, suggesting that FHIT can be used as a biomarker for this cancer type. In another report, allelic loss at 3p and 9p21 was related with elevated risk of malignant transformation of the premalignant lesions in head and neck cancer [90]. Similarly LOH at 8p was a predictor for long-term survival in hepatocellular carcinoma [91].

Another study highlighted the prognostic role of p16 in predicting the recurrence-free probability in patients affected by low-grade urothelial bladder by using p16 expression and LOH at 9p21 and proved the fact that the method is likely to be used in everyday urologic clinical practice to better describe the natural history of urothelial bladder carcinomas [92]. LOH at 16q23.2 was shown to be a predictor of disease-free survival in prostate cancer [93]. Our group has recently demonstrated that deletion at chromosome 14q was associated with poor prognosis in head and neck squamous cell carcinomas [1]. We also showed that frequent deletion of ING2 locus at 4q35.1 associates with advanced tumor stage in head and neck squamous cell carcinoma [67]. Interestingly, in our study, deletion at Dickkopf (dkk)-3 locus (11p15.2) was detected to be related with lower lymph node metastasis and better prognosis in head and neck squamous cell carcinomas, suggesting the different nature of this gene, yet its potential use as a prognostic biomarker [94].

Detection of a gradual increase of mRNA expression of the DNA replication-initiation proteins from epithelial dysplasia (from mild through severe) to squamous cell carcinoma of the tongue has been used as biomarker to distinguish precancerous dysplasia from SCC and is useful for early detection and diagnosis of SCC as an adjunct to clinicopathological parameters [95]. In a recent work, we demonstrated downregulation of TESTIN and its association with cancer history and a tendency toward poor survival in head and neck squamous cell carcinoma [96]. The increased serum midkine concentrations were strongly associated with poor survival in early-stage oral squamous cell carcinoma, suggesting it as a useful marker not only for cancer screening but also for predicting prognosis of OSCC patients [97].

Information on human genome project provided that many gene including cancer-associated genes show alternative splicing. In such a study, deregulation of survivin splicing isoforms has been shown to influence significant implications in tumor aggressiveness and prognosis [98]. In ING family genes, some of the members also have splicing variants. Although we don't have detail study for these variants, their deregulation may have an impact for carcinogenesis. In our work, two major variants of ING1 (p33ING1 and p24ING1) revealed different expression patterns. Our researches indicated alternative splicing variants for ING1, ING3, ING4 and ING5 [13-15,25]. For ING2, a recent study reported 2 splicing variants [31,32]. Though both of them showed decreased expression in head and neck cancer tissues as compared to the normal counterparts, methylation analysis demonstrated that only p33ING1 variant was associated with methylation (Gunduz *et al.* unpublished data).

Not only single gene alterations associated with clinical outcome but also genome-wide or microarray studies were also examined. In such as study, genome-wide transcriptomic profiles obtained for 53 primary oral cancer and 22 matching normal tissues exhibited up-regulated genes and down-regulated genes. In conclusion, this study provided a transcriptomic signature for oral cancer that may lead to a diagnosis or screen tool [99]. In a recent study, the expression levels of ITGA3, ITGB4, and ITGB5 with functional normalization by desmosomal or cytoskeletal molecule genes were shown as candidate biomarkers for cervical lymph node metastasis or for the outcome of death in oral cancer [100].

Another recent study identified allelic deletion of ING1 as a novel genomic marker as related progression to glioblastoma by using comparative genomic hybridization and DNA microarray [101]. In another study, low levels of ING1 mRNA have been reported to be significantly associated with poor prognosis in neuroblastoma [102]. The expression level of ING1 was also closely related to survival. These results suggest that decreased level of ING1 mRNA and/or protein expression could be an indicator of poor prognosis in advanced stages and/or poor survival of various human tumors. On the other hand, an association between p33ING1b protein expression and clinical outcome in colorectal cancer demonstrated that although patients with decreased p33ING1b protein expression in the tumor have a shorter overall and metastasis-free survival rate as compared with patients with normal p33ING1b protein expression, no statistical significance was achieved [103].

However a significant association between p53 mutation status and overall and metastasis-free survival has been found.

Regarding with ING2 gene, its reduced mRNA as well as protein expressions were shown to be associated with tumor progression and shortened survival time in HCC [48]. Recently, our group reported that high LOH frequency in ING2 locus at 4q35.1 was significantly associated with advanced tumor stage in HNSCC, suggesting that ING2 LOH might occur in later stages during HNSCC progression [67]. Hence, the relevance of ING2 in HNSCC carcinogenesis and the potential prognostic significance of ING2 are promising results for future studies.

Several recent studies examined correlation between ING3 protein expression and clinicopathological variables [52,54]. Interestingly, significant reduction of nuclear ING3 was detected in human malignant melanoma, indicating the status of ING3 as a prognostic and therapeutic marker for melanoma [52]. As it has been shown for ING2, decreased nuclear ING3 protein expression was also associated with a poorer 5-year survival rate. The survival rate was 93% for the patients with strong nuclear ING3 staining, whereas it decreased to 44% for the patients with negative-to-moderate nuclear staining. We have recently reported mRNA expression of ING3 in HNSCC and compared the clinicopathological characteristics to evaluate its prognostic value as a biomarker [14,68]. This study revealed that down-regulation of ING3 was more evident in late-stage tumors as compared with early stage cases. Analyses have also showed that down-regulation of ING3 could be used as an independent prognostic factor for poor overall survival and low levels of ING3 may indicate an aggressive nature of HNSCC.

Recently the correlation of the ING4 with patient survival and metastasis was revealed to be as a potential prognostic marker in melanoma [56]. It has been found that ING4 expression was significantly decreased in malignant melanoma compared with dysplastic nevi, and overexpression of ING4 inhibited melanoma cell invasion compared with the control.

4.1.3 ING genes as chemosensitivity marker

Overall survival of head and neck squamous cell carcinoma patients has not improved in the decades. Currently treatment strategies for this cancer are based on the tumor-node-metastasis (TNM) classification. However, due to the extreme biological heterogeneity of the cancer cells, treatment planning especially for chemoradiotherapy is quite difficult and chemotherapy is an important therapeutic modality for cancer, and identification of the genes that predict the response of cancer cells to these agents is critical to treat the patients more efficiently. Although clinical determinants such as TNM classification will be still important, it is now becoming possible, by molecular markers, to elucidate biological information about host and tumor, to break through the molecular heterogeneity and eventually to optimize the choice of treatment [104].

In a recent analysis for prediction of chemosensitivity, it has been reported that examining the TP to DPD ratio of their tumors could identify HNSCC patients, who would most benefit from capecitabine-based chemotherapy. Moreover, the potential role of TP gene therapy in TP to DPD ratio manipulation to optimize the tumoricidal effect of capecitabine has been demonstrated [105]. In another similar study, acquired (10-fold) resistance of

Cal27, a tongue cancer cell line, against cisplatin has been shown to be associated with decreased DKK1 expression and this resistance could partially be reversed by DKK1 overexpression, thus suggesting DKK1 and the WNT signaling pathway as a marker and target for cisplatin chemosensitivity [106].

Recent findings suggest that the ING genes might also have a role in regulating the response of cancer cells to chemotherapeutic agents. In an osteosarcoma cell line, U2OS cells, one of the ING1 splicing variant p33ING1b, prominently enhanced etoposide-induced apoptosis through p53-dependent pathways [107]. In another study of the authors, ectopic expression of p33ING1b was shown to upregulate p53, p21WAF1 and bax protein levels and activate caspase-3 in taxol-treated U2OS cells. Thus the study demonstrated that p33ING1b increased taxol-induced apoptosis through p53-dependent pathway in human osteosarcoma cells, suggesting that p33ING1b may be an important marker and/or therapeutic target in the prevention and treatment of osteosarcoma [108].

Tallen et al. [39] questioned whether p33ING1 mRNA expression correlates with the chemosensitivity of brain tumor cells. They found that, unlike other tumor types, ING1 levels were higher in glioma cell lines than in normal control cells. Medulloblastoma cells revealed the lowest ING1 expression of the lines tested. Comparing all cell lines, p33ING1 gene expression significantly correlated with resistance to vincristine, suggesting that p33ING1 mRNA levels may be used to predict the chemosensitivity of brain tumor cells to vincristine.

The tumor suppressor ING1 shares many biological functions with p53 including cell cycle arrest, DNA repair, apoptosis, and chemosensitivity. To investigate if the p33ING1 isoform is also involved in chemosensitivity, Cheung et al. overexpressed p33ING1 in melanoma cells and examined for cell death after treatment with camptothecin. Results from the survival assay and flow cytometry analysis showed no significant difference among cells transfected with vector, p33ING1, and antisense p33ING1, indicating that p33ING1 does not enhance camptothecin-induced cell death in melanoma cells. Moreover, co-transfection of the p33ING1 and p53 constructs had also no effect on the frequency of cell death. Thus influence of ING1 expression for chemosensitivity may have different depending on the cancer type [109]. In another work, down-regulation of ING1 in the p53-deficient glioblastoma cell line, LN229, increased apoptosis following treatment with cisplatin, indicating that reduced ING1 expression may predict the sensitivity of cancer cells to chemotherapy independent of their p53 status [110]. Although most studies reported that expression of ING genes results in an increase in chemosensitivity, various conditions in different tumors should be tested to predict exact chemotherapy response. These differences could also be related with expression variations of the alternative splicing forms of ING genes.

Another member of ING family, ING4 negatively regulated the cell growth with significant G2/M arrest of cell cycle. Besides overexpression of ING4 enhanced the cell apoptosis triggered by serum starvation in HepG2 cells. Furthermore, the exogenous ING4 upregulated endogenous p21 and Bax in HepG2 cells, but not in p53-deficient Saos-2 cells, suggesting that G2/M arrest induced by ING4 could be mediated by the increased p21 expression in a p53-dependent manner, although there is no significant increase of p53 expression in HepG2 cells. Moreover, HepG2 cells with exogenous ING4 could significantly increase cell death, as exposed to some DNA-damage agents, such as etoposide and doxorubicin, implying that ING4 could enhance chemosensitivity to certain DNA-damage agents in HepG2 cells [111]. In another study, chemopreventive agent curcumin (diferuloyl methane) induced ING4 expression during the cell cycle arrest by a p53-dependent manner in glioma cells (U251) [112]. Therefore ING4 has been suggested for a possible role in the signaling pathways of the chemotherapeutic agents.

4.2 Applications of ING family for gene therapy

Cancer still poses a great treat to human life and classical treatment modalities have still failed to eradicate it. Developments in human genome technology and progress in knowledge of the genes provided us alternative methods such as gene therapy to cure this fatal disease. Currently researchers are working on several basic methods to treat cancer using gene therapy. Some of these methods target healthy cells i.e. immune system cells to enhance their ability to fight cancer. Other approaches directly involve cancer cells, to destroy them or at least to stop their growth. The later method usually involves restoration of the tumor suppressor genes. In tumor cells, ING transcript levels are now known to be often downregulated though mutations are very rare. However, as explained in the above sections, it has been now known that the inactivation of ING family genes at genetic and epigenetic levels has a major role in the carcinogenesis of various neoplasms. Considering involvement of ING tumor suppressors in many cancer types, it can be thought that ING family genes may be of potential target for molecular therapy in human cancer. However, only few preclinical studies exist to evaluate this potential. Thus this section will only give an image and possible speculations for using these genes in cancer therapy.

Regarding the gene therapy of ING family genes in the literature, a few in vitro studies have been reported. In 1999, the introduction of ING1 gene using virus vectors was reported as a pioneer and a promising approach for the treatment of brain tumors [113]. Although adenovirus-mediated introduction of isolated ING1 transcript has inhibited the growth of glioblastoma cells, combined transduction of p33ING1 and p53 synergistically enhanced the apoptosis in these cells [113], suggesting that ING1 may function as a proapoptotic factor as well as enhancing the effect of p53.

Another study has shown similar findings and supported the cooperative role of ING1 and p53 in esophageal cancer [114]. Co-introduction of ING1 and p53 induced more cell death as compared to single use of each gene transcript in esophageal carcinoma cells. Thus, the synergistic effect between p33ING1 and p53 for induction of apoptosis has been suggested for 2 different human cancers, i.e. esophageal carcinoma and glioblastoma. Considering these two in vitro studies, combined gene therapy of one or more ING family members with/without p53 emerged as a promising alternative therapy in those cases with the failure of single use of p53 gene therapy.

Another method in gene therapy could be potentialisation of the introduced gene. In fact, a study showed that one of the ING1 splicing isoforms, p47ING1a, was differentially up-regulated in response to cisplatin in human glioblastoma cells (LN229) that express ING1 proteins and harbor mutated TP53, which might represent a response to protect DNA from this DNA-damaging agent. Thus ING1 down-regulation may sensitize glioblastoma cells with deficient p53 to treatment with cisplatin. It was concluded that the status of p53-independent-ING expression level might predict the relative sensitivity to treatment with cisplatin and HDAC inhibitors in glioblastoma. These studies suggest that molecular therapy of ING1 could be combined with chemotherapeutics in a subset of human cancer.

Interestingly, some of ING family members have additional functions for suppressing the tumor growth such as anti-angiogenesis for ING4. Thus future studies using other members alone or in combination for gene therapy will provide more successful and promising results. In fact, it has been shown that ING4 gene therapy may be effective in human lung carcinoma as a novel anti-invasive and anti-metastatic agent [115]. Adenovirus-mediated ING4 expression suppressed the tumor growth and cell invasiveness in A549 lung cancer cells, suggesting that ING4, as a potent tumor-suppressing agent, present great therapeutic potential. Another interesting study displayed that ING4 inhibited MMP-2 and MMP-9 expressions in melanoma cells, which may contribute to the suppression of melanoma cell invasion [56]. This study demonstrated that overexpression of ING4 significantly decreased melanoma cell invasion by 43% and suppressed cell migration by 63%. Since degradation of basement membrane and extracellular matrix (ECM) is the first step in the invasion and metastasis of malignant tumors, down-regulation of the MMP-2 and MMP-9 expressions with Ad-ING4 may be a potential method in suppressing degradation components of the ECM and basement membrane and thus metastasis. In this respect, association of the ING4 with the MMP pathway may open a new avenue and offer novel opportunities for molecular therapy of cancer. In another recent study, Xie et al. [116] demonstrated that Ad-ING4-mediated transfection of PANC-1 human pancreatic carcinoma cells inhibited cell growth, altered the cell cycle with S-phase reduction and G2/M phase arrest, induced apoptosis, and downregulated interleukin (IL)-6 and IL-8 expression of transfected tumor cells. In athymic mice bearing the PANC-1 human pancreatic tumors, intratumoral injections of Ad-ING4 suppressed the tumor growth, downregulated CD34 expression, and reduced the tumor microvessel formation. Therefore, this study provided a framework for future clinical application of Ad-ING4 in human pancreatic and other carcinoma gene therapies.

In conclusion, these reports suggest that the transfer or forced expression of ING4 into cancer cells by gene therapy also targets its related molecules such as MMPs. Thus combination of ING4 gene therapy with chemicals, which inhibit MMPs, could be a promising treatment method in various cancer types. In this respect, possible applications each member of ING family genes for gene therapy should be tested. A summary of ING gene alterations and their use as possible biomarkers and consequences of the gene restoration in cancer are shown in **Figure 4**.

5. Future aspects

Over a decade of research on the ING family genes has revealed that ING genes are involved in various functions from chromatin remodeling to cell cycle suppression and apoptosis. Moreover ING family genes also cooperate with major tumor suppressor p53 and make complexes with HAT and HDAC. Alterations of these genes occur commonly in many cancer types. Recent studies also suggest that allelic deletion or down-regulation of mRNA

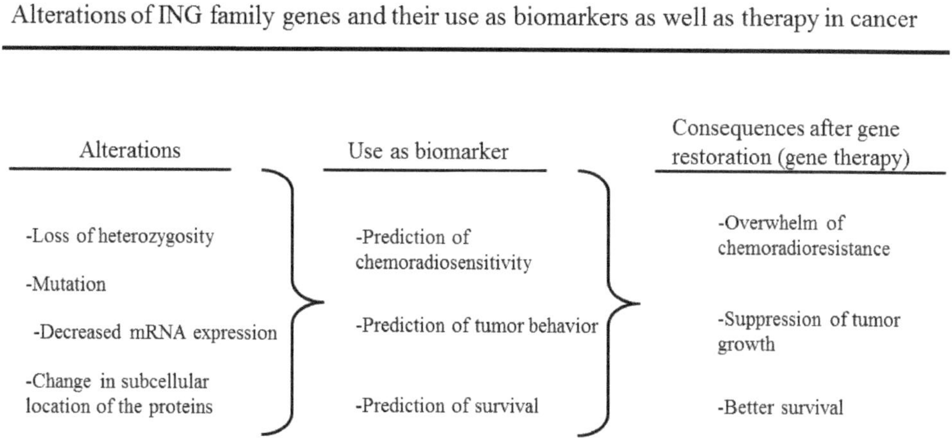

Fig. 4. Alterations of ING family genes and their possible use as biomarker for diagnosis and gene therapy in cancer

expressions as well as change of subcellular localization of proteins of the genes are likely to be used as a prognostic or predictive marker in human cancer. Today many cancer types including head and neck are treated based on clinical staging and findings such as lymph node involvement, TNM stage. However these clinical markers are most time not enough to follow tumor behavior or patients response to the therapy. Thus new methods are warranted to overcome these shortcomings to get a better response to the therapy or to predict which therapeutic method is best for each patient. At this point, involvement of ING genes in p53 tumor suppressor pathways and crosstalk between the variant of a single ING gene need to be clarified for focusing on INGs as diagnostic biomarkers. Progress on the knowledge of functions of ING family genes as well as the relationship with p53 and other unknown molecules will elucidate their roles in the development of human cancers, which will result in their uses in cancer diagnostics as well as therapy.

Cancer today is still one of the most dangerous diseases for human life. So far for treatment of cancer, surgery and chemoradiotherapy are the major therapies. Major difficulty for treatment of the cancer is inefficiency of chemoradiotherapy since each person gives different response to the therapy. So far clinical staging or findings is used to plan for treatment of cancer. However, this is not enough since many patients are resistant to these therapies and there is currently no way to understand efficiency of these methods. Moreover these treatment modalities are not specific and demonstrate high toxicities. Recent developments in human genome and technology provide novel methods for prediction of therapy or tumor behavior as well as tumor-targeted specific therapeutic methods. Thus although development of many molecular biomarkers for prediction of tumor behavior are tested and genetic therapy trials are ongoing, five-year later it is likely to see some of these methods as routine clinical use. For example, LOH of some TSG loci or expression profiles of single or multiple genes or mutation status could direct our therapy and we can have a nearly 100% success for each patient since the treatment will be individualized based on use of multiple molecular biomarkers. Some of these markers could be developed based on the studies on ING family genes. Furthermore, current gene therapies using mostly p53 gene as a tumor suppressor could be expanded to members of ING family genes or combined of various tumor suppressors. Besides gene therapy can also be considered to combine with chemoradiotherapy.

6. Key points

ING family genes are recently identified major tumor suppressor involved in many cancer types.

ING family tumor suppressors have wide functions from cell growth, cell cycle suppression, DNA repair, chromatin remodeling to apoptosis.

ING family genes also cooperate with other tumor suppressors such as p53 and HAT and HDAC.

Alterations of ING genes at genetic and epigenetic level as well as their proteins showed promising results for their use as a molecular biomarker.

These genes are also likely to be used for gene therapy as a single agent or combined with other tumor suppressors.

7. Acknowledgements

This article was partially supported by grants-in-aid from the Scientific and Technological Research Council of Turkey #110S424 to Esra Gunduz.

8. References

[1] Pehlivan D, Gunduz E, Gunduz M, Nagatsuka H, Beder LB, Cengiz B, Rivera RS, Fukushima K, Palanduz S, Ozturk S, Yamanaka N, Shimizu K. Loss of heterozygosity at chromosome 14q is associated with poor prognosis in head and neck squamous cell carcinomas. J Cancer Res Clin Oncol 134(12):1267-76, 2008

[2] Parkin DM, Bray F, Ferlay J, Pisani P. Global cancer statistics, 2002. CA Cancer J Clin 55(2):74-108, 2005

[3] Jemal A, Siegel R, Ward E, Murray T, Xu J, Smigal C, Thun MJ. Cancer statistics, 2006. CA Cancer J Clin 56(2):106-30, 2006

[4] Hinds PW, Weinberg RA. Tumor suppressor genes. Curr Opin Genet Dev 4(1):135-141, 1994

[5] Knudson Jr AG. Mutation and cancer: statistical study of retinoblastoma. Proc Natl Acad Sci USA 68:820-823, 1971

[6] Tang B, Bottinger EP, Jakowlew SB, Bagnall KM, Mariano J, Anver MR, Letterio JJ and Wakefield LM. Transforming growth factor-b1 is a new form of tumor suppressor with true haploid insufficiency. Nat Med 4: 802-807, 1998

[7] Bai F, Pei XH, Godfrey VL and Xiong Y. Haploinsufficiency of p18 (INK4c) sensitizes mice to carcinogen-induced tumorigenesis. Mol Cell Biol 23: 1269-1277, 2003

[8] Mduff FK, Hook CE, Tooze RM, Huntly BJ, Pandolfi PP, Turner SD. Determining the contribution of NPM1 heterozygosity to NPM-ALK-induced lymphomagenesis. Lab Invest. 2011 Jun 27. doi: 10.1038/labinvest.2011.96. [Epub ahead of print]

[9] Huang H, Wei X, Su X, Qiao F, Xu Z, Gu D, Fan H, Chen J. Clinical significance of expression of Hint1 and potential epigenetic mechanism in gastric cancer. Int J Oncol 38:1557-64, 2011

[10] Zhou XZ, Huang P, Shi R, Lee TH, Lu G, Zhang Z, Bronson R, Lu KP. The telomerase inhibitor PinX1 is a major haploinsufficient tumor suppressor essential for chromosome stability in mice. J Clin Invest 121(4):1266-82, 2011

[11] Gunduz M, Gunduz E, Rivera RS, Nagatsuka H. The inhibitor of growth (ING) gene family: potential role in cancer therapy. Curr Cancer Drug Targets 8:275-284, 2008

[12] Gunduz M, Demircan K, Gunduz E, Katase N, Tamamura R, Nagatsuka H. Potential usage of ING family members in cancer diagnostics and molecular therapy. Curr Drug Targets 10(5):465-476, 2009

[13] Gunduz M, Ouchida M, Fukushima K et al. Genomic structure of the human ING1 gene and tumor-specific mutations detected in head and neck squamous cell carcinomas. Cancer Res 60 (12):3143–3146, 2000

[14] Gunduz M, Ouchida M, Fukushima K et al. Allelic loss and reduced expression of the ING3, a candidate tumor suppressor gene at 7q31, in human head and neck cancers. Oncogene 21 (28):4462–4470, 2002

[15] Gunduz M, Nagatsuka H, Demircan K et al. Frequent deletion and down-regulation of ING4, a candidate tumor suppressor gene at 12p13, in head and neck squamous cell carcinomas. Gene 356:109-117, 2005

[16] Soliman MA, Riabowol K. After a decade of study-ING, a PHD for a versatile family of proteins. Trends Biochem Sci 32(11):509-519, 2007

[17] Aguissa-Touré AH, Wong RP, Li G. Cell Mol Life Sci. The ING family tumor suppressors: from structure to function. 68:45-54, 2011

[18] Champagne KS, Kutateladze TG. Structural insight into histone recognition by the ING PHD fingers. Curr Drug Targets 10(5):432-441, 2009

[19] Bienz M. The PHD finger, a nuclear protein-interaction domain. Trends Biochem Sci 31(1):35-40, 2006

[20] Coles AH, Jones SN. The ING gene family in the regulation of the cell growth and tumorigenesis. J Cell Physiol 218:45-57, 2009

[21] Garkavtsev I, Kazarov A, Gudkov A and Riabowol K. Suppression of the novel growth inhibitor p33ING1 promotes neoplastic transformation. Nat Genet 14:415-420, 1996

[22] Feng X, Hara Y and Riabowol K. Different HATS of the ING1 gene family. Trends Cell Biol 12: 532-538, 2002

[23] Aguissa-Touré AH, Wong RP, Li G. Cell Mol Life Sci. The ING family tumor suppressors: from structure to function. 68:45-54, 2011

[24] Cengiz B, Gunduz M, Nagatsuka H *et al.* Fine deletion mapping of chromosome 2q21-37 shows three preferentially deleted regions in oral cancer. Oral Oncol 43(3):241-247, 2007

[25] Cengiz B, Gunduz E, Gunduz M, Beder LB, Tamamura R, Bagci C, Yamanaka N, Shimizu K, Nagatsuka H. Tumor-specific mutation and downregulation of ING5 detected in oral squamous cell carcinoma. Int J Cancer 127:2088-94, 2010

[26] Nagashima M, Shiseki M, Miura K, Hagiwara K, Linke SP, Pedeux R, Wang XW, Yokota J, Riabowol K, Harris CC. DNA damage-inducible gene p33ING2 negatively regulates cell proliferation through acetylation of p53. Proc Natl Acad Sci U S A 98:9671-6, 2001

[27] Nagashima M, Shiseki M, Pedeux RM, Okamura S, Kitahama-Shiseki M, Miura K, Yokota J, Harris CC. A novel PHD-finger motif protein, p47ING3, modulates p53-mediated transcription, cell cycle control, and apoptosis. Oncogene 22:343-50, 2003

[28] Shiseki M, Nagashima M, Pedeux RM, Kitahama-Shiseki M, Miura K, Okamura S, Onogi H, Higashimoto Y, Appella E, Yokota J, Harris CC. p29ING4 and p28ING5 bind to p53 and p300, and enhance p53 activity. Cancer Res 63:2373-8, 2003

[29] Unoki M, Shen JC, Zheng ZM, Harris CC. Novel splice variants of ING4 and their possible roles in the regulation of cell growth and motility. J Biol Chem 281:34677-86, 2006

[30] Unoki M, Kumamoto K, Harris CC. ING proteins as potential anticancer drug targets. Curr Drug Targets 10:442-54, 2009

[31] Unoki M, Kumamoto K, Robles AI, Shen JC, Zheng ZM, Harris CC. A novel ING2 isoform, ING2b, synergizes with ING2a to prevent cell cycle arrest and apoptosis. FEBS Lett 582:3868-74, 2008

[32] Unoki M, Kumamoto K, Takenoshita S, Harris CC. Reviewing the current classification of inhibitor of growth family proteins. Cancer Sci 100:1173-9, 2009

[33] Toyama T, Iwase H, Watson P, Muzik H, Saettler E, Magliocco A, DiFrancesco L, Forsyth P, Garkavtsev I, Kobayashi S, Riabowol K. Suppression of ING1 expression in sporadic breast cancer. Oncogene 18:5187-93, 1999

[34] Tokunaga E, Maehara Y, Oki E, Kitamura K, Kakeji Y, Ohno S, Sugimachi K. Diminished expression of ING1 mRNA and the correlation with p53 expression in breast cancers. Cancer Lett 152:15-22, 2000

[35] Ohmori M, Nagai M, Tasaka T, Koeffler HP, Toyama T, Riabowol K, Takahara J. Decreased expression of p33ING1 mRNA in lymphoid malignancies. Am J Hematol 62:118-9, 1999 Erratum in: Am J Hematol 2000 May;64(1):82.

[36] Oki E, Maehara Y, Tokunaga E, Kakeji Y, Sugimachi K. Reduced expression of p33 (ING1) and the relationship with p53 expression in human gastric cancer. Cancer Lett 147:157-62, 1999

[37] Ito K, Kinjo K, Nakazato T, Ikeda Y, Kizaki M. Expression and sequence analyses of p33(ING1) gene in myeloid leukemia. Am J Hematol 69:141-3, 2002

[38] Hara Y, Zheng Z, Evans SC, Malatjalian D, Riddell DC, Guernsey DL, Wang LD, Riabowol K, Casson AG. ING1 and p53 tumor suppressor gene alterations in adenocarcinomas of the esophagogastric junction. Cancer Lett 192:109-16, 2003

[39] Tallen G, Riabowol K, Wolff JE. Expression of p33ING1 mRNA and chemosensitivity in brain tumor cells. Anticancer Res 23(2B):1631-5, 2003

[40] Tallen G, Kaiser I, Krabbe S, Lass U, Hartmann C, Henze G, Riabowol K, von Deimling A. No ING1 mutations in human brain tumours but reduced expression in high malignancy grades of astrocytoma. Int J Cancer 109:476-9, 2004

[41] Takahashi M, Ozaki T, Todo S, Nakagawara A. Decreased expression of the candidate tumor suppressor gene ING1 is associated with poor prognosis in advanced neuroblastomas. Oncol Rep 12:811-6, 2004

[42] Shen DH, Chan KY, Khoo US, Ngan HY, Xue WC, Chiu PM, Ip P, Cheung AN. Epigenetic and genetic alterations of p33ING1b in ovarian cancer. Carcinogenesis 26:855-63, 2005

[43] Kameyama K, Huang CL, Liu D, Masuya D, Nakashima T, Sumitomo S, Takami Y, Kinoshita M, Yokomise H. Reduced ING1b gene expression plays an important role in carcinogenesis of non-small cell lung cancer patients. Clin Cancer Res 9:4926-34, 2003

[44] Chen L, Matsubara N, Yoshino T, Nagasaka T, Hoshizima N, Shirakawa Y, Naomoto Y, Isozaki H, Riabowol K, Tanaka N. Genetic alterations of candidate tumor suppressor ING1 in human esophageal squamous cell cancer. Cancer Res 61:4345-9, 2001

[45] Bromidge T, Lynas C. Relative levels of alternative transcripts of the ING1 gene and lack of mutations of p33/ING1 in haematological malignancies. Leuk Res 26:631-5, 2002

[46] Krishnamurthy J, Kannan K, Feng J, Mohanprasad BK, Tsuchida N, Shanmugam G. Mutational analysis of the candidate tumor suppressor gene ING1 in Indian oral squamous cell carcinoma. Oral Oncol 37:222-4, 2001

[47] Stark M, Puig-Butille JA, Walker G, Badenas C, Malvehy J, Hayward N, Puig S. Mutation of the tumour suppressor p33ING1b is rare in melanoma. Br J Dermatol 155:94-9, 2006

[48] Zhang HK, Pan K, Wang H, Weng DS, Song HF, Zhou J, Huang W, Li JJ, Chen MS, Xia JC. Decreased expression of ING2 gene and its clinicopathological significance in hepatocellular carcinoma. Cancer Lett 261:183-92, 2008

[49] Okano T, Gemma A, Hosoya Y, Hosomi Y, Nara M, Kokubo Y, Yoshimura A, Shibuya M, Nagashima M, Harris CC, Kudoh S. Alterations in novel candidate tumor suppressor genes, ING1 and ING2 in human lung cancer. Oncol Rep 15:545-9, 2006

[50] Lu F, Dai DL, Martinka M, Ho V, Li G. Nuclear ING2 expression is reduced in human cutaneous melanomas. Br J Cancer 95:80-6, 2006

[51] Kumamoto K, Fujita K, Kurotani R, Saito M, Unoki M, Hagiwara N, Shiga H, Bowman ED, Yanaihara N, Okamura S, Nagashima M, Miyamoto K, Takenoshita S, Yokota J, Harris CC. ING2 is upregulated in colon cancer and increases invasion by enhanced MMP13 expression. Int J Cancer 125:1306-15, 2009

[52] Wang Y, Dai DL, Martinka M, Li G. Prognostic significance of nuclear ING3 expression in human cutaneous melanoma. Clin Cancer Res 13(14):4111-4116, 2007

[53] Borkosky SS, Gunduz M, Beder L, Tsujigiwa H, Tamamura R, Gunduz E, Katase N, Rodriguez AP, Sasaki A, Nagai N, Nagatsuka H. Allelic loss of the ING gene family loci is a frequent event in ameloblastoma. Oncol Res 18:509-18, 2010

[54] Garkavtsev I, Kozin SV, Chernova O, Xu L, Winkler F, Brown E, Barnett GH, Jain RK. The candidate tumour suppressor protein ING4 regulates brain tumour growth and angiogenesis. Nature 428:328-32, 2004

[55] Colla S, Tagliaferri S, Morandi F, Lunghi P, Donofrio G, Martorana D, Mancini C, Lazzaretti M, Mazzera L, Ravanetti L, Bonomini S, Ferrari L, Miranda C, Ladetto M, Neri TM, Neri A, Greco A, Mangoni M, Bonati A, Rizzoli V, Giuliani N. The new tumor-suppressor gene inhibitor of growth family member 4 (ING4) regulates the production of proangiogenic molecules by myeloma cells and suppresses hypoxia-inducible factor-1 alpha (HIF-1alpha) activity: involvement in myeloma-induced angiogenesis. Blood 110:4464-75, 2007. Epub 2007 Sep 11. Erratum in Blood. 2008 Sep 1;112:2170

[56] Li J, Martinka M, Li G. Role of ING4 in human melanoma cell migration, invasion and patient survival. Carcinogenesis 29:1373-9, 2008

[57] Kim S, Chin K, Gray JW, Bishop JM. A screen for genes that suppress loss of contact inhibition: identification of ING4 as a candidate tumor suppressor gene in human cancer. Proc Natl Acad Sci U S A 101:16251-6, 2004

[58] Klironomos G, Bravou V, Papachristou DJ, Gatzounis G, Varakis J, Parassi E, Repanti M, Papadaki H. Loss of inhibitor of growth (ING-4) is implicated in the pathogenesis and progression of human astrocytomas. Brain Pathol 20:490-7, 2010

[59] Nagahama Y, Ishimaru M, Osaki M, Inoue T, Maeda A, Nakada C, Moriyama M, Sato K, Oshimura M, Ito H. Apoptotic pathway induced by transduction of RUNX3 in the human gastric carcinoma cell line MKN-1. Cancer Sci 99:23-30, 2008

[60] Fang F, Luo LB, Tao YM, Wu F, Yang LY. Decreased expression of inhibitor of growth 4 correlated with poor prognosis of hepatocellular carcinoma. Cancer Epidemiol Biomarkers Prev 18:409-16, 2009

[61] Li M, Jin Y, Sun WJ, Yu Y, Bai J, Tong DD, Qi JP, Du JR, Geng JS, Huang Q, Huang XY, Huang Y, Han FF, Meng XN, Rosales JL, Lee KY, Fu SB. Reduced expression and novel splice variants of ING4 in human gastric adenocarcinoma. J Pathol 219:87-95, 2009

[62] Wang QS, Li M, Zhang LY, Jin Y, Tong DD, Yu Y, Bai J, Huang Q, Liu FL, Liu A, Lee KY, Fu SB. Down-regulation of ING4 is associated with initiation and progression of lung cancer. Histopathology 57:271-81, 2010

[63] You Q, Wang XS, Fu SB, Jin XM. Downregulated Expression of Inhibitor of Growth 4 (ING4) in Advanced Colorectal Cancers: A Non-Randomized Experimental Study. Pathol Oncol Res. 2011 May 31. [Epub ahead of print]

[64] Xing YN, Yang X, Xu XY, Zheng Y, Xu HM, Takano Y, Zheng HC. The altered expression of ING5 protein is involved in gastric carcinogenesis and subsequent progression. Hum Pathol 42:25-35, 2011

[65] Zheng HC, Xia P, Xu XY, Takahashi H, Takano Y. The nuclear to cytoplasmic shift of ING5 protein during colorectal carcinogenesis with their distinct links to pathologic behaviors of carcinomas. Hum Pathol 42:424-33, 2011

[66] Krishnamurthy J, Kannan K, Feng J, Mohanprasad BK, Tsuchida N, Shanmugam G. Mutational analysis of the candidate tumor suppressor gene ING1 in Indian oral squamous cell carcinoma. Oral Oncol 37:222–224, 2001

[67] Borkosky SS, Gunduz M, Nagatsuka H, Beder LB, Gunduz E, Ali MA, Rodriguez AP, Cilek MZ, Tominaga S, Yamanaka N, Shimizu K, Nagai N. Frequent deletion of ING2 locus at 4q35.1 associates with advanced tumor stage in head and neck squamous cell carcinoma. J Cancer Res Clin Oncol 135:703-13, 2009

[68] Gunduz M, Beder LB, Gunduz E, Nagatsuka H, Fukushima K, Pehlivan D, Cetin E, Yamanaka N, Nishizaki K, Shimizu K, Nagai N. Downregulation of ING3 mRNA expression predicts poor prognosis in head and neck cancer. Cancer Sci 99:531-8, 2008

[69] Li XH, Kikuchi K, Zheng Y, Noguchi A, Takahashi H, Nishida T, Masuda S, Yang XH, Takano Y. Downregulation and translocation of nuclear ING4 is correlated with tumorigenesis and progression of head and neck squamous cell carcinoma. Oral Oncol 47:217-23, 2011

[70] Li X, Nishida T, Noguchi A, Zheng Y, Takahashi H, Yang X, Masuda S, Takano Y. Decreased nuclear expression and increased cytoplasmic expression of ING5 may be linked to tumorigenesis and progression in human head and neck squamous cell carcinoma. J Cancer Res Clin Oncol 136:1573-83, 2010

[71] Salmena L, Pandolfi PP. Changing venues for tumour suppression: balancing destruction and localization by monoubiquitylation. Nat. Rev. Cancer 7(6):409-413, 2007

[72] Hood JK, Silver PA. Diverse nuclear transport pathways regulate cell proliferation and oncogenesis. Biochim Biophys Acta 1471(1):M31-41, 2000

[73] Tiligada E. Nuclear translocation during the cross-talk between cellular stress, cell cycle and anticancer agents. Curr Med Chem 13(11):1317-1320, 2006

[74] Fabbro M, Henderson BR. Regulation of tumor suppressors by nuclear-cytoplasmic shuttling. Exp Cell Res 282(2):59-69, 2003

[75] Nouman GS, Anderson JJ, Lunec J, Angus B. The role of the tumour suppressor p33 ING1b in human neoplasia. J Clin Pathol 56(7):491-496, 2003

[76] Gunduz E, Gunduz M, Nagatsuka H et al. Epigenetic alterations of BRG1 leads to cancer development through its nuclear-cytoplasmic shuttling abnormalities. Med Hypotheses 67(6):1313-1316, 2006

[77] Nouman GS, Anderson JJ, Mathers ME et al. Nuclear to cytoplasmic compartment shift of the p33ING1b tumour suppressor protein is associated with malignancy in melanocytic lesions. Histopathology 40(4):360-366, 2002

[78] Nouman GS, Anderson JJ, Crosier S et al. Downregulation of nuclear expression of the p33 (ING1b) inhibitor of growth protein in invasive carcinoma of the breast. J Clin Pathol 56(7):507-11, 2003

[79] Nouman GS, Anderson JJ, Wood KM et al. Loss of nuclear expression of the p33 (ING1b) inhibitor of growth protein in childhood acute lymphoblastic leukaemia. J Clin Pathol 55(8):596-601, 2002

[80] Vieyra D, Senger DL, Toyama T et al. Altered subcellular localization and low frequency of mutations of ING1 in human brain tumors. Clin Cancer Res 1:5952-5961, 2003

[81] Scott M, Boisvert FM, Vieyra D, Johnston RN, Bazett-Jones DP, Riabowol K. UV induces nucleolar translocation of ING1 through two distinct nucleolar targeting sequences. Nucleic Acids Res 29:2052–2058, 2001

[82] Leung KM, Po LS, Tsang FC et al. The candidate tumor suppressor ING1b can stabilize p53 by disrupting the regulation of p53 by MDM2. Cancer Res 62:4890–4893, 2002

[83] Nikolaev AY, Li M, Puskas N, Qin J Gu W. Parc: a cytoplasmic anchor for p53. Cell 10:29-40, 2003

[84] Russell MW, Soliman MA, Schriemer D, Riabowol K. ING1 protein targeting to the nucleus by karyopherins is necessary for activation of p21. Biochem Biophys Res Commun 26:490-495, 2008

[85] Wang Y, Dai DL, Martinka M, Li G. Prognostic significance of nuclear ING3 expression in human cutaneous melanoma. Clin Cancer Res 13(14):4111-4116, 2007

[86] Lu F, Dai DL, Martinka M, Ho V, Li G. Nuclear ING2 expression is reduced in human cutaneous melanomas. Br J Cancer 95(1):80-86, 2006

[87] Tsai KW, Tseng HC, Lin WC. Two wobble-splicing events affect ING4 protein subnuclear localization and degradation. Exp Cell Res 314(17):3130-3141, 2008

[88] Shen JC, Unoki M, Ythier D et al. Inhibitor of growth 4 suppresses cell spreading and cell migration by interacting with a novel binding partner, liprin alpha1. Cancer Res 67:2552-2558, 2007

[89] Verri C, Roz L, Conte D et al. Fragile histidine triad gene inactivation in lung cancer: the European Early Lung Cancer project. Am J Respir Crit Care Med 179(5):396-401, 2009

[90] Chang SS, Califano J. Current status of biomarkers in head and neck cancer. J Surg Oncol 97(8):640-643, 2008

[91] Pang JZ, Qin LX, Ren N et al. Loss of heterozygosity at D8S298 is a predictor for long-term survival of patients with tumor-node-metastasis stage I of hepatocellular carcinoma. Clin Cancer Res 13(24):7363-7369, 2007

[92] Bartoletti R, Cai T, Nesi G, Roberta Girardi L, Baroni G, Dal Canto M. Loss of P16 expression and chromosome 9p21 LOH in predicting outcome of patients affected by superficial bladder cancer. J Surg Res 143(2):422-427, 2007

[93] Fromont G, Valeri A, Cher M et al. Allelic loss at 16q23.2 is associated with good prognosis in high grade prostate cancer. Prostate 65(4):341-346, 2005

[94] Katase N, Gunduz M, Beder L et al. Deletion at Dickkopf (dkk)-3 locus (11p15.2) is related with lower lymph node metastasis and better prognosis in head and neck squamous cell carcinomas. Oncol Res 17(6):273-282, 2008

[95] Li JN, Feng CJ, Lu YJ et al. mRNA expression of the DNA replication-initiation proteins in epithelial dysplasia and squamous cell carcinoma of the tongue. BMC Cancer 8:395-402, 2008

[96] Gunduz E, Gunduz M, Beder L et al. Downregulation of TESTIN and its association with cancer history and a tendency toward poor survival in head and neck squamous cell carcinoma. Arch Otolaryngol Head Neck Surg 135(3):254-260, 2009

[97] Ota K, Fujimori H, Ueda M et al. Midkine as a prognostic biomarker in oral squamous cell carcinoma. Br J Cancer 99(4):655-662, 2008

[98] De Maria S, Pannone G, Bufo P et al. Survivin gene-expression and splicing isoforms in oral squamous cell carcinoma. J Cancer Res Clin Oncol 135(1):107-116, 2009

[99] Ye H, Yu T, Temam S, Ziober BL et al. Transcriptomic dissection of tongue squamous cell carcinoma. BMC Genomics 9:69-79, 2008

[100] Kurokawa A, Nagata M, Kitamura N et al. Diagnostic value of integrin alpha3, beta4, and beta5 gene expression levels for the clinical outcome of tongue squamous cell carcinoma. Oral, Maxillofacial Pathology and Surgery Group. Cancer 112(6):1272-1281, 2008

[101] Roversi G, Pfundt R, Moroni RF et al. Identification of novel genomic markers related to progression to glioblastoma through genomic profiling of 25 primary glioma cell lines. Oncogene 25(10):1571-1583, 2006

[102] Takahashi M, Ozaki T, Todo S, Nakagawara A. Decreased expression of the candidate tumor suppressor gene ING1 is associated with poor prognosis in advanced neuroblastomas. Oncol Rep 12:811-816, 2004

[103] Ahmed IA, Kelly SB, Anderson JJ, Angus B, Challen C, Lunec J. The predictive value of p53 and p33 (ING1b) in patients with Dukes'C colorectal cancer. Colorectal Dis 10:344-351, 2008

[104] Almadori G, Bussu F, Paludetti G. Should there be more molecular staging of head and neck cancer to improve the choice of treatments and thereby improve survival? Curr Opin Otolaryngol Head Neck Surg 16(2):117-126, 2008

[105] Saito K, Khan K, Yu SZ et al. The predictive and therapeutic value of thymidine phosphorylase and dihydropyrimidine dehydrogenase in capecitabine (Xeloda)-based chemotherapy for head and neck cancer. Laryngoscope 119(1):82-88, 2009

[106] Gosepath EM, Eckstein N, Hamacher A et al. Acquired cisplatin resistance in the head-neck cancer cell line Cal27 is associated with decreased DKK1 expression and can partially be reversed by overexpression of DKK1. Int J Cancer 123(9):2013-2019, 2008

[107] Zhu JJ, Li FB, Zhu XF, Liao WM. The p33ING1b tumor suppressor cooperates with p53 to induce apoptosis in response to etoposide in human osteosarcoma cells. Life Sci 78(13):1469-1477, 2006

[108] Zhu JJ, Li FB, Zhou JM, Liu ZC, Zhu XF, Liao WM. The tumor suppressor p33ING1b enhances taxol-induced apoptosis by p53-dependent pathway in human osteosarcoma U2OS cells. Cancer Biol Ther 4(1):39-47, 2005

[109] Cheung KJ Jr, Li G. The tumour suppressor p33ING1 does not enhance camptothecin-induced cell death in melanoma cells. Int J Oncol 20(6):1319-1322, 2002

[110] Tallen UG, Truss M, Kunitz F et al. Down-regulation of the inhibitor of growth 1 (ING1) tumor suppressor sensitizes p53-deficient glioblastoma cells to cisplatin-induced cell death. J Neurooncol 86:23–30, 2008

[111] Zhang X, Xu LS, Wang ZQ, Wang KS et al. ING4 induces G2/M cell cycle arrest and enhances the chemosensitivity to DNA-damage agents in HepG2 cells. FEBS Lett 570(1-3):7-12, 2004

[112] Liu E, Wu J, Cao W et al. Curcumin induces G2/M cell cycle arrest in a p53-dependent manner and upregulates ING4 expression in human glioma. J Neurooncol 85(3):263-270, 2007

[113] Shinoura N, Muramatsu Y, Nishimura M et al. Adenovirus-mediated transfer of p33ING1 with p53 drastically augments apoptosis in gliomas. Cancer Res 59(21):5521-5528, 1999

[114] Shimada H, Liu TL, Ochiai T et al. Facilitation of adenoviral wild-type p53-induced apoptotic cell death by overexpression of p33 (ING1) in T.Tn human esophageal carcinoma cells. Oncogene 14:1208-1216, 2002

[115] Xie Y, Zhang H, Sheng W, Xiang J, Ye Z, Yang J. Adenovirus-mediated ING4 expression suppresses lung carcinoma cell growth via induction of cell cycle alteration and apoptosis and inhibition of tumor invasion and angiogenesis. Cancer Lett 18:105-116, 2008

[116] Xie YF, Sheng W, Xiang J, Zhang H, Ye Z, Yang J. Adenovirus-mediated ING4 expression suppresses pancreatic carcinoma cell growth via induction of cell-cycle alteration, apoptosis, and inhibition of tumor angiogenesis. Cancer Biother Radiopharm 24(2):261-269, 2009

5

Cell Signalings and the Communications in Head and Neck Cancer

Yuh Baba[1,2,3], Masato Fujii[2], Yutaka Tokumaru[2] and Yasumasa Kato[3]
[1]*Department of Otolaryngology, Ohtawara Red Cross Hospital, Ohtawara*
[2]*National Institute of Sensory Organs, National Tokyo Medical Center, Tokyo*
[3]*Department of Oral Function and Molecular Biology, Ohu University, Misumido Tomita-machi Koriyama, Japan*

1. Introduction

HNSCC (head and neck squamous cell carcinoma) is the sixth most common neoplasm worldwide (Cripps et al., 2010). Approximately 600,000 new cases are reported each year (Cripps et al., 2010), and in the past 30 years recurrent and/ or metastatic HNSCC has had a poor prognosis (Forastiere et al., 2001; Khuri et al., 2000). More than 50% of newly diagnosed patients do not achieve complete remission, and in approximately 10% of HNSCC cases relapse with metastasis to distant organs has been reported (van Houten et al., 2000). Therefore, research focused on gaining a better understanding of this disease and the development of novel treatment strategies is required.

Epidermal growth factor receptor (EGFR), a ubiquitously expressed transmembrane glycoprotein belonging to the ErbB/HER family of receptor tyrosine kinases (TK), is composed of an extracellular ligand-binding domain, a hydrophobic transmembrane segment and an intracellular TK domain. When ligands bind to EGFR the receptor undergoes a conformational change that promotes homo- or hetero-dimerization with other members of the ErbB/HER family of receptors; subsequent autophosphorylation and activation of the TK domain ensues (Ciardiello & Tortora, 2003). Activation of EGFR leads to activation of intracellular signaling pathways that regulate cell proliferation, invasion, angiogenesis and metastasis.

EGFR is expressed at high levels in the majority of epithelial malignancies including HNSCC. Elevated expression of EGFR in HNSCC correlates with poor prognosis, and it has long been a target of anticancer treatments owing to its critical role in cell survival and proliferation. Numerous tyrosine kinase inhibitors with the Food and Drug Administration (FDA) approval have been developed to target EGFR including gefitinib, erlotinib and lapatinib (Carter et al., 2009). These molecules are reversible competitors, competing with ATP for the tyrosine kinase binding domain of EGFR. By inhibiting receptor activation, downstream signaling pathways are inhibited, leading to a decrease in cell proliferation and survival. EGFR signaling activates a number of downstream effectors including the phosphatidylinositol-3-kinase (PI3Kinase)/ Akt pathway.

2. Rare EGFR mutations in HNSCC

Somatic mutations in the TK domain of the *EGFR* gene (in-frame deletion in exon 19, L858, G719X and L861Q) are associated with increased sensitivity to EGFR tyrosine kinase inhibitors (TKIs) and are present in 10~30% of non-small cell lung carcinoma (NSCLC) cases depending on ethnic origin. These mutant EGFRs selectively activate signal transduction and activator of transcription (STAT) signaling pathways and Akt, which promote cell survival. However, they have no effect on extracellular signal-regulated kinase signaling, which induces proliferation. Furthermore, mutant EGFRs selectively transduce survival signals, and inhibition of those signals by TKIs could contribute to the efficacy of a drug used to treat NSCLC (Sordella et al., 2004). However, molecular analysis of HNSCC tumor samples has not revealed the same spectrum of mutations (Loeffler-Ragg et al., 2006; Ozawa et al., 2009; Taguchi et al., 2008).

A resistance mutation has emerged in EGFR and is known as T790M. It is a missense mutation in the kinase domain that could help to explain resistance to TKIs in NSCLCs exhibiting L858R (Wong, 2008). However, we did not detect this mutation in 86 HNSCC tumor samples (Baba et al., 2011).

3. Inhibition of PI synthesis in HNSCC

3.1 Anti-proliferation

An imbalance between G1 cyclin and CDK (cyclin-dependent kinase) inhibitors (CKIs) contributes to tumorigenesis and tumor progression. Cyclin D1/PRAD1 acts as a positive regulator of the cell cycle via phosphorylaton of pRB (Rb protein), and the formation of a cyclin D1-CDK4 complex. When pRB is hyperphosphorylated by CDKs, pRB release E2F, and E2F is necessary for the activation of a gene expression network that regulates entry and progression through S phase.

CKIs are classified into two groups: members of the Ink4 family (p15, p16, p18, and p19) for cyclin D/CDK4 or cyclin D/CDK6, and the cip/kip family (p21, p27, and p57) for cyclin D/CDK4 and cyclin E/CDK2 (Baba et al., 2000a). Over-expression of cyclin D1 in HNSCC is an important prognostic marker, predicting sensitivity to chemotherapy and radiotherapy (Fujii et al., 2001; Ishiguro et al., 2003; Nishimura et al., 1998). Furthermore, imbalance between cyclin D1 and its inhibitors (p16 and p27) could be critical in the development of HNSCC (Baba et al., 1999, 2001a). Strategies to block cyclin D1 function have been studied extensively; for example, Nakashima et al. (Nakashima & Clayman, 2000) reported that introduction of an antisense cyclin D1 expression vector into cells reduced their growth rate *in vitro* and decreased tumorigenicity in athymic nude mice. We have previously reported that inhibition of PI synthesis caused G1 arrest of HNSCC accompanied by decreased levels of cyclin D1, cyclin E and phosphorylated pRB (Baba et al., 2001b).

3.2 Inhibition of matrix metalloproteinase (MMP) production/ activity

Tumor metastasis is a complex multistep process including growth at the primary site, entry into the circulation (intravasation), adhesion to the basement membranes (BM) of target organs, extravasation and growth at secondary sites. Among these steps, the intravasation and extravasation processes involve degradation of the BM by proteinases, such as some

MMPs. MMP-9/gelatinase B and MMP-2/gelatinase A have specificity for type IV collagen, which acts as the backbone of BM, and therefore probably play a major role in degrading the BM. In HNSCC, MMP-2 and MMP-9 are associated with metastatic potential. Indeed, inhibition of MMP-2 and MMP-9 production lead to repress invasive activity of HNSCC cells (Baba et al., 2000b). Therefore, MMPs are attractive therapy targets and many drugs have been developed to prevent their extracellular matrix-degrading activities during metastasis and angiogenesis.

3.3 Anti-angiogenesis

Angiogenesis, the formation of new blood vessels from pre-existing capillaries or incorporating bone marrow-derived endothelial precursor cells into growing vessels, is associated with the malignant phenotype of cancer. In addition, it also plays a role in diverse diseases such as diabetic retinopathy, age-related macular degeneration, rheumatoid arthritis, psoriasis, atherosclerosis and restenosis (Cherrington et al., 2000). Clinical association of tumor vascularity with tumor aggressiveness has been demonstrated in a wide variety of tumor types including HNSCC. Therefore, determining microvessel density in tumor tissues can be useful in the estimation of a patient's prognosis. Inhibition of angiogenesis can repress the growth rate of tumor cells and lead to cell death resulting from reduced nutrition and oxygen supply to the tumor. VEGF (vascular endothelial growth factor), which plays a major role in many angiogenic processes, binds to its receptor Flk-1/KDR in order to stimulate endothelial cell (EC) proliferation through the phospholipase Cγ-protein kinase C-ERK (extracellular signal-regulated kinase) pathway, but not via Ras (Takahashi et al., 1999). In addition, VEGF stimulates EC migration through p38 MAPK (mitogen-activated kinase) independently of ERK (Rousseau et al., 1997). Therefore, these two major MAPK pathways are eligible targets for therapeutic reduction of angiogenesis in HNSCC.

Most clinical trials concerning anti-angiogenic agents have been conducted in patients with advanced disease that had become resistant to conventional therapies. Phase III trials of these agents have compared the efficacy of standard chemotherapy alone and in combination with an experimental angiogenesis inhibitor (Gotink & Verheul, 2010). The results of some studies were negative or controversial, but several recent clinical trials in which VEGF signaling was blocked demonstrated a significant clinical benefit (Ho & Kuo, 2007). SU11248, a tyrosine kinase inhibitor of the Flk-1/KDR receptor (VEGF receptor) and bevacizumab, a monoclonal antibody to VEGF, have been approved by FDA (Ho & Kuo, 2007). Furthermore, we have demonstrated that the inhibition of PI abrogated stimulation by VEGF on the growth and migration of human umbilical vein ECs through the ERK-cyclin D1 and p38 pathways, respectively (Baba et al., 2004). Because increased PI synthase expression is an early event in HNSCC (Kaur et al., 2010), inhibition of PI synthesis could be a potent therapeutic strategy for HNSCC (Baba et al., 2010).

4. Resistance to EGFR TKIs

In a phase II trial gefitinib was administered to patients with recurrent or metastatic HNSCC and the overall response rate was 11% (Cohen et al., 2003). Furthermore, in a similar study carried out on patients with recurrent and /or metastatic HNSCC, the response rate to erlotinib was 4% (Soulieres et al., 2004). This is suggesting that multiple intracellular signaling pathways are involving to associate tumor survival, growth, and the other malignant phenotype.

4.1 Ras mutations

Previous reports have indicated that activating K-ras mutations could induce activation of the Ras/mitogen activated protein kinase (MAPK) pathway independent of EGFR, which in turn induces resistance to TKIs (Eberhard et al., 2005). The data suggest that K-ras mutation causes insensitivity to TKIs. In HNSCC, H-ras mutations are more common than K-ras mutations and may play an important role in resistance to EGFR-targeted therapies (Anderson et al., 1994).

4.2 Epithelial-Mesenchymal Transition (EMT)

EMT, a change in the morphology and motility of cells that is indicated by increased vimentin expression, decreased expression of E-cadherin and increased expression of claudins 4 and 7, has been associated with gefitinib resistance in HNSCC (Frederick et al., 2007).

4.3 Upregulation of cyclin D1

Upregulation of cyclin D1 in HNSCC cell lines is specifically associated with resistance to gefitinib; retinoblastoma protein (pRb) is hyperphosphorylated by cyclin D1-cyclin dependent kinase 4 (CDK4) (Kalish et al., 2004).

4.4 Cortactin

Recently, increased expression of cortactin, a protein that increases the formation of actin networks critical to cell motility and receptor-mediated endocytosis, has been associated with gefitinib resistance and increased metastasis in HNSCC (Timpson et al., 2007).

Akt has been implicated in EMT by integrin-linked kinase (ILK). The PI3Kinase/Akt pathway not only regulates the transcriptional activity of cyclin D1, but also increases its accumulation by inactivating glycogen synthase kinase-3 (GSK3), which targets cyclin D1 for proteasomal degradation. The effect of cortactin on cancer cell proliferation is associated with increased activation of Akt (Timpson et al., 2007). Therefore, factors related to resistance to EGFR TKIs are associated with the PI3kinase/Akt pathway.

5. PI3kinase/Akt pathway

5.1 Activation of the PI3kinase/Akt pathway

Signaling through the PI3kinase/Akt pathway can be initiated by several mechanisms, all of which increase activation of the pathway in cancer cells. Once activated, the PI3kinase/Akt pathway can be propagated to various substrates including mTOR, a master regulator of protein translation. The pathway is initially activated at the cell membrane, where the signal for activation is propagated through class IA PI3kinase. Activation of PI3kinase can occur through tyrosine kinase receptor for EGF and insulin-like growth factor-1 (IGF-1). Integrins and G-protein-coupled receptors (GPCRS) are also known to activate it. PI3kinase catalyzes phosphorylation of the D3 position on phosphoinositides to generate the biologically active moieties phosphatidylinositol-3,4,5-triphosphate (PI(3,4,5)P3) and phosphatidylinositol-3,4-bisphosphate (PI(3,4)P2). PI(3,4,5)P3 binds to the pleckstrin homology (PH) domains of PDK-1 (3′-phosphoinositide-dependent kinase 1) and Akt, resulting in the proteins being translocated to the cell membrane where they are subsequently activated. The tumor suppressor PTEN (phosphatase and tensin homolog deleted on chromosome ten) antagonizes PI3kinase by dephosphorylating PI (3,4,5)P3 and (PI(3,4)P2), thereby preventing activation of Akt and PDK-1. Akt exists as three structurally similar isoforms, Akt1, Akt2 and Akt3, which are expressed in most tissues. Activation of Akt1 occurs through two crucial phosphorylation events. The first, carried out by PDK-1, occurs at T308 in the catalytic domain. Full activation requires a subsequent phosphorylation at S473 in the hydrophobic motif, which can be mediated by several kinases including PDK-1, ILK, Akt itself, DNA-dependent protein kinase and mTOR; phosphorylation of homologous residues in Akt2 and Akt3 occurs by the same mechanism. Phosphorylation of Akt at S473 is controlled by a recently described phosphatase, PHLPP (PH domain leucine-rich repeat protein phosphatase), that has two isoforms that preferentially decrease activation of specific Akt isoforms (Brognard et al., 2007). Amplification of Akt1 has been described in human gastric adenocarcinoma, and amplification of Akt2 has been described in ovarian, breast and pancreatic carcinoma (Bellacosa et al., 1995; Cheng et al., 1996). Although Akt mutations are rare, Carpten *et al.* (Carpten et al., 2007) recently described somatic mutations occurring in the PH domain of Akt1 in a small percentage of human breast, ovarian and colorectal cancers.

5.2 Downstream substrates of activated Akt

Akt recognizes and phosphorylates the consensus sequence RXRXX (S/T) when it is surrounded by hydrophobic residues. This sequence is present in many proteins resulting in numerous Akt substrates being identified and validated. These substrates control key cellular processes such as apoptosis, cell cycle progression, transcription and translation. For example, Akt phosphorylates the FoxO subfamily of forkhead family transcription factors, inhibiting transcription of several pro-apoptotic genes including Fas-L, IGF Binding Protein1 (IGFBP1) and Bim. Additionally, Akt can directly regulate apoptosis by phosphorylating and inactivating pro-apoptotic proteins such as BAD, which controls the release of cytochrome c from mitochondria, and apoptosis signal-regulating kinase-1 (ASK1), a mitogen-activated protein kinase kinase involved in stress- and cytokine-induced cell death. In contrast, Akt can phosphorylate IkappaBalpha kinase (IKK), which indirectly increases the activity of nuclear factor kappa B (NFκB) and stimulates the transcription of pro-survival genes. Cell cycle progression can also be affected by Akt; inhibitory phosphorylation of the cyclin-dependent kinase inhibitors p21 and p27, and inhibition of GSK3β by Akt, stimulates cell cycle progression by stabilizing cyclin D1 expression. A novel pro-survival Akt substrate, PRAS40 (proline-rich Akt substrate of 40kDa), has been described recently (Vander Haar et al., 2007). Phosphorylation of PRAS40 by Akt attenuates its ability to inhibit mTORC1 kinase activity. It has been suggested that PRAS40 could be a specific substrate of Akt3 (Madhunapantula et al., 2007). Therefore, Akt inhibition could have pleiotropic effects on cancer cells that contribute to an anti-tumor response. The most-studied downstream substrate of Akt is the serine/threonine kinase mTOR (mammalian target of rapamycin). Akt can directly phosphorylate and activate mTOR, and indirectly activate it by phosphorylating and inactivating TSC2 (tuberous sclerosis complex 2, also called tuberin), which normally inhibits mTOR through the GTP binding protein Rheb (Ras homolog enriched in brain) (Inoki et al., 2003). When TSC2 is inactivated by phosphorylation, the GTPase Rheb is maintained in its GTP-bound state, allowing increased activation of mTOR (Inoki et al., 2005). mTOR exists in two complexes: the TORC1 complex, in which mTOR is bound to Raptor; and the TORC2 complex, in which mTOR is bound to Rictor. In the TORC1 complex, mTOR signals to its downstream effectors S6 kinase/ribosomal protein and 4EBP-1/eIF-4E, to control protein translation (Inoki et al., 2005). mTOR is generally considered to be a downstream substrate of Akt, but it can phosphorylate Akt when bound to Rictor in TORC2 complexes (Sarbassov et al., 2005), and this could provide positive feedback in the pathway. In addition, the downstream mTOR effector S6 kinase-1 (S6K1) can regulate the pathway by catalyzing an inhibitory phosphorylation on insulin receptor substrate (IRS) proteins. This prevents IRS proteins from activating PI3kinase, thereby inhibiting activation of Akt (Harrington et al., 2004).

5.3 Rationale for targeting the PI3kinase/Akt pathway

In addition to preclinical studies, clinical observations support the targeting of the PI3kinae/Akt/mTOR pathway in human cancer (Vogt et al., 2009). Immunohistochemical studies using antibodies that recognize Akt phosphorylated at S473 have demonstrated that activated Akt is detectable in cancers including head and neck cancer (Gupta et al., 2002). Tsurutani *et al.* (Tsurutani et al., 2006) recently extended these studies using antibodies against S473 and T308, two sites of Akt phosphorylation. This study demonstrated that Akt activation is selective for NSCLC versus normal tissue, and that phosphorylation of Akt at both sites is a better predictor of poor prognosis in NSCLC than phosphorylation of S473 alone. In addition, amplification of Akt isoforms has been observed in some cancers, albeit at a lower frequency. Another frequent genetic event occurring in human cancer is loss of function of the tumor suppressor PTEN. PTEN normally suppresses activation of the PI3kinase/Akt/mTOR pathway by functioning as a lipid phosphatase. Loss of PTEN function in cancer can occur through mutation, deletion or epigenetic silencing. In tumor types where PTEN mutations are rare such as lung cancer, epigenetic silencing can occur (Forgacs et al., 1998). Several studies have demonstrated the prognostic significance of PTEN loss in multiple human cancers where mutation, deletion or epigenetic silencing of PTEN correlates with poor prognosis and reduced survival (Bertram et al., 2006). Collectively, these studies have established that the loss of PTEN is a common mechanism for activation of the PI3kinase/Akt/mTOR pathway and led to poor prognostic factor in human cancer. Activation of PI3Kinase has been described in human cancers. It can result from amplification, over-expression, or mutations in the p110 catalytic or p85 regulatory subunits. Amplification of the 3q26 chromosomal region, which contains the gene PI3KCA that encodes the p110α catalytic subunit of PI3K, occurs in 40% of ovarian and 50% of cervical carcinomas (Ma et al., 2000; Shayesteh et al., 1999). Somatic mutations of this gene have been detected in several cancer types and result in increased kinase activity of mutant PI3K relative to wild-type PI3K (Samuels & Ericson, 2006). Mutations in the regulatory p85 subunit have also been detected. Any of the aforementioned alterations in individual components would result in activation of the PI3 kinase/Akt pathway, and studies suggest that pathway activation is one of the most frequent molecular alterations that occur in cancer (Samuels & Ericson, 2006).

6. Cross talk between the IGF1 receptor (IGF1R) and EGF receptor (EGFR) pathways through PI3 kinase/Akt

The phenomenon of growth factors switching from one pathway to another has an adaptive component, which could be induced by blocking the dominant growth factor receptor pathway. Blockade of EGFR signaling has been demonstrated to result in the enhancement of the growth promoting effects of the peptide growth factor ligands basic fibroblast growth factor and IGF-1 in DU145 and PC-3 human prostate cancer cells, respectively (Jones et al., 1997). More recently, the substantial growth inhibitory effects of the EGFR-selective tyrosine kinase inhibitor gefitinib on EGFR-positive MCF-7-derived tamoxifen-resistant breast cancer cells, has been demonstrated. Furthermore, this effect can be subverted by additionally exposing cells to non-EGF ligands such as heregulin-β and IGF-II (Knowlden et al., 2005). The reversal of the anti-tumor effects of gefitinib by IGF-II, acting through the IGF-1R, is accompanied by a reactivation of the previously reduced activity of Akt and extracellular-regulated kinase (ERK); ERK signaling contributes to the re-establishment of tumor cell growth. Therefore, in the presence of a dominant growth pathway, cancer cells are capable of responding to other growth factors that are present, thereby compromising the anti-tumor activity of agents designed specifically to inhibit EGFR. Importantly, a previous study demonstrated that following blockade of EGFR signaling, switching to the IGF-1R pathway is a common mechanism used to promote resistance to anti-EGFR treatment (Choi et al., 2010). For example, gefitinib initially inhibited the growth of the EGFR-positive cell lines DU145 (prostate cancer cells) and MCF-7-derived tamoxifen- and fulvestrant resistant breast cancer cell lines, but chronic challenge with the inhibitor resulted in the development of gefitinib-resistant variant sub-lines, all of which presented with up-regulation of multiple IGF-1R signaling components when compared with the parental cell lines (Jones et al., 2004). This resulted in increased production and elevated expression of the IGF-1R ligand IGF-II, increased activity of IGF-1R and increased levels of Akt activity. In addition, the A549 lung cancer cell line, which displays a partial sensitivity to gefitinib, was chronically challenged with the inhibitor; the resistant variant that emerged presented with a marked adaptive increase in the activity of elements of the IGF-1R pathway. The importance of IGF-1R signaling in these various cell types with acquired gefitinib resistance was further supported by the observation that they demonstrated an enhanced dependency on IGF-1R signaling; they were subsequently more sensitive to growth inhibition by IGF-1R-selective tyrosine kinase inhibitors (Jones et al., 2004). Therefore, the dominance of the EGFR pathway in parental cells is replaced by the elevated use of the IGF-1R in gefitinib resistant cells. However, such growth factor pathway switching can not only result from changes occurring during the development of acquired resistance, but also, critically, can occur rapidly and modulate initial sensitivity to EGFR-blockade resulting in *de novo* or intrinsic resistance to anti-EGFR agents such as gefitinib. Indeed, although the EGFR and

IGF-1R pathways are classically regarded as separate entities, promoting growth utilizing overlapping downstream signal transduction molecules indicates that these receptors can affect each other's signaling abilities, although the precise mechanisms involved in this crosstalk have not been fully elucidated. For example, gefitinib only partially blocks EGFR activity in A549 lung cancer cells and this is accompanied by a dramatic increase in the activity but not the expression of IGF-1R. Moreover, in these cells IGF-1R can transphosphorylate EGFR, maintaining EGFR activity in the presence of gefitinib. Therefore, gefitinib limits its own efficacy by facilitating IGF-1R activity in these cells. Interestingly, it was observed that in de novo gefitinib-resistant LoVo colorectal cancer cells, which are defective in terms of ability to produce mature IGF-1R and predominantly express insulin receptor-isoform A (InsR-A), a close family member of the IGF-1R, insulin receptor activity is increased and downstream activated Akt levels are elevated in the presence of gefitinib (Jones et al., 2006). Furthermore, InsR can modulate and maintain EGFR phosphorylation in these cells. Such rapid and dynamic interplay between EGFR and IGF-1R or InsR could play an important role in limiting the anti-tumor activity of gefitinib; partial and de novo resistance to the inhibitor has been demonstrated in A549 and LoVo cells, respectively.

In HNSCC, it has been found that the use of the combination of both IGF-1R and EGFR antibodies was more effective than either single agent alone at reducing cancer cell growth (Barnes et al., 2007). There may be a potential benefit in the use of combined anti-tyrosine kinase receptor directed therapies to treat HNSCC. Slomiany *et al.* also demonstrated the potential for the co-targeting of both IGF-1R and EGFR signaling in HNSCC (Slomiany et al., 2007). Furthermore, Rebucci *et al.* reported that the combination of cetuximab with a PI3K inhibitor could be a good therapeutic option in HNSCC (Rebucci et al., 2011).

7. Cross talk between the NFκB and STAT3 signaling pathways

Of interest, whereas the activation of EGFR leads to the rapid tyrosine phosphorylation of STAT3 in tyrosine705 and the consequent activation of STAT3-dependent gene expression, it was observed that STAT3 tyrosine phosphorylation and the formation of active STAT3 DNA-binding complexes are insensitive to the inhibition of EGFR in a large fraction of HNSCC cell lines (Sriuranpong et al., 2003). Indeed, 9 of 10 cell lines form a representative panel of HNSCC-derived cells showing increased tyrosine phosphorylation and activity of STAT3, but constitutive activity of EGFR was present in only 3 of them (Sriuranpong et al., 2003). In search for the mechanism responsible for the EGFR-independent activation of STAT3 in HNSCC cells, it was observed that the activation of the gp130 cytokine receptor subunit promoted the phosphorylation of STAT3 in tyrosine 705 through the activation of intracellular tyrosine kinases of the JAK family. Suprisingly, the activation of gp 130 was found to be primarily initiated by IL-6, which, on its secretion and release on the cell surface of HNSCC cells in an autocrine fashion. These findings suggest that the persistent activation of STAT3 in HNSCC can result from the deregulated activity of EGFR or from the autocrine activation of STAT3 by tumor-released cytokines in an EGFR-independent fashion. Furthermore, it was found that overexpression of IL-6 in HNSCC cells involves increased transcription from the IL-6 promoter, which is dependent on the presence of an intact NFκB response element located 63 to 75 bp upstream of the IL-6 transcriptional initiation site. Furthermore, inhibition of NFκB led to a remarkable downregulation of IL-6 gene and protein expression, concomitant with a decreased release of other inflammatory cytokines, such as IL-8, IL-10, granulocyte-macrophage colony-stimulating factor (GM-CSF), and granulocyte colony-stimulating factor (G-CSF). Surprisingly, the blockade of NFκB led also to a drastic inhibition of the constitutive STAT3 activity in HNSCC cells, as reflected by the reduced tyrosine phosphorylation of STAT3. Interestingly, interfering with NFκB function also prevented the autocrine/paracrine activation of STAT3 in HNSCC cells (Squarize et al., 2006). These findings support a cross-talk between the NFκB and the STAT3 signaling systems. This cross-talk is initiated by the release of IL-6 as a consequence of the NFκB-dependent activation of the IL-6 promoter, and the subsequent tyrosine phosphorylation of STAT3 by the autocrine/paracrine activation of IL-6 receptors in tumor cells.

8. Future prospects

Signaling of multiple receptor tyrosine kinases (RTKs) is propagated through Akt. Therefore, simultaneous inhibition of EGFR with pathway components such as Akt or mTOR could circumvent the feedback activation observed with either approach alone. The most extensive data concerning proximal and distal signaling inhibition relates to combining PI3kinase/Akt/mTOR pathway inhibitors with EGFR antagonists. Several PI3kinase inhibitors can restore sensitivity to EGFR inhibitors. For example, the selective pI3kinase inhibitor PX-866 and p110α can abolish gefitinib resistance in NSCLC xenografts (Ihle et al., 2005). Synergistic effects of rapamycin and EGFR TKIs have been observed in several *in vitro* systems including glioblastoma multiforme, prostate cancer, pancreatic cancer, squamous cell carcinoma, renal cell carcinoma, leukemia, cervical carcinoma and NSCLC (Birle & Hedley, 2006; Buck et al., 2006; Costa et al., 2007; Hjelmeland et al., 2007; Jimeno et al., 2007; Mohi et al., 2004). Several studies extended efficacy of these combinations in the xenograft experiments. Buck *et al.* (Buck et al., 2006) showed re-sensitization and synergistic growth inhibition with the combination of rapamycin and erlotinib in cell lines that were previously resistant to erlotinib. Li *et al.* noted significant regression of lung tumors in transgenic mice possessing the secondary resistance mutation T790M when treated with a combination of rapamycin and the irreversible EGFR TKI, HKI-272 (Li et al., 2007). In human glioma cell lines with mutant PTEN, addition of the dual PI3kinase/mTOR inhibitor PI-103 to erlotinib was necessary to induce growth arrest (Fan et al., 2007), suggesting that activation of the PI3kinase/Akt/mTOR pathway by EGFR-independent mechanisms confers resistance to EGFR inhibitors, which can nonetheless be overcome by the addition of pathway inhibitors. Collectively, these data suggest that the use of EGFR antagonists with PI3kianse/Akt pathway inhibitors could be beneficial to patients that have developed resistance to EGFR TKIs.

However, we think that the use of EGFR antagonists with PI3kinase/Akt pathway inhibitors might allow the activation of TNFR and/or IL-1R-NFκB-IL6-STAT3 signaling (Fig1). Therefore, we recommend the use of EGFR antagonists with PI3kinase/Akt pathway inhibitors and NFκB-IL6-STAT3 pathway inhibitors.

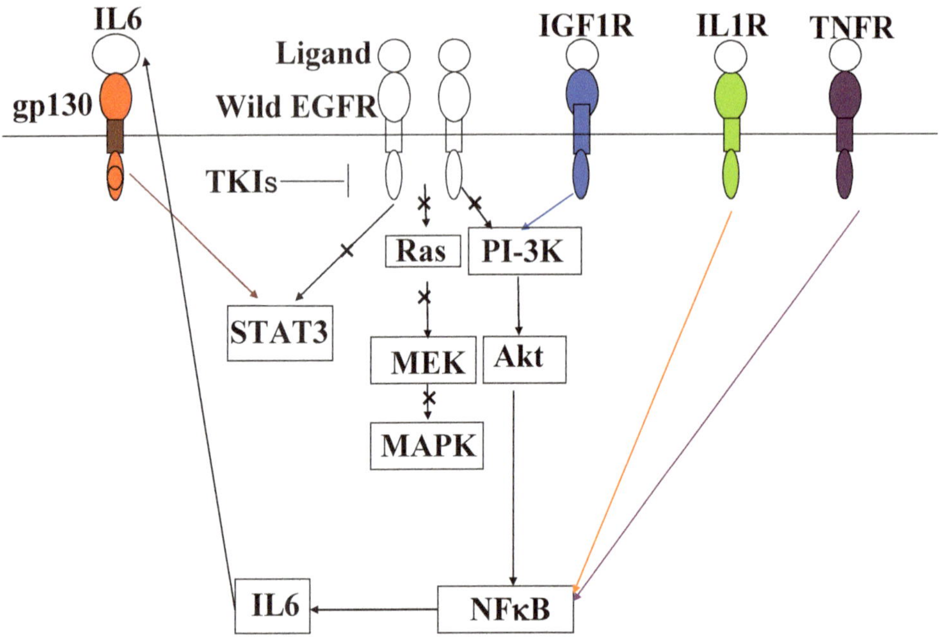

Fig. 1. Cell signalings and the communications in head and neck cancer.

9. Conclusions

EGFR is expressed at a high level in HNSCC but EGFR inhibitor monotherapy has limited success. Previous studies have demonstrated that EGFR mutations are extremely rare inHNSCC; inhibition of PI synthesis provides anti-proliferative, anti-invasive and anti-angiogenesis effects on HNSCC. The PI3kinase/Akt pathway is responsible for cellular survival and there is molecular cross-talk between EGFR and IGF1R signaling through PI3kinase/Akt in HNSCC. Furthermore, there is molecular cross-talk between the NFκB and STAT3 signaling pathways. Therefore, combination therapy targeting PI3kinase/Akt, NFκB/STAT3, and EGFR signaling pathways should provide clinical benefit for patients suffering with HNSCC (Fig. 1). Although various Akt and/or NFκB specific inhibitors have been developed, we recommend using a combination of an EGFR antagonist with numerous chemo-preventive compounds that inhibit the activation of both Akt and NFκB , as natural compounds have little side effect. Resveratrol, trans-3,5,4-trihydroxystibene, was first isolated in 1940 as a constituent of the root of white hellebore (Veratrum grandiflorum O. Loes), but has since been found in various plants including grapes, berries and peanuts. In addition to cardioprotective effects, resveratrol exhibits anticancer properties as suggested by its ability to suppress proliferation of a wide variety of tumor cells. The growth-inhibitory effects of resveratrol are mediated through cell-cycle arrest: up-regulation of p21, p53 and Bax, and down-regulation of survivin, cyclin D1, cyclin E, Bcl-2, Bcl-xl and cIAPs, and activation of caspases. Resveratrol suppresses the activation of several protein kinases including Akt (Banerjee et al., 2010), and limited data from humans suggest that it is pharmacologically safe. Furthermore, resveratrol suppresses TNF-induced activation of NFκB (Manna et al., 2000). Another chemopreventive agent whose effects on Akt signaling have been studied in some detail is the rotenoid deguelin. Deguelin is a rotenoid from the African plant Mundulea sericea (Leguminosae), which was identified as a potent chemopreventive agent on the basis of its action against chemically induced preneoplastic lesions in a mammary organ culture, and its inhibition of papillomas in a two-stage mouse skin carcinogenesis model (Nair et al., 2006). Furthermore, deguelin suppresses the formation of carcinogen-induced aberrant crypt foci in mouse colon (Murillo et al., 2003). More recently, this rotenoid was shown to suppress cigarette smoke-induced lung carcinogenesis (Lee et al., 2005), and it enhances the sensitivity of leukemia cells to chemotherapeutic agents (Bortul et al., 2005). How deguelin mediates its chemopreventive and chemosensitizing effects is not yet fully understood, but various mechanisms have been proposed including suppression of the PI3kinase/Akt pathway (Chen et al., 2009). In Akt-inducible transgenic mice, deguelin was competent at suppressing Akt activation in the lung. At doses achievable in vivo, it reduced pAkt levels, induced apoptosis and suppressed proliferation of premalignant and malignant human bronchial epithelial cells; minimal effects were observed in normal bronchial cells (Chun et al., 2003). Blockade of Akt activation is likely to contribute to the pro-apoptotic actions of deguelin in breast cancer cell lines and anti-angiogenic effects in vitro. Deguelin inhibited formation of murine lung tumors in conjunction with suppression of Akt activation in vivo (Hecht, 2005). Furthermore, deguelin suppresses NFκB activation induced by various carconogens and inflammatory stimuli including TNF and IL-1β (Nair et al., 2006). The cruciferous vegetable component indole-3-carbinol has chemopreventive activity that could be associated with down-regulation of Akt signaling (Chinni & Sarkar, 2002). Furthermore, indole-3-carbinol suppresses NFκB activation induced by various carconogens and inflammatory stimuli including TNF and IL-1β (Takada et al., 2005). Honokiol, used as a muscle relaxant, is derived from the stem and bark of the plant Magnolia officinalis, which is used in traditional Chinese and Japanese medicine. Extensive research has demonstrated that honokiol inhibits skin tumor promotion, nitric oxide synthesis, TNF expression and inhibits invasion. Furthermore, it down-regulates the anti-apoptotic protein bcl-xl, inhibits angiogenesis and tumor growth *in vivo*, induces caspase-dependent apoptosis in B-cell chronic lymphocytic leukemia cells through down-regulation of the anti-apoptotic protein Mcl-1, and overcomes drug resistance in multiple myeloma. Honokiol blocks TNF-induced NFκB activation (Ahn et al., 2006). Indeed, Honokiol inhibits EGFR signaling involving Akt and STAT3, and enhances the antitumor effects of EGFR inhibitors (Leeman-Neill et al., 2010). In conclusion, the combination of an EGFR antagonist with these chemo-preventive compounds that inhibit the activation of both Akt and NFκB may overcome the resistance to EGFR antagonist in HNSCC.

10. Acknowledgement

We thank Dr. Masaya Imoto (Keio University, Japan) for the generous gift of inostamycin. This study was supported in part by a grant-in-aid from the Ministry of Education, Culture, Sports, Science and Technology of Japan (to Y.B.).

11. References

Ahn KS, Sethi G, Shishodia S, Sung B, Arbiser JL & Aggarwal BB. (2006). Honokiol potentiates apoptosis, suppresses osteoclastogenesis, and inhibits invasion through modulation of nuclear factor kappaB activation pathway. *Mol Cancer Res,* Vol.4, No.9, (September 2006), pp. 621-633.

Anderson JA, Irish JC, Mclachlin CM & Ngan BY. (1994). H-ras oncogene mutation and human papillomavirus infection in oral carcinomas. *Arch Otolaryngol Head Neck Surg,* Vol.120, No.7, (July 1994), pp. 755-760.

Baba Y, Tsukuda M, Kagata H, Kato Y & Nagashima Y. (1999). Alteration of p16INK4a and cyclinD1 in head and neck carcinoma cell lines. *Med Sci Res,* Vol.27, (1999), pp. 479-484.

Baba Y, Tsukuda M, Kagata H, Kato Y, Nakatani Y, Ehara M, Nagashima Y, Taki A & Aoki I. (2000a). Nasal natural killer/T cell lymphoma: case report with molecular biologic examination on Epstein-Barr virus and cell cycle regulatory p16, cyclin D1, Rb, and p53 genes. *J Otolaryngol,* Vol.29, No.2, (April 2000a), pp. 121-125.

Baba Y, Tsukuda M, Mochimatsu I, Furukawa S, Kagata H, Nagashima Y, Sakai N, Koshika S, Imoto M & Kato Y. (2000b). Inostamycin, an inhibitor of cytidine5'-diphosphate1, 2-diacyl-sn-glycerol (CDP-DG): inositol transferase, suppresses invasion ability by reducing productions of matrix metalloproteinase-2 and -9 and cell motility in HSC-4 tongue carcinoma cell line. *Clin Exp Metastasis,* Vol.18, No.3, (2000b), pp. 273-279.

Baba Y, Tsukuda M, Mochimatsu I, Furukawa S, Kagata H, Satake K, Koshika S, Nakatani Y, Hara M, Kato Y & Nagashima Y. (2001a). Reduced expression of p16 and p27 proteins in nasopharyngeal carcinoma. *Cancer Detect Prev,* Vol.25, No.5, (2001a), pp. 414-419.

Baba Y, Tsukuda M, Mochimatsu I, Furukawa S, Kagata, H., Nagashima Y, Koshika S, Imoto M & Kato Y. (2001b). Cytostatic effect of inostamycin, an inhibitor of cytidine5'-diphosphate1, 2-diacyl-sn-glycerol(CDP-DG): inositol transferase, on oral squamous cell carcinoma cell lines. *Cell Biol Int,* Vol.25, No.7, (2001b), pp. 613-620.

Baba Y, Kato Y, Mochimatsu I, Nagashima Y, Kurihara M, Kawano T, Taguchi T, Hata R & Tsukuda M. (2004). Inostamycin suppresses vascular endothelial growth factor-stimulated growth and migration of human umbilical vein endothelial cells. *Clin Exp Metastasis,* Vol. 21, No.5, (2004), pp. 419-425.

Baba Y, Kato Y & Ogawa K. (2010). Inostamycin prevents malignant phenotype of cancer: inhibition of phosphatidylinositol synthesis provides a therapeutic advantage for head and neck squamous cell carcinoma. *Cell Biol Int,* Vol. 34, No.2, (January 2010), pp. 171-175.

Baba Y, Fujii M, Tokumaru Y & Kato Y. (2011). New strategy in Head and Neck Cancer: combination therapy targeting the PI3Kinase/Akt and EGFR signaling pathways. *Hypotheses in Clinical Medicine,* (2011), in press.

Banerjee Mustafi S, Chakraborty PK & Raha S. (2010). Modulation of Akt and ERK1/2 pathways by resveratrol in chronic myelogenous leukemia (CML) cells results in the downregulation of Hsp70. *PLoS One,* Vol.5, No.1, (January 2010), e8719.

Barnes CJ, Ohshiro K, Rayala SK, El-Naggar AK & Kumar R. (2007). Inulin-like growth factor receptor as a therapeutic target in head and neck cancer. *Clin Cancer Res,* Vol.13, No.14, (July 2007), pp. 4291-4299.

Bellacosa A, de Feo D, Godwin AK, Bell DW, Cheng JQ, Altomare DA, Wan M, Dubeau L, Scambia G, Masciullo V, Ferrandina G, Benedetti Panici P, Mancuso S, Neri G & Testa JR. (1995). Molecular alterations of the AKT2 oncogene in ovarian and breast carcinomas. *Int J Cancer,* Vol.64, No.4, (August 1995), pp. 280-285.

Bertram J, Peacock JW, Fazli L, Mui AL, Chung SW, Cox ME, Monia B, Gleave ME & Ong CJ. (2006). Loss of PTEN is associated with progression to androgen independence. *Prostate,* Vol.66, No.9, (June 2006), pp. 895-902.

Birle DC & Hedley DW. (2006). Signaling interactions of rapamycin combined with erlotinib in cervical carcinoma xenografts. *Mol Cancer Ther,* Vol.5, No.10, (October 2006), pp. 2494-2502.

Bortul R, Tazzari PL, Billi AM, Tabellini G, Mantovani I, Cappellini A, Grafone T, Martinelli G, Conte R & Martelli AM. (2005). Deguelin, A PI3K/AKT inhibitor, enhances chemosensitivity of leukaemia cells with an active PI3K/AKT pathway. *Br J Haematol,* Vol.129, No. 5, (June 2005), pp. 677-686.

Brognard J, Sierecki E, Gao T & Newton AC. (2007). PHLPP and second isoform, PHLPP2, differentially attenuate the amplitude of Akt signaling by regulating distinct Akt isoforms. *Mol Cell,* Vol.25, No. 6, (March 2007), pp. 917-931.

Buck E, Eyzaguirre A, Brown E, Petti F, McCormack S, Haley JD, Iwata KK, Gibson NW & Griffin G. (2006). Rapamycin synergizes with the epidermal growth factor receptor inhibitor erlotinib in non-small-cell lung, pancreatic, colon, and breast tumors. *Mol Cancer Ther,* Vol. 5, No. 11, (November 2006), pp. 2676-2684.

Carpten JD, Faber AL, Horn C, Donoho GP, Briggs SL, Robbins CM, Hostetter G, Boguslawski S, Moses TY, Savage S, Uhlik M, Lin A, Du J, Qian YW, Zeckner DJ, Tucker-Kellogg G, Touchman J, Patel K, Mousses S, Bittner M, Schevitz R, Lai MH, Blanchard KL & Thomas JE. (2007). A transforming mutation in the pleckstrin homology domain of AKT1 in cancer. *Nature,* Vol.448, No.7152, (July 2007), pp. 439-444.

Carter CA, Kelly RJ & Giaccone G. (2009). Small-molecule inhibitors of the human epidermal receptor family. *Expert Opin Investig Drugs,* Vol. 18, No. 12, (December 2009), pp. 1829-1842.

Chen Y, Wu Q, Cui GH, Chen YQ & Li R. (2009). Deguelin blocks cells survival signal pathways and induces apoptosis of HL-60 cells in vitro. *Int J Hematol,* Vol. 89, No. 5, (June 2009), pp. 618-623.

Cheng JQ, Ruggeri B, Klein WM, Sonoda G, Altomare DA, Watson DK & Testa JR. (1996). Amplification of AKT2 in human pancreatic cells and inhibition of AKT2 expression and tumorigenicity by antisense RNA. *Proc Natl Acad Sci USA,* Vol.93, No.8, (April 1996), pp. 3636-3641.

Cherrington JM, Strawn LM & Shawver LK. (2000). New paradigms for the treatment of cancer: the role of anti-angiogenesis agents. *Adv Cancer Res,* Vol. 79, (2000), pp. 1-38.

Chinni SR & Sarkar FH. (2002). Akt inactivation is a key event in indole-3-carbinol-induced apoptosis in PC-3 cells. *Clin Cancer Res,* Vol. 8, No. 4, (April 2002), pp. 1228-1236.

Choi YJ, Rho JK, Jeon BS, Choi SJ, Park SC, Lee SS, Kim HR, Kim CH & Lee JC. (2010). Combined inhibition of IGFR enhances the effects of gefitinib in H1650: a lung cancer cell line with EGFR mutation and primary resistance to EGFR-TK inhibitors. *Cancer Chemother Pharmacol,* Vol. 66, No. 2, (July 2010), pp. 381-388.

Chun KH, Kosmeder JW2nd, Sun S, Pezzuto JM, Lotan R, Hong WK & Lee HY. (2003). Effects of deguelin on the phosphatidylinositol3-kinase/Akt pathway and apoptosis in premalignant human bronchial epithelial cells. *J Natl Cancer Inst,* Vol. 95, No. 4, (February 2003), pp. 291-302.

Ciardiello F & Tortora G. Epidermal growth factor receptor (EGFR) as a target in cancer therapy: understanding the role of receptor expression and other molecular determinants that could influence the response to anti-EGFR drugs. (2003). *Eur J Cancer,* Vol. 39, No. 10, (July 2003), pp. 1348-1354.

Cohen EE, Rosen F, Sadler WM, Recant W, Stenson K, Huo D & Vokes EE. (2003). Phase II trial of ZD1839 in recurrent or metastatic squamous cell carcinoma of the head and neck. *J Clin Oncol,* Vol. 21, No. 10, (May 2003), pp. 1980-1987.

Costa LJ, Gemmill RM & Drabkin HA. (2007). Upstream signaling inhibition enhances rapamycin effect on growth of kidney cancer cells. *Urology,* Vol. 69, No. 3, (March 2007), pp. 596-602.

Cripps C, Winquist E, Devries MC, Stys-Norman D & Gilbert R. (2010). Epidermal growth factor receptor targeted therapy in stages III and IV head and neck cancer. *Curr Oncol,* Vol. 17, No. 3, (June 2010), pp. 37-48.

Eberhard DA, Johnson BE, Amler LC, Goddard AD, Heldens SL, Herbst RS, Ince WL, Janne PA, Januario T, Johnson DH, Klein P, Miller VA, Ostland MA, Ramies DA, Sebisanovic D, Stinson JA, Zhang YR, Seshagiri S & Hillan KJ. (2005). Mutations in the epidermal growth factor receptor and in KRAS are predictive and prognostic indicators in patients with non-small-cell lung cancer treated with chemotherapy alone and in combination with erlotinib. *J Clin Oncol,* Vol. 23, No. 25, (September 2005), pp. 5900-5909.

Fan QW, Cheng CK, Nicolaides TP, Hackett CS, Knight ZA, Shokat KM & Weiss WA. (2007). A dual phosphoinositide-3-kinase alpha/mTOR inhibitor cooperates with blockade of epidermal growth factor receptor in PTEN-mutant glioma. *Cancer Res,* Vol. 67, No. 17, (September 2007), pp. 7960-7965.

Forastiere A, Koch W, Trotti A & Sidransky D. (2001). Head and neck cancer. *N Engl J Med,* Vol. 345, No. 26, (December 2001), pp. 1890-1900.

Forgacs E, Biesterveld EJ, Sekido Y, Fong K, Muneer S, Wistuba II, Milchgrub S, Brezinschek R, Virmani A, Gazdar AF & Minna JD. (1998). Mutation analysis of the PTEN/MMAC1 gene in lung cancer. *Oncogene,* Vol.17, No.12, (September 1998), pp. 1557-1565.

Frederick BA, Helfrich BA, Coldren CD, Zheng D, Chan D, Bunn PA Jr & Raben D. (2007). Epithelial to mesenchymal transition predicts gefitinib resistance in cell lines of head and neck squamous cell carcinoma and non-small cell lung carcinoma. *Mol Cancer Ther,* Vol. 6, No. 6, (June 2007), pp. 1683-1691.

Fujii M, Ishiguro R, Yamashita T & Tashiro M. (2001). Cyclin D1 amplification correlates with early recurrence of squamous cell carcinoma of the tongue. *Cancer lett,* Vol.172, No.2, (October 2001), pp. 187-192.

Gotink KJ & Verheul HM. (2010). Anti-angiogenic tyrosine kinase inhibitors: what is their mechanism of action? *Angiogenesis,* Vol. 13, No. 1, (March 2010), pp. 1-14.

Gupta AK, Mckenna WG, Weber CN, Feldman MD, Goldsmith JD, Mick R, Machtay M, Rosenthal DI, Bakanauskas VJ, Cerniglia GJ, Bernhard EJ, Weber RS & Muschel RJ. (2002). Local recurrence in head and neck cancer: relationship to radiation resistance and signal transduction. *Clin Cancer Res,* Vol.8, No.3, (March 2002), pp. 885-892.

Harrington LS, Findlay GM, Gray A, Tolkacheva T, Wigfield S, Rebholz H, Barnett J, Leslie NR, Cheng S, Shepherd PR, Gout I, Downes CP & Lamb RF. (2004). The TSC1-2 tumor suppressor controls insulin-PI3K signaling via regulation of IRS proteins. *J Cell Biol,* Vol.166, No.2, (July 2004), pp. 213-223.

Hecht SS. (2005). Deguelin as a chemopreventive agent in mouse lung tumorigenesis induced by tobacco smoke carcinogens. *J Natl Cancer Inst,* Vol. 97, No. 22, (November 2005), pp. 1634-1635.

Hjelmeland AB, Lattimore KP, Fee BE, Shi Q, Wickman S, Keir ST, Hjelmeland MD, Batt D, Bigner DD, Friedman HS & Rich JN. (2007). The combination of novel low molecular weight inhibitors of RAF (LBT613) and target of rapamycin (RAD001) decreases glioma proliferation and invasion. *Mol Cancer Ther,* Vol. 6, No. 9, (September 2007), pp. 2449-2457.

Ho QT & Kuo CJ. (2007). Vascular endothelial growth factor: biology and therapeutic applications. *Int J Biochem Cell Biol,* Vol. 39, No. 7-8, (2007), pp. 1349-1357.

Ihle NT, Paine-Murrieta G, Berggren MI, Baker A, Tate WR, Wipf P, Abraham RT, Kirkpatrick DL & Powis G. (2005). The phosphatudylinositol-3-kinase inhibitor PX-866 overcomes resistance to the epidermal growth factor receptor inhibitor gefitinib in A-549 human non-small cell lung cancer xenografts. *Mol Cancer Ther,* Vol. 4, No. 9, (September 2005), pp. 1349-1357.

Inoki K, Li Y, Xu T & Guan KL. (2003). Rheb GTPase is a direct target of TSC2 GAP activity and regulates mTOR signaling. *Genes Dev,* Vol.17, No.15, (August 2003), pp. 1829-1834.

Inoki K, Ouyang H, Li Y & Guan KL. (2005). Signaling by target of rapamycin proteins in cell growth control. *Microbiol Mol Biol Rev,* Vol.69, No.1, (March 2005), pp. 79-100.

Ishiguro R, Fujii M, Yamashita T, Tashiro M, Tomita T, Ogawa K & Kameyama K. (2003). CCND1 amplification predicts sensitivity to chemotherapy and chemoradiotherapy in head and neck squamous cell carcinoma. *Anticancer Res,* Vol.23, No.6D, (November-December 2003), pp. 5213-5220.

Jimeno A, Kulesza P, Wheelhouse J, Chan A, Zhang X, Kincaid E, Chen R, Clark DP, Forastiere A & Hidalgo M. (2007). Dual EGFR and mTOR targeting in squamous cell carcinoma models, and development of early markers of efficacy. *Br J Cancer,* Vol. 96, No. 6, (March 2007), pp. 952-959.

Jones HE, Dutkowski CM, Barrow D, Harper ME, Wakeling AE & Nicholson RI. (1997). New EGF-R selective tyrosine kinase inhibitor reveals variable growth responses in prostate carcinoma cell lines PC-3 and DU-145. *Int J Cancer,* Vol. 71, No. 6, (June 1997), pp. 1010-1018.

Jones HE, Goddard L, Gee JM, Hiscox S, Rubini M, Barrow D, Knowlden JM, Williams S, Wakeling AE & Nicholson RI. (2004). Insulin-like growth factor-I receptor signaling and acquired resistance to gefitinib (ZD1839; Iressa) in human breast and prostate cancer cells. *Endocr Relat Cancer,* Vol. 11, No. 4, (December 2004), pp. 793-814.

Jones HE, Gee JM, Barrow D, Tonge D, Holloway B & Nicholson RI. (2006). Inhibition of insulin receptor isoform-A signaling restores sensitivity to gefitinib in previously de novo resistant colon cancer cells. *Br J Cancer,* Vol. 95, No. 2, (July 2006), pp. 172-180.

Kalish LH, Kwong RA, Cole IE, Gallagher RM, Sutherland RL & Musgrove EA. (2004). Deregulated cyclin D1 expression is associated with decreased efficacy of the selective epidermal growth factor receptor tyrosine kinase inhibitor gefitinib in head and neck squamous cell carcinoma cell lines. *Clin Cancer Res,* Vol. 10, No. 22, (November 2004), pp. 7764-7774.

Kaur J, Sawhney M, Dattagupta S, Shukla NK, Srivastava A & Ralhan R. (2010). Clinical significance of Phosphatidyl Inositol Synthase overexpression in oral cancer. *BMC Cancer,* Vol. 10, No. 168, (April 2010), pp. 1-11.

Khuri FR, Shin DM, Glisson BS, Lippman SM & Hong WK. (2000). Treatment of patients with recurrent or metastatic squamous cell carcinoma of the head and neck: current status and future directions. *Semin Oncol,* Vol. 27, No.4, (August 2000), pp. 25-33.

Knowlden JM, Hutcheson IR, Barrow D, Gee JM & Nicholson RI. (2005). Insulin-like growth factor-I receptor signaling in tamoxifen-resistant breast cancer: a supporting role to the epidermal growth factor receptor. *Endocrinology,* Vol. 146, No. 11, (November 2005), pp. 4609-4618.

Lee HY, Oh SH, Woo JK, Kim WY, Van Pelt CS, Price RE, Cody D, Tran H, Pezzuto JM, Moriarty RM & Hong WK. (2005). Chemopreventive effects of deguelin, a novel Akt inhibitor, on tobacco-induced lung tumorigenesis. *J Natl Cancer Inst,* Vol. 97, No. 22, (November 2005), pp. 1695-1699.

Leeman-Neill RJ, Cai Q, Joyce SC, Thomas SM, Bhola NE, Neill DB, Arbiser JL & Grandis JR. (2010). Honokiol inhibits epidermal growth factor receptor signaling and enhances the antitumor effects of epidermal growth factor receptor inhibitors. *Clin Cancer Res,* Vol. 16, No. 9, (May 2010), pp. 2571-2579.

Li D, Shimamura T, Ji H, Chen L, Haringsma HJ, McNamara K, Liang MC, Perera SA, Zaghlul S, Borgman CL, Kubo S, Takahashi M, Sun Y, Chirieac LR, Padera R F, Lindeman NI, Janne PA, ThomasRK, Meyerson ML, Eck MJ, Engelman JA, Shapiro GI & Wong KK.(2007). Bronchial and peripheral murine lung carcinomas induced by T790M-L858R mutant EGFR respond to HKI-272 and rapamycin combination therapy. *Cancer Cell,* Vol. 12, No. 1, (July 2007), pp. 81-93.

Loeffler-Ragg J, Witsch-Baumgartner M, Tzankov A, Hilbe W, Schwentner I, Sprinzl GM, Utermann G & Zwierzina H. (2006). Low incidence of mutations in EGFR kinase domain in Caucasian patients with head and neck squamous cell carcinoma. *Eur J Cancer,* Vol. 42, No. 1, (January 2006), pp. 109-111.

Ma YY, Wei SJ, Lin YC, Lung JC, Chang TC, Whang-Peng J, Liu JM, Yang DM, Yang WK & Shen CY. (2000). PI3CA as an oncogene in cervical cancer. *Oncogene,* Vol.19, No.23, (May 2000), pp. 2739-2744.

Madhunapantula SV, Sharma A & Robertson GP. (2007). PRAS40 deregulates apoptosis in malignant melanoma. *Cancer Res,* Vol.67, No.8, (April 2007), pp. 3626-3636.

Manna SK, Mukhopadhyay A & Aggarwal BB. (2000). Resveratrol suppresses TNF-induced activation of nuclear transcription factors NF-kappaB, activator protein-1, and apoptosis: potential role of reactive oxygen intermediates and lipid peroxidation. *J Immunol,* Vol. 164, No. 12, (June 2000), pp. 6509-6519.

Mohi MG, Boulton C, Gu TL, Sternberg DW, Neuberg D, Griffin JD, Gilliland DG & Neel BG. (2004). Combination of rapamycin and protein tyrosine kinase (PTK) inhibitors for the treatment of leukemias caused by oncogenic PTKs. *Proc Natl Acad Sci USA,* Vol. 101, No. 9, (March 2004), pp. 3130-3135.

Murillo G, Kosmeder JW 2nd, Pezzuto JM & Mehta RG. (2003). Deguelin suppresses the formation of carcinogen-induced aberrant crypt foci in the colon of CF-1 mice. *Int J Cancer,* Vol. 104, No. 1, (March 2003), pp. 7-11.

Nair AS, Shishodia S, Ahn KS, Kunnumakkara AB, Sethi G & Aggarwal BB. (2006). Deguelin, an Akt inhibitor, suppresses IkappaBalpha kinase activation leading to suppression of NF-kappaB-regulated gene expression, potentiation of apoptosis, and inhibition of cellular invasion. *J Immunol,* Vol. 177, No. 8, (October 2006), pp. 5612-5622.

Nakashima T & Clayman GL. (2000). Antisense inhibition of cyclin D1 in human head and neck squamous cell carcinoma. *Arch Otolaryngol Head Neck Surg,* Vol. 126, No. 8, (August 2000), pp. 957-961.

Nishimura G, Tsukuda M, Zhou L, Furukawa S & Baba Y. (1998). CyclinD1 expression as a prognostic factor in advanced hypopharyngeal carcinoma. *J Laryngol Otol,* Vol.112, No.6, (1998), pp. 552-555.

Ozawa S, Kato Y, Ito S, Komori R, Tsukinoki K, Ozono S, Maehata Y, Taguchi T, Imagawa-Ishiguro Y, Tsukuda M, Kubota E & Hata R. (2009). Restoration of BRAK/CXCL14 gene expression by gefitinib is associated with antitumor efficacy of the drug in head and neck squamous cell carcinoma. *Cancer Sci,* Vol. 100, No. 11, (November 2009), pp. 2202-2209.

Rebucci M, Peixoto P, Dewitte A, Wattez N, De Nuncques MA, Rezvoy N, Vautravers-Dewas C, Buisine MP, Guerin E, Peyrat JP, Lartigau E & Lansiaux A. (2011). Mechanisms underlying resistance to cetuximab in the HNSCC cell line: role of AKT inhibition in bypassing this resistance. *Int J Oncol,* Vol. 38, No. 1, (January 2011), pp. 189-200.

Rousseau S, Houle F, Landry J & Huot J. (1997). P38MAP kinase activation by vascular endothelial growth factor mediates actin reorganization and cell migration in human endothelial cells. *Oncogene,* Vol. 15, No. 18, (October 1997), pp. 2169-2177.

Samuels Y & Ericson K. (2006). Oncogenic PI3K and its role in cancer. *Curr Opin Oncol,* Vol.18, No.1, (January 2006), pp. 77-82.

Sarbassov DD, Guertin DA, Ali SM & Sabatini DM. (2005). Phosphorylation and regulation of Akt/PKB by the rector-mTOR complex. *Science,* Vol.307, No.5712, (February 2005), pp. 1098-1101.

Shayesteh L, Lu Y, Kuo WL, Baldocchi R, Godfrey T, Collins C, Pinkel D, Powell B, Mills GB & Gray JW. (1999). PIK3CA is implicated as an oncogene in ovarian cancer. *Nat Genet,* Vol.21, No.1, (January 1999), pp. 99-102.

Slomiany MG, Black LA, Kibbey MM, Tingler MA, Day TA & Rosenzweig SA. (2007). Insulin-like growth factor-1 receptor and ligand targeting in head and neck squamous cell carcinoma. *Cancer Lett,* Vol. 248, No. 2, (April 2007), pp. 269-279.

Sordella R, Bell DW, Haber DA & Settleman J. (2004). Gefitinib-sensitizing EGFR mutations in lung cancer activate anti-apoptotic pathways. *Science,* Vol. 305, No. 5687, (August 2004), pp. 1163-1167.

Soulieres D, Senzer NN, Vokes EE, Hidalgo M, Agarwala SS & Siu LL. (2004). Multicenter phase II study of erlotinib, an oral epidermal growth factor receptor tyrosine kinase inhibitor, in patients with recurrent or metastatic squamous cell cancer of the head an neck. *J Clin Oncol,* Vol. 22, No. 1, (January 2004), pp. 77-85.

Squarize CH, Castilho RM, Sriuranpong V, Pinto DS Jr & Gutkind JS. (2006). Molecular cross-talk between the NFkappaB and STAT3 signaling pathways in head and neck squamous cell carcinoma. *Neoplasia,* Vol. 8, No. 9, (September 2006), pp. 733-746.

Sriuranpong V, Park JI, Amornphimoltham P, Patel V, Nelkin BD & Gutkind JS. (2003). Epidermal growth factor receptor-independent constitutive activation of STAT3 in head and neck squamous cell carcinoma is mediated by the autocrine/paracrine stimulation of the interleukin 6/gp130 cytokine system. *Cancer Res,* Vol. 63, No. 11, (June 2003), pp. 2948-2956.

Taguchi T, Tsukuda M, Imagawa-Ishiguro Y, Kato Y & Sano D. (2008). Involvement of EGFR in the response of squamous cell carcinoma of the head and neck cell lines to gefitinib. *Oncol Rep,* Vol. 19, No. 1, (January 2008), pp. 65-71.

Takada Y, Andreeff M & Aggarwal BB. (2005). Indole-3-carbinol suppresses NF-kappaB and IkappaBalpha kinase activation, causing inhibition of expression of NF-kappaB-regulated antiapoptotic and metastatic gene products and enhancement of apoptosis in myeloid and leukemia cells. *Blood,* Vol. 106, No. 2, (July 2005), pp. 641-649.

Takahashi T, Ueno H & Shibuya M. (1999). VEGF activates protein kinase C-dependent, but Ras-independent Raf-MEK-MAP kinase pathway for DNA synthesis in primary endothelial cells. *Oncogene,* Vol. 18, No. 13, (April 1999), pp. 2221-2230.

Timpson P, Wilson AS, Lehrbach GM, Sutherland RL, Musgrove EA & Daly RJ. (2007). Aberrant expression of cortactin in head and neck squamous cell carcinoma cells is associated with enhanced cell proliferation and resistance to the epidermal growth factor receptor inhibitor gefitinib. *Cancer Res,* Vol. 67, No. 19, (October 2007), pp. 9304-9314.

Tsurutani J, Fukuoka J, Tsurutani H, Shih JH, Hewitt SM, Travis WD, Jen J & Dennis PA. (2006). Evaluation of two phosphorylation sites improves the prognostic significance of Akt activation in non-small-cell lung cancer tumors. *J Clin Oncol,* Vol.24, No.2, (January 2006), pp. 306-314.

van Houten VM, van den Brekel MW, Denkers F, Colnot DR, Westerga J, van Diest PJ, Snow GB & Brakenhoff RH. (2000). Molecular diagnosis of head and neck cancer. *Recent Results Cancer Res,* Vol. 157, (2000), pp. 90-106.

Vander Haar E, Lee SI, Bandhakavi S, Griffin TJ & Kim DH. (2007). Insulin signaling to mTOR mediated by the Akt/PKB substrate PRAS40. *Nat Cell Biol,* Vol.9, No.3, (March 2007), pp. 316-323.

Vogt PK, Gymnopoulos M & Hart JR. (2009). PI3-kinase and cancer: changing accents. *Curr Opin Genet Dev,* Vol.19, No.1, (February 2009), pp. 12-17.

Wong KK. (2008). Searching for a magic bullet in NSCLC: the role of epidermal growth factor receptor mutations and tyrosine kinase inhibitors. *Lung Cancer,* Vol. 60, No. Suppl 2, (June 2008), pp. 10-18.

6

Arachidonic Acid Metabolism and Its Implication on Head and Neck Cancer

Sittichai Koontongkaew[1,2] and Kantima Leelahavanichkul[1]
[1]*Faculty of Dentistry, Thammasat University, Pathumthani*
[2]*Medicinal Herb Research Unit, Thammasat University, Pathumthani*
Thailand

1. Introduction

Most of head and neck cancer (HNC) are squamous cell carcinoma. Recent advances in molecular biology have documented significant genetic differences between head and neck squamous cell carcinoma (HNSCC) cells and normal cells, leading to the development of potential new therapeutics and chemoprevention (Choi & Myers, 2008). Historically, the association between inflammation and cancer has been recognized. More recently, a number of chronic inflammatory diseases have been shown to be associated with a variety of human cancers, including HNC (Conroy *et al.*, 2010; Fitzpatrick & Katz, 2010). The relationship between oral health and cancer has been examined for a number of specific cancer sites. Several studies have reported associations between periodontal disease or tooth loss and risk of oral, upper gastrointestinal, lung, and pancreatic cancer in different populations (Meyer *et al.*, 2008). Cumulating evidences support the view that inflammatory mediators, some of that may downregulate DNA repair pathways directly or indirectly. Certain inflammatory mediators may affect on cell cycle checkpoints that result in the accumulation of random genetic alterations. These in turn lead to a genomically heterogenous population of expanding cells naturally selected for their ability to proliferate, invade and evade hose defenses (Colotta *et al.*, 2009).

Molecular studies of the well-known relationship between polyunsaturated fatty acid metabolism and carcinogenesis provide novel molecular targets for cancer chemoprevention and treatments. Several classes of agents have shown promise as chemopreventive agents, including the nonsteroidal anti-inflammatory drugs (NSAIDs), which posses a valid scientific basis for the prevention of multiple cancers, including HNC. Because NSAIDs are well-accepted inhibitors of cyclooxygenase (COX) and prostaglandin (PG) production, research work initially focused on COX-and PG-dependent mechanism of NSAIDs actions. Polyunsaturated fatty acid, including arachidonic and linoleic acids, can enhance tumorigenesis (Shureiqi & Lippman, 2001). Aberrant arachidonic acid (AA) metabolism, especially COX-2 and 5-lipoxygenase (5-LOX) pathways, are activated during oral carcinogenesis, and can be targeted for cancer prevention (el-Hakim & Langdon, 1991). Recently, we found that inhibition of AA metabolism caused a decrease in HNSCC cell invasion and matrix metalloproteinase (MMP) activities. Our findings suggest the contributory roles of COX and LOX in HNC development and progression (Koontongkaew *et al.*, 2010).

This review will briefly summarize the implication of AA metabolism in HNC. We will discuss what are known of COX and LOX in tumorigenesis of HNC. Possible mechanisms of action of COX and LOX and potential roles for AA inhibitors in the prevention and therapy of this cancer will be documented in this review.

2. Arachidonic acid cascade

AA is a long chain polyunsaturated fatty acid containing 20 carbons. It can be stored in membrane phospholipids and released from nuclear envelop or plasma membrane by cytosolic phospholipase A2 (cPLA2), either constitutively or in respond to a variety of cell specific stimuli, including growth factors, hormones, cytokines, signaling molecules, or cell trauma. Free AA can be subsequently metabolized by three key enzymes, COX, LOX, or cytochrome P450 (CYP450) to generate lipid mediators, eicosanoids, which involved in various biological function, inflammation regulation, and more recently, tumor progression (Funk, 2001; Wang *et al.*, 2007; Hyde & Missailidis, 2009). COX metabolism generates prostanoids, including prostaglandins (PGs) and thromboxanes (TXs). LOX generates leukotrienes (LTs), lipoxin (LXs) and hepoxillins (HOs). CYP450 metabolic pathway gives a family of lipoxygenase-like hydroeicosatetraenoic acids (HETEs), epoxyeicosatrienoic acids (EETs) and ω-HETEs (Capdevila *et al.*, 2000).

2.1 The COX pathway

In the COX pathway, COX first oxidized AA to form prostaglandin G2 (PGG_2), and is then metabolized into an intermediate prostaglandin H_2 (PGH_2) by peroxidase activity (Figure 1). PGH_2 is an unstable endoperoxide, which is catalyzed to five primary prostanoids, including PGD_2, PGE_2, $PGF_{2\alpha}$, PGI_2 and thromboxane A_2 by specific synthases.

Three isoforms of COX have been identified, COX-1, COX-2 and COX-3 (Williams *et al.*, 1999; Wang *et al.*, 2007). COX-1 and COX-2 are similar in structure and catalytic activity. Both enzymes have the same molecular weight and share a 61% amino acid sequence homology. COX-3 is the splice variants of COX-1, which retains intron 1 and has a frameshift mutation (Wang *et al.*, 2007). COX-3 was constitutively highest expressed in the cerebral cortex and heart tissue (Chandrasekharan *et al.*, 2002). COX-1 is constitutively expressed in almost all tissues and resident inflammatory cells. It generates PGs that control homeostasis. COX-2 is normally undetectable. Constitutive COX-2 expression is well recognized in brain, kidney and the female reproductive tract. However, COX-2 is the most important regulator in the respond to inflammation and many types of cancers. COX-2 can be induced by multiple cytokines and growth factors, via activation of transcription factors that act on the promoter region, including TATA box, and NF-IL6 motif, two AP-2 sites, three Sp1 sites, two NF-κB sites, a CRE motif and an E-box (Park *et al.*, 2006).

The PGEs subclass, including cytosolic PGE synthase (cPGEs) and membrane-bound PGE synthases (mPGEs), is also involved in inflammation and carcinogenesis. Once the various PGs are synthesized, they are exported into the extracellular microenvironment and bind to the specific G-protein coupled receptors (GPCRs) that can be activated by autocrine and paracrine fashions in the tumor microenvironment (Sugimoto & Narumiya, 2007).

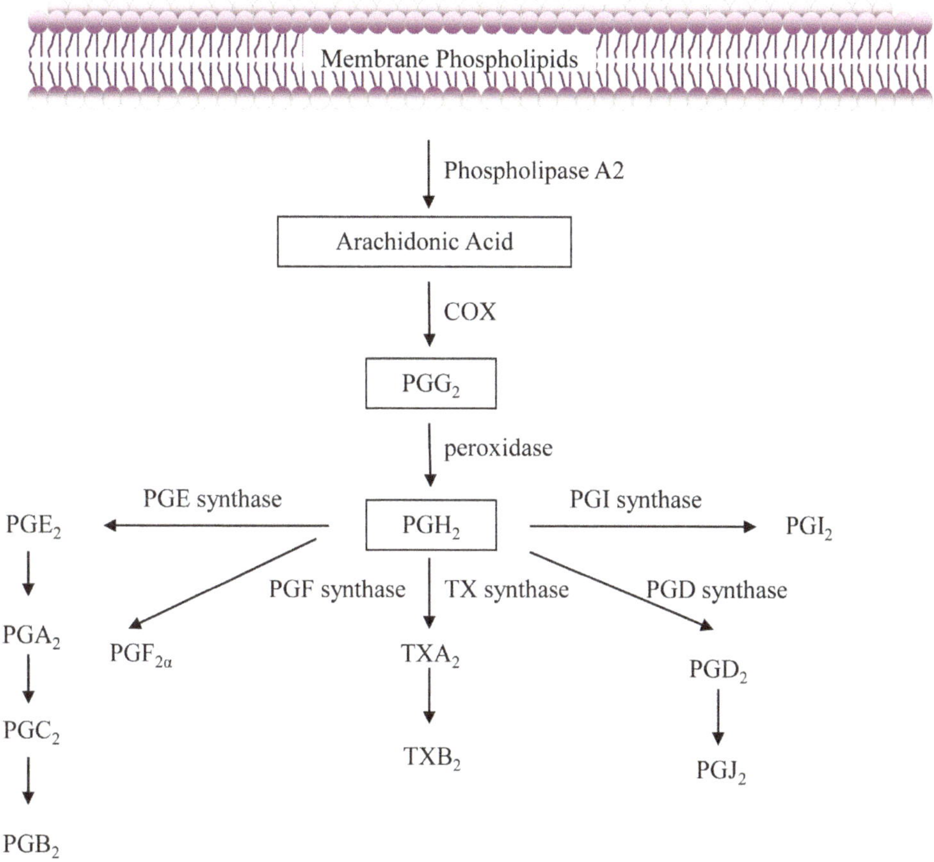

Fig. 1. Main products and enzymes of the COX pathway. COX: cyclooxygenase; PG: prostaglandin; TX: thromboxane.

3. COX and HNC

In the last decade inflammation and cancer had been linked together as biomarkers and novel targets of cancer therapy in a large number of cancers, including HNC. Overexpressions of COX-2 and prostanoids have been shown in various forms of human cancers, including HNC, and they can be linked with cancer progression and metastasis (Lee *et al.*, 2001; Krysan *et al.*, 2004; Huh *et al.*, 2009). COX-2 expression was correlated with shorter survival in non-small cell lung cancer and poor survival in prostate cancer and gliomas patients (Khuri *et al.*, 2001; Shono *et al.*, 2001; Khor *et al.*, 2007). Upregulation of COX-2 has been reported in human tissues and cell lines as well as in serum of patients with HNC. The increased levels of COX-2 were associated with the risk of tobacco- and betel nut-related cancers, advance clinical stage, survival and lymph node metastasis (Tang *et al.*, 2003; Molinolo *et al.*, 2007; Chiang *et al.*, 2008; Husvik *et al.*, 2009; Saba *et al.*, 2009; Kapoor *et al.*, 2010; Mittal *et al.*, 2010). In addition, PGE_2 receptors are widely expressed in a variety of HNSCC cell lines as well as in tumor tissues (Abrahao *et al.*, 2010).

Several studies showed the effects of COX inhibitors on cancer cell proliferation, invasion and proliferation, invasion and metastasis. Selective COX-2 inhibitors decreased viability, invasion and adhesion of HNSCC cells by down-regulated MMP-2, MMP-9 and vascular endothelial growth factor (VEGF) secretion (Kim *et al.*, 2010; Koontongkaew *et al.*, 2010; Li *et al.*, 2010). Moreover, suppression of COX-2 expression by small RNAs reduced cancer cell proliferation and invasion by decreased VEGF production (Park *et al.*, 2010; Wang *et al.*, 2010). Selective COX-1 inhibitor also decreased cancer cell proliferation (Koontongkaew *et al.*, 2010). However, little is known about the molecular mechanism of the COX-2 pathway in the regulation of HNSCC cell growth. Molecular mechanism of cell apoptosis by COX-2/PGE_2 through phosphatidylinositol 3-kinase (PI3K)/AKT pathway has been suggested in human epidermoid carcinoma cells (Agarwal *et al.*, 2009).

COX-2 is expressed in tumor neovasculature as well as in tumor tissues. The proangiogenic factors of COX-2 are TXA_2, PGI_2 and PGE_2. Selective inhibitor of COX-2 has been shown to suppress angiogenesis *in vitro* and *in vivo* by reduced VEGF production (Williams *et al.*, 2000). This suggests a role of COX in the process of angiogenesis, which might have an effect in HNSCC cell proliferation.

3.1 COX and ERK pathway

Upregulation of epidermal growth factor receptor (EGFR) has been suggested as a major pathway involved in HNSCC progression (Le Tourneau *et al.*, 2007; Molinolo *et al.*, 2009). Activation of EGFR has been shown to induce increased COX-2 expression in various normal and cancer cell lines, including HNSCC cells. However, the signaling pathway involved in COX-2 via EGFR varies depending on the type of cells and inducers, but the ras/ raf/ mitogen-activated protein kinases (MAPKs) signaling pathways mainly contribute to both increased transcriptional and posttranscriptional controls. On the other hand, COX-2 could induce transactivation or upregulate EGFR expression (Choe *et al.*, 2005; Husvik *et al.*, 2009).

Selective COX-2 inhibitors have been shown to decrease PGE_2 production *in vitro* and *in vivo* (Hoshikawa *et al.*, 2009; Abrahao *et al.*, 2010). This implies that upregulated PGE_2 in tumor microenvironment by COX-2 overexpression may promote the growth of HNSCC cells in an autocrine and/or paracrine effects by acting on widely expressed PGE_2 receptors in HNSCC cells. Additionally, p53, a tumor suppressor, play an inhibitory role in AA metabolism. It downregulates COX-2 expression and leads to tumor cell apoptosis (Subbaramaiah *et al.*, 1999).

3.2 COX and PI3K/AKT pathway

The PI3K/AKT pathway plays critical roles in the control of cancer cell survival and apoptosis in many cancers, including HNC (Jiang & Liu, 2008; Cohen *et al.*, 2011). It has been recognized that protein kinase B (Akt/PKB) activity is implicated in K-Ras-induced expression of COX-2, and the mRNA stability of COX-2 partially depends on the activation of AKT (Sheng *et al.*, 2001). Indomethacin, a NSAID, has been found to induce apoptosis in renal cell carcinoma cells by activating AKT and MAPK signaling (Ou *et al.*, 2007). Celecoxib, a selective COX-2 inhibitor, had been shown to induce apoptosis through (PI3K)/AKT and the COX-2 signaling pathway in various cancers, including non-small cell lung carcinoma, prostate and gastric cancers (Kulp *et al.*, 2004; Zhu *et al.*, 2004; Fan *et al.*, 2006). In HNC, however, the mechanism of COX-2 upregulation is not fully understood. There was reported that COX alone did not effect on pEGFR, pERK1/2 and pAKT. However, inhibition of combination of COX and EGFR reduced the AKT activities of HNSCC cells (Chen *et al.*, 2004b).

3.3 COX and tumor invasion

It is well documented that COX inhibitors reduce cancer cell migration, cell adhesion and tumor invasiveness (Lin *et al.*, 2002). Increased invasiveness has been associated with activation of MMPs. MMPs are a family of proteolytic enzymes linked to several malignant properties of a variety of tumor cells, including HNSCC cells (Rosenthal & Matrisian, 2006). Therefore, it is possible that COX-2 enhances tumor cell invasion through the upregulated MMP activities. To date, however, a few studies have investigated the importance of COX-2 in modulating the invasive properties of HNSCC cells. Recently, we found that COX-1 and COX-2 inhibitors reduced cell viability, MMP-2 and MMP-9 activities, and *in vitro* invasion of primary and metastatic HNSCC cells (Koontongkaew *et al.*, 2010). Our findings are consistent with other studies that demonstrated the inhibitory effects of COX inhibitors on MMP activities in breast (Larkins *et al.*, 2006), prostate (Attiga *et al.*, 2000), colon (Ishizaki *et al.*, 2006) and lung cancer cells (Karna & Palka, 2002). Regarding the role of COX-2 in the metastasis and invasion of HNSCC cells, the precise mechanism remains obscure, but a decrease of COX-2 dependent PGE_2 may downregulate MMP production through PGE_2 receptors (Dohadwala *et al.*, 2002).

4. Inhibition of COX

NSAIDs, non-selective inhibitors for COX, are over-the-counter drugs and widely use as analgesics, anti-inflammations, antipyretic and chemoprevention in cardiovascular diseases and other disorders. Experimental tumor model studies show that NSAIDs impair the growth and development of HNSCC, indicating potential as a chemopreventive agent (Cornwall *et al.*, 1983; Lin *et al.*, 2002; Mohan & Epstein, 2003). Moreover, both non-selective and selective of COX prevented 4-nitroquinoline- oxide (NQO)-induced tumorigenesis in rats (McCormick *et al.*, 2010). Regular use of aspirin has been shown to reduce the risk of colon cancer (Dube *et al.*, 2007). Celecoxib is approved for the chemoprevention of colon cancer in patients with familial adenomatous polyposis. This COX-2 inhibitor has also been shown to reduce the incidence of various cancers *in vivo* (Grosch *et al.*, 2006). To date, however, no definitive conclusion on the effect of NSAIDs/aspirin use on the risk of HNSCC is well documented (Wilson *et al.*, 2011). Although NSAIDs or aspirin may have protective effect on HNSCC, further large-scale studies are required.

Selective COX-2 inhibitors were reported to enhance treatment responds to radiotherapy or combination of radiotherapy and chemotherapy, suggesting that the inhibitors can improve the response of various cancers to conventional cancer therapies (Liao *et al.*, 2003; Komaki *et al.*, 2004). To date, several concurrent clinical trial studies of HNC are using a combination of standard treatment with a selective COX-2 inhibitor and the others, such as EGFR inhibitor, which has been shown to improve survival in patients with non-small cell lung cancer (Fidler *et al.*, 2008). A combination of EGFR-selective tyrosine kinase inhibitor with a COX-

2 inhibitor (celecoxib) induced cell cycle arrest and apoptosis in HNSCC cells. The combination showed strong reduction of EGFR, ERK1/2 and AKT activations (Chen *et al.*, 2004b). The phase 1 clinical trial, using a combination of an EGFR inhibitor (erlotinib), a selective COX-2 inhibitor (celecoxib) and reirradiation showed a feasible and clinically active regimen for recurrent HNC patients (Kao *et al.*, 2011). During and after radiotherapy in combination with celecoxib, significant decrease of the plasma levels of VEGF were observed in patients with advanced HNC who had high COX-2 expression in their tumor tissues (Halamka *et al.*, 2011).

5. The LOX pathway

In human cells, generally, four types of LOXs have been identified, namely 5-, 12- and 15-LOX-1 and LOX-2. Collectively, they catalyze the oxygenation of AA into hydroperoxyeicosatetraenoic acids (HPETEs) (Figure 2). Ultimately, this is followed by their conversion to their corresponding hydroeicosatetraenoic acids (HETEs), leading to the formation of LTs, LXs and HOs. The metabolism of linoleic acid preferentially results in the formation of hydroxyloctadecadienoic acids (HODEs). 5-LOX catalyzes the first step in the oxygenation of AA to produce 5-HPETE, and the subsequent metabolism of 5-HPETE to 5-HETE and LTs. LTs belong to a key group of pro-inflammatory mediators that are synthesized from AA via the 5-LOX pathway. The activity of 5-LOX leads to the formation of unstable LTA4, which can be converted into LTB4 or cysteinyl LTs (LTC4, LTD4 and LTE4) Platelet-type 12-LOX (*p*12-LOX) exclusively uses AA released from glycerol-phospholipid pools to synthesize 12S-HPETE and 12S-HETE, whereas leukocyte-type 12-LOX can also synthesize 15S-HETE and 12S-HETE. In addition to leukocytes and platelets, the expression of 12-LOX isozymes has been observed in various types of cells, including smooth muscle cells, endothelial cells and keratinocytes. 15-lipoxygeases (15-LOX) can be subdivided into two isoforms, namely 15-LOX-1 and 15-LOX-2. 15-LOX-1 is mainly expressed in reticulocytes, eosinophils and airway epithelial cells, as well as in macrophages. In terms of enzymatic characteristics, 15-LOX-1 preferentially metabolizes linoleic acid primarily to 13S-HODE, but also metabolizes AA to 15S-HETE. 15-LOX-2, on the other hand, converts AA to 15S-HETE and poorly metabolizes linoleic acid (Romano & Claria, 2003).

The products of LOX metabolism represent either intermediary products such as HPETE, which are transformed enzymatically into secondary products, including LTs, LXs, HOs and HETEs, which can act as signaling molecules in their own right or give rise to the production of reactive oxygen species (ROS). Signaling of LOX-derived products can occur through either G protein coupled cell-surface receptors, in the case of LOs and LTs, or through activation of nuclear receptors such as peroxisome proliferator activated receptors (PPARs) in the case of HETEs and HODEs (Pidgeon *et al.*, 2007).

6. LOX and HNC

Early tumorigenesis studies in animals demonstrated the contributory roles of AA and linoleic acid in tumorigenesis. Various LOX products have been linked to tumorigenesis *in vitro* and also *in vivo* in animal models. In addition, the modulation of LOX metabolism has anticarcinogenic effects on tumor development. Therefore, it suggests that LOX modulation has been targeted for developing anticarcinogenic agents (Shureiqi & Lippman, 2001).

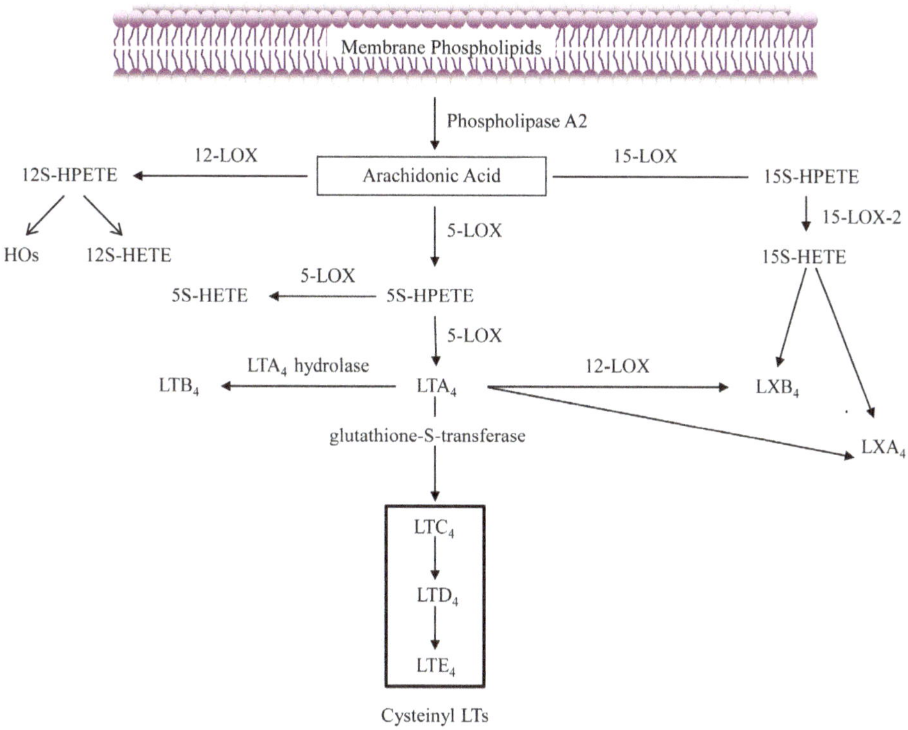

Fig. 2. Main products and enzymes of the LOX pathway. LOX: lipoxygenase; HPETE: hydroperoxyeicosatetraenoic acid; HETE: hydroxyeisatetraenoic acid; HOs: Hepoxillins; LXs: lipoxins; LT: leukotriene.

5-LOX, 12-LOX, 15-LOX-1 and 15-LOX-2 were detected in HNSCC cell lines derived from primary and metastatic tumors. Therefore, it is not surprised that LOX metabolites, including 5-HETE, 12-HETE, 15-HETE and 13-HODE were found in primary and metastatic HNSCC cells. However, there was no correlation between LOX isoforms and their metabolites in HNSCC cells (Schroeder *et al.*, 2004). The level of LTB4, a metabolite of the 5-LOX pathway, was found to be higher in oral cancer lesions in human and hamsters (el-Hakim *et al.*, 1990; Li *et al.*, 2005). This enzyme was also upregulated in other cancers, including prostate (Gupta *et al.*, 2001), pancreatic (Hennig *et al.*, 2002), colon (Ohd *et al.*, 2003) and esophageal cancers (Chen *et al.*, 2004a). Previous studies in 7,12-dimethylbenz[*a*]anthracene (DMBA)-induced hamster oral cancer demonstrated overexpression of 5-LOX in the stromal inflammatory cells and epithelial cells at the early stages of oral squamous cell carcinogenesis. Moreover, zileuton, a specific 5-LOX inhibitor and celecoxib (a specific COX-2 inhibitor), either alone or in combination, had an inhibitory effect on the incidence of oral tumor in DMBA-treated animals. Zileuton seems even more effective than celecoxib. These findings suggest that the 5-LOX pathway of AA metabolism plays an important role in inflammation-associated oral cancer (Li *et al.*, 2005).

Recently, studies in the mouse model showed that the expression of 5-LOX and COX-2 was increased in dysplasia and squamous cell carcinoma of 4-nitroquinoline-1-oxide (4NQO)-

treated tongues, and further enhanced by ethanol. Fewer tumors were induced in Alox5-/- mice, as were cell proliferation, inflammation, and angiogenesis in the tongue, as compared with Alox5+/+ mice. COX-2 expression was induced by ethanol in knockout mice, while 5-LOX and LTA4H expression and LTB4 biosynthesis were dramatically reduced. Moreover, ethanol enhanced expression and nuclear localization of 5-LOX and stimulated LTB4 biosynthesis in human tongue squamous cell lines. These findings suggest that the activation of the 5-LOX pathway of AA metabolism involves in oral carcinogenesis (Guo *et al.*, 2011).

Inhibition of AA metabolism (COX-2 and 5-LOX) by curcumin has also been suggested as a key mechanism of its anticarcinogenic action in DMBA-induced hamster oral carcinoma (Li *et al.*, 2002; Bengmark, 2006). Zyflamed, a product containing 10- concentrate herbal extracts significantly reduced infiltration of inflammatory cells, incidence of hyperplasia and dysplastic lesions, cell proliferation as well as number of tumors in the DMBA-induced hamster cheek pouch model. Furthermore, it was shown that zyflamed reduced LTB4 formation compared with that of the control (Yang *et al.*, 2008).

In a long-term carcinogenesis study, topical application of LTB4 enhanced oral carcinogenesis by increasing the incidence and sizes of tumors. LTB4 inhibitors significantly inhibited oral carcinogenesis, and the anticarcinogenesis as such correlated with reduced levels of LTB4 (Sun *et al.*, 2006). An *in-vitro* study demonstrated that addition of LTB4 to RBL-1 cells, a rat leukemia cell line expressing high levels of 5-LOX, could counteract the inhibition of cell proliferation produced by a LOX inhibitor (zyflamed) (Yang *et al.*, 2008).

LOX products were indentified in human mixed saliva and in saliva fractions obtained from a parotid or submandibular gland. In glandular saliva, only linoleic acid was detected at levels of 20-30 ng/ml. In contrast, mixed saliva showed a linoleic acid concentration of around 300 ng/ml, AA levels of around 30 ng/ml, HODE levels between 5 and 10 ng/ml, and HETE levels up to 25 ng/ml. By far the most abundant HETE was 12-HETE, and incubation experiments with AA showed the presence of a substantial 12-LOX activity in human mixed saliva, but not in saliva fractions. Investigating mixed saliva and glandular saliva of patients with squamous cell carcinoma in the upper aerodigestive tract and of controls; most patients showed elevated levels of free AA and elevated HETE levels. Besides a moderate increase in 12-HETE levels, markedly elevated concentrations of 5-HETE and 15-HETE were observed for the carcinoma patients. Therefore, it is proposed that the level of free AA, and the quantitative HETE profile appear to be good markers for the inflammatory processes occurring in the oral mucosa and in saliva in response to the development of squamous cell carcinoma (Metzger *et al.*, 1995).

6.1 Molecular mechanisms of LOX-mediated HNC development

As mentioned above, substantial evidence supports a functional role for LOX-catalyzed AA metabolism in HNC development. Pharmacologic and natural inhibitors of LOX have been shown to suppress carcinogenesis and tumor growth in a number of experimental models. In recent years participation of LOX in the regulation of cell proliferation, apoptosis and angiogenesis has emerged. Many cell pathways are involved in the process by which cells choose between growth arrest, apoptosis or survival. The crosstalk of LOX derived products with different growth factor receptor-induced signaling cascades is involved in the stimulation of tumor cell growth.

The aberrant activation of multiple signaling pathways, including EGFR, *ras*, NFκB, STAT, Wnt/β-catenin, TGF-β and PI3K/AKT were observed in HNSCC (Molinolo *et al.*, 2009). Oncogenic events in HNC associated with abnormal activation of the PI3K/AKT pathway include mutations, allelic loss, or the promoter methylation of the negative regulator phosphatase and tensin homolog (PTEN) (Cohen *et al.*, 2011). LOX metabolites may exert their biological effects in an intracrine manner, through the activation of transcription factors of the PPAR family, or they may interact with specific trans-membrane G protein-couple cell surface receptors in an autocrine or paracrine manner (Pidgeon *et al.*, 2007). LOX metabolites may involve in ERK1/2, PI3K/AKT cascade, and STAT signaling pathways in HNSCC cells (Pidgeon *et al.*, 2007). PTEN may be oxidized and inactivated during AA metabolism in cancer cells. Oxidation of PTEN resulted in a decrease of its phosphatase activity, favoring increased PI-3, 4, 5-trisphosphate (PIP_3) production, activation of AKT and phosphorylation of downstream AKT targets. Such activation leads to cell cycle induction during HNC development (Covey *et al.*, 2007; Jiang & Liu, 2008).

Tumor growth does not only depend on increased cell proliferation but also on prolonged cell survival through the inhibition of cell death or apoptosis. LOX inhibition has been shown to induce apoptosis in cancer cells (Lepage *et al.*, 2010). LOX metabolites may enhance cancer cell survival through an increase in Bcl-2. In addition, they can upregulate the p-ERK and p-AKT levels, suggesting the involvement of ERK and AKT pathways in the LOX-mediated regulation of growth in cancer cells (Agarwal *et al.*, 2009). However, it was found that metabolism of AA by 5-LOX activity promotes survival of cancer cells via signaling through PKCε, a pro-survival serine/threonine kinase which is not dependent on the AKT and ERK-pathway (Sarveswaran *et al.*, 2011).

In addition to its role in neoplastic transformation, 5-LOX and its AA metabolite had shown to be involved in angiogenesis. 12S-HETE has been shown to be a mitogenic factor for microvascular endothelial cells and stimulates endothelial cell migration. Moreover, 12S-HETE has an ability to induce the expression of VEGF, an important proangiogenic factor, at both protein and promoter levels (Pidgeon *et al.*, 2007).

However, little is known about the role of LOX in HNC cell metastasis. The process of tumor invasion by cancer cells involves degradation of the underlying basement membrane, which largely made up of collagen IV. MMP-2 and MMP-9 showed substrate specificity toward type IV and V collagen and a number of studies have demonstrated a strong correlation between MMP expression and metastatic potential (Rosenthal & Matrisian, 2006). Recently, our findings demonstrated the inhibitory effects of NDGA (nordihydroguaiaretic acid, the selective LOX inhibitor) and ETYA (5, 8, 11, 14-eicosatetraynoic acid, the COX and LOX inhibitor) on cell proliferation, MMP activity and invasion in primary and metastatic HNSCC cells (Koontongkaew *et al.*, 2010). It is possible that LOX inhibitors activate PPARγ activity and subsequent reduction in MMP-9 signaling (Hyde & Missailidis, 2009).

The ability of tumor cells to generate 12S-HETE is positively correlated to their metastatic potential and the increased expression of *p*12-LOX enhanced the metastatic potential of cancer cells. Moreover, 12S-HETE has been found to modulate multi steps of the metastatic process encompassing tumor cell and endothelial cell interactions, tumor cell motility, proteolysis and invasion (Furstenberger *et al.*, 2006). Moreover, LOX may promote tumor cell migration through FAK (focal adhesion kinase) activation (Navarro-Tito *et al.*, 2008).

It should be noted that the role of LOX in HNC development is thought to be more complex, compared with that of COX because 6 LOX genes have been identified in human and different profiles of LOX were found in studies on human tumor biopsies and experimentally induced animal tumor models. The inverse expression pattern of individual LOX isoenzymes in normal versus malignant tissues and the biological effects of the corresponding LOX products propose the important role of dynamic balance among LOX isoenzymes in tumorigenesis. It has been shown a dynamic balance among LOX shifting toward the procarcinogenic 5- and *p*12-LOX and away from anticarcinogenic LOXs such as 15-LOX-1, 15-LOX-2, 8-LOX and epidermal-type 12-LOX (*e*12-LOX) during prostate and colon cancer development (Menna *et al.*, 2010). However, at present little is known about modulation of carcinogenesis through pro-and anticarcinogenic LOX isoforms in HNC development and progression.

7. Converging pathways of COX and LOX in HNC

The AA-metabolizing enzymes are overexpressed during animal and human carcinogenesis and AA metabolites such as PGE_2, 5-HETE and LTB4 had been implicated in HNC development. COX-2 and 5-LOX play important roles in inflammation and inflammation-associated tumorigenesis. It is evident that COX and LOX display similarities in expression and functions in HNC. In particular, the COX-2 and 5-LOX pathways are activated together during inflammation, and blocking one pathway may activate the other. It was shown that inhibition of COX-2 might lead to a shunt of AA metabolism towards the LT pathway in HNC. Suppressing PGE_2 levels by a COX-2 inhibitors, celecoxib, leads to an increase in the activity of 5-LOX, 12-LOX and 15-LOX-2 and results in the increase of their products, including, 5-HETE, 12-HETE and 15-HETE (Schroeder *et al.*, 2004). A study in the mouse model of HNC, demonstrated an increase of LTB4 in tumor tissues in mice treated with PGE_2. In contrast, LTB4 could not decrease tumor tissue levels of PGE_2 (Scioscia *et al.*, 2000). Therefore, simultaneous blocking of each enzyme may be required to achieve substantial elevation in free AA levels and prevent the shunting of metabolism to another active pathway.

Taken together, COX-2 and 5-LOX may have redundant function in HNC pathobiology. First, COX-2 and 5-LOX enhance tumor cell proliferation. Second, both COX-2 and 5-LOX are proangiogenic with a convergent targeting on VEGF, FGF and MMPs. Third, COX-2 as well as 5-LOX inhibitors, arrest cell cycle progression and induce apoptotic cell death in HNSCC cells. Fourth, both COX-2 and 5-LOX enhance HNSCC cell invasion and tumor metastasis. In addition, active COX2 and 5-LOX are localized in the nucleus, and they may function as endogenous ligands for nuclear receptors such as the PPARs (Menna *et al.*; Romano & Claria, 2003) (Figure 3).

8. Future prospects and conclusions

The summarized findings contained in this review support the contributory role of chronic inflammation in the pathogenesis of HNC. A hallmark of the inflammatory process is the synthesis of inflammatory cytokines and AA metabolites. Two major AA metabolic routes, *i.e.*, the COX and LOX pathways control the biosynthesis of eicosanoid. COX-derived eicosanoids comprise PG and TXA_2, whereas HPETE and LTs are products of LOX-catalyzed arachidonic acid metabolism. In HNC, COX-2 and LOX are coexpressed and upregulated in tumor cell lines, experimentally induced animal tumor models and human tumor biopsies. Currently, the underlying mechanisms for the tumorigenic effects of COX and LOX remain somewhat undefined. A number of studies of HNC have suggested the involvement of COX-2 and/ or 5-LOX in tumor cell proliferation, apoptosis, angiogenesis and metastasis.

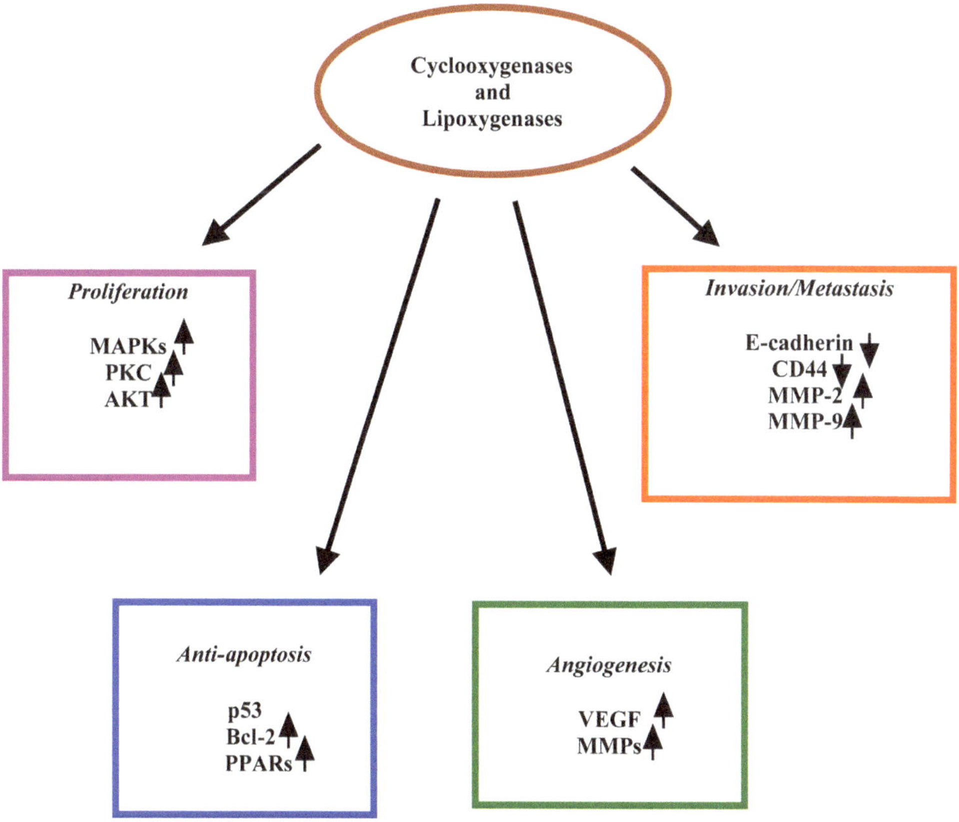

Fig. 3. Effects of COXs and LOXs on tumerigenesis. Both COXs and LOXs stimulate proliferation, inhibit apoptosis, induce angiogenesis, and enhance invasion and metastasis in cancer cells. MAPKs: mitogen activated protein kinases; PKC: protein kinase C; Bcl-2: B-cell lymphoma2; PPARs: peroxisome proliferator-activated receptor; VEGF: vascular endothelial growth factor; MMP: matrix metalloproteinase.

COX and/ or LOX inhibitors in many instances demonstrate potent anticancer effects. Manipulation of AA metabolism, therefore, represents a promising approach to develop HNC therapy. However, in spite of extensive research in COX and LOX inhibitors, their combined use for chemoprevention is still in its development stage. Further investigations are indeed necessary to develop appreciate chemopreventive strategies in HNC. First, the mechanism by which COX and LOX pathways are deregulated, interacted with each other, or contribute to head and neck tumorigenesis must be more clarified. Second, more clinical studies are critical to evaluate the effectiveness of COX and LOX inhibitors and to understand their mechanisms of action a single agent and in combination in HNC, specifically. Eventually, possible drug toxicity from a combined use must be evaluated over the long term.

9. References

Abrahao AC, Castilho RM, Squarize CH, Molinolo AA, dos Santos-Pinto D, Jr. & Gutkind JS (2010) A role for COX2-derived PGE2 and PGE2-receptor subtypes in head and neck squamous carcinoma cell proliferation. *Oral Oncol* 46, 880-887.

Agarwal S, Achari C, Praveen D, Roy KR, Reddy GV & Reddanna P (2009) Inhibition of 12-LOX and COX-2 reduces the proliferation of human epidermoid carcinoma cells (A431) by modulating the ERK and PI3K-Akt signalling pathways. *Exp Dermatol* 18, 939-946.

Attiga FA, Fernandez PM, Weeraratna AT, Manyak MJ & Patierno SR (2000) Inhibitors of prostaglandin synthesis inhibit human prostate tumor cell invasiveness and reduce the release of matrix metalloproteinases. *Cancer Res* 60, 4629-4637.

Bengmark S (2006) Curcumin, an atoxic antioxidant and natural NFκB, cyclooxygenase-2, lipooxygenase, and inducible nitric oxide synthase inhibitor: a shield against acute and chronic diseases. *JPEN J Parenter Enteral Nutr* 30, 45-51.

Capdevila JH, Falck JR & Harris RC (2000) Cytochrome P450 and arachidonic acid bioactivation. Molecular and functional properties of the arachidonate monooxygenase. *J Lipid Res* 41, 163-181.

Chandrasekharan NV, Dai H, Roos KL, Evanson NK, Tomsik J, Elton TS & Simmons DL (2002) COX-3, a cyclooxygenase-1 variant inhibited by acetaminophen and other analgesic/antipyretic drugs: cloning, structure, and expression. *Proc Natl Acad Sci U S A* 99, 13926-13931.

Chen X, Wang S, Wu N, Sood S, Wang P, Jin Z, Beer DG, Giordano TJ, Lin Y, Shih WC, Lubet RA & Yang CS (2004a) Overexpression of 5-lipoxygenase in rat and human esophageal adenocarcinoma and inhibitory effects of zileuton and celecoxib on carcinogenesis. *Clin Cancer Res* 10, 6703-6709.

Chen Z, Zhang X, Li M, Wang Z, Wieand HS, Grandis JR & Shin DM (2004b) Simultaneously targeting epidermal growth factor receptor tyrosine kinase and cyclooxygenase-2, an efficient approach to inhibition of squamous cell carcinoma of the head and neck. *Clin Cancer Res* 10, 5930-5939.

Chiang SL, Chen PH, Lee CH, Ko AM, Lee KW, Lin YC, Ho PS, Tu HP, Wu DC, Shieh TY & Ko YC (2008) Up-regulation of inflammatory signalings by areca nut extract and role of cyclooxygenase-2 -1195G>a polymorphism reveal risk of oral cancer. *Cancer Res* 68, 8489-8498.

Choe MS, Zhang X, Shin HJ, Shin DM & Chen ZG (2005) Interaction between epidermal growth factor receptor- and cyclooxygenase 2-mediated pathways and its implications for the chemoprevention of head and neck cancer. *Mol Cancer Ther* 4, 1448-1455.

Choi S & Myers JN (2008) Molecular pathogenesis of oral squamous cell carcinoma: implications for therapy. *J Dent Res* 87, 14-32.

Cohen Y, Goldenberg-Cohen N, Shalmon B, Shani T, Oren S, Amariglio N, Dratviman-Storobinsky O, Shnaiderman-Shapiro A, Yahalom R, Kaplan I & Hirshberg A (2011) Mutational analysis of PTEN/PIK3CA/AKT pathway in oral squamous cell carcinoma. *Oral Oncol,* 47, 946-950.

Colotta F, Allavena P, Sica A, Garlanda C & Mantovani A (2009) Cancer-related inflammation, the seventh hallmark of cancer: links to genetic instability. *Carcinogenesis* 30, 1073-1081.

Conroy H, Mawhinney L & Donnelly SC (2010) Inflammation and cancer: macrophage migration inhibitory factor (MIF)--the potential missing link. *QJM* 103, 831-836.

Cornwall H, Odukoya O & Shklar G (1983) Oral mucosal tumor inhibition by ibuprofen. *J Oral Maxillofac Surg* 41, 795-800.

Covey TM, Edes K & Fitzpatrick FA (2007) Akt activation by arachidonic acid metabolism occurs via oxidation and inactivation of PTEN tumor suppressor. *Oncogene* 26, 5784-5792.

Dohadwala M, Batra RK, Luo J, Lin Y, Krysan K, Pold M, Sharma S & Dubinett SM (2002) Autocrine/paracrine prostaglandin E2 production by non-small cell lung cancer cells regulates matrix metalloproteinase-2 and CD44 in cyclooxygenase-2-dependent invasion. *J Biol Chem* 277, 50828-50833.

Dube C, Rostom A, Lewin G, Tsertsvadze A, Barrowman N, Code C, Sampson M & Moher D (2007) The use of aspirin for primary prevention of colorectal cancer: a systematic review prepared for the U.S. Preventive Services Task Force. *Ann Intern Med* 146, 365-375.

el-Hakim IE & Langdon JD (1991) Arachidonic acid cascade and oral squamous cell carcinoma. *Clin Otolaryngol Allied Sci* 16, 563-573.

el-Hakim IE, Langdon JD, Zakrzewski JT & Costello JF (1990) Leukotriene B4 and oral cancer. *Br J Oral Maxillofac Surg* 28, 155-159.

Fan XM, Jiang XH, Gu Q, Ching YP, He H, Xia HH, Lin MC, Chan AO, Yuen MF, Kung HF & Wong BC (2006) Inhibition of Akt/PKB by a COX-2 inhibitor induces apoptosis in gastric cancer cells. *Digestion* 73, 75-83.

Fidler MJ, Argiris A, Patel JD, Johnson DH, Sandler A, Villaflor VM, Coon Jt, Buckingham L, Kaiser K, Basu S & Bonomi P (2008) The potential predictive value of cyclooxygenase-2 expression and increased risk of gastrointestinal hemorrhage in advanced non-small cell lung cancer patients treated with erlotinib and celecoxib. *Clin Cancer Res* 14, 2088-2094.

Fitzpatrick SG & Katz J (2010) The association between periodontal disease and cancer: a review of the literature. *J Dent* 38, 83-95.

Funk CD (2001) Prostaglandins and leukotrienes: advances in eicosanoid biology. *Science* 294, 1871-1875.

Furstenberger G, Krieg P, Muller-Decker K & Habenicht AJ (2006) What are cyclooxygenases and lipoxygenases doing in the driver's seat of carcinogenesis? *Int J Cancer* 119, 2247-2254.

Grosch S, Maier TJ, Schiffmann S & Geisslinger G (2006) Cyclooxygenase-2 (COX-2)-independent anticarcinogenic effects of selective COX-2 inhibitors. *J Natl Cancer Inst* 98, 736-747.

Guo Y, Wang X, Zhang X, Sun Z & Chen XL (2011) Ethanol promotes chemically induced oral cancer in mice through activation of the 5-lipoxygenase pathway of arachidonic acid metabolism. *Cancer Prev Res (Phila)*, 4, 1863-1872.

Gupta S, Srivastava M, Ahmad N, Sakamoto K, Bostwick DG & Mukhtar H (2001) Lipoxygenase-5 is overexpressed in prostate adenocarcinoma. *Cancer* 91, 737-743.

Halamka M, Cvek J, Kubes J, Zavadova E, Kominek P, Horacek J, Dusek L & Feltl D (2011) Plasma levels of vascular endothelial growth factor during and after radiotherapy in combination with celecoxib in patients with advanced head and neck cancer. *Oral Oncol* 47, 763-767.

Hennig R, Ding XZ, Tong WG, Schneider MB, Standop J, Friess H, Buchler MW, Pour PM & Adrian TE (2002) 5-Lipoxygenase and leukotriene B(4) receptor are expressed in human pancreatic cancers but not in pancreatic ducts in normal tissue. *Am J Pathol* 161, 421-428.

Hoshikawa H, Goto R, Mori T, Mitani T & Mori N (2009) Expression of prostaglandin E2 receptors in oral squamous cell carcinomas and growth inhibitory effects of an EP3 selective antagonist, ONO-AE3-240. *Int J Oncol* 34, 847-852.

Huh JW, Kim HR, Lee JH & Kim YJ (2009) Comparison of cyclooxygenase-2 and CD44 mRNA expression in colorectal cancer and its relevance for prognosis. *Virchows Arch* 454, 381-387.

Husvik C, Khuu C, Bryne M & Halstensen TS (2009) PGE2 production in oral cancer cell lines is COX-2-dependent. *J Dent Res* 88, 164-169.

Hyde CA & Missailidis S (2009) Inhibition of arachidonic acid metabolism and its implication on cell proliferation and tumour-angiogenesis. *Int Immunopharmacol* 9, 701-715.

Ishizaki T, Katsumata K, Tsuchida A, Wada T, Mori Y, Hisada M, Kawakita H & Aoki T (2006) Etodolac, a selective cyclooxygenase-2 inhibitor, inhibits liver metastasis of colorectal cancer cells via the suppression of MMP-9 activity. *Int J Mol Med* 17, 357-362.

Jiang BH & Liu LZ (2008) PI3K/PTEN signaling in tumorigenesis and angiogenesis. *Biochim Biophys Acta* 1784, 150-158.

Kao J, Genden EM, Chen CT, Rivera M, Tong CC, Misiukiewicz K, Gupta V, Gurudutt V, Teng M & Packer SH (2011) Phase 1 trial of concurrent erlotinib, celecoxib, and reirradiation for recurrent head and neck cancer. *Cancer* 117, 3173-3181.

Kapoor V, Singh AK, Dey S, Sharma SC & Das SN (2010) Circulating cycloxygenase-2 in patients with tobacco-related intraoral squamous cell carcinoma and evaluation of its peptide inhibitors as potential antitumor agent. *J Cancer Res Clin Oncol* 136, 1795-1804.

Karna E & Palka JA (2002) Inhibitory effect of acetylsalicylic acid on metalloproteinase activity in human lung adenocarcinoma at different stages of differentiation. *Eur J Pharmacol* 443, 1-6.

Khor LY, Bae K, Pollack A, Hammond ME, Grignon DJ, Venkatesan VM, Rosenthal SA, Ritter MA, Sandler HM, Hanks GE, Shipley WU & Dicker AP (2007) COX-2 expression predicts prostate-cancer outcome: analysis of data from the RTOG 92-02 trial. *Lancet Oncol* 8, 912-920.

Khuri FR, Wu H, Lee JJ, Kemp BL, Lotan R, Lippman SM, Feng L, Hong WK & Xu XC (2001) Cyclooxygenase-2 overexpression is a marker of poor prognosis in stage I non-small cell lung cancer. *Clin Cancer Res* 7, 861-867.

Kim YY, Lee EJ, Kim YK, Kim SM, Park JY, Myoung H & Kim MJ (2010) Anti-cancer effects of celecoxib in head and neck carcinoma. *Mol Cells* 29, 185-194.

Komaki R, Liao Z & Milas L (2004) Improvement strategies for molecular targeting: Cyclooxygenase-2 inhibitors as radiosensitizers for non-small cell lung cancer. *Semin Oncol* 31, 47-53.

Koontongkaew S, Monthanapisut P & Saensuk T (2010) Inhibition of arachidonic acid metabolism decreases tumor cell invasion and matrix metalloproteinase expression. *Prostaglandins Other Lipid Mediat* 93, 100-108.

Krysan K, Merchant FH, Zhu L, Dohadwala M, Luo J, Lin Y, Heuze-Vourc'h N, Pold M, Seligson D, Chia D, Goodglick L, Wang H, Strieter R, Sharma S & Dubinett S (2004) COX-2-dependent stabilization of survivin in non-small cell lung cancer. *FASEB J* 18, 206-208.

Kulp SK, Yang YT, Hung CC, Chen KF, Lai JP, Tseng PH, Fowble JW, Ward PJ & Chen CS (2004) 3-phosphoinositide-dependent protein kinase-1/Akt signaling represents a major cyclooxygenase-2-independent target for celecoxib in prostate cancer cells. *Cancer Res* 64, 1444-1451.

Larkins TL, Nowell M, Singh S & Sanford GL (2006) Inhibition of cyclooxygenase-2 decreases breast cancer cell motility, invasion and matrix metalloproteinase expression. *BMC Cancer* 6, 181-192.

Le Tourneau C, Faivre S & Siu LL (2007) Molecular targeted therapy of head and neck cancer: review and clinical development challenges. *Eur J Cancer* 43, 2457-2466.

Lee LM, Pan CC, Cheng CJ, Chi CW & Liu TY (2001) Expression of cyclooxygenase-2 in prostate adenocarcinoma and benign prostatic hyperplasia. *Anticancer Res* 21, 1291-1294.

Lepage C, Liagre B, Cook-Moreau J, Pinon A & Beneytout JL (2010) Cyclooxygenase-2 and 5-lipoxygenase pathways in diosgenin-induced apoptosis in HT-29 and HCT-116 colon cancer cells. *Int J Oncol* 36, 1183-1191.

Li N, Chen X, Liao J, Yang G, Wang S, Josephson Y, Han C, Chen J, Huang MT & Yang CS (2002) Inhibition of 7,12-dimethylbenz[a]anthracene (DMBA)-induced oral carcinogenesis in hamsters by tea and curcumin. *Carcinogenesis* 23, 1307-1313.

Li N, Sood S, Wang S, Fang M, Wang P, Sun Z, Yang CS & Chen X (2005) Overexpression of 5-lipoxygenase and cyclooxygenase 2 in hamster and human oral cancer and chemopreventive effects of zileuton and celecoxib. *Clin Cancer Res* 11, 2089-2096.

Li WZ, Huo QJ, Wang XY & Xu F (2010) Inhibitive effect of celecoxib on the adhesion and invasion of human tongue squamous carcinoma cells to extracellular matrix via down regulation of MMP-2 expression. *Prostaglandins Other Lipid Mediat* 93, 113-119.

Liao Z, Milas L, Komaki R, Stevens C & Cox JD (2003) Combination of a COX-2 inhibitor with radiotherapy or radiochemotherapy in the treatment of thoracic cancer. *Am J Clin Oncol* 26, S85-91.

Lin DT, Subbaramaiah K, Shah JP, Dannenberg AJ & Boyle JO (2002) Cyclooxygenase-2: a novel molecular target for the prevention and treatment of head and neck cancer. *Head Neck* 24, 792-799.

McCormick DL, Phillips JM, Horn TL, Johnson WD, Steele VE & Lubet RA (2010) Overexpression of cyclooxygenase-2 in rat oral cancers and prevention of oral carcinogenesis in rats by selective and nonselective COX inhibitors. *Cancer Prev Res (Phila)* 3, 73-81.

Menna C, Olivieri F, Catalano A & Procopio A (2010) A Lipoxygenase inhibitors for cancer prevention: promises and risks. *Curr Pharm Des* 16, 725-733.

Metzger K, Angres G, Maier H & Lehmann WD (1995) Lipoxygenase products in human saliva: patients with oral cancer compared to controls. *Free Radic Biol Med* 18, 185-194.

Meyer MS, Joshipura K, Giovannucci E & Michaud DS (2008) A review of the relationship between tooth loss, periodontal disease, and cancer. *Cancer Causes Control* 19, 895-907.

Mittal M, Kapoor V, Mohanti BK & Das SN (2010) Functional variants of COX-2 and risk of tobacco-related oral squamous cell carcinoma in high-risk Asian Indians. *Oral Oncol* 46, 622-626.

Mohan S & Epstein JB (2003) Carcinogenesis and cyclooxygenase: the potential role of COX-2 inhibition in upper aerodigestive tract cancer. *Oral Oncol* 39, 537-546.

Molinolo AA, Amornphimoltham P, Squarize CH, Castilho RM, Patel V & Gutkind JS (2009) Dysregulated molecular networks in head and neck carcinogenesis. *Oral Oncol* 45, 324-334.

Molinolo AA, Hewitt SM, Amornphimoltham P, Keelawat S, Rangdaeng S, Meneses Garcia A, Raimondi AR, Jufe R, Itoiz M, Gao Y, Saranath D, Kaleebi GS, Yoo GH, Leak L, Myers EM, Shintani S, Wong D, Massey HD, Yeudall WA, Lonardo F, Ensley J & Gutkind JS (2007) Dissecting the Akt/mammalian target of rapamycin signaling network: emerging results from the head and neck cancer tissue array initiative. *Clin Cancer Res* 13, 4964-4973.

Navarro-Tito N, Robledo T & Salazar EP (2008) Arachidonic acid promotes FAK activation and migration in MDA-MB-231 breast cancer cells. *Exp Cell Res* 314, 3340-3355.

Ohd JF, Nielsen CK, Campbell J, Landberg G, Lofberg H & Sjolander A (2003) Expression of the leukotriene D4 receptor CysLT1, COX-2, and other cell survival factors in colorectal adenocarcinomas. *Gastroenterology* 124, 57-70.

Ou YC, Yang CR, Cheng CL, Raung SL, Hung YY & Chen CJ (2007) Indomethacin induces apoptosis in 786-O renal cell carcinoma cells by activating mitogen-activated protein kinases and AKT. *Eur J Pharmacol* 563, 49-60.

Park JY, Pillinger MH & Abramson SB (2006) Prostaglandin E2 synthesis and secretion: the role of PGE2 synthases. *Clin Immunol* 119, 229-240.

Park SW, Kim HS, Hah JH, Kim KH, Heo DS & Sung MW (2010) Differential effects between cyclooxygenase-2 inhibitors and siRNA on vascular endothelial growth factor production in head and neck squamous cell carcinoma cell lines. *Head Neck* 32, 1534-1543.

Pidgeon GP, Lysaght J, Krishnamoorthy S, Reynolds JV, O'Byrne K, Nie D & Honn KV (2007) Lipoxygenase metabolism: roles in tumor progression and survival. *Cancer Metastasis Rev* 26, 503-524.

Romano M & Claria J (2003) Cyclooxygenase-2 and 5-lipoxygenase converging functions on cell proliferation and tumor angiogenesis: implications for cancer therapy. *FASEB J* 17, 1986-1995.

Rosenthal EL & Matrisian LM (2006) Matrix metalloproteases in head and neck cancer. *Head Neck* 28, 639-648.

Saba NF, Choi M, Muller S, Shin HJ, Tighiouart M, Papadimitrakopoulou VA, El-Naggar AK, Khuri FR, Chen ZG & Shin DM (2009) Role of cyclooxygenase-2 in tumor progression and survival of head and neck squamous cell carcinoma. *Cancer Prev Res (Phila)* 2, 823-829.

Sarveswaran S, Thamilselvan V, Brodie C & Ghosh J (2011) Inhibition of 5-lipoxygenase triggers apoptosis in prostate cancer cells via down-regulation of protein kinase C-epsilon. *Biochim Biophys Acta*, 1813, 2108-2117.

Schroeder CP, Yang P, Newman RA & Lotan R (2004) Eicosanoid metabolism in squamous cell carcinoma cell lines derived from primary and metastatic head and neck cancer and its modulation by celecoxib. *Cancer Biol Ther* 3, 847-852.

Scioscia KA, Snyderman CH, D'Amico F, Comsa S, Rueger R & Light B (2000) Effects of arachidonic acid metabolites in a murine model of squamous cell carcinoma. *Head Neck* 22, 149-155.

Sheng H, Shao J & Dubois RN (2001) K-Ras-mediated increase in cyclooxygenase 2 mRNA stability involves activation of the protein kinase B1. *Cancer Res* 61, 2670-2675.

Shono T, Tofilon PJ, Bruner JM, Owolabi O & Lang FF (2001) Cyclooxygenase-2 expression in human gliomas: prognostic significance and molecular correlations. *Cancer Res* 61, 4375-4381.

Shureiqi I & Lippman SM (2001) Lipoxygenase modulation to reverse carcinogenesis. *Cancer Res* 61, 6307-6312.

Subbaramaiah K, Altorki N, Chung WJ, Mestre JR, Sampat A & Dannenberg AJ (1999) Inhibition of cyclooxygenase-2 gene expression by p53. *J Biol Chem* 274, 10911-10915.

Sugimoto Y & Narumiya S (2007) Prostaglandin E receptors. *J Biol Chem* 282, 11613-11617.

Sun Z, Sood S, Li N, Ramji D, Yang P, Newman RA, Yang CS & Chen X (2006) Involvement of the 5-lipoxygenase/leukotriene A4 hydrolase pathway in 7,12-dimethylbenz[a]anthracene (DMBA)-induced oral carcinogenesis in hamster cheek pouch, and inhibition of carcinogenesis by its inhibitors. *Carcinogenesis* 27, 1902-1908.

Tang DW, Lin SC, Chang KW, Chi CW, Chang CS & Liu TY (2003) Elevated expression of cyclooxygenase (COX)-2 in oral squamous cell carcinoma--evidence for COX-2 induction by areca quid ingredients in oral keratinocytes. *J Oral Pathol Med* 32, 522-529.

Wang MT, Honn KV & Nie D (2007) Cyclooxygenases, prostanoids, and tumor progression. *Cancer Metastasis Rev* 26, 525-534.

Wang YH, Wu MW, Yang AK, Zhang WD, Sun J, Liu TR & Chen YF (2010) COX-2 Gene increases tongue cancer cell proliferation and invasion through VEGF-C pathway. *Med Oncol*, doi:10.1007/s12032-12010-19737-12033

Williams CS, Mann M & DuBois RN (1999) The role of cyclooxygenases in inflammation, cancer, and development. *Oncogene* 18, 7908-7916.

Williams CS, Tsujii M, Reese J, Dey SK & DuBois RN (2000) Host cyclooxygenase-2 modulates carcinoma growth. *J Clin Invest* 105, 1589-1594.

Wilson JC, Anderson LA, Murray LJ & Hughes CM (2011) Non-steroidal anti-inflammatory drug and aspirin use and the risk of head and neck cancer: a systematic review. *Cancer Causes Control* 22, 803-810.

Yang P, Sun Z, Chan D, Cartwright CA, Vijjeswarapu M, Ding J, Chen X & Newman RA (2008) Zyflamend reduces LTB4 formation and prevents oral carcinogenesis in a 7,12-dimethylbenz[alpha]anthracene (DMBA)-induced hamster cheek pouch model. *Carcinogenesis* 29, 2182-2189.

Zhu J, Huang JW, Tseng PH, Yang YT, Fowble J, Shiau CW, Shaw YJ, Kulp SK & Chen CS (2004) From the cyclooxygenase-2 inhibitor celecoxib to a novel class of 3-phosphoinositide-dependent protein kinase-1 inhibitors. *Cancer Res* 64, 4309-4318.

Part 3

Therapeutic Options

7

Nasopharyngeal Carcinoma: The Role for Chemotherapeutics and Targeted Agents

Jared Knol[1], Tiffany King[2] and Mark Agulnik[3]
[1]*Department of Medicine, Feinberg School of Medicine, Northwestern University, Chicago, Illinois*
[2]*Division of Hematology/Oncology, Northwestern Medical Faculty Foundation, Chicago, Illinois*
[3]*Division of Hematology/Oncology, Department of Medicine, Feinberg School of Medicine, Northwestern University, Robert H. Lurie Comprehensive Cancer Center, Chicago, Illinois*
USA

1. Introduction

Nasopharyngeal carcinoma (NPC) is a distinguishing and rare form of head and neck cancer whose predominant tumor type arises in the nasopharynx, the narrow tubular passage behind the nasal cavity. The disease is classified into three histopatholigical types by The World Health Organization (WHO): Keratinizing squamous cell carcinoma (SCC, WHO Type I), Nonkeratinizing carcinoma: differentiated (WHO Type II) and undifferentiated (WHO Type III) and basaloid squamous cell carcinoma[1]. Worldwide, there are 80,000 incident cases and 50,000 deaths annually,[2] however the disease is vastly more common in certain regions in Asia and Africa than anywhere else in the world. In the United States, the incidence ranges from 0.2 and 0.5 cases per 100,000 population, which constitutes roughly 0.02% of all cancers, compared with endemic areas such as areas in Asia, where NPC might represent 25% of all cancers[3]. In fact, it is sometimes referred to as Cantonese cancer because it occurs in about 25 cases per 100,000 people in this region, 25 times higher than the rest of the world[4].

Making it distinct is the fact that it differs from other head and neck squamous cell carcinomas (HNSCCs) in epidemiology, histology, natural history, and response to treatment. The remarkable geographic and demographic variation of NPC incidence suggests a multifactorial etiology of NPC. In endemic populations, the risk of NPC appears to be related to an interaction of these factors, namely Epstein-Barr virus (EBV) infection; genetic predisposition; and environmental factors such as the traditionally high intake of preserved foods[5-7].

2. RT and chemotherapy for locally advanced disease

The radiosensitizing properties of systemic chemotherapy are firmly established for head and neck tumors[8], and NPC is inherently more chemosensitive than other head and neck malignancies[9]. Therefore, it follows intuitively that adding systemic chemotherapy or targeted therapies to radiotherapy could provide NPC patients with additional clinical benefit. This hypothesis was tested in the late 1990s, and the utility of platinum-based chemotherapy in addition to radiation (RT) in locally advanced NPC was clearly demonstrated in 1998 when the Intergroup 0099 trial was terminated prematurely due to a clear survival benefit in the chemotherapy with radiotherapy arm[10]. Since that time several randomized trials have been published, all varying in their chemotherapy regimens and timing of chemotherapy in relation to RT (Tables 1 and 2).

Trial	No. of pts	Treatment Arms
Neoadjuvant + RT vs RT alone		
VUMCA (1996)	a: 171	a: Bleomycin/Epirubicin/Cisplatin → RT
	b: 168	b: RT
Chua et al (1998)	a: 167	a: Cisplatin/Epirubicin → RT
	b: 167	b: RT
Ma et al (2001)	a: 224	a: Cisplatin/Bleomycin/5-FU → RT
	b: 225	b: RT
Hareyama et al (2002)	a: 40	a: Cisplatin/5-FU → RT
	b: 40	b: RT
Concurrent + RT vs RT alone		
Lin et al (2003)	a: 141	a: Cisplatin/5-FU + RT
	b: 143	b: RT
Chan et al (2002, 2004)	a: 174	a: Cisplatin + RT
	b: 176	b: RT
Zhang et al (2005)	a: 59	a: Oxaliplatin + RT
	b: 56	b: RT
Adjuvant + RT vs RT alone		
Rossi et al (1988)	a: 113	a: RT → Vincristine/Cyclophosphamide/Adriamycin
	b: 116	b: RT
Chi et al (2002)	a: 77	a: RT → Cisplatin/Fluorouracil/Leucovorin
		b: RT
Neoadjuvant + Adjuvant + RT vs RT alone		
Chan et al (1995)	a: 37	a: Cisplatin/Fluorouracil → RT → Cisplatin/5-FU
	b: 40	b: RT
Concurrent + Adjuvant + RT vs RT alone		
Al-Sarraf et al (1998, 2001)	a: 93	a: Cisplatin + RT → Cisplatin/5-FU
	b: 92	b: RT
Wee et al (2005)	a: 111	a: Cisplatin + RT → Cisplatin/5-FU
	b: 110	b: RT
Lee et al (2005, 2010)	a: 172	a: Cisplatin + RT → Cisplatin/5-FU
	b: 176	b: RT
Lee et al (2006)	a: 51	a: Cisplatin + RT → Cisplatin/5-FU
	b: 44	b: Cisplatin + AF RT → Cisplatin/5-FU
	c: 52	c: AF RT
	d: 42	d: RT
Kwong et al (2004)	a1: 57	a1: Uracil-Tegafur + RT → Cisplatin/5-FU,Vincristine/Bleomycin/MTX
	a2: 53	a2: Uracil-Tegafur + RT
	a3: 54	a3: RT → Cisplatin/5-FU, Vincristine/Bleomycin/MTX
	b: 55	b: RT
Chen et al (2008)	a: 158	a: Cisplatin + RT → Cisplatin/5-FU
	b: 158	b: RT

Table 1. Randomized Trials of Chemotherapy with RT vs RT alone in locally advanced NPC

Trial	Treatment Arm	OS	DFS	Median F/U (mo)
Neoadjuvant + RT vs RT alone				
VUMCA (1996)	a	3yr – 60%	3yr – 52%*	49
	b	54%	32%	
Chua et al (1998)	a	3yr – 78%	3yr – 48%	30
	b	71%	42%	
Ma et al (2001)	a	5yr – 63%	5yr – 59%*	62
	b	56%	49%	
Hareyama et al (2002)	a	5yr – 60%	5yr – 55%	49
	b	48%	43%	
Chua (2005)	a	5yr – 62%	5yr – 51%*	67
	b	58%	43%	
Concurrent + RT vs RT alone				
Lin et al (2003)	a	5yr – 72%*	5yr – 72%*	65
	b	54%	53%	
Chan et al (2002, 2004)	a	NR	2yr – 76%	33
	b	NR	69%	
	a	5yr – 70%	5yr – 60%	65
	b	59%	52%	
Zhang et al (2005)	a	2yr – 100%*	2yr – 96%*	24
	b	77%	83%	
Adjuvant + RT vs RT alone				
Rossi et al (1998)	a	5yr – 55%	5yr – 54%	49.5
	b	61%	50%	
Chi et al (2002)	a	4yr – 59%	4yr – 58%	43
	b	67%	56%	
Neoadjuvant + Adjuvant + RT vs RT alone				
Chan et al (1995)	a	2yr – 80%	2yr – 68%	28.5
	b	81%	72%	
Concurrent + Adjuvant + RT vs RT alone				
Al-Sarraf et al (1998, 2001)	a	3yr – 76%*	3yr – 66%*	32.4
	b	46%	26%	
	a	5yr – 67%*	5yr – 58%*	60
	b	37%	29%	
Wee et al (2005)	a	2yr – 85%*	3yr – 80%*	38.4
	b	78%	65%	
Lee et al (2005, 2010)	a	3yr – 77%	3yr – 69%	25
	b	76%	61%	
	a	5yr – 68%	5yr – 62%*	70.8
	b	64%	53%	
	a	8yr – 61%	NR	
	b	54%	NR	
Lee et al (2006)	a	3yr – 87%	3yr – 73%	33
	b	88%	88%	
	c	73%	63%	
	d	83%	65%	
Kwong et al (2004)	a1	3yr – 89%	3yr – 70%	32.5
	a2	84%	69%	
	a3	71%	54%	
	b	83%	61%	
Chen et al (2008)	a	2yr – 90%*	2yr – 85%*	29
	b	80%	73%	

* statistically significant result

Table 2. OS and DFS of randomized trials of chemotherapy with RT vs. RT alone in locally advanced NPC

2.1 Neoadjuvant chemotherapy

Four trials have assessed the role of neoadjuvant chemotherapy followed by RT versus RT alone. The VUMCA study[11], active from 1989-1993, was a multi-center phase II trial of 339 patients, in which 171 patients were randomized to receive neoadjuvant bleomycin, epirubicin, and cisplatin (BEC). The remaining 168 patients received RT alone. After a median followup of 49 months the authors noted increased disease free survival (DFS) in the chemotherapy with RT arm (52% vs 32%). However, no difference in overall survival (OS) was seen, and the trial was notable for an 8% rate of treatment-related death in the experimental arm versus 1% among patients treated with RT alone.

A small study of 80 patients, active from 1991-1998, was published by Hareyama et al[12]. Forty patients were randomized to cisplatin and 5-fluorouracil prior to RT, and the control arm received RT alone. A trend toward both OS and DFS at three years was seen in the neoadjuvant arm (60% and 55% vs 48% and 43%, respectively), though this did not reach statistical significance. In 1998, Chua et al published the results of a trial active from 1989-1993, in which 334 patients were randomized to either cisplatin and epirubicin with RT or RT alone[13]. Intention to treat analysis at three years revealed a trend toward improved DFS and OS in the chemoradiotherapy arm (58% and 80% vs 46% and 72%, respectively), however the results did not reach statistical significance.

In 2001 Ma et al reported a trial, active from 1993-1994, in which 449 patients were randomized to two to three cycles of cisplatin, 5-fluorouracil, and bleomycin with RT versus RT alone[14]. Intention to treat analysis at five years revealed a statistically significant improvement in DFS (59% vs 49%), however, while a trend toward improved OS was noted this did not reach statistical significance. In 2005, Chua published an analysis of pooled data from the latter two trials, which together included 784 patients with a median follow up of 67 months[15]. This analysis revealed a statistically significant DFS benefit in the neoadjuvant arm (51% vs 43%). However, consistent with the other trials, a trend toward OS (62% vs 58%) did not reach statistical significance. In summary, four trials of neoadjuvant platinum-based chemotherapy in addition to RT have revealed, at best, modest improvement in DFS and a trend toward improved overall survival. However to date no trial has shown a clear and statistically significant survival benefit with the neoadjuvant strategy.

2.2 Concurrent chemotherapy

To date, three trials have assessed the strategy of concurrent chemotherapy and RT as compared to RT alone. In 2002, Chan et al reported a trial, active from 1994-1997, of 350 patients randomized to weekly low-dose cisplatin plus RT versus RT alone[16]. Notably, the study population in this trial had relatively advanced disease: 90% of patients were Ho's stage III or IV, and over 70% were AJCC stage III or IV. A trend toward improved DFS at two years was seen (76% vs 69%), however this did not reach statistical significance. Updated data published in 2005 revealed modestly improved DFS and OS for the chemotherapy arm at five years: DFS was 60% and 52% ($p = 0.06$) and OS was 70% and 59% ($p = 0.05$) for the chemotherapy + RT and RT alone arms, respectively[17]. A subgroup analysis of this data revealed that patients with more advanced disease (T3 and T4) derived the most benefit. Lin et al reported data in 2003 from a 1993-1999 study of concurrent cisplatin and 5-fluorouracil plus

RT vs RT alone[18]. All patients in this trial had AJCC stage III or IV disease. The study revealed statistically significant improvement in both DFS and OS with concurrent chemotherapy: 5-year OS rates for the chemotherapy arm were 72% compared with 54% in the control arm, and the 5-year DFS rates were 72 versus 53%, respectively. Of note, significantly more toxicity was noted in the chemotherapy arm. In 2005, Zhang et al published a trial, active from 2001-2003, of 115 patients randomized to six doses of weekly oxaliplatin plus concurrent RT versus RT alone[19]. Consistent with the earlier cisplatin-based trials, this study revealed a significant DFS and OS benefit for patients treated with concurrent platinum-based chemotherapy. For the chemotherapy + RT and RT alone arms, respectively, two year OS was 100% versus 77% and two year DFS was 96% versus 83%. In summary, three trials of concurrent platinum-based chemotherapy plus radiotherapy have revealed statistically significant improvements in DFS and OS as compared to radiotherapy alone. In these trials, the benefit was greatest in patients with advanced disease.

2.3 Adjuvant chemotherapy

The first trial that addressed the question of adding chemotherapy to RT for patients with NPC used an adjuvant strategy. In 1988, Rossi et al published the results of a 4 year multi-center trial, active from 1979-1983, in which 229 patients were randomized to either adjuvant vincristine, cyclophosphamide, and adriamycin following RT or RT alone[20]. Follow up at four years did not reveal a statistically significant difference in DFS or OS between the two groups. Notably, no platinum agent was used in this trial, and therefore the lack of benefit must be interpreted in light of subsequent studies which have established platinum-based chemotherapy as the cornerstone of chemotherapy plus RT strategies in this disease. However, a later study of adjuvant chemotherapy, which did include cisplatin, was published in 2002 by Chi et al and revealed no significant DFS or OS benefit[21]. Between 1994 and 1999, 157 patients were randomized to either adjuvant cisplatin with 5-fluorouriacil and leucovorin plus RT versuss RT alone. At five years, the DFS rates were 54.4% vs 49.5% and the OS rates were 60.5% and 54.5%, respectively, for the chemotherapy and RT arms. Neither of these differences reached statistical significance. In summary, two trials have addressed the strategy of adjuvant chemotherapy following RT, one of which was published prior to the Intergroup 0099 trial and as such did not include a platinum agent. Neither study revealed a statistically significant improvement in survival with adjuvant chemotherapy following RT as compared to RT alone.

2.4 Neoadjuvant plus adjuvant chemotherapy

To date, only one study has assessed the effect of combined neoadjuvant and adjuvant chemotherapy in addition to RT. In 1995, Chan et al reported a study of 82 patients randomized to two cycles of neoadjuvant and four cycles of adjuvant chemotherapy (both with cisplatin) plus RT vs RT alone[22]. No difference in either DFS or OS was noted after two years follow up. In summary, the single published trial of combined neoadjuvant and adjuvant chemotherapy (cisplatin) plus RT revealed no benefit of this strategy as compared to RT alone.

2.5 Concurrent plus adjuvant chemotherapy

To date, the most influential study to address the question of chemotherapy plus RT in locally advanced NPC utilized a combined concurrent and adjuvant platiunum-based chemotherapy strategy, and, consequently, this approach has subsequently received the most research attention. In 1998, Al-Sarraf et al published the results of the Intergroup 0099 study, active between 1989 and 1995, in which 193 patients were randomized to either RT alone or a chemotherapy arm[10]. Patients in the chemotherapy group were treated with cisplatin on days 1, 22 and 43 of the concurrent RT, and three adjuvant cycles of cisplatin with 5-fluorouracil were given monthly after completion of chemoradiotherapy. At 3 years, DFS was 69% in the chemotherapy group and 24% in the RT alone arm. Overall survival at 3 years was 78 *vs* 47%, favoring chemotherapy. These results prompted early closure of the study, given the clear benefit demonstrated with concurrent plus adjuvant cisplatin. Updated analysis at 5 years confirmed the benefit of treatment, with 5-year DFS rates of 58 *vs* 29% and 5-year OS rates of 67 *vs* 37%, both favoring the combined therapy arm[23]. Analysis of the National Cancer database since the first published results of the Intergroup 0099 study data in 1998 has demonstrated that this study has led to a demonstrable change in NPC management. Of all patients enrolled in the database and matching the eligibility criteria of the Intergroup 0099 study, only 38% received chemotherapy along with RT prior to 1997, while since the publication of the data, 65% of these patients have received concurrent and adjuvant chemotherapy[24].

One-quarter of all patients treated on the Intergroup 0099 protocol had World Health Organization (WHO) stage I histology (keratinizing squamous cell carcinoma). A phase III randomized trial active from 1997-2003, using a similar chemotherapy and RT plan but restricted to patients with WHO type IIa (nonkeratinising squamous cell carcinoma) and IIb (undifferentiated carcinoma) histologies was published by Wee et al in 2005[25]. The two and three year DFS and OS rates were statistically significant and favored the use of chemotherapy, confirming the findings of the Intergroup 0099 trial. Of note, the chemotherapy regimen used in the Wee et al study differed slightly from the Intergroup 0099 trial in that the dose of cisplatin was given in divided doses rather than one dose, however, the total dose remained the same. Lee et al have published data from the Hong Kong NPC Study Group in which the Intergroup 0099 regimen was applied to patients with nonkeratinizing or undifferentiated NPC[26]. Preliminary results published in 2004 suggested a trend toward improved DFS in the chemotherapy arm. Long term follow up data published in 2010 confirmed the trend toward improved DFS seen on the initial analysis (62% vs 53% favoring chemotherapy). However, while five-year analysis showed a clear reduction death due to disease progression in the chemotherapy arm (28% vs 38% favoring chemotherapy, $p = 0.08$), the five-year overall survival data revealed only a modest trend favoring chemotherapy (68% vs 64%, $p = 0.22$)[27]. The discrepancy between a clear decreased in disease-associated death and nearly identical five-year overall survival was attributed to an increase in non-cancer deaths among patients in the chemotherapy arm.

A similar trial, also published by Lee et al, utilized the identical chemotherapy as IG-0099, but assessed both the therapeutic gain with concurrent and adjuvant chemotherapy and/or accelerated RT[28]. Four arms were evaluated, conventional RT vs. accelerated fraction RT vs. conventional RT with concurrent and adjuvant chemotherapy vs. accelerated fraction RT with concurrent and adjuvant chemotherapy. After 189 patients were randomized, the study was closed due to poor accrual. Preliminary data after a median follow-up of 2.9 years, showed no statistically significant change in either OS or DFS at 3-years.

In 2008, Chen et al published the results of a study of 316 patients performed between 2002 and 2005, in which subjects randomized to the chemotherapy arm received weekly cisplatin concurrent with RT, followed by cisplatin and 5-fluorouracil every four weeks for three cycles following completion of RT[29]. Preliminary analysis after two years revealed a statistically significant difference in both overall (89.8% vs 79.7%) and disease free (84.6% vs 72.5%) survival, favoring chemotherapy, at the expense of increased toxicity in the chemotherapy arm.

Finally, a factorial study of four different regimens was published by Kwong et al in 2004[30]. This study assessed the combination of RT alone *vs* three other schemas: RT with adjuvant chemotherapy, concurrent chemoradiotherapy and lastly, concurrent chemoradiotherapy followed by adjuvant chemotherapy. UFT (uracil an tegafur in a 4:1 molar ratio) was given concurrent with RT, while the adjuvant therapy consisted of alternating cycles of cisplatin/5-fluorouracil and vincristine/bleomycin/methotrexate.

Although a trend towards improved DFS and OS was noted with the addition of concurrent chemotherapy, it did not reach statistical significance at 3 years. In assessing distant metastases rates, a significant reduction was attributable to concurrent chemotherapy. In this study, adjuvant chemotherapy did not improve outcome.

3. Chemotherapy for recurrent and metastatic disease

The management of recurrent and metastatic NPC remains challenging. Several studies have evaluated the use of platinum drugs in combination with various other chemotherapeutic agents including gemcitabine [31,32], bleomycin-5FU[33], 5FU[34], capecitabine[35], bleomycin/epirubicin/5FU[36], paclitaxel[37], and docetaxel[38]. Given the known chemosensitivity of NPC, it is not surprising that these regimens are associated with good overall response rates, ranging from 56% - 79%. However, the duration of response is short, and median overall survival in these trials was on average approximately one year (range: 11 - 25 mo). Two trials of non-platinum based monotherapy (gemcitabine[39] and capecitabine[40]) were associated with worse overall response rates (28% and 37%, respectively) and similar median overall survival (7.2 and 14 months, respectively). Adding vinorelbine to gemcitabine for patients with platinum-resistant disease yielded an overall response rate of 36% with a median overall survival of 11.9 months[41]. Irinotecan used as monotherapy in heavily pretreated patients has been associated with an overall response rate of 14% (all partial responses) and median overall survival of 11.4 months[42]. The poor clinical outcomes associated with traditional chemotherapeutic agents underscores the urgent need for new and more effective therapeutic options in the locally advanced and metastatic setting.

4. Targeted therapy

Given the poor clinical outcomes associated with chemotherapeutics in the metastatic setting, evaluation of targeted therapies become of utmost importance (Table 3).

Epidermal growth factor receptor (EGFR) expression in NPC has been correlated with decreased survival, increased rates of locoregional failure, and more aggressive disease [43,44]. Drawing on those findings, Chan et al published a study in 2005 evaluating the anti-EGFR

Table 3. Targeted therapy in NPC

Reference	Targeted Tx	Other Tx	# of patients/ # evaluable	Disease Status	Overall Response	Median Overall Survival	Grade 3/4 Toxicity
Chan (2005)	Cetuximab	Carboplatin	60/59	Recurrent/Metastatic	11.7% (1)	233 days	51.7%
Ma (2007)^	Cetuximab	Cisplatin + IMRT	20/12	Locally advanced	83%	NR	85% (2)
Elser (2007) (3)	Sorafenib	None	7/NR	NR	N/A (4)	7.7 months	NR
Chua (2008)	Gefitinib	None	19/NR	Recurrent/Metastatic	0%	19 months	0%
Ma (2008)	Gefitinib	None	16/15	Recurrent/Metastatic	0%	12 months	? (6)
You (2009)^	Erlotinib	Cisplatin/Carboplatin + Gemcitabine (5)	20/11	Recurrent/Metastatic	0%	NR	NR

(1)All partial responses
(2)No composite grade 3/4 toxicity data reported. Reports that 85% of patients experienced grade 3/4 leukopenia and 85% experienced grade 3/4 mucositis.
(3)This study included both SCCHN and NPC patients. Data is presented here only for the 7 NPC patients enrolled.
(4)One of 26 evaluable SCCHN/NPC patients had a partial response. However, it is not reported whether this patient had SCCHN or NPC.
(5)Erlotinib was given as maintenance after completion of 6 cycles platinum + gemcitabine or as 2nd line therapy after progression on chemotherapy
(6)Reports grade 3/4 toxicity as "rare", most common was rash in (33%)
^ Abstract

monoclonal antibody, cetuximab, in combination with carboplatin[45]. This multi-center phase II trial enrolled 60 patients, all of who had evidence of disease progression within 12 months of platinum-based chemotherapy. Notably, 93.3% of patients in this trial had stage IV disease at the time of enrollment, and 85% had distant metastases. The treatment protocol consisted of carboplatin infused every three weeks for a maximum of eight cycles, along with cetuximab 400mg/m2 followed by 250mg/m2 weekly. The median number of cetuximab infusions completed was 10, with a range of 1-30. Only 53.3% of the patients received at least 3 carboplatin infusions. Of patients enrolled, 11.7% had a partial response to therapy; no complete responses were observed in this study and 48.3% of patients had stable disease. Median time to progression was 81 days, and median overall survival was 233 days. Grade 3 or 4 toxicity was observed in 51.7% of patients, 31.7% of whom had toxicity that was attributed to cetuximab. A subsequent trial of cetuximab in combination with cisplatin-IMRT was reported in abstract form by Ma et al in 2008[46]. The 20 patients in this trial differed from those in Chan et al in that all subjects had untreated, non-metastatic disease. The cetuximab dosing was the same (400mg/m2 initially, followed by 250mg/m2 weekly). Cisplatin was administered at 30mg/m2 weekly, along with weekly IMRT. Ninety percent of patients received at least 5 doses of cetuximab, and 80% received at least 5 cisplatin infusions. Preliminary analysis at 3 months revealed promising results: of 12 patients evaluable for response, 10 had a complete response and the remaining two had stable disease.

Two studies have evaluated the use of the small molecule EGFR tyrosine kinase inhibitor, gefitinib, as monotherapy in advanced platinum-resistant NPC. In 2008 Chua et al reported a single-center phase II study of 19 patients with relapsed or progressive despite at least two prior chemotherapy regimens (one of which included a platinum drug)[47]. In contrast to the previously mentioned trials, this study protocol assessed response to anti-EGFR therapy alone without any concurrent chemotherapeutic agent. Patients in the study received gefitinib 250mg daily until disease progression, unacceptable toxcitiy, or patient refusal. Median treatment duration was 10 weeks; 63% of patients were taken off study due to disease progression, and the remaining patients expressed a preference not to continue treatment. The regimen was well tolerated, with no grade 3 or 4 toxicity reported. Unfortunately, no patients in this study achieved either partial or complete response. Similar disappointing results were reported by Ma et al in 2008[48]. In that trial, 16 patients with progressive disease after prior platinum-based therapy were treated with oral gefitinib 500 mg/day. Three patients achieved stable disease (range: 2.8 - 8.5 months), and the drug was generally well tolerated. However, consistent with the results reported by Chua et al, no patient achieved a partial or complete response. In 2009, You et al presented data in abstract form reporting their study of the EGFR tyrosine kinase inhibitor, erlotinib[49]. In that small trial of 20 patients, subjects were first treated with up to 6 cycles of gemcitabine + a platinum agent (either cisplatin or carboplatin), followed by erlotinib 150 mg/day as maintenance (if stable disease) or 2nd line therapy (if progressive disease prior to 6 chemotherapy cycles). Of the 11 patients evaluable for response to erlotinib, three had stable disease that was maintained for 3, 4, and 7 months.

Sorafenib, a multi-kinase inhibitor with activity against VEGFR-2, VEGFR-3, PDGFR, FLT-3, c-kit, and the Raf isoforms c-Raf and b-Raf, was evaluated in a 2007 study published by Elser et al.[50] Of particular theoretical interest is the anti-angiogenesis activity of sorafenib mediated by its activity against the vascular endothelium growth factor receptor (VEGFR), given the known VEGF overexpression in NPC[51-53]. Notably, this study was not limited to NPC and also enrolled patients with SCCHN; of 27 patients enrolled, only 7 had NPC. Patients received sorafenib 400 mg twice daily as monotherapy, and therapy was generally well tolerated with few grade 3 or 4 toxicities. Although the reported response data for the entire patient cohort was promising (9 of 26 evaluable patients had stable disease, and one had a partial response), response data specific to the NPC subgroup was not separately reported. Median time to progression for the 7 patients with NPC was 3.2 months, and median overall survival was 7.7 months.

In addition to monoclonal antibody and small molecule targeted therapy, immunotherapy may play a role in the future management of NPC. This approach has great theoretical appeal in NPC, given the strong association with Epstein-Barr virus (EBV). NPC cells express two distinct EBV latent membrane proteins, LMP-1 and LMP-2, and these proteins represent targets for adoptive immunotherapy[54]. In a phase I study published by Straathof et al in 2005, 10 patients with advanced NPC were treated with EBV-specific cytotoxic T lymphocytes (CTL)[55]. Four patients were in remission at the time of enrollment, and all remained disease-free 19–27 months after infusion. Of the remaining 6 patients, all with relapsed or refractory disease, 2 had complete responses, 1 had a partial response, 1 had stable disease and 2 had no response. CTL was well tolerated in this study. Follow up data from the same group was published in 2010, and this again demonstrated clinical benefit following CTL infusion[56]. Of 23 patients in this study (all with a history of relapsed/refractory NPC), 8 were in remission and 15 were not. Of the 8 patients in remission, 5 remained disease free at the time of publication (range: 17-75 months post-infusion). Furthermore, CTL infusion was associated with a 48.7% overall response rate in patients with active disease, though for the subset of patients with metastatic disease the overall response rate was only 10%.

5. Conclusion

In summary, the anti-EGFR monoclonal antibody, cetuximab, has been associated with a small but significant overall response in patients with recurrent/metastatic disease who progressed despite platinum-based therapy. Furthermore, nearly half of the patients in that study achieved stable disease. Preliminary data in the locally advanced setting are more promising, with one small trial reporting an 83% overall response. In both of these trials, cetuximab was given in combination with platinum-based chemotherapy. Treatment with small molecule inhibitors has been less successful: two studies of the tyrosine kinase inhibitor, gefitinib, have shown no benefit. Inhibitors of angiogenesis are theoretically attractive subjects of investigation given the documented VEGF overexpression in NPC, and these agents warrant further investigation. Finally, the clear association between NPC and EBV represents a disease-specific biologic property that may be exploited via immunotherapy, and early work with EBV-specific cytotoxic T lymphocytes has produced promising results.

6. References

[1] Thompson L: World Health Organization classification of tumours: pathology and genetics of head and neck tumours. Ear Nose Throat J 85:74, 2006

[2] Parkin DM, Bray F, Ferlay J, et al: Global cancer statistics, 2002. CA Cancer J Clin 55:74-108, 2005
[3] Phillips CA, Hendershot DM: Functional electrical stimulation and reciprocating gait orthosis for ambulation exercise in a tetraplegic patient: a case study. Paraplegia 29:268-76, 1991
[4] Chang ET, Adami HO: The enigmatic epidemiology of nasopharyngeal carcinoma. Cancer Epidemiol Biomarkers Prev 15:1765-77, 2006
[5] Yuan JM, Wang XL, Xiang YB, et al: Preserved foods in relation to risk of nasopharyngeal carcinoma in Shanghai, China. Int J Cancer 85:358-63, 2000
[6] Farrow DC, Vaughan TL, Berwick M, et al: Diet and nasopharyngeal cancer in a low-risk population. Int J Cancer 78:675-9, 1998
[7] Liebowitz D: Nasopharyngeal carcinoma: the Epstein-Barr virus association. Semin Oncol 21:376-81, 1994
[8] Seiwert TY, Salama JK, Vokes EE: The chemoradiation paradigm in head and neck cancer. Nat Clin Pract Oncol 4:156-71, 2007
[9] Chan AT, Teo PM, Leung TW, et al: The role of chemotherapy in the management of nasopharyngeal carcinoma. Cancer 82:1003-12, 1998
[10] Al-Sarraf M, LeBlanc M, Giri PG, et al: Chemoradiotherapy versus radiotherapy in patients with advanced nasopharyngeal cancer: phase III randomized Intergroup study 0099. J Clin Oncol 16:1310-7, 1998
[11] Preliminary results of a randomized trial comparing neoadjuvant chemotherapy (cisplatin, epirubicin, bleomycin) plus radiotherapy vs. radiotherapy alone in stage IV(> or = N2, M0) undifferentiated nasopharyngeal carcinoma: a positive effect on progression-free survival. International Nasopharynx Cancer Study Group. VUMCA I trial. Int J Radiat Oncol Biol Phys 35:463-9, 1996
[12] Hareyama M, Sakata K, Shirato H, et al: A prospective, randomized trial comparing neoadjuvant chemotherapy with radiotherapy alone in patients with advanced nasopharyngeal carcinoma. Cancer 94:2217-23, 2002
[13] Chua DT, Sham JS, Choy D, et al: Preliminary report of the Asian-Oceanian Clinical Oncology Association randomized trial comparing cisplatin and epirubicin followed by radiotherapy versus radiotherapy alone in the treatment of patients with locoregionally advanced nasopharyngeal carcinoma. Asian-Oceanian Clinical Oncology Association Nasopharynx Cancer Study Group. Cancer 83:2270-83, 1998
[14] Ma J, Mai HQ, Hong MH, et al: Results of a prospective randomized trial comparing neoadjuvant chemotherapy plus radiotherapy with radiotherapy alone in patients with locoregionally advanced nasopharyngeal carcinoma. J Clin Oncol 19:1350-7, 2001
[15] Chua DT, Ma J, Sham JS, et al: Long-term survival after cisplatin-based induction chemotherapy and radiotherapy for nasopharyngeal carcinoma: a pooled data analysis of two phase III trials. J Clin Oncol 23:1118-24, 2005
[16] Chan AT, Teo PM, Ngan RK, et al: Concurrent chemotherapy-radiotherapy compared with radiotherapy alone in locoregionally advanced nasopharyngeal carcinoma: progression-free survival analysis of a phase III randomized trial. J Clin Oncol 20:2038-44, 2002

[17] Chan AT, Leung SF, Ngan RK, et al: Overall survival after concurrent cisplatin-radiotherapy compared with radiotherapy alone in locoregionally advanced nasopharyngeal carcinoma. J Natl Cancer Inst 97:536-9, 2005

[18] Lin JC, Jan JS, Hsu CY, et al: Phase III study of concurrent chemoradiotherapy versus radiotherapy alone for advanced nasopharyngeal carcinoma: positive effect on overall and progression-free survival. J Clin Oncol 21:631-7, 2003

[19] Zhang L, Zhao C, Peng PJ, et al: Phase III study comparing standard radiotherapy with or without weekly oxaliplatin in treatment of locoregionally advanced nasopharyngeal carcinoma: preliminary results. J Clin Oncol 23:8461-8, 2005

[20] Rossi A, Molinari R, Boracchi P, et al: Adjuvant chemotherapy with vincristine, cyclophosphamide, and doxorubicin after radiotherapy in local-regional nasopharyngeal cancer: results of a 4-year multicenter randomized study. J Clin Oncol 6:1401-10, 1988

[21] Chi KH, Chang YC, Guo WY, et al: A phase III study of adjuvant chemotherapy in advanced nasopharyngeal carcinoma patients. Int J Radiat Oncol Biol Phys 52:1238-44, 2002

[22] Chan AT, Teo PM, Leung TW, et al: A prospective randomized study of chemotherapy adjunctive to definitive radiotherapy in advanced nasopharyngeal carcinoma. Int J Radiat Oncol Biol Phys 33:569-77, 1995

[23] Al-Sarraf M: Superiority of Five Year Survival with Chemo-Radiotherapy (CT-RT) vs Radiotherapy in Patients (Pts) with Locally Advanced Nasopharyngeal Cancer (NPC). Intergroup (0099) (SWOG 8892, RTOG 8817, ECOG 2388) Phase III Study: Final Report. Proc Am Soc Clin Oncol 20:abstract 905, 2001

[24] Hoffman H CJ, Weber R, Ang K, Porter K, Langer C.: Changing patterns of practice in the management of nasopharynx carcinoma (NPC): Analysis of the National Cancer Database (NCDB). ASCO Meeting Abstracts Sept 3:5501, 2004

[25] Wee J, Tan EH, Tai BC, et al: Randomized trial of radiotherapy versus concurrent chemoradiotherapy followed by adjuvant chemotherapy in patients with American Joint Committee on Cancer/International Union against cancer stage III and IV nasopharyngeal cancer of the endemic variety. J Clin Oncol 23:6730-8, 2005

[26] Lee AW, Lau WH, Tung SY, et al: Preliminary results of a randomized study on therapeutic gain by concurrent chemotherapy for regionally-advanced nasopharyngeal carcinoma: NPC-9901 Trial by the Hong Kong Nasopharyngeal Cancer Study Group. J Clin Oncol 23:6966-75, 2005

[27] Lee AW, Tung SY, Chua DT, et al: Randomized trial of radiotherapy plus concurrent-adjuvant chemotherapy vs radiotherapy alone for regionally advanced nasopharyngeal carcinoma. J Natl Cancer Inst 102:1188-98, 2010

[28] Lee AW, Tung SY, Chan AT, et al: Preliminary results of a randomized study (NPC-9902 Trial) on therapeutic gain by concurrent chemotherapy and/or accelerated fractionation for locally advanced nasopharyngeal carcinoma. Int J Radiat Oncol Biol Phys 66:142-51, 2006

[29] Chen Y, Liu MZ, Liang SB, et al: Preliminary results of a prospective randomized trial comparing concurrent chemoradiotherapy plus adjuvant chemotherapy with radiotherapy alone in patients with locoregionally advanced nasopharyngeal carcinoma in endemic regions of china. Int J Radiat Oncol Biol Phys 71:1356-64, 2008

[30] Kwong DL, Sham JS, Au GK, et al: Concurrent and adjuvant chemotherapy for nasopharyngeal carcinoma: a factorial study. J Clin Oncol 22:2643-53, 2004
[31] Ngan RK, Yiu HH, Lau WH, et al: Combination gemcitabine and cisplatin chemotherapy for metastatic or recurrent nasopharyngeal carcinoma: report of a phase II study. Ann Oncol 13:1252-8, 2002
[32] Ma BB, Hui EP, Wong SC, et al: Multicenter phase II study of gemcitabine and oxaliplatin in advanced nasopharyngeal carcinoma--correlation with excision repair cross-complementing-1 polymorphisms. Ann Oncol 20:1854-9, 2009
[33] Boussen H, Cvitkovic E, Wendling JL, et al: Chemotherapy of metastatic and/or recurrent undifferentiated nasopharyngeal carcinoma with cisplatin, bleomycin, and fluorouracil. J Clin Oncol 9:1675-81, 1991
[34] Au E, Ang PT: A phase II trial of 5-fluorouracil and cisplatinum in recurrent or metastatic nasopharyngeal carcinoma. Ann Oncol 5:87-9, 1994
[35] Li YH, Wang FH, Jiang WQ, et al: Phase II study of capecitabine and cisplatin combination as first-line chemotherapy in Chinese patients with metastatic nasopharyngeal carcinoma. Cancer Chemother Pharmacol 62:539-44, 2008
[36] Taamma A, Fandi A, Azli N, et al: Phase II trial of chemotherapy with 5-fluorouracil, bleomycin, epirubicin, and cisplatin for patients with locally advanced, metastatic, or recurrent undifferentiated carcinoma of the nasopharyngeal type. Cancer 86:1101-8, 1999
[37] Yeo W, Leung TW, Chan AT, et al: A phase II study of combination paclitaxel and carboplatin in advanced nasopharyngeal carcinoma. Eur J Cancer 34:2027-31, 1998
[38] Chua DT, Sham JS, Au GK: A phase II study of docetaxel and cisplatin as first-line chemotherapy in patients with metastatic nasopharyngeal carcinoma. Oral Oncol 41:589-95, 2005
[39] Foo KF, Tan EH, Leong SS, et al: Gemcitabine in metastatic nasopharyngeal carcinoma of the undifferentiated type. Ann Oncol 13:150-6, 2002
[40] Chua D, Wei WI, Sham JS, et al: Capecitabine monotherapy for recurrent and metastatic nasopharyngeal cancer. Jpn J Clin Oncol 38:244-9, 2008
[41] Wang CC, Chang JY, Liu TW, et al: Phase II study of gemcitabine plus vinorelbine in the treatment of cisplatin-resistant nasopharyngeal carcinoma. Head Neck 28:74-80, 2006
[42] Poon D, Chowbay B, Cheung YB, et al: Phase II study of irinotecan (CPT-11) as salvage therapy for advanced nasopharyngeal carcinoma. Cancer 103:576-81, 2005
[43] Chua DT, Nicholls JM, Sham JS, et al: Prognostic value of epidermal growth factor receptor expression in patients with advanced stage nasopharyngeal carcinoma treated with induction chemotherapy and radiotherapy. Int J Radiat Oncol Biol Phys 59:11-20, 2004
[44] Leong JL, Loh KS, Putti TC, et al: Epidermal growth factor receptor in undifferentiated carcinoma of the nasopharynx. Laryngoscope 114:153-7, 2004
[45] Chan AT, Hsu MM, Goh BC, et al: Multicenter, phase II study of cetuximab in combination with carboplatin in patients with recurrent or metastatic nasopharyngeal carcinoma. J Clin Oncol 23:3568-76, 2005
[46] Ma BB KM, Hui EP, King AD, Chan SL, Yu BK, Chiu SK, Lee FH, Chan AT.: A phase II study of concurrent cetuximab-cisplatin and intensity-modulated radiotherapy (IMRT) in locoregionally advanced nasopharyngeal carcinoma (NPC) with

correlation using dynamic contrast-enhanced magnetic resonance imaging (DCE-MRI). JCO Abstract, 2008
[47] Chua DT, Wei WI, Wong MP, et al: Phase II study of gefitinib for the treatment of recurrent and metastatic nasopharyngeal carcinoma. Head Neck 30:863-7, 2008
[48] Ma B, Hui EP, King A, et al: A phase II study of patients with metastatic or locoregionally recurrent nasopharyngeal carcinoma and evaluation of plasma Epstein-Barr virus DNA as a biomarker of efficacy. Cancer Chemother Pharmacol 62:59-64, 2008
[49] You B CE, Chin SF, Wang L, Jarvi A, Bharadwaj RR, Kamel-Reid S, Perez-Ordonez B, Siu LL: A phase II trial of erlotinib after gemcitabine plus platinum-based chemotherapy in patients (pts) with recurrent and/or metastatic nasopharyngeal carcinoma (NPC) European Journal of Cancer Supplements, 2009
[50] Elser C, Siu LL, Winquist E, et al: Phase II trial of sorafenib in patients with recurrent or metastatic squamous cell carcinoma of the head and neck or nasopharyngeal carcinoma. J Clin Oncol 25:3766-73, 2007
[51] Krishna SM, James S, Balaram P: Expression of VEGF as prognosticator in primary nasopharyngeal cancer and its relation to EBV status. Virus Res 115:85-90, 2006
[52] Montag M, Dyckhoff G, Lohr J, et al: Angiogenic growth factors in tissue homogenates of HNSCC: expression pattern, prognostic relevance, and interrelationships. Cancer Sci 100:1210-8, 2009
[53] Segawa Y, Oda Y, Yamamoto H, et al: Close correlation between CXCR4 and VEGF expression and their prognostic implications in nasopharyngeal carcinoma. Oncol Rep 21:1197-202, 2009
[54] Lee SP, Tierney RJ, Thomas WA, et al: Conserved CTL epitopes within EBV latent membrane protein 2: a potential target for CTL-based tumor therapy. J Immunol 158:3325-34, 1997
[55] Straathof KC, Bollard CM, Popat U, et al: Treatment of nasopharyngeal carcinoma with Epstein-Barr virus--specific T lymphocytes. Blood 105:1898-904, 2005
[56] Louis CU, Straathof K, Bollard CM, et al: Adoptive transfer of EBV-specific T cells results in sustained clinical responses in patients with locoregional nasopharyngeal carcinoma. J Immunother 33:983-90, 2010

8

Advanced Radiation Therapy for Head and Neck Cancer: A New Standard of Practice

Putipun Puataweepong
Ramathibodi Hospital, Mahidol University
Thailand

1. Introduction

Radiation therapy plays an important role in head and neck cancer management, including in the definitive nonsurgical setting, in postoperative patients with high-risk features and in recurrent setting. Because head and neck cancer can be very aggressive with a high tendency to recur locally, it is important to adequately irradiate all local-regional cancer cells (both gross disease and microscopic disease) to doses sufficient for tumor control. At the same time, many of the normal tissues in the head and neck area are very sensitive to radiation; such anatomic structures as the salivary glands, larynx, and constrictor muscles can be particularly damaged by treatment resulting in long-term sequelae.

The radiation oncologist was placed in the difficult situation of attempting to provide high doses of radiation to tumor and target volumes and minimal doses of radiation to normal structures. New technologies along with increased clinical familiarity and experience with these technologies have allowed the practice of radiotherapy to increase the distance between tumor dose and normal tissue dose, which in turn improves the ratio of cancer cure to treatment morbidity. The evolution in radiation therapy techniques over the last 30 years began from 2 dimensional (2D) radiation therapy using coplanar beams, usually in single or opposing pairs: e.g., right and left lateral or anterior field in head-and-neck cancer (Figure 1).

During the late 1980s, advancements in imaging and computer technology introduced the new methods to identify the targets on CT scans and display the radiation beams in three dimensions relative to the anatomy. In addition, radiation therapy by modern computer planning and multileaf collimators became available. The result was the introduction of Three Dimensional Conformal Radiotherapy (3D-CRT), which allowed better precision of irradiation delivery to image-based targets and some improvements in the sparing of noninvolved critical tissue. Another step forward was the development of Intensity Modulated Radiation Therapy (IMRT), which facilitated a higher degree of dose conformality and offered opportunities for additional clinical gains. More recently, Imaging-Guided Radiotherapy (IGRT) has emerged, making the better precision of patient setup with the ability for tracking of tumor regression and anatomical changes in the surrounding tissue during the whole course of radiation therapy. The other different techniques have evolved in head and neck cancer treatment. Stereotactic irradiation, gamma knife unit or linear

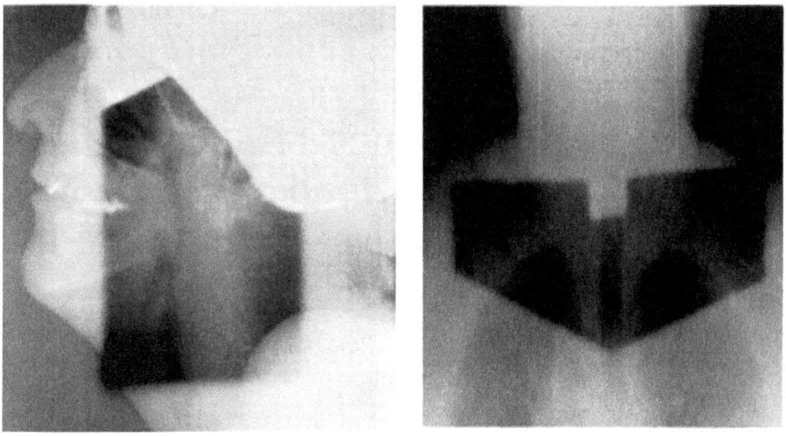

Fig. 1. Example of radiotherapy field using conventional - 2D radiation therapy, usually in single or opposing pairs: e.g., right and left lateral or anterior field in head-and-neck cancer

accelerator (LINAC)-based, is one method used in radiation therapy treatment. The radiation delivered has a sharp dose fall-off between the target and the surrounding normal tissue, thus allowing very precise delivery of radiation beam to the tumor while sparing and minimizing the radiation dose delivered to the surrounding organs. Lastly, other technical approaches such as proton beam radiotherapy or the CyberKnife are also used in this setting.

2. Intensity Modulated Radiation Therapy (IMRT)

IMRT is a form of 3D-CRT that implies the use of multiple radiation fields whose intensity varies across the field, depending on the thickness of the target and the existence of critical organs or critical noninvolved tissue. IMRT allows a relatively uniform dose in an irregularly shaped target while avoiding a high dose to the surrounding structures. The major differences between IMRT and more traditional radiotherapy techniques are the introduction of computer-controlled multileaf collimators, and the computer planning software (inverse planning) that allow for the intensity modulation of the various radiotherapy beamlets. Due to the relative ease of implementation of this technology (eg, compared with proton beam irradiation) and the obvious theoretic benefits, IMRT has quickly become standard for many cancers, including head and neck.

2.1 Imaging for treatment planning

Most of the case, the simulation contrast-enhanced CT is the only imaging modality required for the delineation of the targets. Magnetic resonance imaging (MRI) is a necessary adjunct to CT because it provides better detail of tumor extension and surround normal organ such as the tumors located close to the base of skull and the parapharyngeal and retropharyngeal spaces (Som,1997; Schechter et al., 2001) (Figure 2) Another potential imaging modality for this purpose is fluorodeoxyglucose-positron emission tomography (FDG-PET). However, in a series of HNCs in which CT, MRI, and FDG-PET were obtained, and surgery was then performed to validate the primary tumor extent and lymph node involvement, a rather limited benefit of FDG-PET over CT and MRI was found. (Schechter et al., 2001). PET-derived gross tumor volumes were smaller than those derived from CT and MRI, and surgical specimens were even smaller. However, when examined in detail, despite overestimation in most dimensions, all three imaging modalities actually underestimated the mucosal extent of disease (Schechter et al., 2001). Therefore, physical examination and laryngoscopy findings should be part of the definition in addition to image modalities such as CT and PET.

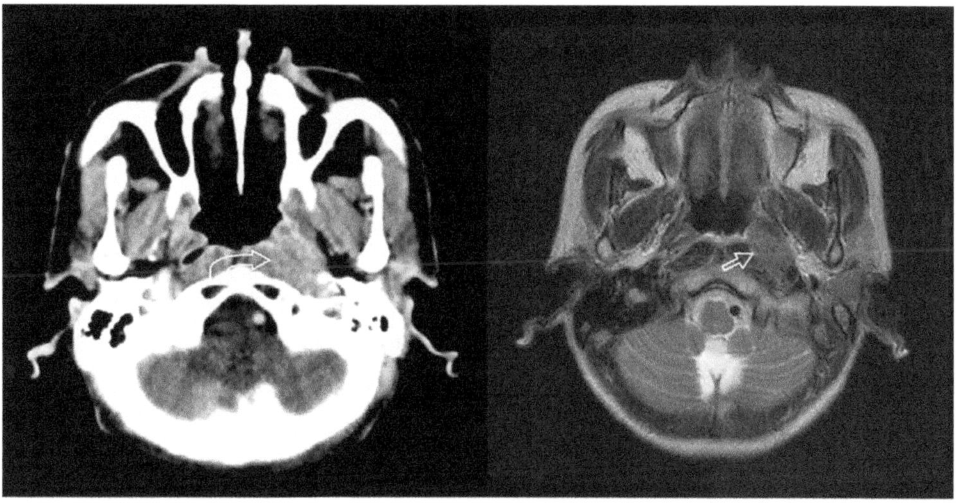

Fig. 2. CT (left) and MRI (right) scan of nasopharyngeal cancer . MRI provides information in prevertebral muscle invasion better than CT scan (arrow)

2.2 Delineating tumor and target volume

ICRU 50 defines five volumes of interest related to treatment. The following definition are illustrated in Figure 3.

2.2.1 Gross tumor volume (GTV): The GTV is the volume that contains the gross palpable or visible extent and location of malignant growth. The GTV may be identified on physical examination, a radiograph, or sectional images.

2.2.2 Clinical target volume (CTV): The CTV is the volume that contains the GTV and any suspected microscopic disease. The CTV is the volume that must receive the prescribed dose to effect cure or palliation.

2.2.3 Planning Target Volume (PTV): The PTV is a volume that contains the GTV and CTV and that is defined to account for the irradiation geometry and all uncertainties in treatment, such as organ and patient motions and set-up errors. The PTV is a volume that, when covered by the prescription dose, will ensure the delivery of the prescription dose to the CTV. The PTV includes a margin for motion and set-up error but not for microscopic disease. The PTV is a function of treatment geometry, because the number of beams and their orientations may impose limitations on the PTV's shape or scope.

2.2.4 Treated volume (TV): The TV is the volume enclosed by a selected (prescribed) isodose surface and is a function of the treatment geometry required for planning the PTV. For an acceptable plan, the TV is greater than the PTV, although an ideal TV/PTV ratio would be 1.0, indicating perfect conformation (assuming the locations of the volumes were identical).

2.2.5 Irradiated volume (IV): The IV is a volume that receives a significant dose; significance is determined by morbidity or other measures.

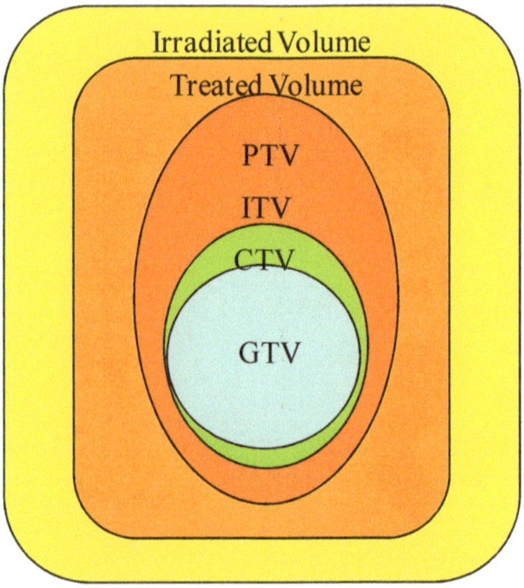

Fig. 3. The Internatinal Commission on Radiation Units and Measurement Report 50 (ICRU 50) defines five volmes of interest related to treatment.

In the routine practice, once the GTVs and CTVs are outlined on the axial CT scans, a expansion of CTV is performed to obtain the PTVs that accommodate setup uncertainties. Typically the magnitude of the margin is 3 to 5 mm, which means that an extra 5-mm ring of normal tissue around the target receives full dose. In a region with critical targets and organs at risk is close to the tumor, reducing this margin can potentially reduce treatment-related toxicity. An example of the delineation of the targets and noninvolved structures in a case of nasopharyngeal cancer is provided in Figure 4.

2.3 Dose prescription

The delivery of a single IMRT plan throughout the course of treatment provides better dose conformality than the use of several consecutive plans common in conventional radiotherapy, which consist of initial fields encompassing all targets followed with a boost to the gross tumor. Generally, when a single plan is prescribed, the PTV of gross tumor receives both a higher dose per fraction and total dose than the PTVs of the subclinical disease. Therefore, with a standard IMRT plan, the GTV would receive 70 Gy over 35 fractions , and the PTV of subclinical disease would receive lower fraction doses, usually 63 Gy to the high-risk and 56 to 59Gy to lesser-risk elective targets, over 35 fractions (1.8 Gy and 1.6-1.7 Gy) . Figure 5 shows isodose distribution in oropharygeal cancer compared between 3D-CRT and IMRT technique.

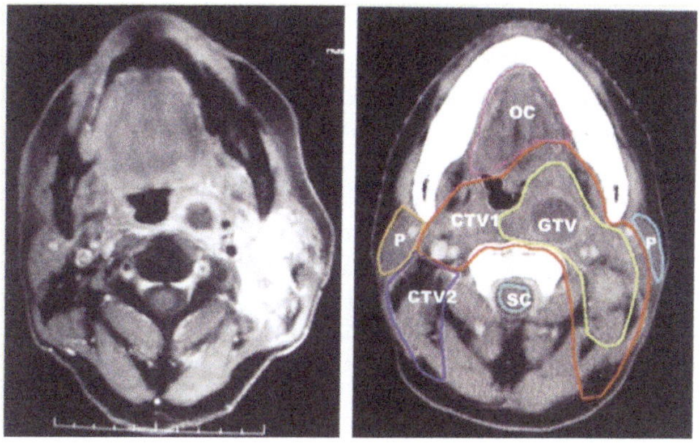

P represents the parotid gland; *red* represents CTV1 (high risk area) ; *purple* represent CTV 2 (low risk area) ; *yellow* represents GTV.

Fig. 4. Delineation of the targets and noninvolved structures in a case of nasopharyngeal cancer.

Radiation Therapy Oncology Group protocol H-0022 specified the prescription dose as the dose that encompasses at least 95% of the PTV. No more than 20% of the PTV can receive more than 110%, and no more than 1% of the PTV can receive less than 93%, of the prescribed dose.

Dose constraints regarding critical organs are usually stated in terms of the maximal dose. Commonly applied constraints in the head and neck are maximal doses of 45 Gy to the spinal cord, 54 Gy to the brainstem, 70Gy to the mandible, 50 to 55Gy to the optic pathway and maintain the mean dose to the contralateral parotids less than 26 Gy.

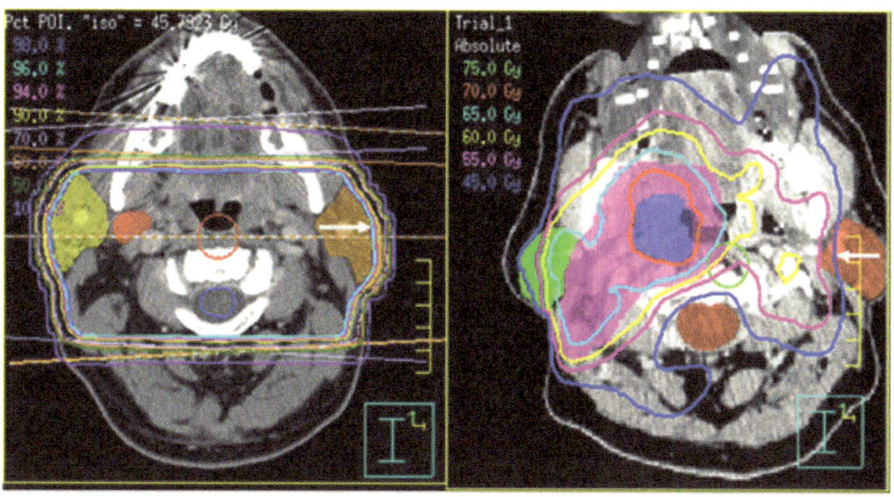

Fig. 5. Isodose distributions contrasting conventional (left) and IMRT (right) H&N treatment plans. Significant reduction of dose to the left parotid gland is achieved with the IMRT plan.

2.4 Clinical results in head and neck cancer treated with IMRT

In general the main intent in IMRT planning is preservation of function. One of the main issues is reducing xerostomia. Other potential functional gains from IMRT compared with conventional RT include reduced long-term dysphagia. Sparing of pharyngeal constrictors and the glottic and supraglottic larynx may be beneficial in this regard. (Eisbruch et al., 2004) . Most studies comparing IMRT with conventional treatments are retrospective and therefore have a potential selection bias. The only one randomized study from England (PARSPORT trial) (Christopher et al., 2011) was compared IMRT and conventional radiation in term of the incidence of xerostomia in head and neck cancer patient. At 24 months, grade 2 or worse xerostomia was significantly less common with IMRT (29%) than with conventional radiotherapy (83%) (p<0.0001). At 12 and 24 months, significant benefits were seen in recovery of saliva secretion with IMRT compared with conventional radiotherapy, as were clinically significant improvements in dry- mouth-specific and global quality of life scores. Until now, it still has no standard criteria to select which patients were more suitable for IMRT treatment. Many different selection factors were used to each institute. Generally, in patients who have poor performance status, cannot tolerate lengthy treatment, to be too sick to benefit from complex therapy, requiring urgent start of therapy, more simple, conventional treatment may be selected. Therefore the comparison of IMRT with conventional RT in such situations would be very difficult. We summarized the clinical result of IMRT in head and neck cancer as describe below.

2.5.1 Nasopharynx

The use of IMRT for the nasopharynx represents opportunities to spare many critical noninvolved structures and to improve tumor coverage, as detailed previously. These improvements have been demonstrated in several treatment planning exercises in nasopharyngeal and oropharyngeal tumors, in which IMRT plans were compared with "standard 3D" plans in the same patients.(De et al., 1999; Yao et al.,2005). The available level I evidence (two randomized prospective trials) to document the efficacy of IMRT involves nasopharyngeal cancer (NPC). Similar in design, each trial randomized patients between conventional radiation and IMRT along with concurrent chemotherapy(Pow et al., 2006; Kam et al., 2007). The results were that salivary gland (parotid) function was significantly and dramatically improved in both studies. Regarding to Pow and coworkers study (Pow et al., 2006), they found an improvement in stimulated saliva flow with IMRT and also found that patients treated with IMRT had an improvement in patient-reported quality of life scores. Similarly, Kam and coworkers (Kam et al., 2007) found a reduction in observer-rated xerostomia from 82.1% with conventional radiotherapy to 39.3% with IMRT along with improvements in measured parotid flow rates. The primary end point for both studies was parotid function; neither trial was powered or intended to examine the role of IMRT in disease control or overall survival. Although there is no level I evidence proving that IMRT is equal to or superior to conventional radiation therapy in terms of disease control, several large retrospective series have been reported. A large clinical series of IMRT of nasopharyngeal cancer has been reported by investigators at the University of California in San Francisco (Sultanem et al., 2000). They reported in 67 patients treated in the years 1995 to 2000. This regimen yielded excellent locoregional tumor control: The rate was 97% at median follow-up of 31 months, with reasonable rates of acute toxicity. Another large clinical series from the memorial Sloan-Kettering (Wolden et al., 2006) reported on 74 patients with newly diagnosed, nonmetastatic nasopharyngeal cancer were treated with IMRT. Most of the patients received concurrent and adjuvant platinum-based chemotherapy. At the median follow-up of 35 months, the 3-year actuarial rate of local control is 91%, and regional control is 93%; freedom from distant metastases, progression-free survival, and overall survival at 3 years are 78%, 67%, and 83%, respectively. There was 100% local control for Stage T1/T2 disease, compared to 83% for T3/T4 disease (p = 0.01). There is a trend for improved local control with IMRT when compared to local control of 79% for 35 patients treated before 1998 with three-dimensional planning and chemotherapy (P= 0.11). Rates of severe (Grade 3-4) ototoxicity and xerostomia are low with IMRT as a result of normal-tissue protection.

2.5.2 Paranasal sinuses

The proximity of the optic apparatus is the main obstacle to adequate irradiation of tumors in the locally advanced paranasal sinuses. In these cases, IMRT can provide adequate target coverage while sparing the optic pathways. The clinical series of IMRT in paranasal sinus cancer has been reported from the UCSF (Daly et al., 2007). In this study, 36 patients with malignancies of the sinonasal region were treated with IMRT. The 2-year and 5-year estimates of local control were 62% and 58%, respectively. One patient developed isolated distant metastasis, and none developed isolated regional failure. The 5-year rates of disease-free and overall survival were 55% and 45%, respectively. The incidence of ocular toxicity was minimal with no patients reporting decreased vision. The another study from University Hospitals Leuven in Belgium (Dirix et al., 2010) was compared the results of IMRT and convention radiotherapy for paranasal sinus cancer. From this study, 40 patients with cancer of the paranasal sinuses (n = 34) or nasal cavity (n = 6) received postoperative IMRT to a dose of 60 Gy or 66 Gy. Treatment outcome and toxicity were retrospectively compared with that of a previous patient group (n = 41) who were also postoperatively treated to the same doses but with three-dimensional conformal radiotherapy. Two-year local control, overall survival, and disease-free survival were 76%, 89%, and 72%, respectively. Compared to the three-dimensional conformal radiotherapy treatment, IMRT resulted in significantly improved disease-free survival (60% vs. 72%; p = 0.02). The use of IMRT significantly reduced the incidence of acute as well as late side effects, especially regarding skin toxicity, mucositis, xerostomia, and dry-eye syndrome. The largest clinical series of IMRT for paranasal sinuses was reported from Ghent University Hospital in Belgium (Madani et al., 2008). In this study, 84 patients with sinonasal tumors were treated with IMRT. The median follow-up of living patients was 40 months. The 5-year local control, overall survival, disease-specific survival, disease-free survival, and freedom from distant metastasis rate was 70.7%, 58.5%, 67%, 59.3%, and 82.2%, respectively. No difference was found in local control and survival between patients with primary or recurrent tumors. On multivariate analysis, invasion of the cribriform plate was significantly associated with lower local control (p = 0.0001) and overall survival (p = 0.0001). One patient developed Grade 3 radiation-induced retinopathy and neovascular glaucoma. Nonocular late radiation-induced toxicity comprised complete lacrimal duct stenosis in 1 patient and brain necrosis in 3 patients. Osteoradionecrosis of the maxilla and brain necrosis were detected in 1 of the 5 reirradiated patients.

2.5.3 Oropharynx

In general, all series investigating IMRT for oropharyngeal cancer have reported outstanding locoregional control rates. (Clavel et al., 2011; Setton et all, 2010; Lok et al., 2011). These series reported 2-year locoregional tumor control rates of 90% to 98% for patient populations who mainly had stage III or IV tumors. Clavel et al ((Clavel et al., 2011) was compared the toxicity and efficacy of IMRT vs. conventional radiotherapy (CRT) in patients treated with concomitant carboplatin and 5-fluorouracil for locally advanced oropharyngeal cancer. From this study, 249 patients were treated with definitive chemoradiation. One hundred patients had 70 Gy in 33 fractions using IMRT, and 149 received CRT at 70 Gy in 35 fractions. Median follow-up was 42 months. Three-year actuarial rates for locoregional control, disease-free survival, and overall survival were 95.1% vs. 84.4% ($P = 0.005$), 85.3% vs. 69.3% ($p = 0.001$), and 92.1% vs. 75.2% ($p < 0.001$) for IMRT and CRT, respectively. IMRT was associated with less acute dermatitis and less xerostomia. This study suggests that IMRT is associated with favorable locoregional control and survival rates with less xerostomia and acute dermatitis than CRT when both are given concurrently with chemotherapy. The largest series of OPC treated with IMRT was reported from the Memorial Sloan-Kettering Cancer (Setton et al., 2010). In this study, 442 patients with histologically confirmed OPC underwent IMRT. Most of the patients (91%) received chemotherapy. Median follow-up was 36.8 months. The 3-year cumulative incidence of local failure, regional failure, and distant metastasis was 5.4%, 5.6%, and 12.5%, respectively. The 3-year OS rate was 84.9%. The incidence of late dysphagia and late xerostomia ≥Grade 2 was 11% and 29%, respectively. The further study from MSKCC was reported (Lok et al., 2011). In this update study, the 2-year cumulative incidence of LF, RF and DF was 6.1%, 5.2%, and 12.2%, respectively. The 2-year OS rate was 88.6%. In their cohort study, Gross tumor volume was found to be associated with overall survival, local failure, and distant metastatic failure.

2.5.4 Larynx and hypopharynx

IMRT can improve target dose homogeneity for laryngeal and hypopharyngeal SCC while reducing the dose to the normal tissues at risk (Daly et al., 2011; Studer et al., 2010; Huang et al., 2010). Clinical data on IMRT for laryngeal and hypopharyngeal SCC are scarce, however, and include limited numbers of patients within large heterogeneous series of multiple HN tumor sites (Sultanem et al., 2000; Huang et al., 2010). In general, Hypopharyngeal tumors, which fare worse than laryngeal tumors, warrant investigation of more aggressive treatment. For example, at Stanford university (Daly et al., 2011), 42 patients with squamous cell carcinoma of the hypopharynx (n = 23) and larynx (n = 19) underwent IMRT .Three local failures occurred within the high-dose region and 3 occurred in regional nodes. Seven patients developed distant metastasis as the initial failure. Three-year actuarial estimates of locoregional control, freedom from distant metastasis, and overall survival rates were, respectively, 80%, 72%, and 46%.The largest series was reported from Studer et al (Studer et al., 2010). In this study, 65 hypopharyngeal, 31 supraglottic, and 27 locoregionally advanced glottic tumor patients underwent definitive IMRT (with simultaneous chemotherapy in 86%). The 2-year local, nodal, and locoregional control rates for the entire cohort were 82%, 90%, and 77%, respectively; the disease-free and overall survival rates were 75% and 83%, respectively. The ultimate 2-year LRC rate, including salvage surgery, was 86%.

Although the benefits of IMRT warrant its widespread use, there are some disadvantages to this technology such as the planning process and treatment delivery for IMRT is much more consume a higher time and cost than traditional radiotherapy planning. This prolonged treatment planning time can occasionally delay treatment initiation, which has been shown to be detrimental in the setting of head and neck cancer. (Ang et al., 2001). In addition to IMRT is a relatively new technology, the physician or dosimetrist might need very high conformal dose distribution and spare normal tissue as much as possible. But too tight of dose constraint on normal organs can result in inadequate treatment of the cancer. A recent report (Cannon & Lee, 2008) describes three cases in which patients had a recurrence near the parotid gland, which was spared using IMRT technology. It is possible that these recurrences may have been avoided with conventional radiotherapy that did not attempt to reduce the radiation dose to the parotid glands. Finally, some of the long-term effects of IMRT are unknown. The increased of number of beam and radiation output from IMRT results in an increased the other normal structure and total body dose of irradiation to the patient. Some studies (Rosenthal et al., 2008; Lee et al., 2002) describe the increased dose to several normal structures, such as brainstem, cochlea, scalp, mucous membrane and skin. For increasing in total body radiation dose, this is unavoidable because of radiation that leaks out from the linear accelerator head during long treatment times. In addition to this increased scatter radiation, IMRT exposes a larger volume of normal tissue to low-dose radiation in an effort to avoid high doses of radiation to one or more critical structures. The combined effects of increased scatter and low-dose radiation have a theoretic risk of increased secondary malignancies.

3. Image-Guided Radiotherapy

Image-guided radiotherapy (IGRT) is a broad term of radiation therapy technique that is incorporation of multidimensional imaging modalities into the planning and implementation of radiotherapy. The aim of IGRT was for minimizing setup uncertainties, enable to reduce the PTV margins, and assessing anatomic changes in tumor and critical tissue during the whole course of therapy. Imaging has always been used in the design of radiotherapy fields, previously in the form of fluoroscopy, two-dimensional planning films, and more recently the routine use of CT simulation. With the much improvements in diagnostic radiology, three-dimensional imaging, such as positron emission tomography (PET) and MRI, are now readily available as is the ability to obtain daily CT scans and four-dimensional imaging (with time as the fourth dimension) that allows even greater precision and accuracy for radiotherapy treatments. IGRT can be divided into three separate areas. The first is the use of IGRT in treatment planning including the integration of diagnostic radiology information into treatment field design before the patient starts treatment. Second is the use of various technologies (eg, Linac-mounted cone-beam CT [CBCT] scan devices) for improved treatment precision and correction of daily set-up variables. The third form of IGRT combines the first two and uses available technology to replan and adjust the radiotherapy throughout the course of treatment (adaptive radiotherapy).

3.1 Use of diagnostic radiology

One form of IGRT is in using diagnostic technology to better define treatment volumes. 18-Flurodeoxyglucose (FDG) PET scans, especially with incorporation of a diagnostic CT scan

(PET-CT scans) and Magnetic Resonance Imaging (MRI) are increasingly used in radiotherapy planning. FDG-PET scans use a radioactive glucose that is specific uptake at a higher rate by tumor and involved lymph nodes than by normal tissues. The difference in uptake rate between tumor cell and normal tissue allow the clinician easily define which is tumor or normal structures. PET scans can also help discover tumors areas that appear normal on CT scan but have significantly increased metabolic activity (and likely contain malignancy) as shown in Figure 6. Clinical experience is growing regarding the ability of PET scans better to define gross disease and nodal volumes.(Heron et al., 2004; Scarfone et al., 2004; Nishioka et al., 2002; Koshy et al., 2005; Wang et al., 2006; Vernon et al., 2006). For example, Heron and coworkers (Heron et al., 2004) reported on the use of integrated PET-CT radiotherapy planning versus conventional CT planning and found that the CT-based planning overestimated the tumor volume by 150% compared with PET-CT-based planning.

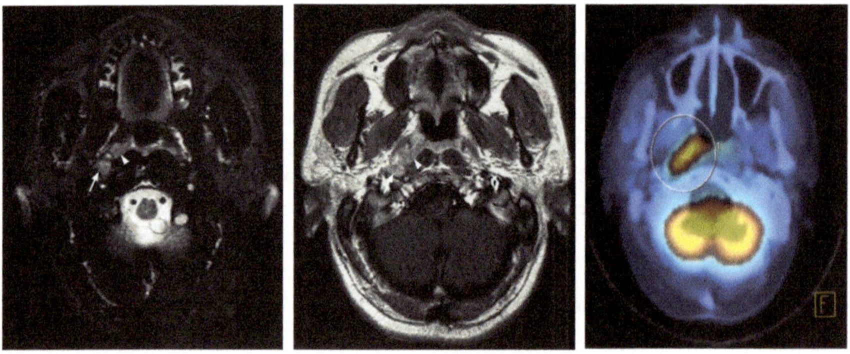

Fig. 6. CT scan (left, middle) and PET scans (right). PET scans can discover tumors areas that appear normal on CT scan but have significantly increased metabolic activity

3.2 Technologies for improved treatment precision and correction of daily set-up variables

Several target localization technologies can be used for monitor the patient's position during treatment delivery. For example, surface markers and optimal tracking, megavoltage Electronic Portal Imaging (EPIDs), implanted radioplaque markers, kilovoltage imaging, ultrasound and in-room CT systems. There is an emerging shift from localization inferred from surface marks or radiographs, to the more direct use of implantable markers and soft tissue localized via volumetric imaging in the treatment room. The classic method for patient set-up is to immobilize the patient using a face mask. Markings are made on this mask and before the daily radiotherapy treatments; radiation therapy technologists use the mask marks to position the patient. The positioning is typically confirmed by taking a two-dimensional radiograph (portal film) before the first radiation treatment and then periodically (different institutions have different policies on how often these verification films are taken; once per week is a commonly accepted standard). If the verification films show an obvious displacement, the patient is repositioned before treatment. These two-dimensional verification films are capable of detecting most large errors (>5–10 mm), but have limitations because they only use two dimensions and can lead to missing potential set-up inaccuracy. They are also highly dependent on bony rather than soft tissue and tumor geometry. The method to reduce daily set-up error that may not be noticed on traditional two-dimensional verification films is the use of CT imaging in the treatment room. The common system is cone beam CT (CBCT) (Figure 7). A CBCT scan is essentially a CT scanner built into the linear accelerator. The CBCT is used to obtain a CT scan of the patient in the anatomic area of interest (eg, the head and neck region) after the patient has been positioned on the treatment table. After the CBCT has been taken, a computer algorithm aligns the CBCT to the initial planning CT scan and adjustments, if required, can be made before the start of treatment. Several authors have reported on the use of CBCT in head and neck radiotherapy (Hong et al., 2005; Li et al., 2008). Hong and coworkers (Hong et al., 2005) analyzed the magnitude of difference between two- and three-dimensional patient set-ups, finding that substantial set-up errors could be discovered when all six degrees of freedom were registered. This set-up error was then used to calculate dosimetric consequences of not correcting these errors, finding that the planning tumor volume could be underdosed by as much as 20% to 30%. Others (Sharpe et al., 2005; vakilha et al., 2007) have found reductions in the parotid and spinal cord dose with the use of daily imaging for position verification. CBCTs have the potential to increase set-up accuracy, and this could allow reduction in the tumor margins that would increase the distance from the high-dose radiation areas to the normal structures. Even small changes in margin can have significant effects on normal tissue doses and outcomes. The increasing of radiation dose to the patient associated with CBCT might be concern regarding to the complication especially in the risk of secondary malignancy. Most CBCT systems add the extra patient-received radiation dose about 3 cGy (Islam et al., 2006; Sykes et al., 2005), whereas the typical daily radiation treatment dose is 180 to 200 cGy. The daily CBCT represents 1% to 1.5% of the daily radiation dose. It should be mentioned, however, that unlike the daily radiation dose, the dose from the CBCT involves significantly more normal tissue and has higher skin dose.

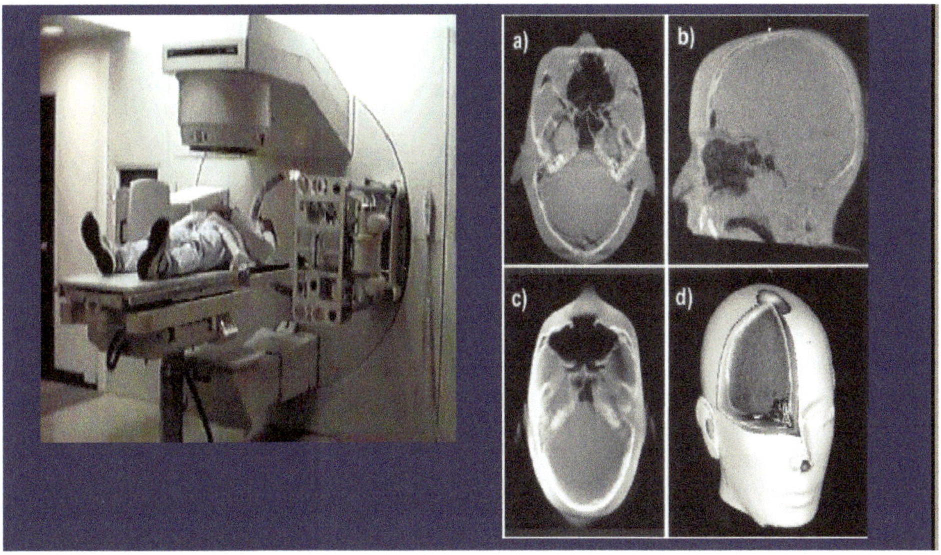

Fig. 7. Cone beam imaging at Linac unit can provide daily set up

3.3 Technology to replan and adjust the radiotherapy throughout the course of treatment (adaptive radiotherapy)

With advancement of IGRT and available volumetric information, it has become evident that a single pretreatment planning CT cannot represent the patient's anatomy for the entire treatment course, particularly for head and neck cancer patients. The patient anatomy changes from day to day (interfractional organ motion) and even during the dose delivery process (intrafractional organ motion) due to patient setup inaccuracy and voluntary or involuntary physiologic processes of the patient. For example, organ motion happens involuntarily for structures that are part of or adjacent to the digestive or urinary systems, Changes in the patient's condition, such as weight gain or loss and rapid changes in the tumor volumes due to the treatment response, can also affect the relative position of the clinical target volume. An alternative way that IGRT can be used is in replanning radiotherapy or adaptive radiotherapy. Repeating a CT-simulation scan at one or more time points during the course of therapy, a second treatment plan, using the patient's altered anatomy, can be used to increase the accuracy of the radiotherapy. Realization of the anatomic changes and subsequent radiotherapy replanning can result in improved dose to both tumor and normal structures. Several authors(Hansen et al., 2006; Dogan, 2007; Han et al., 2008) found that without replanning, tumor coverage and dosimetry decreases (despite the typical decrease in tumor volume size during therapy), whereas at the same time spinal cord dose is increased by up to 10%.

4. Proton therapy

Interest in the use of charged particle radiation has been primarily stimulated by the superior dose distributions that can be achieved with these particles compared with those produced by standard photon. Charged particles deposit energy in tissue through multiple interaction of energy is also transferred to tissue through collisions with the nuclei of atoms the energy loss per unit path length is relatively small and constant until near the end of the range, where the residual energy is lost over a short distance, resulting in a steep rise in the absorbed dose. This portion of the particle track, where energy is rapidly lost over a short distance, is known as the Bragg peak (Figure 8). The proton dose distribution is still characterized by a lower dose region in normal tissue proximal to the tumor, a uniform high-dose region in the tumor, and zero dose beyond the tumor.

With the use of inverse planning, intensity-modulated proton therapy (IMPT) can further improve the therapeutic index of radiotherapy. Several groups have published treatment planning comparisons of (photon) IMRT with IMPT. Using IMPT, mean doses to the organs at risk such as parotid glands, mandible, larynx, spinal cord and brain stem have been reduced by as much as 50%. The earliest published from Simon and colleage (Simon et al., 2011) showed significantly lowered the maximum doses to the spinal cored, brainstem and mean doses to the larynx and parotid glands of IMPT compared to IMRT and adaptive IMRT. A systematic review in the benefit of PT in head and neck cancer with respect to normal tissue sparing was reported (Water et al., 2011). There were 14 studies were identified and included in this review. Four studies included paranasal sinus cancer cases, three included nasopharyngeal cancer cases, and seven included oropharyngeal, hypopharyngeal, and/or laryngeal cancer cases. Seven studies compared the most sophisticated photon and proton techniques: intensity-modulated photon therapy versus

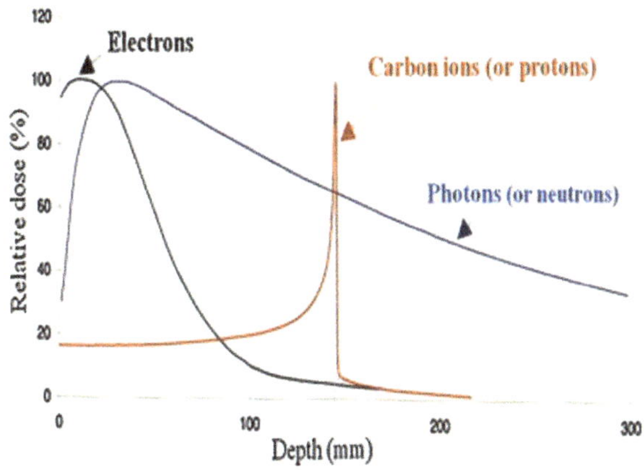

Fig. 8. Bragg peak in proton therapy radiation: comparison of deep dose distribution with other types of radiation treatment

intensity-modulated proton therapy (IMPT). Four studies compared different proton techniques. All studies showed that protons had a lower normal tissue dose, while keeping similar or better target coverage. Two studies found that these lower doses theoretically translated into a significantly lower incidence of salivary dysfunction. This result concluded that that PT have the potential for a significantly lower normal tissue dose, while keeping similar or better target coverage. IMPT probably offers the most advantage and will allow for a substantially lower probability of radiation-induced side effects. The areas in the head and neck such as paranasal sinus and nasopharynx that close to optic apparatus and brain and some radioresistant tumors such as uveal melanoma, chordoma, and chondrosarcoma could have clinical gain from proton therapy. However, the use of proton therapy in head and neck cancers requires special considerations in the simulation and treatment planning process, and currently available PT technology may not permit realization of the maximum potential benefits of proton therapy. Figure 9 shows a comparison of IMRT plan and a Proton therapy.

4.1 Clinical experience of proton therapy for head and neck cancers

Proton therapy in head and neck cancer is relatively new, so there still have few clinical data of proton therapy in head and neck cancer. The previous reports usually are small sample size and do not provide enough information to support the actual benefits in the therapeutic ratio from proton therapy compared with photon based radiation.

4.1.1 Nasopharyngeal carcinoma

The report from Massachusetts General Hospital on 17 patients treated with a combination of protons and photon untreated T4N0-N3 nasopharyngeal carcinoma and followed for a median of 43 months(Chan & Liebach' 2008) The median dose to the gross target volume was 73.6 Gy. The three-year outcomes were as follows: local-regional control, 92%; relapse-free survival, 79%; and overall survival, 74%. Toxicity was not described, so it is difficult to assess the therapeutic ratio, but the high disease control rates are very promising.

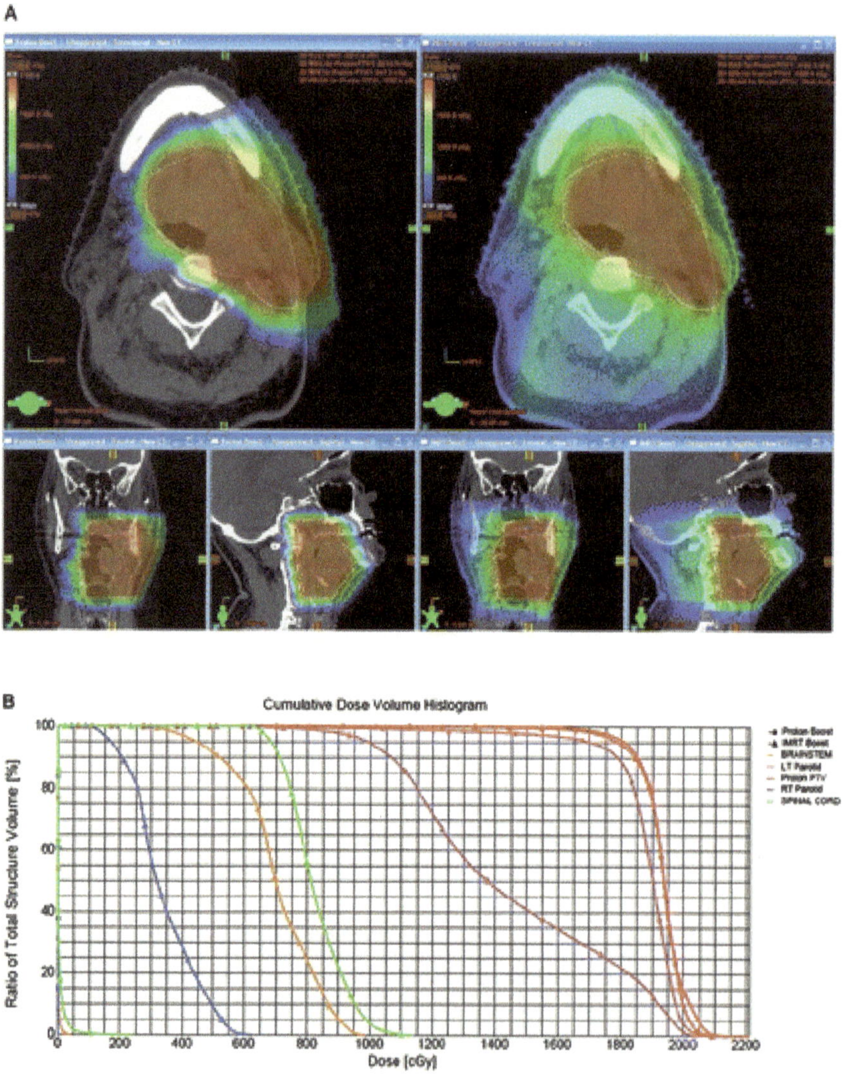

Fig. 9. (A) The dose distributions achieved with the PT plan (left) and the IMRT plan (right). There is greater integral dose with the IMRT plan. (B) The dose-volume histogram (DVH) comparison between the two plans; as apparent from the curves on the far right, the target coverage was the same for the two plans, but the PT plan delivered a significantly lower dose to the optic structures, including the chiasm, the lacrimal glands, the retina, and the optic nerves as well as the brainstem and parotids.

4.1.2 Oropharyngeal carcinoma

The reported from Loma Linda University Medical Center (Slater et al., 2005) on 29 patients with stage II-IV oropharyngeal cancer treated with a combination of protons and photons to 75.9 Gy/CGE in 45 fractions over 5.5 weeks. The 5-year actuarial locoregional control rate was 84%. The actuarial 2-year disease-free survival rate was 81%; at 5 years, it was 65%.Late Grade 3 toxicity was seen in 3 patients (10%).

4.1.3 Nasal cavity and paranasal sinuses

Chan and Liebsch reported on 102 patients with paranasal sinus cancers treated between 1991 and 2002 with PT to a median dose of 71.6 Gy at the Massachusetts General Hospital and followed for a median of 6.6 years (Chan & Liebach, 2008). Only 20% of patients had a complete resection prior to RT. The five-year local control rate was 86%; no toxicity information was offered in this report. Another study from MGH experience reported on 36 patients treated with proton/photon accelerated fractionated RT for paranasal sinus cancers to a median dose of 69.6 Gy (Weber et al., 2006), the median follow-up was 52 months. Thirteen patients developed late visual toxicity including cataracts in three patients.Late Effect Normal Tissue complication (LENT) grade I vascular retinopathy in one patient, LENT grade 1 optic neuropathy in one patient, lacrimal duct stenosis in three patients and dry-eye syndrome in five patients. No patients were reported to have lost vision. These excellent outcomes suggest the possibility of achieving both high rates of tumor control and low rates of severe toxicity with PT in sinonasal tumors.

4.1.4 Adenoid cystic carcinoma

The report from Massachusetts General Hospital (Pommier et al., 2006) on 23 patients treated for adenoid cystic cancer with skull base extension with photon/proton RT. The median follow-up was 64 months. Twenty patients (87%) had gross disease at the time of RT. The local control rate at 5 years was 93%. The rate of freedom from distant metastasis at 5 years was 62%. The disease-free and overall survival rates at 5 years were 56% and 77%, respectively. In multivariate analysis, significant adverse factors predictive for overall survival were change in vision at presentation (p= .02) and involvement of sphenoid sinus and clivus (p = .01).One patient developed grade 4 retinopathy. Three patients developed grade 3 complications requiring surgery including dacrocystorhinostomy in one patient, surgery for ectropion in one patient, and lens replacement for a cataract in one patient. These results suggest the possibility of both high rates of disease control and low rates of severe toxicity with PT alone in adenoid cystic cancer.

5. Stereotactic radiation: LINAC-based and gamma knife

Stereotactic Radiosurgery and radiotherapy are techniques to administer precisely directed, high-dose irradiation that tightly conforms to target to create a desired radiobiological response while minimizing radiation dose to surrounding normal tissue. In the case of radiosurgery (SRS), all of the radiation is done in a single session or fraction, while in stereotactic radiotherapy (SRT), more than one fraction of irradiation is administered. Stereotactic technique combines stereotactic localization with multiple cross-fired beams from a highly collimated high-energy radiation source.

5.1 Radiosurgery devices

Radiosurgery can be performed using various devices, including the GammaKnife, modified linear accelerators (Linacs) or particle beam devices.

5.1.1 Gamma knife radiosurgery

The source of GammaKnife come from Cobalt-60, this radioisotope decay and give high energy gamma ray for radiation treatment. The first prototype unit of Gamma Knife was created by Leksell and Larson in 1967. It uses a relatively hemispherical array of multiple fixed cobalt-60 201 sources, that are create small, relatively spherical treatment volumes of varied diameter with sharp dose falloff (Figure 10).

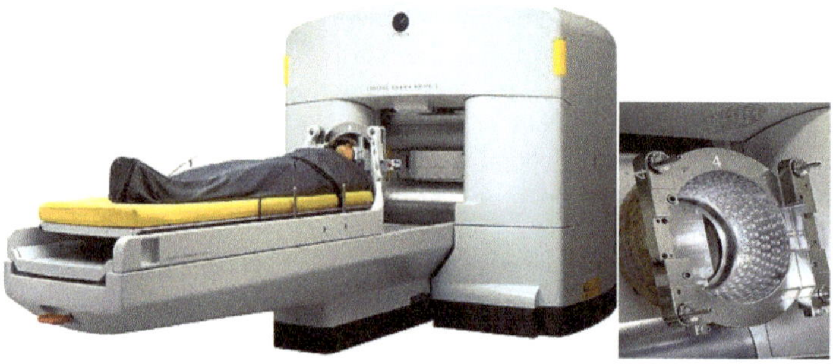

Fig. 10. GammaKnife unit and helmet for cobalt-60 201 sources

5.1.2 Linear accelerator based stereotactic radiotherapy (X-knife)

Linear accelerators (Linacs) (Figure 11)can be used for radiosurgery. Most early Linac-based radiosurgery techniques used multiple radiation arcs with circular collimators to create spherical dose distributions for three dimensional targets. Improved hardware and advanced planning software have been developed to enhance conformity. These include beam shaping with micromultileaf collimators, intensity modulation with inverse treatment planning algorithms.

5.1.3 Particle beam radiosurgery

The advantage of proton radiosurgery is that the beams stop at a depth related to the beam's energy (Bragg peak). The lack of an exit dose and the sharp beam profile of protons allow target irradiation with lower integral doses than are delivered with photon irradiation.

5.2 Clinical experience for stereotactic radiosurgery in head and neck cancer

More recently, stereotactic radiosurgery ncers both in primary cases (Kawaguchi et al., 2009) and in recurrent cases(Pai et al., 2002; Low et al., 2006; Roh et al., 2009) The complete response rates for these studies vary from 8.6-54% with 2-year overall survival rates ranging from 14.3-41% and 1-year overall survival rates of 18-52.1%. As the ranges of these outcomes suggest, the heterogeneity between these various studies is large. Various factors, including tumor stage, tumor volume, adequate irradiation dose, prior treatment, and anatomical site

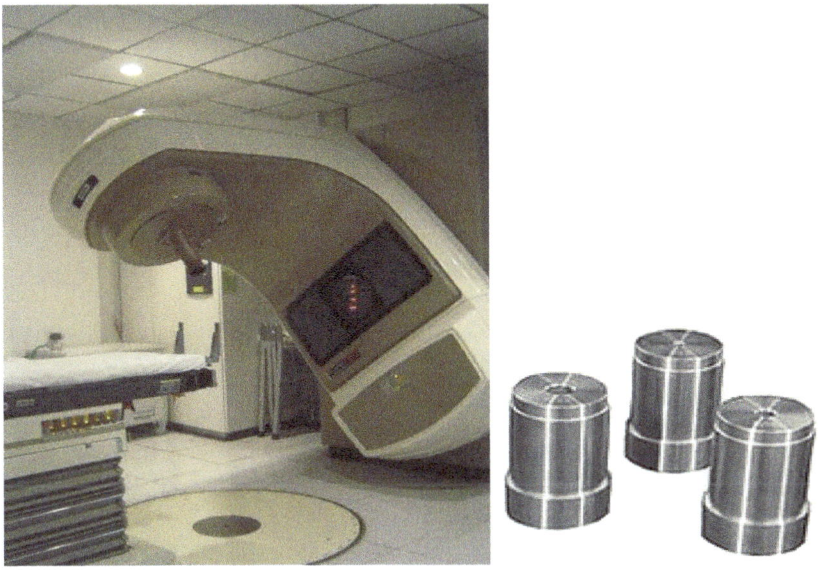

Fig. 11. Linac-based radiosurgery machine and circular collimators

complexly, influenced these reported outcomes. Kawaguchi et al (Kawaguchi et al., 2010) reported on 22 patients with advanced, recurrent head and neck carcinoma were treated with stereotactic radiosurgery with the marginal doses of 20-42 Gy delivered in two to five fractions. At an overall median follow-up of 24 months, for the 14 locally recurrent patients without lymph node metastases, 9 patients (64.3%) had a complete response (CR), 1 patient (7.1%) had a partial response (PR), 1 patient (7.1%) had stable disease (SD), and 3 patients (21.4%) had progressive disease (PD). For the 8 patients with lymph node metastases, 1 patient with a single retropharyngeal (12.5%) had CR; the remaining 7 patients (87.5%) all progressed. The overall actuarial 2-year survival for the patients with and without lymph node metastases is 12.5% and 78.6%, respectively.

6. Robotic radiosurgery (CyberKnife)

The CyberKnife (Accuray, Sunnyvale, CA, USA) is a frameless robotic radiosurgery system that has been utilized by numerous clinicians around the world to treat intracranial and extracranial tumors (Tate et al., 1999; Voynov et al., 2006; Le et al., 2003; Jansen et al., 2000). The CyberKnife system consists of a small and compact 6 MV Linac coupled to a multijointed robotic manipulator with 6 degree of freedom (Figure 12). The current generation of CyberKnife consists of two precisely calibrated diagnostic x-ray tubes fixed to the ceiling of the treatment room and two orthogonal flat-panel detector located under the floor. The CyberKnife depends on a co-registration of digitally reconstructed radiographs that are generated from CT images and x-ray projections that are captured during the treatment session. Changes in target position are relayed to the robotic arm, which adjusts pointing of the treatment beam. The robotic arm moves through a sequence of positions (nodes). At each node, a pair of images is obtained, the patient position is determined, and adjustment are made. CyberKnife was based on tracking of the skeletal anatomy of the skull and spine. For treatment soft tissue lesion in the body such as lung, liver and prostate, implanted fiducial was need for target localization and respiratory tracking. The advantages of the CyberKnife include the ability to deliver radiation without a frame, the feature of increased fractionation flexibility, and the ability to treat extracranial lesions. Figure 13 shows isodose distribution in nasopharyngeal cancer treated with CyberKnife.

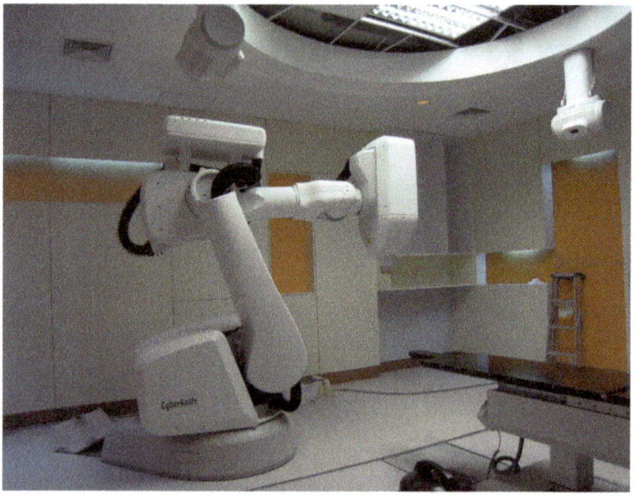

Fig. 12. CyberKnife Robotic Radiosurgery system

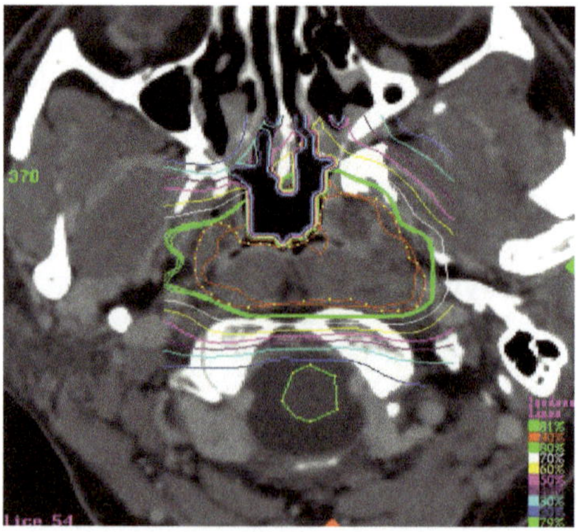

Fig. 13. Isodose distribution for nasopharygeal CA treated with CyberKnife.

6.1 Clinical experience of CyberKnife for head and neck cancer

The use of CyberKnife for head and neck cancer is relatively new. Cengiz and colleage (Cengiz et al., 2010) reported 46 recurrent, unresectable, and previously irradiated head-and-neck cancer patients treated with CyberKnife. The local disease control was achieved in

31 patients (83.8%). The median overall survival was 11.93 months and the median progression free survival was 10.5 months. One-year progression-free survival and overall survival were 41% and 46%, respectively. In this study, 8 (17.3%) patients had carotid blow-out syndrome, and 7 (15.2%) patients died of bleeding from carotid arteries. The author discovered that this fatal syndrome occurred only in patients with tumor surrounding carotid arteries and carotid arteries receiving all prescribed dose. Another report from Korea (Seo et al., 2009) shown 35 patients with locally recurrent NPC treated using CyberKnife. The overall survival (OS) rate, local failure-free survival (LFFS) rate, and disease progression-free survival (DPFS) rate at 5 years were 60%, 79%, and 74%, respectively. Twenty-three patients achieved complete response after CyberKnife. Only T stage at recurrence was an independent prognostic factor for OS and DPFS. Five patients exhibited severe late toxicity (Grade 4 or 5).

7. Conclusion

Modern in Radiation therapy has significant considerable promise to improve cancer treatment. The benefit of these technologies is able to deliver more radiation to the tumor and better spares normal tissue and critical structure. It is expected that these modern radiation therapy will yield improvements in all important outcomes including overall survival, disease free survival, local control and quality of life for patients. However, most modern technologies have not been proven to change patients' ultimate outcome. In addition, modern radiation therapy may be associated with significant increases in cost to the patients and the medical system. Therefore, continued careful studied and quantification of the effects of modern radiation therapy on treatment outcomes is needed so that definitive statements may be made about its necessity in everyday radiotherapy.

8. References

[1] Som PM: The present controversy over the imaging method of choice for evaluating the soft tissues of the neck. *AJNR Am J Neuroradiol* 1997; 18:1869-1872.

[2] Schechter NR, Gillenwater AM, Byers RM, et al: Can positron emission tomography improve the quality of care for head and neck cancer patients?. *Int J Radiat Oncol Biol Phys* 2001; 51:4-9.

[3] Schechter NR, Gillenwater AM, Byers RM, et al: Can positron emission tomography improve the quality of care for head and neck cancer patients?. *Int J Radiat Oncol Biol Phys* 2001; 51:4-9.

[4] Rouviere H: *Lymphatic Systems of the Head and Neck*. [Tobias MJ, trans]Ann Arbor, MI, Edwards Brothers, 1938.

[5] Mukherji SK, Armao D, Joshi VM: Cervical nodal metastases in squamous cell carcinoma of the head and neck: what to expect. *Head Neck* 2001; 23:995-1005.

[6] Lindberg RD: Distribution of cervical lymph node metastases from squamous cell carcinoma of the upper respiratory and digestive tracts. *Cancer* 1972; 29:1446-1449.

[7] Byers RM, Wolf PF, Ballantyne AJ: Rationale for elective modified neck dissection. *Head Neck Surg* 1988; 10:160-167.

[8] Shah JP: Patterns of cervical lymph node metastasis from squamous carcinomas of the upper aerodigestive tract. *Am J Surg* 1990; 160:405-409.

[9] Robbins KT, Medina JE, Wolfe GT, et al: Standardizing neck dissection terminology. Official report of the Academy's Committee for Head and Neck Surgery and Oncology. *Arch Otolaryngol Head Neck Surg* 1991; 117:601-605.

[10] Robbins KT: Integrating radiological criteria into the classification of cervical lymph node disease. *Arch Otolaryngol Head Neck Surg* 1999; 125:385-387.

[11] Eisbruch A, Marsh LH, Dawson LA, et al: Recurrences near the base of the skull following IMRT of head and neck cancer: implications for target delineation in the high neck, and for parotid sparing. *Int J Radiat Oncol Biol Phys* 2004; 59:28-42.

[12] van Asselen B, Dehnad H, Raaijmakers CP, et al: The dose to the parotid glands with IMRT for oropharyngeal tumors: the effect of reduction of positioning margins. *Radiother Oncol* 2002; 64:197-204.

[13] Mohan R, Wu Q, Manning M, et al: Radiobiological considerations in the design of fractionation strategies for intensity modulated radiation therapy of the head and neck. *Int J Radiat Oncol Biol Phys* 2000; 46:619-630.

[14] Wu Q, Manning M, Schmidt-Ullrich R, et al: The potential for sparing of parotids and escalation of biologically equivalent dose with intensity modulated radiation treatments of head and neck cancers: a treatment design study. *Int J Radiat Oncol Biol Phys* 2000; 46:195-205.

[15] De Neve W, De Gersem W, Derycke S: Clinical delivery of IMRT for relapsed or second-primary head and neck cancer using a multileaf collimator with dynamic control. *Radiother Oncol* 1999; 50:301-314.

[16] Yao M, Dornfeld KJ, Buatti JM, et al: Intensity modulated treatment for head and neck squamous cell carcinoma: the University of Iowa experience. *Int J Radiat Oncol Biol Phys* 2005; 63:410-421.

[17] Kam MK, Leung SF, Zee B, et al: Prospective randomized study of intensity-modulated radiotherapy on salivary gland function in early-stage nasopharyngeal carcinoma patients. *J Clin Oncol* 2007; 25:4873-4879.

[18] Pow EHN, Kwong DLW, McMillan AS, et al: Xerostomia and quality of life after intensity modulated radiotherapy vs conventional radiotherapy for early stage nasopharyngeal carcinoma: initial report on a randomized controlled trial. *Int J Radiat Oncol Biol Phys* 2006; 66:981-991.

[19] Sultanem K, Shu HK, Xia P, et al: Three-dimensional intensity-modulated radiotherapy in the treatment of nasopharyngeal carcinoma: the University of California-San Francisco experience. *Int J Radiat Oncol Biol Phys* 2000; 48:711-722.

[20] Wolden S.L., Chen W.C., Pfister D.G., et al: Intensity-modulated radiation therapy (IMRT) for nasopharyngeal cancer: update of the memorial Sloan-Kettering experience. *Int J Radiat Oncol Biol Phys* 64. 57-62.200

[21] Daly ME, Chen AM, Bucci MK, El-Sayed I, Xia P, Kaplan MJ, Eisele DW. Intensity-modulated radiation therapy for malignancies of the nasal cavity and paranasal sinuses. Int J Radiat Oncol Biol Phys. 2007 Jan 1;67(1):151-7.

[22] Dirix P, Vanstraelen B, Jorissen M, Vander Poorten V, Nuyts S. Intensity-modulated radiotherapy for sinonasal cancer: improved outcome compared to conventional radiotherapy.15;78(4):998-1004, 2010.

[23] Madani I, Bonte K, Vakaet L, Boterberg T, De Neve W. Intensity-modulated radiotherapy for sinonasal tumors: Ghent University Hospital update..2009 Feb 1;73(2):424-32. 2008.

[24] Clavel S, Nguyen DH, Fortin B, Després P, Khaouam N, Donath D, Soulières D, Guertin L, Nguyen-Tan PF. Simultaneous Integrated Boost Using Intensity-Modulated Radiotherapy Compared with Conventional Radiotherapy in Patients Treated with Concurrent Carboplatin and 5-Fluorouracil for Locally Advanced Oropharyngeal Carcinoma.. Int J Radiat Oncol Biol Phys. 2011 . Int J Radiat Oncol Biol Phys. 2010 Dec 16.

[25] Setton J, Caria N, Romanyshyn J, Koutcher L, Wolden SL, Zelefsky MJ, Rowan N, Sherman EJ, Fury MG, Pfister DG, Wong RJ, Shah JP, Kraus DH, Shi W, Zhang Z, Schupak KD, Gelblum DY, Rao SD, Lee NY. Intensity-Modulated Radiotherapy in the Treatment of Oropharyngeal Cancer: An Update of the Memorial Sloan-Kettering Cancer Center Experience.

[26] Lok BH, Setton J, Caria N, Romanyshyn J, Wolden SL, Zelefsky MJ, Park J, Rowan N, Sherman EJ, Fury MG, Ho A, Pfister DG, Wong RJ, Shah JP, Kraus DH, Zhang Z, Schupak KD, Gelblum DY, Rao SD, Lee NY. Intensity-Modulated Radiation Therapy in Oropharyngeal Carcinoma: Effect of Tumor Volume on Clinical Outcomes. Int J Radiat Oncol Biol Phys. 2011 Jun 1

[27] Daly ME, Le QT, Jain AK, Maxim PG, Hsu A, Loo BW Jr, Kaplan MJ, Fischbein NJ, Colevas AD, Pinto H, Chang DT. Intensity-modulated radiotherapy for locally advanced cancers of the larynx and hypopharynx. Head Neck. 2011 Jan; 33(1):103-11.

[28] Studer G, Peponi E, Kloeck S, Dossenbach T, Huber G, Glanzmann C. Surviving hypopharynx-larynx carcinoma in the era of IMRT. Int J Radiat Oncol Biol Phys. 2010 Aug 1;77(5):1391-6. Epub 2010 Jan 7.

[29] Huang WY, Jen YM, Chen CM, Su YF, Lin CS, Lin YS, Chang YN, Chao HL, Lin KT, Chang LP. Intensity modulated radiotherapy with concurrent chemotherapy for larynx preservation of advanced resectable hypopharyngeal cancer. Radiat Oncol. 2010 May 15;5:37.

[30] Lee N, O'Meara W, Chan K, et al. Concurrent chemotherapy and intensity-modulated radiotherapy for locoregionally advanced laryngeal and hypopharyngeal cancers. *Int J Radiat Oncol Biol Phys* 2007; 69:459-468.

[31] Eisbruch A, Ten Haken R, Kim HM, et al: Dose, volume and function relationships in parotid glands following conformal and intensity modulated irradiation of head and neck cancer. *Int J Radiat Oncol Biol Phys* 1999; 45:577-587.

[32] Eisbruch A, Schwartz M, Rasch C, et al: Dysphagia and aspiration after chemoradiotherapy for head-and-neck cancer: which anatomic structures are affected and can they be spared by IMRT?. *Int J Radiat Oncol Biol Phys* 2004; 60:1425-1433.

[33] Ang K.A., Trotti A., Brown B.W., et al. Randomized trial addressing risk features and time factors of surgery plus radiotherapy in advanced head-and-neck cancer. *Int J Radiat Oncol Biol Phys* 51. (3): 571-578.2001.

[34] Cannon D.M., Lee N.Y. Recurrence in region of spared parotid gland after definitive intensity-modulated radiotherapy for head and neck cancer. *Int J Radiat Oncol Biol Phys* 70. 660-665.2008;

[35] Rosenthal D.I., Chambers M.S., Fuller C.D., et al: Beam path toxicities to non-target structures during intensity-modulated radiation therapy for head and neck cancer. *Int J Radiat Oncol Biol Phys* 69. (3): S1.2008;

[36] Lee N., Chuang C., Quivey J.M., et al. Skin toxicity due to intensity-modulated radiotherapy for head-and-neck carcinoma. *Int J Radiat Oncol Biol Phys* 53. (3): 630-637.2002;

[37] Heron D.E., Andrade R.S., Flickinger J., et al. Hybrid PET-CT simulation for radiation treatment planning in head-and-neck cancers: a brief technical report. *Int J Radiat Oncol Biol Phys* 60. 1419-1424. 2004.

[38] Scarfone C., Lavely W.C., Cmelak A.J., et al. Prospective feasibility trial of radiotherapy target definition for head and neck cancer using 3-dimensional PET and CT imaging. *J Nucl Med* 45. 543-552.2004.

[39] Nishioka T., Shiga T., Shirato H., et al. Image fusion between 18 FDG-PET and MRI/CT for radiotherapy planning of oropharyngeal and nasopharyngeal carcinomas. *Int J Radiat Oncol Biol Phys* 53. 1051-1057.2002.

[40] Koshy M., Paulino A.C., Howell R., et al. F-18 PET-CT fusion in radiotherapy treatment planning for head and neck cancer. *Head Neck* 27. 494-502.2005.

[41] Wang D., Schultz C.J., Jursinic P.A., et al. Initial experience of FDG-PET/CT guided IMRT of head-and-neck carcinoma. *Int J Radiat Oncol Biol Phys* 65. 143-151.2006.

[42] Vernon M.R., Maheshwari M., Schultz C.J., et al. Clinical outcomes of patients receiving integrated PET/CT-guided radiotherapy for head and neck carcinoma. *Int J Radiat Oncol Biol Phys* 70. 678-684.2006.

[43] Smitsmans M.H., de Bois J., Sonke J.J., et al. Automatic prostate localization on cone-beam CT scans for high precision image-guided radiotherapy. *Int J Radiat Oncol Biol Phys* 63. (4): 975-984.2005.

[44] Hong T.S., Wolfgang A.T., Chappell R.J., et al. The impact of daily setup variations on head-and-neck intensity-modulated radiation therapy. *Int J Radiat Oncol Biol Phys* 61. 779-788.2005.

[45] Li H., Zhu X.R., Zhang L., et al. Comparison of 2D radiographic images and 3D cone beam computed tomography for positioning head-and-neck radiotherapy patients. *Int J Radiat Oncol Biol Phys* 71. (3): 916-925.2008.

[46] Sharpe M., Brock K., Rehbinder H., et al. Adaptive planning and delivery to account for anatomical changes induced by radiation therapy of head and neck cancer. *Int J Radiat Oncol Biol Phys* 63. S3.2005;

[47] Vakilha M., Hwang D., Breen S.L.: Changes in position and size of parotid glands assessed with daily cone-beam CT during image-guided IMRT for head and neck cancer: implications for dose received. *Int J Radiat Oncol Biol Phys* 69. (3): S1.2007;

[48] van Asselen B., Dehnad H., Raaijmakers C.P., et al. The dose to the parotid glands with IMRT for oropharyngeal tumors: the effect of reduction of positioning margins. *Radiother Oncol* 64. (2): 197-204.2002.

[49] Islam M.K., Purdie T.G., Norrlinger B.D., et al. Patient dose from kilovoltage cone beam computed tomography imaging in radiation therapy. *Med Phys* 33. 1573-1582.2006.

[50] Sykes J.R., A Amer, Czajka J., et al. A feasibility study for image guided radiotherapy using low dose, high speed, cone beam X-ray volumetric imaging. *Radiat Oncol* 77. 45-52.2005;

[51] Brenner D.J., Hall E.J.: Computed tomography: an increasing source of radiation exposure. *N Engl J Med* 357. 2277-2284.2007.

[52] Einstein A.J., Henzolva M.J., Rajagopalan S. Estimating risk of cancer associated with radiation exposure from 64-slice computed tomography coronary angiography. *JAMA* 298. (3): 317-323.2007.

[53] Hansen E.K., Bucci M.K., Quivev J.M., et al. Repeat CT imaging and replanning during the course of IMRT for head-and-neck cancer. *Int J Radiat Oncol Biol Phys* 64. (2): 355-362.2006.

[54] Barker J.L., Garden A.S., Ang K.K., et al. Quantification of volumetric and geometric changes occurring during fractionated radiotherapy for head-and-neck cancer using an integrated CT/linear accelerator system. *Int J Radiat Oncol Biol Phys* 59. (4): 960-970.2004.

[55] Dogan N. Improvements of head and neck IMRT patient plans via repeat CT imaging and re-planning. *Int J Radiat Oncol Biol Phys* 69. (3): S1.2007;

[56] Han C., Yi-Jen C., Liu A., et al. Actual dose variation of parotid glands and spinal cord for nasopharyngeal cancer patients during radiotherapy. *Int J Radiat Oncol Biol Phys* 70. 1256-1262.2008.

[57] Yeung AR, Malyapa RS, Mendenhall WM, et al: Dosimetric comparison of IMRT and proton therapy for head and neck tumors. *Int J Radiat Oncol Biol Phys* 2006; 66:S412.

[58] Mock U, Georg D, Bogner J, et al: Treatment planning comparison of conventional, 3D conformal, and intensity-modulated photon (IMRT) and proton therapy for paranasal sinus carcinoma. *Int J Radiat Oncol Biol Phys* 2004; 58:147-154.

[59] Simone CB 2nd, Ly D, Dan TD, Ondos J, Ning H, Belard A, O'Connell J, Miller RW, Simone NL. Comparison of intensity-modulated radiotherapy, adaptive radiotherapy, proton radiotherapy, and adaptive proton radiotherapy for treatment of locally advanced head and neck cancer. Radiother Oncol. 2011 Jun 12.

[60] Lomax AJ, Goitein M, Adams J: Intensity modulation in radiotherapy: photons versus protons in the paranasal sinus. *Radiother Oncol* 2003; 66:11-18.

[61] Lunsford LD. Lars Leksell. Notes at the side of a raconteur. Stereotact Funct Neurosurg. 1996;67:153–168.

[62] Ammar A. Lars Leksell's vision—radiosurgery. Acta Neurochir Suppl (Wien). 1994;62:1–4.

[63] Radiosurgery Update. New York, Elsevier, 1992, pp 3-9.

[64] Tate DJ, Adler JR Jr, Chang SD. Stereotactic radiosurgical boost following radiotherapy in primary nasopharyngeal carcinoma: impact on local control. *Int J Radiat Oncol Biol Phys.* 1999;45:915–921.

[65] Kawaguchi K, Yamada H, Horie A, Sato K. Radiosurgical treatment of maxillary squamous cell carcinoma. *Int J Oral Maxillofac Surg.* 2009;38:1205–1207.

[66] Pai PC, Chuang CC, Wei KC. Stereotactic radiosurgery for locally recurrent nasopharyngeal carcinoma. *Head Neck.* 2002;24:748–753.

[67] Low JS, Chua ET, Gao F, Wee JT. Stereotactic radiosurgery plus intracavitary irradiation in the salvage of nasopharyngeal carcinoma. *Head Neck.* 2006;28:321–329.

[68] Voynov G, Heron DE, Burton S. Frameless stereotactic radiosurgery for recurrent head and neck carcinoma. *Technol Cancer Res Treat.* 2006;5:529–535.

[69] Roh KW, Jang JS, Kim MS. Fractionated stereotactic radiotherapy as reirradiation for locally recurrent head and neck cancer. *Int J Radiat Oncol Biol Phys.* 2009;74:1348–1355.

[70] Heron DE, Ferris RL, Karamouzis M. Stereotactic Body Radiotherapy for Recurrent Squamous Cell Carcinoma of the Head and Neck: Results of a Phase I Dose-Escalation Trial. *Int J Radiat Oncol Biol Phys.* 2009.

[71] Le QT, Tate D, Koong A. Improved local control with stereotactic radiosurgical boost in patients with nasopharyngeal carcinoma. *Int J Radiat Oncol Biol Phys.* 2003;56:1046–1054.

[72] Jansen EP, Keus RB, Hilgers FJ. Does the combination of radiotherapy and debulking surgery favor survival in paranasal sinus carcinoma? *Int J Radiat Oncol Biol Phys.* 2000;48:27–35.

[73] Fu D, Kuduvalli G. A fast, accurate, and automatic 2D-3D image registration for image-guided cranial radiosurgery. *Med Phys.* 2008;35:2180–2194.

[74] Cengiz M, Ozyiğit G, Yazici G, Doğan A, Yildiz F, Zorlu F, Gürkaynak M, Gullu IH, Hosal S, Akyol F. Salvage Reirradiaton With Stereotactic Body Radiotherapy for Locally Recurrent Head-and-Neck Tumors.Int J Radiat Oncol Biol Phys. 2011 Sep 1;81(1):104-9.

[75] Seo Y, Yoo H, Yoo S, Cho C, Yang K, Kim MS, Choi C, Shin Y, Lee D, Lee G. Robotic system-based fractionated stereotactic radiotherapy in locally recurrent nasopharyngeal carcinoma. Radiother Oncol. 2009 Dec;93(3):570-4.

9

Novel Chemoradiotherapy Regimens Incorporating Targeted Therapies in Locally Advanced Head and Neck Cancers

Ritesh Rathore
Roger Williams Medical Center, Boston University School of Medicine
USA

1. Introduction

Head and neck squamous cell carcinoma (HNSCC) is the sixth most common cancer worldwide. The majority of cases present with locally advanced, non-metastatic HNSCC for which the survival rates are approximately 50% at 5 years. Primary surgery followed by chemoradiotherapy (CRT) or definitive platinum-containing CRT are the standard therapeutic approaches utilized in locally advanced HNSCC. In the updated MACH-NC meta-analysis, CRT resulted in an absolute 8% improvement in overall survival (OS) at 5 years (Pignon et al., 2007; Pignon et al., 2009). However, despite incremental therapeutic advances, the problems of locoregional recurrences, distant metastases, organ preservation, and toxicity amelioration remain a significant challenge.

Several molecular pathways are deregulated and activated in HNSCC making it attractive area for the evaluation of the recently available and in-development molecular targeted therapies. Among the pathways implicated in the development of HNSCC are the epidermal growth factor receptor (EGFR) pathway and the vascular endothelial growth factor (VEGF) receptor pathway. In this chapter we will review the current data with completed and ongoing trials with molecular targeted therapies in the management of locally advanced HNSCC.

2. Epidermal growth factor receptor inhibitors

EGFR is a member of the human epidermal growth factor receptor family of receptor tyrosine kinases that is overexpressed in most HNSCC cases. Signal activation with natural ligand fixation to EGFR leads to receptor homodimerization or heterodimerization with other HER receptors occurs which in turn leads to the activation of downstream signaling molecular pathways. These pathways, including the Ras/Raf/Mek/Erk and the phosphatidylinositol-3-kinase/protein kinase B (PI3K/AKT) pathways, are involved in tumor proliferation, apoptosis, angiogenesis, and cell migration/invasion. Increased EGFR expression as well as a high EGFR gene copy number are associated with worsened survival outcomes (Grandis et al., 1998; Ang et al., 2002). EGFR inhibition is a promising strategy in HNSCC since it results in inhibition of tumor cell proliferation, potentiation of apoptotsis and antiangiogenic effects (Ciardiello, 2005; Hirata et al., 2002). Currently available anti-EGFR therapeutic agents can be classified into monoclonal antibodies (mAbs) and tyrosine kinase inhibitors (TKIs).

2.1 Monoclonal antibodies against EGFR

Monoclonal antibodies directed against EGFR inhibit activation of distinct EGFR signaling pathways and inhibit tumor growth through cell cycle arrest, pro-apoptotic effect, and inhibition of angiogenesis, invasion and metastasis, and possibly immune mechanisms (Baselga et al., 2000; Mendelsohn & Baselga, 2003). Moreover, anti-EGFR antibodies can augment the antitumor activity of RT and chemotherapy (Huan & Harari, 2000; Milas et al., 2004; Baselga et al., 1993; Fan et al., 1993).

Characteristic	Cetuximab	Nimotuzumab	Zalutumab	Panitumumab
Ig subclass	IgG1	IgG1	IgG1	IgG2
Type	Chimeric	Humanized	Fully human	Fully human
Status	Phase III	Phase III	Phase III	Phase III

Table 1. Current EGFR antibodies in evaluation in head and neck cancers

2.1.1 Cetuximab

Cetuximab is a chimeric human-murine monoclonal antibody that binds competitively to the EGFR with a higher affinity than its endogenous ligands. It has been studied extensively in HNSCC in several phase II and III studies and was approved by the FDA, in combination with RT for the treatment of patients with locally advanced head and neck cancer.

2.1.1.1 Cetuximab and radiotherapy alone

Bonner et al have published updated 5-year survival results of their pivotal phase III study which compared RT alone (n = 213 patients) with cetuximab plus RT (n = 211 patient) in patients locally advanced HNSCC of the oropharynx, hypopharynx, or larynx (Bonner et al., 2010). Patients were stratified by their Karnofsky performance score (60-80 versus 90-100), Tumor stage (T1-3 versus T4), N stage (N0 versus N1-3), and radiotherapy fractionation. The primary endpoint of the trial was duration of locoregional control and the secondary endpoints were quality of life and overall survival.

The updated median OS for patients treated with cetuximab and radiotherapy was 49 months versus 29.3 months in the RT alone group (p= 0.018). The 5-year OS rates for the cetuximab-RT and RT-alone groups were 45.6 months and 36.4 mmonths, respectively. Patients treated with cetuximab had a 26% reduction in the risk of death (hazard ratio [HR], 0.74%; 95% confidence interval [CI], 0.57-0.97) and a 9% absolute benefit in OS rate at 5 years. Though locoregional disease control was positively impacted with the addition of cetuximab (HR, 0.68; p = 0.005) there was no such impact upon distant disease control. In subgroup analysis, median OS values for patient receiving cetuximab-RT versus RT alone were statistically significantly different for primary tumor T1-T3 stage (69.5 months versus 41.4 months), N1-3 neck nodes (53 versus 26.9 months), stage II-III patients (69.5 months versus 46.9 months), and stage IV patients (43.2 months versus 24.2 months).

A forest plot analysis was done to assess whether certain patient groups benefitted with the addition of cetuximab to RT. In this analysis, factors which were associated with a potential increased benefit included presence of oropharyngeal tumors, concomitant boost RT, early T stage (T1-T3), high Karnofsky performance score (90%-100%), male sex, and age < 65 years. These results are provocative but given that the trial was not powered for this subgroup analysis, they should be interpreted with caution.

Patients who received cetuximab commonly developed an acneiform rash (83.7%); the severity of the rash was grade 3-4 in 16.8% patients. Infusion-related reactions were also seen in 15.4% patients; in 3.9% patients these were of grade 3/4 severity. However, in-field toxicities, such as mucositis, dermatitis, and dysphagia did not significantly increase with the addition of cetuximab to RT. Quality-of-life parameters were not adversely affected by the addition of cetuximab. This study allowed different RT fractionation regimens which may have impacted results and survival outcomes.

Based on the results of this study, the combination of cetuximab with RT is considered an alternative to platinum-based CRT for the treatment of locally advanced HNSCC and has been included in the National Comprehensive Cancer Network (NCCN) guidelines as an option for the treatment of locoregionally advanced HNSCC since 2007.

2.1.1.2 Cetuximab and chemoradiotherapy

The favorable results with the use of cetuximab plus RT have led to the adoption of this regimen in locally advanced HNSCC. A natural progression has been the evaluation of integration of cetuximab into existing chemoradiotherapy, typically involving platinum-based regimens. Several phase II studies from various groups have been conducted. Larger randomized trials have been launched and more recently the preliminary results of a randomized study evaluating the combination of cisplatin, cetuximab, and RT in this setting have been presented.

Multiple phase II studies have investigated the integration of cetuximab with standard platinum-based CRT regimens. A pilot study from the Memorial Sloan Kettering group evaluated 22 patients treated with accelerated fractionation by concomitant boost RT and cisplatin (100 mg/m2 on weeks 1 and 4) plus weekly cetuximab (Pfister et al., 2006). In this study, acute toxicities were typical of cisplatin-RT and cetuximab was related to grade 3/4 acneiform rash (10%) and infusion reactions (5%). However, the trial was closed prematurely due to significant adverse events including 2 deaths (one due pneumonia, one unknown cause), one myocardial infacrction, one bacteremia, and one atrial fibrillation. The 3-year PFS and OS rates were 76% and 56%, respectively.

In other studies, the combination of cisplatin and cetuximab concurrently with standard RT has not shown such an adverse event profile. This combination was evaluated in a phase II study by the Eastern Cooperative Oncology Group (ECOG) in patients with unresectable locally advanced HNSCC (E3303) (Langer et al., 2008). Cisplatin (75 mg/m2 every 3 weeks for 3 doses) was combined with weekly cetuximab followed by maintenance cetuximab for 6 months in responding patients with tolerable toxicity. Of 61 patients actually treated on study, the overall response rate was 48% with stable disease in 31% patients. The major grade 3/4 toxicities included neutropenia (26%), rash (28%), dermatitis (15%), mucositis (55%) and one death (neutropenic fever). The CR rate was 36.7% and maintenance cetuximab could be given in 74.6% patients. The 2-year PFS was 44% and the median PFS was 17.4 months. The 2-year OS was 66% with a median OS of 34.2 months. The patterns of relapse included distant (54.2%), regional (16.6%), both distant and regional (8.3%), local and regional (8.3%) and local only in 1 patient (4.2%).

In a randomized phase II study from the Radiation Therapy Oncology Group, 238 high-risk patients with resected HNSCC were randomized to receive weekly cetuximab with either weekly cisplatin 30 mg/m2 or weekly docetaxel 15 mg/m2 with 60 Gy RT over a 6-week period (RTOG 0234) (Kies et al., 2009). Patients were considered high-risk based on positive margins, $\geq$ 2 involved lymph nodes or extracapsular nodal spread. Data were available on 203 patients, 97 in the cisplatin arm and 106 in the docetaxel arm. Major grade 3/4 toxicities in the cispaltin and docetaxel arms included neutropenia (28% and 14%), mucositis (37% and 33%) and dermatitis (33% each) in the cisplatin and docetaxel groups, respectively. The 2-year OS in the cisplatin and docetaxel arms were 69% and 79%, respectively. Likewise, the 2-year DFS in the cisplatin and docetaxel arms were 57% and 66%, respectively. The 2-years distant metastasis rates with docetaxel and cisplatin were 26% and 13%, respectively and this in turn was most likely responsible for the improvement in DFS in the docetaxel arm.

In an Italian study, Merlano et al have evaluated the combination of 3 cycles of every 3-weeks cisplatin (20 mg/m2/day X 5 days) and 5-fluorouracil (200 mgm2/day X 5 days) with weekly cetuximab and rapidly alternated to 3 split courses of RT (70 Gy) (Merlano et al., 2011). In 45 patients treated, the overall RR was 91% with a CR rate of 71%. Major grade 3/4 toxicities included stomatitis (65%), neutropenia (40%), thrombocytopenia (15%), and grade 3 radiodermatitis (74%) with 3 patients dying during therapy. The median PFS and OS were reported at 21+ months and 32.6+ months, respectively.

The combination of amifostine, cetuximab, weekly cisplatin (30 mg/m2) along with conformal/hypofractionated RT (2.7 Gy/fraction, total 21 fractions in 4 weeks) was evaluated in a Greek study by Koukourakis et al. (Koukourakis et al., 2010). In this study, 43 patients were treated with the dosing of amifostine individualized according to tolerance. High dose and standard dose amifostine were tolerated by 41.8% and 34.9% patients, respectively and high dose amifostine was linked to reduced RT delays. Grade 3/4 mucositis occurred in 16.2% patients, fungal infections occurred in 41.8% patients, and cetuximab interruptions due to acneiform rash were necessary in 23.3% of patients. The complete response rate was 68.5% and the 2-year local control and survival rates were 72.3% and 91% respectively.

Suntharalingam et al from the University of Maryland group evaluated cetuximab with weekly carboplatin (AUC 2), paclitaxel (40 mg/m2) and 70.2 Gy RT in 43 patients with unresectable disease (Suntharalingham et al., 2011). The planned cetuximab and chemotherapy cycles were completed in 70% and 56% patients, respectively. Major toxicities included grade 3 mucositis (79%), dysphagia (21%), radiodermatitis (16%), rash (9%), and grade 3/4 neutropenia (21%). The CR rate was 84% at end of therapy and the estimated 3-year locoregional control rate was 72%. Local and distant recurrences were seen in 6 and 10 patients, respectively. The 3-year actuarial OS and DFS rates were 59% and 58%, respectively.

Birnbaum et al from the Brown University Oncology Group have evaluated a short 4-week cetuximab "induction" period followed by cetuximab with weekly carboplatin (AUC 1), paclitaxel (40 mg/m2) and concurrent RT to 66-72 Gy in 32 patients (Birnbaum et al., 2010). Patients were stratified by operable or inoperable disease. Patients with potentially resectable disease underwent interim tumor biopsy after 5 weeks CRT; positive biopsy patients underwent salvage surgery and the others completed CRT. Grade 3/4 radiodermatitis occurred in 53% patients which was increased compared to the prior experience with the chemotherapy regimen alone by these investigators. With a minimum follow-up of 3 years, the updated analysis shows the PFS and OS to be 53% and 59%, respectively. The rates of local, distant and combined recurrences were 22%, 15%, and 7%, respectively. The investigators detected no improvement in local control or distant metastasis free survival compared to their prior results with chemotherapy-RT alone.

Kao et al have evaluated the addition of cetuximab to the well-described non-platinum FHX regimen consisting of 5-fluorouracil, hydroxyurea, and hyperfractionated intensity modulated radiotherapy in 33 patients with locally advanced HNSCC (Kao et al., 2011). Prior organ-conserving surgery was allowed. RT was administered in 1.5 Gy fractions twice daily during weeks 1, 3, 5, and 7 to a median dose of 72 Gy. Grade 3 toxicity consisted of mucositis (33%), radiodermatitis (15%),neutropenia (12%) and thrombocytopenia (3%). The 2-year rates of locoregional control, DFS, and OS were 83%, 69%, and 86%, respectively. There were no grade 4 events and 64% patients completed treatment without requiring a feeding tube.

A large randomized phase III study was completed by the RTOG that compared accelerated fractionation RT by concomitant boost and cisplatin with or without cetuximab in patients with previously untreated, locally advanced HNSCC (Ang et al., 2011). A total of 940 patients with stage III-IV oropharynx, hypopharynx, and larynx cancers with Zubrod performance scores 0-1 were randomized to one either the experimental arm of cisplatin (100 mg/m2 every 3 weeks x 2 doses), weekly cetuximab and RT (42 fractions, total dose 70-72 Gy) over 6 weeks or the same regimen without cetuximab. Of 895 evaluable patients, 497 patients were randomized to the experimental arm and 448 patients to the standard arm. The primary tumor sites were oropharynx (70%) and larynx (23%). Among the experimental and standard arms, the distribution of stage IV disease (85% vs. 87%), T3-4 stage (60% vs. 62%) and node-positive disease (88% vs. 90%) were fairly well balanced.

The primary endpoint of this study was PFS and the secondary endpoints were OS, toxicity and early mortality. Interim analyses were planned at 108, 217, and 325 events and a planned subgroup analysis for interaction of p16 status with treatment outcomes was conducted. With a target accrual of 940 patients, the study was powered at 84% to detect a HR of 0.75. The trial was ended early after the third interim analysis showed that it was unlikely to meet its primary endpoint.

The cetuximab-containing arm had higher rates of grade 3/4 mucositis (43% versus 33%, $p=0.003$), in-field skin toxicity (25% versus 15%, $p<0.001$), out-of-field skin reactions (19% versus 1%, $p < 0.001$) but grade 3/4 dysphagia rates were similar (62% versus 66%, $p=0.27$). The rates of 30-day mortality were similar (2% versus 1.8%) as were the total grade 3-5 adverse event rates (92% versus 90%).

With a median follow-up of 2.4 years for surviving patients, there were no significant differences in 2-year PFS rates (63.4% versus 64.3%) or OS (82.6% versus 79.7%). The risk of distant metastases was numerically reduced in the experimental arm by 26% (HR 0.74, p = 0.7) while the risk of locoregional progression was numerically higher in the cetuximab arm (HR 1.21, p=0.92). In a planned subgroup analysis, 321 of 628 patients with oropharynx cancer were evaluated for HPV p16 status. The p16 positivity rate was 73% (235 patients) and both PFS and OS did not differ according to the PFS status.

Treatment Regimen	Patients (n)	Responses	Toxicity	Reference
CETUXIMAB AND CRT ALONE				
CRT: cisplatin (2 cycles), cetuximab and RT over 6 weeks	22	RR: 94% 3-year PFS and OS: 56% and 76%	Major grade 3/4 cetuximab-related toxicities were rash (10%) and hypersensitivity (5%); study closed due to significant adverse events.	Pfister et al, 2006
CRT: cisplatin, cetuximab and RT Maintenance: cetuximab x 6 months (E3303)	61(unresectable)	RR: 48%2-year PFS and OS: 44% and 66%	Major grade 3/4 toxicities were neutropenia (26%), rash (28%), dermatitis (15%), mucositis (55%); one patient death	Langer et al, 2008
CRT:cetuximab, RT, plus weekly cisplatin or weekly docetaxel (RTOG 0234)	203 (postoperative)	2-year DFS: 57% (cisplatin) and 66% (docetaxel)	Major grade 3/4 toxicities were: radiodermatitis (39% each) and mucositis (37% vs. 33%)	Kies et al, 2009
CRT: cisplatin & 5-FU x 3 cycles, weekly cetuximab and split-course RT	45(unresectable)	RR: 91 CR: 71%% PFS: 21+ mths OS: 32.6+ mths	Major grade 3/4 toxicities were neutropenia (40%), stomatitis (65%)and radiodermatitis (73%); 3 patient deaths	Merlano et al, 2011
CRT:amifostine, cetuximab, weekly cisplatin, and RT	43	CR: 68.5% 2-year OS: 91%	Major grade 3/4 toxicities were mucositis (16%), fungal infections (42%); cervical strictures in (33%)	Koukourakis et al, 2010

Treatment Regimen	Patients (n)	Responses	Toxicity	Reference
CETUXIMAB AND CRT ALONE				
CRT: weekly carboplatin, paclitaxel, RT and cetuximab	43 (unresectable)	CR: 84% 3-year OS and DFS: 59% and 58%	Major toxicities were grade 3 mucositis (79%), dysphagia (21%), radiodermatitis (16%), rash (9%), and grade 3/4 neutropenia (21%)	Suntharalingam et al, 2011
CRT: cetuximab, 5-FU, hydroxyurea, hypefractionated RT	32	3-year OS and PFS: 54% and 53%	Major grade 3/4 toxicities were mucositis (69%); radiodermatitis (53%), acneiform rash (9%)	Birnbaum et al, 2010
CRT: weekly carboplatin, paclitaxel, RT and cetuximab	33	2-year DFS and OS: 69% and 86%	Major grade 3 toxicities were mucositis (33%), radiodermatitis (15%), and neutropenia (12%)	Kao et al, 2011

CRT: chemoradiotherapy; RT: radiotherapy; RR: response rate; CR; complete response; PFS: progression free survival; DFS: disease free survival; OS: overall survival

Table 2. Selected Trials Incorporating Cetuximab with Chemotherapy and Radiotherapy

2.1.1.3 Induction chemotherapy prior to cetuximab and radiotherapy

A French randomized phase II study (TREMPLIN) evaluated IC with 3 cycles of the TPF regimen followed by either every 3-week 100 mg/m2 cisplatin with RT (arm A) or cetuximab with RT (arm B) in patients with laryngeal or hypopharyngeal cancer. (Lefebvre et al., 2011) Patients with a less than 50% response to IC underwent salvage surgery while responding patients were randomized to either of the 2 combined modality regimens. The primary end point was laryngeal preservation. Of 153 enrolled patients, 116 patients could be randomized, 60 to arm A and 56 to arm B. There was no difference between cisplatin-RT and cetuximab-RT in terms of 3-month or 18-month larynx function preservation. At 32 months mean follow-up, there were more local failures in the cetuximab-RT arm (12 versus 5); however, 7 patients could be effectively salvaged in the cetuximab arm leading to equivalent ultimate local failure rates. The rates for OS for arm A and arm B were 85% and 85%; respectively. The cetuximab-RT arm was better tolerated leading to improved treatment delivery (71% versus 43%).

A Swedish phase II has evaluated has similarly evaluated 2 cycles of IC with TPF chemotherapy followed by cetuximab-RT in patients with locally advanced unresectable

HNSCC (Mercke et al., 2011). Among 90 patients enrolled upon this study, the 1-year DFS rate was 86%. This approach was associated with mostly acute toxicities but there were few long-term toxicities.

2.1.1.4 Cetuximab as part of Induction Chemotherapy (IC) regimens

In recurrent or metastatic HNSCC, cetuximab can augment the efficacy of chemotherapy. In a randomized study, 442 patients with recurrent or metastatic HNSCC were randomly assigned to therapy with platinum- containing doublet chemotherapy with or without cetuximab (Vermorken et al., 2008). The addition of cetuximab improved response rates by 16% and the median overall survival by 2.7 months, with a reduction in the risk of death of 20% (HR, 0.80); (p = 0.04). Consequently, cetuximab has been evaluated as part of induction therapy in a number of CRT trials in HNSCC.

The University of Pittsburgh group has published results evaluating IC consisting of docetaxel, cisplatin, and cetuximab (TPE) followed by RT, cisplatin, and cetuximab (XPE) which was followed by maintenance cetuximab for 6 months in 39 patients (Argiris et al., 2010). Among 37 evaluable patients, the overall objective response was 86% after IC and 100% after CRT. Using positron emission tomography scanning, the primary site complete response rates after IC and CRT were 59% and 77%, respectively. With a median follow-up of 36 months, the 3-year PFS and OS were 70% and 74%; respectively. Relapses were seen in locoregional sites (8 patients), distant (3 patients) or both (1 patient). Significant grade 3/4 hematologic toxicity was common during TPE, including neutropenia in 77% and febrile neutropenia in10%. Human paplilloma virus (HPV) positivity was not associated with treatment efficacy. This regimen was deemed was highly effective with promising long-term survival and was recommended for further testing in larger trials.

In a multicenter phase II study, the Eastern Cooperative Oncology Group (ECOG) evaluated a short 6-week IC regimen with weekly carboplatin, paclitaxel, and cetuximab (E2303) in operable locally advanced HNSCC (Wanebo et al., 2010). Induction was followed by CRT consisting of weekly doses of same agents. Primary site biopsies were done after completion of IC if if there was a clinical response. After the first 5 weeks of CRT (50 Gy), repeat primary site biopsy was done in all patients. At this point, biopsy-negative patients continued to receive CRT to a final dose of 68-72 Gy, whereas patients with biopsy-positive results underwent salvage surgery. Maintenance cetuximab was then administered to all patients for 6 months. Seventy patients underwent IC, 68 patients underwent CRT; 63 patients are available for analysis. Of 41 patients undergoing biopsy after IC, the pathologic complete response rate was 59%. After 5 weeks CRT, 60 patients underwent re-biopsies among whom the pathologic complete response rates were 95%. Of the 63 patients eligible for analysis, the pathologic complete response rate was 91%. Local, regional, and distant recurrence rates were 11%, 8% and 8%, respectively. At 2 years, primary site disease control was 83%, PFS was 66% and OS was 82%. HPV status did not correlate with responses or survival (Psyrri et al., 2011). These preliminary findings suggest that this approach produces high primary site pathologic complete response rates and survival rates. This approach of selective organ preservation has been previously tested by the authors using a similar regimen without cetuximab but is not standard practice (Ready et al., 2011; Wanebo et al., 2010).

Treatment Regimen	Patients (n)	Responses	Toxicity	Reference
IC: docetaxel, cisplatin, and cetuximab x 3 cycles CRT: cisplatin, cetuximab and RT Maintenance: 6 mths cetuximab	39 (resectable patients= 33)	RR: 86% after IC and 100% after CRT CR: 5% after IC and 24% after CRT 3-year PFS and OS: 70% and 74%	During IC: major grade 3/4 toxicities were neutropenia 77%, febrile neutropenia 10% During CRT: major grade 3/4 toxicities were mucositis 54%, dermatitis 27%, neutropenia 36%, thrombocytopenia 12%, febrile neutropenia 6%	Argiris et al, 2010
IC: paclitaxel, carboplatin , and cetuximab x 6 weeks CRT: paclitaxel, carboplatin, cetuximab and RT Maintenance: 6 mths cetuximab (E2303)	70 (operable patients)	Pathologic CR: 63% after IC and 97% after CRT 2-year DFS and OS: 62% and 82%	During CRT: major grade 3/4 toxicities were mucositis (32%) , neutropenia (31%), rash (9%), radiation dermatitis (13%); one patient death	Wanebo et al, 2010
IC: paclitaxel, carboplatin , and cetuximab x 6 weeks Follow-up therapy: surgery, RT or CRT	47 (resectable)	RR: 96% after IC CR: 19% after IC 3-year DFS and OS: 87% and 91%	During IC: grade 3 rash (45%), grade 3/4 neutropenia (21%), no deaths during IC	Kies et al, 2010
IC: docetaxel, cisplatin, 5-FU and cetuximab x 4 cycles CRT: cetuximab, RT	50 (unresectable patients)	RR: 78% after IC CR: 24% after IC 2-year DFS and OS: 42% and 60%	During IC: febrile neutropenia (26%); 2 deaths During CRT: grade 3/4 toxicities mucositis (56%), dermatitis (10%)	Mesia et al, 2010
IC: carboplatin, paclitaxel, cetuximab x 2 cycles CRT: either RT plus CetuxFHX (cetuximab, 5-FU, hydroxyurea) OR CetuxPX (cetuximab, cisplatin)	110	RR: 91.8% after IC 2-year OS: 89.5% with CetuxFHX and 91.4% with CetuxPX	During IC: major grade 3/4 toxicities were rash (16%) and neutropenia (36%) During CRT: major grade 3/4 toxicities in CetuxFHX were mucositis (91%), dermatitis (82%) and in Cetux PX were mucositis (94%) and dermatitis (50%)	Seiwert et al, 2011

Treatment Regimen	Patients (n)	Responses	Toxicity	Reference
IC: docetaxel, cisplatin, 5-FU (TPF) CRT: cisplatin plus RT versus cetuximab plus RT (TREMPLIN)	153 (resectable; 116 went on to CRT arms)	OS: 85% in both arms at 32 mths	More treatment delivery in cetuximab arm (71%) vs cisplatin arm (43%)	Lefebvre et al, 2011
IC: docetaxel, cisplatin, 5-FU (TPF) CRT: cetuximab, RT	90 (unresectable)	RR: 58% after IC DFS: 86% at 1-year	Grade 3 radiodermatitis 4%, cetuximab delays 20%, mostly acute toxicities	Mercke et al, 2011

IC: induction chemotherapy; CRT: chemoradiotherapy; RT: radiotherapy; RR: response rate; CR; complete response; PFS: progression free survival; DFS: disease free survival; OS: overall survival

Table 3. Selected Trials of Induction Chemotherapy Regimens incorporating Cetuximab.

The MD Anderson Cancer Center group has published results of their phase II study of dose-dense weekly IC regimen consisting of paclitaxel, carboplatin, and cetuximab for 6 weeks along with G-CSF. IC was followed by locoregional therapy with either surgery, RT alone, or cisplatin-RT. This regimen was highly active with a CR and OR rate of 19% and 96%, respectively. Six patients had relapses; locoregional in 4 patients, distant in 1 patient and both in 1 patient. The 3-year PFS and OS rates were 87% and 91%, respectively; HPV status was found to correlate with both PFS and OS (Kies et al., 2010).

The combination of docetaxel, cisplatin, 5-Fluorouracil plus cetuximab (TPF-C) as IC has been investigated in a Spanish multicenter phase II study (Mesia et al., 2009). Fifty patients with unresectable HNSCC were treated with 4 cycles of TPF-C chemotherapy along with G-CSF and antibiotic prophylaxis, followed by accelerated boost RT with concurrent cetuximab alone. The ORR after IC and end of CRT were 78% and 72%, respectively (intent-to-treat population) with only 86% patients starting CRT. Locoregional disease control at 1-year was 44%. With a median follow-up of 19 months, actuarial disease free survival and overall survival at 2 years were 42% and 60%, respectively.

Another approach as practiced by the University of Chicago group, has been to evaluate IC containing cetuximab, carboplatin, paclitaxel for 2 cycles followed by randomization to one of 2 CRT approaches: concurrent cetuximab, 5-fluorouracil, hydroxyurea and hyperfractionated RT (CetuxFHX) or cetuximab, cisplatin, and accelerated RT with concomitant boost (CetuxPX) (Seiwert et al., 2011). In the preliminary report, 110 patients had a overall response rate of 91.8% with IC. After end of all treatment, the 2-year OS in the CetuxFHX and CetuxPX arms was 89.5% and 91.4%, respectively. The 2-year PFS for CetuxFHX and CetuxPX was 82.3% and 89.7%, respectively. Even though the trial was marked by high rates of severe rash, dermatitis, mucositis, and neutropenia 95% of patients were able to complete all therapy. Survival outcomes between the two CRT arms were not significantly different.

2.1.2 Panitumumab

Panitumumab is a fully human IgG2 antibody that binds with high affinity to the EGFR and is approved in the setting of recurrent colorectal cancer. Panitumumab has been evaluated in preclinical studies for HNSCC (Lopez-Albaitero & Ferris, 2007; Kruser et al., 2008) which showed a favorable interaction between panitumumab and RT.

Wirth et al have conducted a phase I study of panitumumab in combination with CRT for which the preliminary results have been presented (Wirth et al., 2008). In this study, 19 patients with locally advanced HNSCC received IMRT (70 Gy) with concurrent weekly dosing of carboplatin (AUC 1.5) plus panitumumab (2.5 mg/kg) plus paclitaxel (2 dose levels, 15 and 30 mg/m^2) over a 7-week period. At the higher paclitaxel dose level 1 patient developed febrile neutropenia which was considered a dose limiting event. Major toxicities included grade 3 dysphagia (95%), grade 3 radiodermatitis (42%), and grade 3/4 mucositis (89%). Among evaluable patients, the primary site CR rate was 87%.

Panitumumab is being evaluated in the postoperative setting in resected locally advanced HNSCC with high-risk features (extracapsular nodal spread, > 2 nodes involved, perineural or angiolymphatic invasion, or < 1mm margins) (Ferris et al., 2010). The treatment consisted of RT (60-66 Gy) over 6-7 weeks concurrent with weekly panitumumab (2.5 mg/kg) and cisplatin (30 mg/m2). The planned accrual is 47 patients and final results of this study are awaited. Other trials with panitumumab in combination with CRT are currently ongoing.

2.1.3 Nimotuzumab

Nimotuzumab is a humanized IgG1 monoclonal antibody against EGFR developed in Cuba. This was originally a mouse IgG2a antibody (R3) which was humanized and the resulting antibody (h-R3) inhibits EGFR by binding to domain III of the extracellular domain. Nimotuzumab partially blocks the EGF binding site as well as stabilizes a receptor-protein configuration that is unfavorable for dimer formation. In pre-clinical evaluation, nimotuzumab reduced tumor proliferation, increased apoptosis, and had a lower binding affinity to EGFR than cetuximab.

2.1.3.1 Nimotuzumab and radiotherapy alone

Several early studies have been conducted with nimotuzumab as a single agent in combination with RT alone in locally advanced HNSCC. It is well tolerated as a single agent at weekly doses up to 400 mg and is associated with a very low incidence of rash (Boku et al., 2009).

In a phase I/II trial conducted in Cuba, Crombet et al enrolled 24 patients with unresectable HNSCC who received 6 weekly infusions of nimotuzumab administered concurrently with RT to a total dose of 60-66 Gy (Crombet et al., 2004). Initially, nimotuzumab doses were escalated from 50 mg to 400 mg weekly and the last 10 patients were treated at 200 mg or 400 mg weekly only. This combination was well tolerated without the development of skin toxicities while common adverse events were infusion reactions, grade 3 radiodermatitis (12.5%), grade 3 mucositis (20.8%), and grade 3 dysphagia (12.5%). The overall RR was 87.5% among 16 evaluable patients responded and the CR rate was 56%. The OS appeared to correlate with the administered dose level, with the 3-year survival rate ranging from 16.7% for the 2 lower doses to 66.7% for the 2 higher doses. Based on serum levels, the nimotuzumab dose of 200 mg/week was selected for further clinical testing.

In a follow-up study by the same group, Rodriguez et al performed a randomized phase II study in which they evaluated the combination of 6 weekly doses of nimotuzumab and RT (60-66 Gy) to patients treated with placebo plus RT in locally advanced unresectable HNSCC (Rodriguez et al., 2010). A total of 106 patients were enrolled; 54 on the nimotuzumab arm and 51 in the standard arm. Grade 1/2 events attributable to nimotuzumab included asthenia (14.6%), fever (9.8%), headache (9.8%), chills (7.8%), and anorexia (7.8%). Consistent with other reports, no acneiform skin rash was observed, differentiating nimotuzumab from other anti-EGFR antibodies. There was no significant exacerbation of adverse events with the addition of nimotuzumab to RT. Among 75 patients evaluable for response, the CR rates for the nimotuzumab and placebo groups were 59.5% and 34.2%, respectively. In the intent to treat analysis, the median OS differed significantly between the nimotuzumab and placebo arms at 12.5 months and 9.5 months, respectively. In a subset analysis, patients with at least weak EGFR-expression had an improvement in median OS compared to EGFR-negative patients (16.5 months versus 7.2 months, p=0.0038)

In a small Spanish study, Rojo et al evaluated nimotuzumab (200 mg and 400 mg doses) plus RT in 10 patients with advanced HNSCC felt to be unsuitable for CRT (Rojo et al., 2008). The overall response rate was 80% and median OS was 7.2 months. Nimotuzumab was well tolerated and no skin rash was observed again. Pharmacodynamic studies were conducted in this study which showed that nimotuzumab inhibited EGFR phopshorylation; molecular downstream effects included decrease of p-ERK and upregulation of p-AKT in tumor but not in the skin. There were no associations between doses or responses and pharmacodynamic effects in this study.

2.1.3.2 Nimotuzumab and chemoradiotherapy

In an open-label, phase IIb randomized study from India, Babu et al evaluated nimotuzumab in patients with locally advanced, inoperative HNSCC (Babu et al., 2010). Of 113 screened patients, 92 were randomized to receive a) RT alone, b) RT plus nimotuzumab, c) RT plus cisplatin, and d) RT plus cisplatin plus nimotuzumab. The nimotuzumab dose was 200 mg/week x 6 weeks, the cisplatin dose was 50 mg/week, and RT was given to a total dose of 60-6 Gy all over 6 weeks. Of 76 evaluable patients, the locoregional response rates were as follows: RT (37%), RT plus nimotuzumab (76%), RT plus cisplatin (70%), and RT plus cisplatin plus nimotuzumab (100%). Similarly, after 48 months follow-up the median OS rates were as follows: RT (12.7 months), RT plus nimotuzumab (14.3 months), RT plus cisplatin (21.9 months), and RT plus cisplatin plus nimotuzumab (not reached). The addition of nimotuzumab to CRT resulted in this small population resulted in significant reduction in the risk of death (HR 0.35, p=0.01).

Preliminary results of another study from India were reported by Gupta et al in which 17 patients with locally advanced HNSCC were treated with weekly doses of nimotuzumab 200 mg plus cisplatin 40 mg/m2 concurrent with RT (66 Gy in 33 fractions) (Gupta et al., 2010). All patients completed planned nimotuzumab treatments and were evaluated for the primary endpoint of responses and safety. No grade 3/4 adverse events were reported. The overall RR was 76% (CR 59%) while 2 patients progressed after therapy (one patient each in the 5th and 6th month). Additional clinical trials, including a randomized phase III evaluation in the postoperative treatment setting is planned.

2.2 EGFR tyrosine kinase inhibitors

EGFR tyrosine kinase inhibitors (EGFR-TKIs) are a class of oral drugs which bind intracellularly to EGFR and competitively inhibit the receptor activity resulting in inhibition of downstream signaling pathways (Steeghs et al., 2007). In HNSCC, the EGFR-TKIs which have been evaluated are erlotinib, gefitinib, and lapatinib.

2.2.1 Erlotinib

Erlotinib is an approved drug in advanced non-small cell lung cancer as monotherapy and in advanced pancreatic cancer in combination with gemcitabine. In recurrent or metastatic HNSCC, erlotinib has been evaluated as monotherapy and in combination with other chemotherapeutic agents.

In a phase I trial Savvides et al combined erlotinib with docetaxel and RT in locally advanced HNSCC (Savvides et al., 2006). The regimen consisted of weekly docetaxel (15 to 20 mg/m2) plus daily erlotinib (50 to 150 mg) with concurrent RT (70 Gy) followed by maintenance erlotinib for up to 2 years. One patient developed dose-limiting toxicities at each of the first 3 levels but no dose-limiting toxicity was observed at the 4th dose level. The CR rate was 83% (15 of 18 evaluable patients) and full dose erlotinib and docetaxel 20 mg/m^2 weekly were the recommended for phase II evaluation.

Herchenhorn et al conducted a phase I/II study in Brazil which evaluated the combination of erlotinib (50 to 150 mg), cisplatin (100 mg/m2 every 3 weeks x 3 doses), and RT (70.2 Gy) in 37 patients with locally advanced HNSCC (Herchenhorn et al., 2007). The phase II dosing of erlotinib at 150 mg dose was evaluated in 31 patients. The CR rate in these patients was 74%. Major grade 3/4 toxicities were radiodermatitis (51%), nausea (48%), mucositis (29%), dysphagia (35%), and vomiting (39%) were the most common adverse events (Herchenhorn et al., 2007). With a median follow-up of 37 months, the 3-year PFS and OS rates were 61% and 72%, respectively.

In a Spanish phase I study, de la Vega et al evaluated combination of erlotinib, weekly cisplatin, and RT (up to 63 Gy) in resected patients with locally advanced HNSCC (Arias de la Vega et al., 2011). Thirteen patients were treated and the recommended phase II evaluation dose was full dose erlotinib (150 mg) with weekly cisplatin (30 mg/m2) for 6 weeks. Further studies with erlotinib in patients with locally advanced HNSCCHN are ongoing.

2.2.2 Gefitinib

Gefitinib is an oral EGFR-TKI with modest single-agent activity in recurrent or metastatic HNSCC (Cohen et al., 2003; Cohen et al., 2005; Kirby et al., 2006). However, 2 phase III randomized trials did not show survival benefit of single-agent gefitinib over standard methotrexate (Stewart et al., 2009) or of docetaxel plus gefitinib versus docetaxel plus placebo in patients with recurrent or metastatic HNSCC (Argiris et al., 2009). Multiple studies of the combination of gefitinib with RT or CRT in locally advanced HNSCC have been conducted.

Rodriguez et al conducted a phase II trial of multiagent CRT including daily gefitinib (250 mg) with 2 cycles of infusional 96-hours of cisplatin and 5-fluorouracil, and concurrent hyperfractionated RT (72-74 Gy) followed by maintenance gefitinib for 2 years (Rodriguez et al., 2009). Acute toxicities, including transient renal dysfunction and hospital admissions were significantly increased with the addition of gefitinib compared to historical controls. The 3-year estimates of freedom from recurrence and OS were 72% and 68%, respectively. Less than half the patients were projected to complete maintenance gefitinib. The investigators concluded that this regimen increased toxicity without improving efficacy.

The combination of weekly cisplatin (40 mg/m2) and gefitinib (250 mg) plus concomitant boost accelerated radiation (72 Gy) was evaluated by Rueda et al in 46 patients with unresectable locally advanced HNSCC (Reuda et al., 2007). Grade 3/4 toxicity included mucositis (47%), radiodermatitis (14%), rash (5%), diarrhea (2%), and grade 3 neutropenia (5%). Response evaluation at 3 months post therapy completion showed a RR of 63% and CR rate of 52%. With a median follow-up of 23 months, the 2-year PFS and OS were 47% and 56%, respectively.

A large, double blind, randomized phase II study was reported by Gregoire et al from Belgium (Gregoire et al., 2011). In this study, 226 patients with locally advanced HNSCC were randomized to gefitinib (250 mg or 500 mg) with cisplatin and RT followed by maintenance gefitinib or placebo. The primary objective was 2-year local disease control rate. The addition of gefitinib did not improve 2-year local control rates when given concurrently with CRT (32.7% versus 33.6%) or as maintenance (28.8% versus 37.4%).

Treatment Regimen	Patients (n)	Responses	Toxicity	Reference
Erlotinib and CRT				
CRT: weekly docetaxel, erlotinib and RT Maintenance: erlotinib x 2 years	23	CR: 83%	Mostly acute toxicities; one patient death	Savvides et al, 2006
CRT: cisplatin x 3 cycles, daily erlotinib and RT	37(unresectable)	CR: 74% 3-year PFS and OS: 61% and 72%	Major grade 3/4 toxicities were nausea (48%), vomiting (39%), radiodermatitis (52%), and mucositis (29%)	Herchenhorn et al, 2010
Gefitinib and CRT				
CRT: 2 cycles cisplatin and 5-FU, daily gefitinib and RT Maintenance: gefitinib x 2 years	60	3-year FFR and OS : 72% and 67%	Transient renal dysfunction (28%), re-hospitalization (83%), 5 patient deaths, increased diarrhea and rash with gefitinib	Rodriguez et al, 2009

Treatment Regimen	Patients (n)	Responses	Toxicity	Reference
CRT: weekly cisplatin, gefitinib, and RT	46 (unresectable)	RR: 63% CR: 52% 2-year PFS and OS: 47% and 56%	Major grade 3/4 toxicties were: mucositis (47%), rash (5%), radiodermatitis (14%).	Rueda et al, 2007
CRT: cisplatin, gefitinib (250mg vs. 500 mg) or placebo, and RT Maintenance: gefitinib x 1 year	226 (randomized phase II)	2-year LDCR: 33% each for gefitinib vs. no gefitinib	Increase in serious adverse events in gefitnib arms	Gregoire et al, 2011
IC: carboplatin, paclitaxel x 2 cycles CRT: RT, 5-FU, hydroxyurea, and gefitinib Maintenance: gefitinib x 2 years	69	CR: 90% after CRT 4-year PFS and OS: 72% and 74%	Major grade 3/4 toxicties during CRT were: neutropenia (16%), mucositis (85%), radiodermatitis (33%), infection (17%)	Cohen et al, 2010
IC: docetaxel, 5-FU, carboplatin, and gefitinib x 2 cycles CRT: docetaxel, gefitinib and RT Maintenance: gefitinib x 2 years	62	RR: 80% CR: 36% 3- year PFS and OS: 41% and 54%	Major grade 3/4 toxicties were: radiodermatitis (9%), mucositis (57%), hospitalizations (42%); one patient death	Hainsworth et al, 2009

IC: induction chemotherapy; CRT: chemoradiotherapy; RT: radiotherapy; RR: response rate; CR; complete response; PFS: progression free survival; DFS: disease free survival; OS: overall survival

Table 4. Selected Trials incorporating EGFR-TKI's in Chemoradiotherapy Regimens

Gefitinib was well tolerated during both phases but no efficacy improvement was noted.

Cohen et al have reported the University of Chicago experience with the addition of gefitinib to IC and subsequent CRT in a phase II trial (Cohen et al., 2010). Sixty-nine patients with locally advanced HNSCC were treated with 2 cycles of carboplatin and paclitaxel followed by fluorouracil, hydroxyurea, gefitinib, and twice daily RT followed by maintenance gefitinib for 2 years. Major grade 3/4 toxicity during CRT included mucositis (85%), radiodermatitis (33%), neutropenia (16%), and infection (17%). The CR rate was 90% after completion of CRT. After a median follow-up of 3.5 years, the 4-year PFS and OS s were 72% and 74%, respectively.

Finally, Hainsworth et al from the Sarah Cannon group treated 62 patients with locally advanced HNSCC with an IC regimen of 2 cycles of docetaxel (60 mg/m2) and carboplatin (AUC 5) every 3 weeks plus 6 weeks of daily infusional 5-FU (200 mg/m2) and gefitinib (250 mg) (Hainsworth et al., 2009). CRT consisted of RT (68.4 Gy) with weekly docetaxel (20 mg/m2) and daily gefitinib 250 mg/d followed by maintenance gefitinib for up to 2 years. IC resulted in major grade 3 mucositis (27%) and diarrhea (16%) as well as grade 3/4 neutropenia (30%). During CRT, the major grade 3/4 toxicities were mucositis (59%) and radiodermatitis (9%). The RR after IC and CRT was 46% and 80%, respectively. With a median follow-up of 33 months, the 3-year PFS and OS rates were 41% and 54%, respectively, which were not superior to survival results reported with CRT alone by the same group.

2.2.3 Lapatinib

Lapatinib is a dual-inhibitor which targets EGFR and HER-2 and may inhibit their dimerization as a result. In preclinical models, lapatinib has synergistic activity with chemotherapy and RT (Montemurro et al., 2007). Harrington et al have reported results of a phase I trial of the combination of lapatinib (500 mg, 1000 mg, 1500 mg), cisplatin (100 mg/m2 every 3 weeks x 3 cycles), and RT (66-70 Gy) in 31 patients (Harrington et al., 2009). No DLT's were observed in this evaluation and the recommended lapatinib dose of for phase II evaluation was determined as 1500 mg daily. The overall RR was 81% while radiodermatitis, mucositis, lymphopenia, and neutropenia were the most common side effects.

Harringtpon et al have also presented preliminary results of their phase II randomized evaluation of lapatinib or placebo, cisplatin, and RT as per the recommended schedule above followed by maintenance lapatinib or placebo (Harrington et al., 2010). In 67 patients randomized to lapatinib or placebo, the grade 3/4 toxicities were balanced with grade 3 rash and diarrhea being more common in the lapatinib arm. The CR rates in the lapatinib and standard arms were 53% and 36%, respectively. CRT dose intensities were not adversely impacted by lapatinib. Early data showed hazard ratios for PFS and OS by independent review of 0.71 and 0.70, respectively.

2.3 Predictors of outcome after treatment with EGFR inhibitors

The level of EGFR expression as detected by immunohistochemistry (IHC) has been evaluated as a potential biomarker of cetuximab efficacy in HNSCC. In patients with metastatic HNSCC, EGFR expression as determined using the DAKO assay with staining intensity graded on an ordinal scale 0-3 and staining density assessed according to the percentage of cells stained (Kies et al., 2007). High expression was defined as staining intensity 3 + on 80% of cells. EGFR expression was not predictive of response to cetuximab nor was there any association with survival.

The University of Pittsburgh group has reported results of evaluation of baseline serum biomarkers in their study evaluating cetuximab in locally advanced HNSCC (Ferris et al., 2009). A panel consisting of 31 cytokines were measured before and after 3 cycles of induction cetuximab-containing chemotherapy. Low baseline VEGF and IL-6 levels were potentially associated with complete response among patients evaluated by PET imaging post-therapy.

Fountzilas et al evaluated genetic biomarkers in patients undergoing cetuximab containing radiation in locally advanced HNSCC (Fountzilas et al., 2009). In this report, tumor EGFR, MET, ERCC1, and p-53 protein and/or gene expression were not associated with treatment response. However, a high level of matrix metalloproteinase MMP9 mRNA expression was found to be significantly associated with objective response.

Tumors of patients treated with cisplatin-chemotherapy with or without cetuximab on the phase III EXTREME registration study were evaluated for EGFR gene copy number FISH (Licitra et al., 2009). Tumors were classified as FISH positive or FISH negative using the Colorado scoring system. Patients with FISH positive tumors were evenly distributed across both arms. The FISH scores had no influence on the response rate in the cetuximab-containing arm and no effect on survival on either; thus EGFR gene copy number was not predictive of cetuximab efficacy in this setting. In patients treated with gefitnib, cisplatin and radiotherapy in locally advanced HNSCC, EGFR protein expression, FISH and mutation status did not predict for response or survival (Tan et al., 2011).

The most common adverse event associated with anti-EGFR agents that occurs in more than two-thirds of patients is skin rash which usually occurs in the first 3 weeks of treatment. It is likely related to EGFR expression in the skin and the severity of rash is associated with efficacy. Several studies in HNSCC have shown a direct correlation between the development of rash and better patient outcome after EGFR inhibitor therapy (Soulieres et al., 2004; Cohen et al., 2003; Baselga et al., 2005; Burtness et al., 2005; Herbst et al., 2005). In the Bonner study, patients with a grade 2 or greater rash had a significantly lower risk of death (Bonner et al., 2010). Patients with a prominent rash had significantly longer overall survival than those patients who had a mild rash (68.8 months vs. 25.6 months; HR 0.49; p=0.002). It is possible that occurrence of acneiform rash is a biomarker of an immunological response that is conducive for optimal outcome. It thus seems that currently occurrence of a high-grade rash may be the only biomarker predictive of favorable outcome with cetuximab containing therapy.

3. Vascular endothelial growth factor pathway inhibitors

VEGF was associated with an increased risk of death in HNSCC in a recent meta-analysis of 12 studies (Kyzas et al., 2005). In HNSCC, both VEGF and the VEGF receptor are upregulated and are important for tumor cell survival in hypoxic conditions (Moriyama et al., 1997; Denhart et al., 1997; Inoue et al., 1997; Petruzzelli et al., 1997). Pre-clinical studies have demonstrated that blockage of the VEGF pathways by anti-angiogenic drugs increases the anti-tumor effects of radiation. As such targeting the VEGF pathway through monoclonal antibodies and receptor tyrosine kinase inhibitors is a promising therapeutic approach in HNSCC. The currently available data with the use of bevacizumab in locally advanced HNSCC is reviewed below.

3.1 Bevacizumab

The humanized monoclonal antibody bevacizumab binds VEGF-A and is currently approved for clinical use in many advanced solid tumors, including colorectal cancer, non-small cell lung cancer, renal cell carcinoma, and glioblastomas. Bevacizumab inhibits angiogenesis and also facilitates chemotherapy delivery into tumors (Shirai & O'Brien, 2007;

Olsson et al., 2006). Antiangiogenic agents, in preclinical studies appear to overcome resistance and potentiate the effect of traditional therapies such as radiotherapy and chemotherapy (Seiwert & Cohen, 2008).

3.1.1 Bevacizumab and chemoradiotherapy

Various combinations of bevacizumab and radiotherapy have been evaluated in phase I/II trials in locally advanced HNSCC. Seiwert et al from the University of Chicago group have published results of a phase I evaluation of bevacizumab, 5-fluorouracil, hydroxyurea, and radiation (BFHX). In this study, 43 patients with recurrent, previously irradiated or poor prognosis, treatment-naïve HNSCC were treated with every 2-week regimen of bevacizumab (escalating doses from 2.5 to 10 mg/kg), hydroxyurea (500-1000 mg BID), and 5-FU (600-800 mg/m^2 as a continuous infusion for 5 days) in combination with RT (1.8-2 Gy once daily) on a week on-week off schedule (Seiwert et al., 2008). The MTD of the combination was bevacizumab (10 mg/kg), 5-FU (600 mg/m^2) and hydroxyurea (500 mg) and this cohort was expanded to 26 patients. The median OS was 10.3 months. Significant severe late toxicities were observed including development of fistula (5 patients), ulceration or tissue necrosis (4 patients), and thrombosis (3 patients).

Results of a follow-up phase II randomized study by the same group have been reported by Salama et al in which the BFHX regimen was compared to the prior FHX regimen (Salama et al., 2011). In this study, 26 patients with intermediate stage III-IV patients (excluding N2-N3 stage) were enrolled. The study was halted following unexpected locoregional progression in 4 patients with T4 tumors randomized to the BFHX regimen. The incidence of mucositis and dermatitis was not increased with the addition of bevacizumab to CRT. The pathologic CR rate on study was 77%. The 2-year OS was 68% and the DFS for BFHX and FHX were 59% and 89%, respectively. Two patients died during CRT and one patient died within 30 days after post-CRT surgery.

Savvides et al have presented preliminary results of a phase II study evaluating the combination of weekly docetaxel (20 mg/m^2) and every 2-week bevacizumab (5 mg/kg) with daily RT (70.2 Gy) followed by maintenance bevacizumab for up to 1 year (Savvides et al., 2008). Of 23 enrolled patients, 17 patients remained in CR and 4 patients recurred. No unexpected toxicities or severe bleeding episodes were noted while 8 patients required hospitalization during CRT. The estimated 1-year PFS and OS were 78% and 89%, respectively.

Preliminary results of a phase II study from the Sloan Kettering group which investigated the addition of bevacizumab (15 mg/kg every 3 weeks x 3 cycles) to cisplatin (50 mg/m^2 on days 1, 2, 22, 23, 43 and 44) and RT (70 Gy) have been presented by Pfister et al (Pfister et al., 2009). Plans for maintenance bevacizumab were discontinued after the occurrence of a grade 4 pulmonary hemorrhage. Major toxicities included grade 3 mucositis (76%) and grade 3/4 neutropenia (41%). Two patients died within 90 days of last treatment; one had a sudden death and another died from aspiration pneumonia. The estimated 1-year PFS and OS were 83% and 88%, respectively.

Preliminary results of a RTOG phase II trial of bevacizumab and CRT in patients with locally advanced nasopharyngeal carcinoma were reported by Lee et al (Lee et al., 2011). In this study, 44 patients were enrolled and received 3 cycles of bevacizumab (15 mg/kg), cisplatin (100 mg/m2), and IMR (70 Gy) followed by 3 cycles of adjuvant bevacizumab (15 mg/kg), cisplatin (80 mg/m2), and 5-fluorouracil (1000 mg/m2/day x 4 days). The most common grade 4 toxicity was hematologic and grade 3/4 mucositis was seen in 77% cases. The 2-year PFS and OS were 71.7% and 90.9%, respectively. These survival rates were favorable compared to prior RTOG data with regards to OS but not PFS.

3.1.2 Bevacizumab with induction chemotherapy and CRT

In a phase II study, Meluch et al evaluated IC with paclitaxel (200 mg/m2), carboplatin (AUC 6), and 5-FU (200 mg/m2/day x 3 weeks) plus bevacizumab (15 mg/kg) followed by concurrent RT (68.4 Gy) with paclitaxel (50 mg/mw/week), bevacizumab (15 mg/kg), and erlotinib (150 mg daily) in locally advanced HNSCC (Meluch et al., 2009). Of 60 enrolled patients, preliminary results in the first 48 patients showed that the most common grade 3/4 adverse events during IC were neutropenia (46%), neutropenic fever (6%), mucositis (14%), and diarrhea (14%); during CRT grade 3/4 mucositis occurred in 76% patients. The overall RR was 77% after completion of the entire treatment. After a median follow-up of 16 months, the 18-month PFS and OS were 85% and 87%, respectively. No unexpected toxicities were observed with this regimen.

4. Conclusion

The evaluation of targeted therapies in the management of locally advanced head and neck squamous cancers is evolving. Currently, randomized trials data support the use of the anti-EGFR monoclonal antibody cetuximab in combination with radiotherapy in this setting. Conversely, the currently available data do not support the use of cetuximab in combination with chemotherapy and radiotherapy in this setting based on the results of the RTOG 0522 study. As such, the use of combined targeted and chemotherapy regimens outside of a clinical trial is not recommended at present. The challenge in the appropriate use of anti-EGFR therapies is the determination of appropriate patients prospectively through the use of relevant biomarkers. Presently, the development of a high-grade rash is the only potential biomarker of benefit in the use of ant-EGFR therapy.

The clinical trials scenario is replete with ongoing randomized trials evaluating anti-EGFR monoclonal antibodies and tyrosine kinase inhibitors in combination with chemotherapy. Additional trials are investigating the role of anti-VEGF therapies and mTOR inhibitors are in early clinical trials. The results of these trials will shape the future of targeted therapies in this setting.

5. References

Adelstein DJ, Li Y, Adams GL, et al. (2003).An intergroup phase III comparison of standard radiation therapy and two schedules of concurrent chemoradiotherapy in patients with unresectable squamous cell head and neck cancer. *J Clin Oncol* 21(1):92-98.

Adelstein DJ, Lavertu P, Saxton JP, et al. (2000). Mature results of a phase II randomized trial comparing concurrent chemoradiotherapy with radiation therapy alone in patients with stage III and IV squamous cell carcinoma of the head and neck. *Cancer* 88(4): 876-883.

Ahmed S, Cohen EE, Haraf DJ, et al. (2007). Updated results of a phase II trial integrating gefitinib (G) into concurrent chemoradiation (CRT) followed by Gefitinib adjuvant therapy for locally advanced head and neck cancer (HNC). *J Clin Oncol* 25(18S): 6028.

Ang KK, Zhang QE, Rosenthal DI, et al. (2011). A randomized phase III trial (RTOG 0522) of concurrent accelerated radiation plus cisplatin with or without cetuximab for stage III-IV head and neck squamous cell carcinomas (HNC). *J Clin Oncol* 29 (suppl; abstr 5500)

Ang KK, Berkey BA, Tu X, et al. (2002). Impact of epidermal growth factor receptor expression on survival and pattern of relapse in patients with advanced head and neck carcinoma. *Cancer Res* 62(24): p. 7350-7356.

Arias de la Vega F, Contreras J, de Las Heras M, et al. (2011). Erlotinib and chemoradiation in patients with surgically resected locally advanced squamous cell carcinoma of the head and neck: a GICOR phase I trial. *Ann Oncol.* [Epub ahead of print].

Argiris A, Ghebremichael M, Gilbert J, Burtness B, Forastiere A. (2009). A phase III randomized, placebo-controlled trial of docetaxel (D) with or without gefitinib (G) in recurrent or metastatic (R/M) squamous cell carcinoma of the head and neck (SCHNN): A trial of the Eastern Cooperative Oncology Group (ECOG) [ASCO Annual Meeting, abstr 6011]. *J Clin Oncol.* 27:15s.

Argiris A, Heron DE, Smith RP, et al. (2010). Induction docetaxel, cisplatin, and cetuximab followed by concurrent radiotherapy, cisplatin, and cetuximab and maintenance cetuximab in patients with locally advanced head and neck cancer. *J Clin Oncol* 28(36): 5294-00.

Babu KG, Viswanath L, Reddy BK, et al. (2010). An open-label, randomized, study of h-R3mAb (nimotuzumab) in patients with advanced (stage III or IVa) squamous cell carcinoma of head and neck (SCCHN): Four-year survival results from a phase IIb study. *J Clin Oncol* 28:15s, 2010 (suppl; abstr 5530).

Baselga J and Arteaga CL. (2005). Critical update and emerging trends in epidermal growth factor receptor targeting in cancer. *J Clin Oncol* 23(11): p. 2445-2459.

Baselga J, Norton L, Masui H, et al. (1993). Antitumor effects of doxorubicin in combination with anti-epidermal growth factor receptor monoclonal antibodies. *J Natl Cancer Inst.* 85(16):1327-33.

Baselga J, Pfister D, Cooper MR, et al. (2000). Phase I studies of anti-epidermal growth factor receptor chimeric antibody C225 alone and in combination with cisplatin. *J Clin Oncol* 18(4):904-914.

Baselga J, Trigo JM, Bouthis J, et al. (2005). Phase II multicenter study of the antiepidermal growth factor receptor monoclonal antibody cetuximab in combination with platinum-based chemotherapy in patients with platinum-refractory metastatic and/or recurrent squamous cell carcinoma of the head and neck. *J Clin Oncol* 23(24):5568-77.

Bernier J, Domenge C, Ozsahin M, et al. (2004). Postoperative irradiation with or without concomitant chemotherapy for locally advanced head and neck cancer. *N Engl J Med* 350(19):1945-52.

Bernier J, Russi EG, Homey B, et al. (2011). Management of radiation dermatitis in patients receiving cetuximab and radiotherapy for locally advanced squamous cell carcinoma of the head and neck: proposals for a revised grading system and consensus management guidelines. *Ann Oncol* 22(10):2191-200.

Birnbaum A, Dipetrillo T, Rathore R, et al., (2010). Cetuximab, paclitaxel, carboplatin, and radiation for head and neck cancer: a toxicity analysis. *Am J Clin Oncol* 33(2):144-7.

Boku N, Yamazaki K, Yamamoto N, et al. (2009). Phase I study of nimotuzumab, a humanized anti-epidermal growth factor receptor (EGFR) IgG1 monoclonal antibody in patients with solid tumors in Japan. [ASCO Annual Meeting, abstr el4574]. *J Clin Onocol*.27.

Bonner J, Harari PM, Giralt J, et al. (2006). Radiotherapy plus cetuximab for squamous-cell carcinoma of the head and neck. *N Engl J Med* 354(6): 576-78.

Bonner J, Harari PM, Giralt J, et al. (2010). Radiotherapy plus cetuximab for locoregionally advanced head and neck cancer: 5-year survival data from a phase 3 randomized trial, and relation between cetuximab-induced rash and survival. *Lancet* 11: 21-28.

Boze, A, Sudaka A, Fischel JL, et al. (2008). Combined effects of bevacizumab with erlotinib and irradiation: a preclinical study on a head and neck cancer orthotopic model. *Br J Cancer* 99(1): 93-99.

Bozec A, Formento P, Lasalle S, et al. (2007). Dual inhibition of EGFR and VEGFR pathways in combination with irradiation: antitumour supra-additive effects on human head and neck cancer xenografts. *Br J Cancer* 97(1): 65-72.

Budach V, Bernier J, Lefebvre J, et al. (2010). Trends in the treatment of locally advanced squamous cell carcinoma of the head and neck (LA SCCHN) in Europe between 2006 and 2009. *Ann Oncol* 21(8):1031p(abstract).

Burtness B, Goldwasser MA, Flood W, Mattar B, Forastiere A. (2005). Phase III randomized trial of cisplatin plus placebo compared with cisplatin plus cetuximab in metastatic/recurrent head and neck cancer: an Eastern Cooperative Oncology Group study. *J Clin Oncol* 23(34):8646-54.

Chung C, Ely K, MacGavran L, et al. (2006). Increased epidermal growth factor receptor gene copy number is associated with poor prognosis in head and neck squamous cell carcinoma. *J Clin Oncol* 24(25): p. 4170-76.

Ciardiello F. Epidermal growth factor receptor inhibitors in cancer treatment. (2005). *Future Oncol* 1(2):221-234.

Cohen EE, Haraf DJ, Kunnavakkam R, et al. (2010). Epidermal growth factor receptor inhibitor gefitinib added to chemoradiotherapy in locally advanced head and neck cancer. *J Clin Oncol* 10;28(20):3336-43.

Cohen EE, Kane MA, List MA, et al. (2005). Phase II trial of gefitinib 250 mg daily in patients with recurrent and/or metastatic squamous cell carcinoma of the head and neck. *Clin Cancer Res* 11(23):8418-24.

Cohen EE, Rosen F, Stadler WM, et al. (2003). Phase II Trial of ZD1839 in recurrent or metastatic squamous cell carcinoma of the head and neck. *J Clin Oncol* 21(10):1980-7.

Cooper JS, Pajak TF, Forastiere AA, et al. (2004). Postoperative concurrent radiotherapy and chemotherapy for high risk squamous-cell carcinoma of the head and neck. *N Engl J Med* 350(19): 1937-44.

Crombet T, Osorio M, Cruz T, et al. (2004). Use of the humanized anti-epidermal growth factor receptor monoclonal antibody h-R3 in combination with radiotherapy in the treatment of locally advanced head and neck cancer patients. *J Clin Oncol*. 22(9):1646-54.

Denhart BC, Guidi AJ, Tognazzi K, Dvorak HF, Brown LF. (1997). Vascular permeability factor/vascular endothelial growth factor and its receptors in oral and laryngeal squamous cell carcinoma and dysplasia. *Lab Invest*. 77(6):659-64.

Fan Z, Baselga J, Masui H, Mendelsohn J. (1993). Antitumor effect of anti-epidermal growth factor receptor monoclonal antibodies plus cis-diamminedichloroplatnium on well established A431 cell xenografts. *Cancer Res*. 53(19):4637-42.

Ferris R, Feinstein T, Grandis J, et al. (2009). Serum biomarkers as predictors of clinical outcome after cetuximab-based therapy in patients with locally advanced squamous cell carcinoma of the head and neck (SCCHN). *J Clin Oncol* 27:15s (suppl; abstr 6035)

Ferris R, Kotsakis AP, Heron DE, et al. (2010). A phase II trial of postoperative radiotherapy (RT), cisplatin and panitumumab in patients with high-risk, resected locally advanced squamous cell carcinoma of the head and neck (SCCHN). *J Clin Oncol* 28(15S):TPS262.

Forastiere A, Maor M, Weber RS, et al. (2006). Long-term results of intergroup RTOG 91-11: a phase III trial to preserve the larynx-induction cisplatin/5-FU and radiation therapy versus concurrent cisplatin and radiation therapy versus radiation therapy. *J Clin Oncol* 24:185 (abstract 5517).

Fountzilas G, Kalogera-Fountzila A, Lambaki S, et al. (2009). MMP9 but not EGFR, MET, ERCC1, P16, and P-53 is associated with response to concomitant radiotherapy, cetuximab, and weekly cisplatin in patients with locally advanced head and neck cancer. *J Oncol.* 2009:305908. Epub 2009 Dec 29.

Grandis J, Melhem M, Gooding W, et al. (1998). Levels of TGF-a and EGFR protein in head and neck squamous cell carcinoma and patient survival. *J Natl Cancer Inst*; 90(11):824-832.

Gregoire G, Hamoir M, Chen C, et al. (2011). Gefitinib plus cisplatin and radiotherapy in previously untreated head and neck squamous cell carcinoma: A phase II, randomized, double-blind, placebo-controlled study. *Radiother Oncol* 100(1): 62-69.

Gorski D, Beckett MA, Jaskowiak NT, et al. (1999). Blockage of the vascular endothelial growth factor stress response increases the antitumor effects of ionizing radiation. *Cancer Res* 59(14):3374-78.

Gupta M., Madholia V, Gupta N, et al. (2010). Results from a pilot study of nimotuzumab with concurrent chemoradiation in patients with locally advanced squamous cell carcinoma of head and neck. *J Clin Oncol* 28:15s (suppl; abstr 5565)

Hainsworth J, Spigel DA, Burris HA, et al. (2009). Neoadjuvant chemotherapy/gefitinib followed by concurrent chemotherapy/radiation therapy/gefitinib for patients with locally advanced squamous carcinoma of the head and neck. *Cancer.* 115(10):2138-46.

Harrington KJ, El-Hariry IA, Holford CS, et al. (2009). Phase I study of lapatinib in combination with chemoradiation in patients with locally advanced squamous cell carcinoma of the head and neck. *J Clin Oncol* 27(7): 1100-07.

Harrington KJ, Berrier A, Robinson M, et al. (2010). Phase II study of oral lapatinib, a dual-tyrosine kinase inhibitor, combined with chemoradiotherapy (CRT) in patients (pts) with locally advanced, unresected squamous cell carcinoma of the head and neck (SCCHN). *J Clin Oncol* 28:15s, 2010 (suppl; abstr 5505).

Hayes D, Raez LE, Sharma AK, et al. (2010). Multicenter randomized phase II trial of combined radiotherapy and cisplatin with or without erlotinib in patients with locally advanced squamous cell carcinoma of the head and neck (SCCHN): Preliminary toxicity results. *J Clin Oncol* 28:15s (suppl; abstr 5580)

Herbst RS, Arquette M, Shin DM et al. (2005). Phase II multicenter study of the epidermal growth factor response antibody cetuximab and cisplatin for recurrent and refractory squamous cell carcinoma of the head and neck. *J Clin Oncol.* 23(24):5578-87.

Hirata A, Ogawa S, Kometani T, et al. (2002). ZD1839 (Iressa) induces antiangiogenic effects through inhibition of epidermal growth factor receptor tyrosine kinase. *Cancer Res* 62(9):2554-2560

Herchenhorn D, Dias FL, Pineda RM, et al. (2007). Phase II study of erlotinib combined with cisplatin and radiotherapy for locally advanced squamous cell carcinoma of the head and neck (SCCHN) [ASCO Annual Meeting, abstr 6033]. *J Clin Oncol.* 25-18S.

Herchenhorn D, Dias FL, Viegas CM, et al., (2010). Phase I/II study of erlotinib combined with cisplatin and radiotherapy in patients with locally advanced squamous cell carcinoma of the head and neck. *Int J Radiat Oncol Biol Phys* 78(3):696-702. Epub 2010 Apr 24.

Huang S and Harari PM. (2000). Modulation of radiation response after epidermal growth factor receptor blockade in squamous cell carcinomas: inhibition of damage repair, cell cycle kinetics, and tumor angiogenesis. *Clin Cancer Res* 6(6):2166-74.

Inoue K, Ozeki Y, Suganuma T, Sugiura Y, Tanaka S. (1997). Vascular endothelial growth factor expression in primary esophageal squamous cell carcinoma. Association with angiogenesis and tumor progression. *Cancer* 79(2):206-13.

Kao J, Genden EM, Gupta V, et al. (2011). Phase 2 trial of concurrent 5-fluorouracil, hydroxyurea, cetuximab, and hyperfractionated intensity-modulated radiation therapy for locally advanced head and neck cancer. *Cancer* 117(2):318-26.

Kies MS, Holsinger FC, Lee JJ, et al. (2010). Induction chemotherapy and cetuximab for locally advanced squamous cell carcinoma of the head and neck: results from a phase II prospective trial. *J Clin Oncol* 28(1):8-14. Epub 2009 Nov 16.

Kies M, Harris J, Rotman MZ, et al. (2009). Phase II randomized trial of postoperative chemoradiation plus cetuximab for high-risk squamous cell carcinoma of the Head and Neck (RTOG 0234). *Int J Rad Oncol Biol Phys* 75(3s):abstract 29.

Kies MS, Ghebremichael M, Katz TL, Herbst RS, Youssoufian H, Burtness B. (2007). EGFR expression by immunohistochemistry (IHC) and response to chemotherapy and cetuximab in squamous cell carcinoma of the head and neck (SCCHN). *J Clin Oncol* 25(18S):6024 (abstract).

Kirby AM, A'Hern RP, D'Ambrosio C, et al. (2006). Gefitinib (ZD1839, Iressa) as palliative treatment in recurrent or metastatic head and neck cancer. *Br J Cancer*. 94(5):631-6.

Kotsakis A, Heron DE, Kubicek GJ, et al. (2010). Phase II randomized trial of radiotherapy (RT), cetuximab (E) and pemetrexed (Pem) with or without bevacizumab (B) in locally advanced squamous cell carcinoma of the head and neck (SCCHN). *J Clin Oncol* 28:15s (suppl; abstr TPS264).

Koukourakis MI, Tsoutsou PG, Karpouzis A, et al. (2010). Radiochemotherapy with cetuximab, cisplatin, and amifostine for locally advanced head and neck cancer: a feasibility study. *Int J Radiat Oncol Biol Phys* 77(1):9-15.

Koutcher L, Sherman E, Fury M, et al. (2011). Concurrent cisplatin and radiation versus cetuximab and radiation for locally advanced head and neck cancer. *Int J Radiat Oncol Biol Phys*. 81(4):915-22.

Kruser TJ, Armstrong EA, Ghia AJ, et al. (2008). Augmentation of radiation response by panitumumab in models of upper aerodigestive tract cancer. *Int J Radiat Oncol Biol Phys* 72(2):534-42.

Kyzas PA, Cunha IW and Ionnidis JP. (2005). Prognostic significance of vascular endothelial growth factor immunohistochemical expression in head and neck squamous cell carcinoma: a meta-analysis. *Clin Cancer Res* 11(4):1434-40.

Langer C, Lee JW, Patel UA, et al. (2008). Preliminary analysis of ECOG 3303: Concurrent radiation (RT), cisplatin (DDP) and cetuximab (C) in unresectable, locally advanced (LA) squamous cell carcinoma of the head and neck (SCCHN). *J Clin Oncol* 26: (May 20 suppl; abstr 6006)

Lee NY, Zhang QE, Garden AS, et al. (2011). Phase II study of chemoradiation plus bevacizumab (BV) for locally/regionally advanced nasopharyngeal carcinoma (NPC): Preliminary clinical results of RTOG 0615. *J Clin Oncol* 29: (suppl; abstr 5516)

Lefebvre J, Ponitreau Y, Roland F, et al. (2011). Sequential chemoradiotherapy (SCRT) for larynx preservation (LP): Results of the randomized phase II TREMPLIN study. *J Clin Oncol* 29: (suppl; abstr 5501)

Liang K, Ang KK, Milas L, et al. (2003). The epidermal growth factor receptor mediates radioresistance. *Int J Radiat Oncol Biol Phys* 57(1):246-54.

Licitra L, Roland F, Bokemeyer C, et al. (2009). Biomarker potential of EGFR gene copy number by FISH in the phase III EXTREME study: Platinum-based CT plus cetuximab in first-line R/M SCCHN. *J Clin Oncol* 27:15s (suppl; abstr 6005)

Lopez-Albaitero A, Ferris RL. (2007). Immune activation by epidermal growth factor receptor specific monoclonal antibody therapy for head and neck cancer. *Arch Otolaryngol Head Neck Surg* 133(12):1277-81.

Meluch A, Spigel D, Burris HA, et al. (2009). Combined modality therapy with radiation therapy (RT), chemotherapy, bevacizumab, and erlotinib in the treatment of patients (pts) with locally advanced squamous carcinoma of the head and neck. *J Clin Oncol* 27:15s (suppl; abstr 6012)

Mendelsohn J and Baselga J. (2003). Status of epidermal growth factor receptor antagonists in the biology and treatment of cancer. *J Clin Oncol* 21(14):2787-99.

Mercke C, Sjodin H, Haugen H, et al. (2011). Survival, tumor control, and toxicity with TPF before accelerated radiotherapy potentiated with cetuximab for stage III-IV unresectable head and neck cancer: A phase II study. *J Clin Oncol* 29: (suppl; abstr 5552)

Merlano M, Russi E, Benasso M, et al. (2011). Cisplatin-based chemoradiation plus cetuximab in locally advanced head and neck cancer: a phase II clinical study. *Ann Oncol* 22:712-17.

Mesia R, Rueda A, Vera A, et al. (2010). Is there a role for adjuvant cetuximab after radiotherapy (RT) plus cetuximab in patients (pts) with locally advanced squamous cell carcinoma of the oropharynx? A phase II randomized trial. *J Clin Oncol* 28:15s (suppl; abstr 5534)

Mesia R, Vazquez S, Grau JJ, et al. (2009). A single-arm phase II trial to evaluate the combination of cetuximab plus docetaxel, cisplatin, and 5-fluorouracil (TPF) as induction chemotherapy (IC) in patients (pts) with unresectable SCCHN [ASCO Annual Meeting, abst 6015]. *J Clin Oncol* 27:15s.

Milas L, Fan Z, Andratschke NH, Ang KK. (2004). Epidermal growth factor receptor and tumor response to radiation: in vivo preclinical studies. *Int J Radiat Oncol Biol Phys* 58(3): p. 966-971.

Montemurro F, Valabrega G, Aglietta M. (2007). Lapatinib: a dual inhibitor of EGFR and HER2 tyrosine kinase activity. *Expert Opin Ther Pat* 7(2):257-68.

Moriyama M, Kumagai S, Kawashiri S, Kojima K, Kakihara K, Yamamoto E. (1997). Immunohistochemical study of tumour angiogenesis in oral squamous cell carcinoma. *Oral Oncol* 33(5):369-74.

Olsson AK, Dimberg A, Kreuger J, Claesson-Welsh L. (2006). VEGF receptor signaling - in control of vascular function. *Nat Rev Mol Cell Biol.* 7(5):359-71.

Petruzzelli GJ, BenefieldJ, Taitz AD, et al. (1997). Heparin-binding growth factor(s) derived from head and neck squamous cell carcinomas induce endothelial cell proliferations. *Head Neck.* 19(7):576-82.

Pfister D, Su YB, Kraus DH, et al. (2006). Concurrent cetuximab, cisplatin, and concomitant boost radiotherapy for locoregionally advanced, squamous cell head and neck cancer: a pilot phase II study of a new combed modality paradigm *J Clin Oncol* 24(7):1072-78.

Pfister D, Lee NY, Sherman E, et al. (2009). Phase II study of bevacizumab (B) plus cisplatin (C) plus intensity-modulated radiation therapy (IMRT) for locoregionally advanced head and neck squamous cell cancer (HNSCC): Preliminary results. *J Clin Oncol* 27:(15s) (suppl; abstr 6013)

Pignon J, le Maitre A, Maillard E, Bourhis J. (2009). MACH-NC Collaborative Group. Meta-analysis of chemotherapy in head and neck cancer (MACH-NC): an update on 93 randomized trials and 17, 346 patients. *Radiother Oncol* 92(1):4-14.

Pignon JP, le Maître A, Bourhis J. (2007). MACH-NC Collaborative Group. Meta-Analyses of chemotherapy in Head and Neck Cancer (MACH-NC): an update. *Int J Radiat Oncol Biol Phys* 69(2 Suppl):S112-4.

Psyrri A, Ghebremicahel MS, Pectasides E, et al. (2011). P16 protein status and response to treatment in a prospective clinical trial (ECOG 2303) of patients with head and neck squamous cell carcinoma (HNSCC). *J Clin Oncol* 29: (suppl;abstr e 16032).

Ready NE, Rathore R, Johnson TT, et al. (2011). Weekly Paclitaxel and Carboplatin Induction Chemotherapy Followed by Concurrent Chemoradiotherapy in Locally Advanced Squamous Cell Carcinoma of the Head and Neck. *Am J Clin Oncol* [Epub ahead of print].

Rodriguez MO, Rivero TC, del Castillo Bahi R, et al. (2010). Nimotuzumab plus radiotherapy for unresectable squamous-cell carcinoma of the head and neck. *Cancer Biol Ther.* 9(5):343-9. Epub 2010 Mar 20.

Rodriguez CP, Adelstein DJ, Saxton JP, et al. (2009). Multiagent concurrent chemoradiotherapy (MACCRT) and gefitinib in locoregionally advanced head and neck squamous cell cancer (HNSCC) [ASCO Annual Meeting, abstr 6037]. *J Clin Oncol* 27:15s.

Rojo F, Gracias E, Villena N, et al. (2010). Pharmacodynamic trial of nimotuzumab in unresectable squamous cell carcinoma of the head and neck: a SENDO Foundation study. *Clin Cancer Res* 16:2474-82. Epub 2010 Apr 6.

Rojo F, Gracias E, Villena N, et al. (2008). Pharmacodynamic study of nimotuzumab, an anti-epidermal growth factor receptor (EGFR) monoclonal antibody (MAb), in patients with unresectable squamous cell carcinoma of the head and neck (SCCHN): A SENDO Foundation study. *J Clin Oncol* 26: 2008 (May 20 suppl; abstr 6070).

Rueda A, Median JA, Mesia R, et al. (2007). Gefitinib plus concomitant boost accelerated radiation (AFX-CB) and concurrent weekly cisplatin for locally advanced unresectable squamous cell head and neck carcinomas (SCCHN): A phase II study. *J Clin Oncol* 25(185):6031(abstr).

Salama JK, Haraf DJ, Stenson KM, et al. (2011). A randomized phase II study of 5-fluorouracil, hydroxyurea, and twice-daily radiotherapy compared with bevacizumab plus 5-fluorouracil, hydroxyurea, and twice-daily radiotherapy for intermediate-stage and T4N0-1 head and neck cancers. *Ann Oncol* 22(10):2304-9. Epub 2011 Feb 17.

Savvides P, Agarala SS, Greskovich J, et al. (2006) Phase I study of EGFR tyrosimne kinase inhibitor erlotinib in combination with docetaxel and radiation in locally advanced squamous cell cancer of the head and neck (SCCHN). J Clin Oncol 24: (suppl; abstr 5545)

Savvides P, Greskowich J, Bokar JA, et al. (2008). Phase II study of bevacizumab in combination with docetaxel and radiation in locally advanced head and neck squamous cell cancer. *J Clin Oncol* 26: (suppl; abstr 6071).

Seiwert T, Haraf DJ, Cohen EE, et al. (2011). A randomized phase II trial of cetuximab-based induction chemotherapy followed by concurrent cetuximab, 5-FU, hydroxyurea, and hyperfractionated radiation (CetuxFHX) or cetuximab, cisplatin, and accelerated radiation with concomitant boost (CetuxPX) in patients with locoregionally advanced head and neck cancer (HNC). *J Clin Oncol* 29: (suppl; abstr 5519).

Seiwert TY, Cohen EE. (2008). Targeting angiogenesis in head and neck cancer. *Semin Oncol.* 35(3):274-85.

Seiwert TY, Haraf DJ, Cohen EE, et al. (2008). Phase I study of bevacizumab added to fluorouracil- and hydroxyurea-based concomitant chemoradiotherapy for poor-prognosis head and neck cancer. *J Clin Oncol.* 26(10):1732-41.

Shirai K, O'Brien PE. (2007). Molecular targets in squamous cell carcinoma of the head and neck. *Curr Treat Options Oncol* 8(3):239-51.

Soulieres D, Senzer NN, Vokes EE, Hidalgo M, Agarawala SS, Siu LL. (2004). Multicenter phase II study of erlotinib, an oral epidermal growth factor receptor tyrosine kinase inhibitor, in patients with recurrent or metastatic squamous cell cancer of the head and neck. *J Clin Oncol* 22(1):77-85

Steeghs N, Nortier JW, Gelderblom H. (2007). Small molecule tyrosine kinase inhibitors in the treatment of solid tumors: an update of recent developments *Ann Surg Oncol* 14(2):942-53.

Stewart JS, Cohen EE, Licitra L, et al. (2009). Phase III study of gefitinib compared with intravenous methotrexate for recurrent squamous cell carcinoma of the head and neck [corrected]. *J Clin Oncol* 27(11):1864-71.

Suntharalingham M, Kwok Y, Golubeva O, et al. (2011). Phase II study evaluating the addition of cetuximab to the concurrent delivery of weekly carboplatin, paclitaxel, and daily radiotherapy for patients with locally advanced squamous cell carcinomas of the head and neck. *Int J Radiat Oncol Biol Phys* 1-6 (e-pub).

Tan EH, Goh C, Lim WT, et al. (2011). Gefitinib, cisplatin, and concurrent radiotherapy for locally advanced head and neck cancer: EGFR FISH, protein expression, and mutational status are not predictive biomarkers. *Ann Oncol* [Epub ahead of print]

Vermorken JB, Mesia R, Rivera F, et al. (2008). Platinum-based chemotherapy plus cetuximab in head and neck cancer. *N Engl J Med* 359(11):1116-27.

Wachsberger P, Burd R, Dicker AP. (2003). Tumor response to ionizing radiation combined with antiangiogenesis or vascular targeting agents: exploring mechanisms of interaction. *Clin Cancer Res* 9(6):1957-71.

Wanebo HJ, Ghebremichael MS, Burtness B, et al. (2010). Phase II induction cetuximab (C225), paclitaxel (P), and carboplatin (C) followed by chemoradiation with C224, P, C, and RT 68-72Gy for stage III/IV head and neck squamous cancer: Primary site organ preservation and disease control at 2 years (ECOG, E2303). *J Clin Oncol* 28: 15s (suppl; abstr 5513)

Wirth, L., Posner MR, Tishler RB, et al. (2007). Phase I study of panitumumab, chemotherapy and intensity-modulated radiotherapy (IMRT) for head and neck cancer (HNC): Early results. *J Clin Oncol* 25(18S):6083.

Wirth LJ, Posner MR, Tishler RB, et al. (2008). Phase I study of panitumumab + chemoradiotherapy (CRT) for head and neck cancer (HNC). *J Clin Oncol* 26: 2008 (May 20 suppl; abstr 6007).

Part 4

Post-Treatment Considerations

10

DNA Repair Capacity and the Risk of Head and Neck Cancer

Marcin Szaumkessel[1], Wojciech Gawęcki[2] and Krzysztof Szyfter[1,2]
[1]*Institute of Human Genetics, Polish Academy of Sciences, Poznań*
[2]*Dept. of Otolaryngology and Laryngological Oncology, K. Marcinkowski University of Medical Sciences, Poznań, Poland*

1. Introduction

According to the chemical carcinogenesis hypothesis (Husgafvel-Pursiainen, 2004) (Loeb & Harris, 2008) chemical carcinogens exert their activity by penetrating cells, cell nuclei and interact with DNA generating DNA lesions such as single- or double-strand DNA breaks and DNA base modifications (adduction, substitution, base oxidation). DNA lesions when not removed are fixed as DNA mutations. Mutations as alterations of DNA structure are responsible for a change of the genetic information and the same remain the key step in carcinogenic transformation of cells. The whole process of carcinogens metabolism in a cell proceeds under enzymatic control (Fig.1). The first step known as metabolic activation provides changes in carcinogen molecule into better solubility and higher reactivity with detoxifying enzymes. Only few chemical carcinogens can omit this step and react directly with the enzymes. The second step being a detoxification proper consists of enzymatic conjugation of activated carcinogens and removal carcinogen metabolites out of a cell. This step is highly efficient and usually over 90% of exogenous compounds are being removed. At this stage the activated carcinogens are capable to react with DNA but still detoxification remains the main pathway when a reactivity towards DNA is less likely. Generation of DNA lesions is automatically followed by DNA repair.

The process of DNA repair is recognized as the last line of a cell defense against mutagens/carcinogens. DNA repair is carried into effect on separate pathways adjusted to a type and extent of DNA damage, and the cell cycle (Jenkins et al., 2010). A most commonly accepted categorization of DNA repair mechanisms is shown in Table 1. To comment a multitude of DNA repair mechanisms, a direct repair, DNA excision repair and recombination repair are specialized in dealing with various types of DNA lesions at first instance. Mismatch DNA repair pathway works later to remove DNA lesions remaining after processing by the above mentioned mechanisms or emerge late in the cell cycle. Recombination repair is involved both in DNA and chromosome repair. SOS-repair acts only when DNA lesions occur abundantly.

There are roughly 4000 chemical compounds occurring in tobacco smoke. Carcinogenic properties were attributed up to 60 constituents carcinogenic properties. The main carcinogens of tobacco smoke are: polycyclic aromatic compounds (with benzo/a/pyrene as the best known example), aromatic amines, N-nitrosamines and reactive oxygen species (Talhout et al., 2011). The molecular aspects of carcinogenesis generated by tobacco smoke is relatively well recognized (Hecht, 2003; Husgafvel-Pursiainen, 2004). Lesions generated by tobacco smoke carcinogens include single-strand DNA breaks, adducts carcinogen:DNA and oxidative DNA damage. Any preference to a specific DNA sequence was not established. Anyway, guanosine residue was found to be the most sensitive DNA element for carcinogen attack. Regardless a lack of sequence specificity an attention was focused on lesions generated in cancer-related genes. *TP53* lesions and mutation were studied most efficiently. A direct relation between benzo/a/pyrene:guanosine adducts formation generating later on G:C to T:A mutations was proven in the case of *TP53* (Denissenko, 1996). Further, studying cancer-related genes a pattern of mutations derived from tobacco smoke exposure was identified in *TP53* and other genes (Le Calvez et al., 2005).

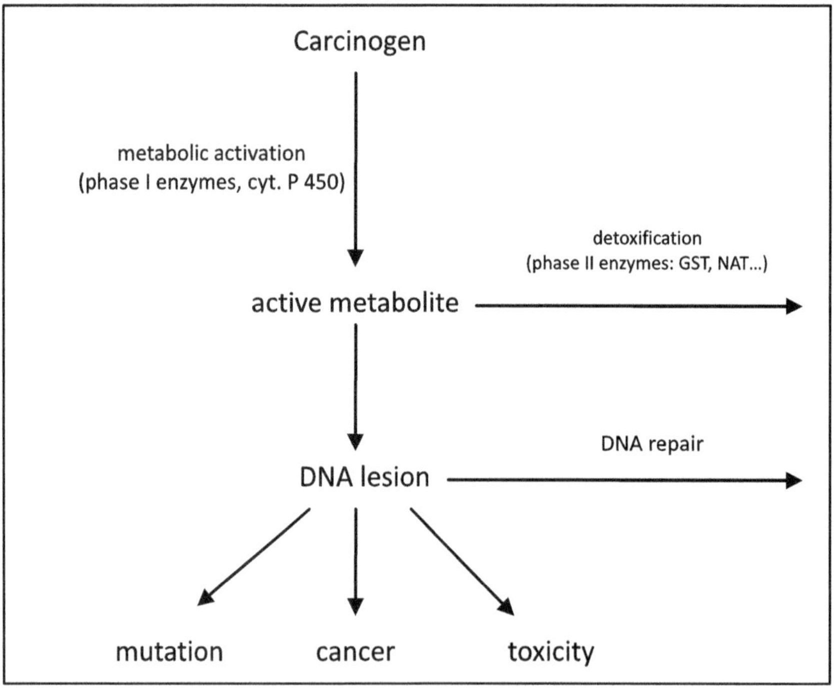

Fig. 1. Carcinogen metabolic pathways and health effects.

An epidemiological evidence for a causative contribution of tobacco smoking to cancer of lung or larynx as well as an increased risk to develop many types of cancers among tobacco smokers has been provided long ago (Vineis et al., 2004). A strong association between tobacco smoking and cancer risk leads to an opinion on predominance of exogenous factors over genetic background (Le Marchand, 2005). On the other hand, only a minority of smokers develop any type of cancer. Hence, it was deduced that a combination of exogenous exposure and individual predisposition is responsible for carcinogenic transformation (Taioli, 2008). An extensive review of cancer genes divided into contributing

Type	Subtype	Comment
Direct repair		restricted to a few lesions
Excision repair	Base excision repair (BER)	removes majority of lesions
	Nucleotide excision repair (NER)	as above
Recombination repair	Homologous end joining	repair of DNA and chromosomes
	Non-homologous end joining	as above
Mismatch repair		specialized in removal mispairing of DNA bases
	Transcription-coupled repair	preference for actively transcribed genes, fast
	Global repair	slow repair of overall genome
SOS repair		mutation-prone system
FA	Homologous recombination	ICL removal

Table 1. Classification of DNA repair pathways.

to cancer risk and connected with cancer progression was written by Vogelstein and Kinzler (2004). An impact of genetic factor on health effects of tobacco smoking was also discussed more specifically in relation to head and neck cancer (Badawy et al., 2008; Rossing, 1998). As such specific genes as *BRCA1* or *APC* involved in breast and colon cancer, respectively, were not discovered in head and neck cancer, an attention was paid on so-called "low-penetration" genes, mainly those involved in carcinogens processing. Within the group of low-penetration genes a potential significance of DNA repair genes was admitted (Livneh et al., 2005). The latter author points at the key function of DNA repair that is removal or by-pass the damaged sites to restore the original structure and function.

2. Genotype versus phenotype

A comparison of tumor cells with normal cells has shown that the level of damage is higher in neoplastic cells. An observation was applicable to various types of damage including single-strand DNA breaks, carcinogen:DNA adducts, DNA mutations, chromosome aberrations and others. Next, an observation was extended also on other cells including peripheral blood lymphocytes derived from cancer subjects compared to those from healthy individuals. The latter observation has got a substantial significance as blood lymphocytes are commonly used as a surrogate material for biological analysis obtainable on non-invasive way (Phillips, 2005). However, the early results concerning a high level of DNA lesions and chromosome aberrations in cancer subjects posed a fundamental question concerning a role of former exposure to carcinogens confronted with an impaired DNA repair. Although some papers ignored an impact of DNA repair, their authors brought into light a differentiation between active and passive smoking as a source of carcinogens (Phillips, 2002), location of an organ exposed (Hainaut, Olivier, & Pfeifer, 2001) or exposure threshold (Jenkins et al., 2010).

On the other hand an early paper from M.R. Spitz group (Wei, Cheng, Hong, & Spitz, 1996) dealed with DNA repair in lung cancer subjects. DNA repair capacity was estimated in peripheral blood lymphocytes using host-cell reactivation assay, which measures cellular reactivation of a reporter gene damage to exposure to activated benzo/a/pyrene. The mean level of DNA repair was significantly lower in subjects than in controls. The final conclusion was that individuals with reduced DNA repair level are at an increased risk to develop lung cancer. Applying the same method the study was repeated on head and neck subjects. A reduced DNA repair capacity was shown when 55 newly diagnosed, untreated head and neck subjects were compared to 61 healthy controls (Cheng et al., 1998).

Following years have provided several papers documenting impairment of DNA repair potential in association with cancer. Alternative methods were shown to be useful to study DNA repair impairment. Schmezer et al. (2001) applied comet assay to study bleomycin-induced damage in peripheral blood lymphocytes. Lung cancer blood donors (100 cases) were found more sensitive for such damage in comparison with healthy donors (110). High mutagen sensitivity in cancer subjects was explained as resulted from significantly reduced DNA repair capacity. The paper contains also interesting technical remarks. The authors demonstrated applicability of cryo-preserved lymphocytes to estimate DNA repair up to 12 months after blood collection. A similar experimental attempt was used in our own studies (Gajecka et al., 2005). A higher level of spontaneous and benzo/a/pyrene-induced was shown by comet assay in peripheral blood lymphocytes derived from laryngeal cancer subjects compared with healthy donors (52 cases v. 54 controls). A level of spontaneous DNA damage tended to increase with tumor grading. The latter result was not confirmed by the analogical study (L. E. Wang et al. 2010) done on much bigger group (744 head and neck subjects v. 753 matched cancer-free controls). The conclusion of Wang et al. was that the reduced removal of tobacco smoke-induced DNA adducts contributes to the risk of head and neck cancer but does not influence tumor characteristics. However, our results taken as "phenotype" were apparent. Then, we attempted to explain them by distribution of so-called "risk" and "protection" genotypes of *XPD*, *XRCC1* and *XRCC3* genotypes of DNA repair genes. The distribution differences did not reach the level of statistical significance that means that phenotype-genotype correlation was poor. Still, phenotypic deficit of DNA repair was only partly confirmed by overrepresentation of "risk" genotypes of the studied DNA repair genes. Again, an impairment of DNA repair was shown in head and neck cancer cells taken from tissue biopsies compared to peripheral blood lymphocytes of healthy controls exposed to hydrogen peroxide treated taken as a model genotoxicant (47 cases v. 38 healthy controls). An advanced comet assay permitted for estimation of single-strand DNA breaks, oxidative lesions and efficiency of DNA repair. Besides, a general deficit of DNA repair, the authors established that H_2O_2-induced lesions were repaired less effectively in cancer cells from patients with metastasis than from those without metastasis (Rusin et al., 2009).

The most direct way to understand a link between DNA repair deficit and head and neck cancer are studies on processing of tobacco smoke lesions and their removal (Hecht, 2003; L. E. Wang et al., 2010; Wei et al., 1996). Polycyclic aromatic hydrocarbons are represented by several compounds present in tobacco smoke and generate a variety of carcinogen: DNA adducts. The structural features of the PHA-adducts play a role in differential repair of these adducts. Although PAH:DNA adducts are repaired dominantly by nucleotide excision repair (NER) pathway, differences in repair efficiency still occur for individual DNA adducts removal (Zhong et al., 2010). At this point it is necessary to remind that DNA lesions not removed fast enough are most harmful for a cell.

It was already mentioned that another type of DNA lesions generated by tobacco smoke is oxidative DNA damage. The major mechanism for repair of oxidized DNA bases represented by 8-oxoguanine is base excision repair (BER), but nucleotide excision repair seems to be involved too. It has been shown in lung cancer that the enzymes involved in recognition of oxidative DNA damage alter their activity and, in turn affect tumor growth because of increased formation of apurinic sites in DNA (Radak et al., 2005). The question of alterations of oxidative DNA damage repair which leads to accumulation of oxidative DNA lesions, mutagenesis and cancer development was reviewed recently (D'Errico, Parlanti, & Dogliotti, 2008).

In head and neck cancer one of the most disregulated genes is epidermal growth factor receptor overexpressed in ca. 90% cases. Reiter et al. (2010) undertook a study to explain a reason of EGFR overexpression in terms of sensitivity to mutagens and DNA repair potential. Oropharyngeal cancer cells were exposed to activated benzo/a/pyrene in vitro. Unexpectingly, an extent of damage was comparable in EGFR gene locus and in chromosome centromere, as well as in non-tumor tissue control. Also DNA repair capacity was comparable in all experiments. It looks, nor EGFR gene amplification, neither DNA repair might have a moderate effect on protein over-expression.

3. Evidence from genetic polymorphism

Variation in DNA repair as a factor in cancer susceptibility was associated early with single nucleotide polymorphism (SNP). Many gene variants are common in human population. Some structural variants decreasing a capacity to repair DNA were found more frequently in cancer cases and could be recognized as "risk" variants. The extreme case of DNA repair deficiency was established in a few rare diseases where DNA repair defect was followed by over-frequent tendency to develop cancer (Tab. 2). Gene variants working opposite way would be known as "protective" variants. Such attribution is not having a universal character because of ethnic differences in gene variants distribution (Becker, Nieters, & Rittgen, 2003; Mohrenweiser & Jones, 1998). Though, the mechanisms dominantly involved in their repair of tobacco smoke-induced lesions are: base-excision repair (BER), nucleotide excision repair (NER) followed by recombination repair and mismatch repair, it was assumed that impairment of DNA repair process, particularly in the key pathways would contribute to the increased risk of head and cancer. This assumption is workable within the hypothesis of chemical carcinogenesis but a connection with the hypothesis on cancer stem cells (Sales, Winslet, & Seifalian, 2007) is not excluded. At this point one had to stress that the working material for studies on genetic polymorphisms are blood cells as all the cells of the organism have the same genetic information not changed throughout their ontology.

Establishing a link between single nucleotide polymorphism, distribution of gene variants and cancer risk was followed by publication of plethora of papers. Very early papers deal usually with an involvement of one repair gene/enzyme. The good example is a paper of

Disease	Main genes identified	Cancer preference
Xeroderma pigmentosum	*XPA*, XPC, *XPD*, *XP-*variant	skin
Ataxia telangiestasia	*ATM*	breast, other sites
Cockayne's syndrome	*ERCC6* (*CSB*), *ERCC8*	
Bloom's syndrome	*BLM*	Broad spectrum of cancer predisposition
Fanconi's Anemia	14 FA genes (listed below)	AML, head and neck, breast, gyneaological cancers
Trichothiodystrophy	*XPD*	skin

Table 2. Major diseases associated with DNA repair deficit.

Sturgis et al., (1999) describing an analysis of X-ray cross-complementing group one (*XRCC1*) gene polymorphism in relation to head and neck risk. The *XRCC1* gene participates in base excision repair (BER) by encoding a protein acting in the repair of single-strand DNA breaks. Two different polymorphisms of *XRCC1* were studied in the group of 203 cancer cases v. 425 controls. Distribution of gene variants did not vary considerably between the groups but *XRCC1* 26304T allele was found as a risk factor. The same group (Ho et al., 2007) studied also polymorphism of the same gene as a risk factor of salivary gland carcinomas. Three groups of samples were collected: 138 salivary gland carcinomas, 50 benign gland tumor and 503 cancer-free controls. It was established that *XRCC1* 1915C allele was associated with a lower risk and *XRCC1* 194Trp allele with a higher risk of salivary gland carcinoma. A much broader character had a study of Hao et al. (2004) on gene polymorphism connected with BER mechanism of DNA repair. There have studied 129 SNPs in the eight BER genes including *ERCC1*. An estimation of distribution of gene variants in Chinese cohort (419 esophageal cancer subjects v. 480 healthy controls) pointed at four gene variants including *XRCC1-77C* allele as predictors of an increased risk. Esophageal cancer does not belong formally to head and neck cancer group but anatomical vicinity and histological classification as squamous cell carcinoma allows for a close analogy. Interestingly, analogical on a large cohort of breast cancer (over 20 000 cases v. comparative number of controls) established only a moderate influence of one of three studied polymorphism on breast cancer in Asians and Africans but not in Caucasians (Y. Huang, Li, & Yu, 2009).

Investigation of gene polymorphism in nucleotide excision repair (NER) attracted many research groups. The studies were focused on *XPD* that is an evolutionary conserved ATP-dependent helicase, responsible for unwinding DNA molecule and removal of bulky carcinogen:DNA adducts. Structure-activity relationship of polymorphic gene variants of *XPD* was already established and described with considerations on its impact of cancer risk (Lunn et al., 2000). Previously shown reduced DNA repair capacity in head and neck cancer subjects together with removal of tobacco smoke-derived DNA adducts by *XPD* allowed to expect a key role of this gene in risk modulation. In line with this expectation Sturgis et al. (2000) studied a distribution of two polymorphisms of *XPD* in 189 head and neck subjects and 496 cancer-free controls. All subjects were non-Hispanic whites. A frequency of *XPD 22541A* variant did not differ enough to influence a relative risk. For *XPD* 39531C a moderate increase of risk was established. The latter polymorphism was studied also on Swedish cohort consisting of 185 lung cancer cases v. 162 matched controls. The conclusion of the study was that the XPD variant alleles may by associated with a reduced repair of aromatic DNA adducts and increase lung cancer risk (Hou et al., 2002). The results of Hou et al. were fully confirmed in another study done on Chinese cohort (135 cancer cases v. 152 controls) targeting for esophageal squamous cell carcinoma (Yu et al., 2004). However, a meta-analysis of genetic polymorphism of three genes involved in NER (namely: *ERCC1*, *XPD* and *XPG*) provided some skepticism about their role. The authors concluded that fluctuation of variant frequency and their association with cancer risk will probably be minimal (Kiyohara & Yoshimasu, 2007). As the published results did not meet expectation it attracted to search for other polymorphism not known yet. An example is the paper by Kumar et al. (Kumar, Angelini, & Hemminki, 2003), who discovered a novel intronic mutation in the *XPD* gene.

Hence, further studies were aiming for a parallel coincidence of gene defect, gene-gene and gene-environment interaction. The genes most commonly studied for a joint effect were *XRCC1*, *XRCC3* and *XPD*, representing different DNA repair pathways, namely: BER, NER and recombination repair, respectively. Such attempt was used by Matullo et al. (2003) to estimate effect of three polymorphisms in *XRCC1* exon 10, *XPD* exon 23 and *XRCC3* exon 7. Distribution of gene variants was assessed in 628 Italian healthy individuals and confronted with the level of aromatic DNA adducts in blood lymphocytes. A dose-response relationship between the number of risk variants and DNA adduct level. The interpretation was that the combined effect of multiple variant alleles modulates DNA repair capacity. The same trio of DNA repair genes supplanted by *MGMT* (enzyme coded by *MGMT* is repairing O^6-alkylguanine adducts) was analyzed in 555 head and neck cancer cases v. 792 controls. Ethnic differences were found. *XRCC1* Gln399Gln was associated with decreased risk in whites, but *XPD* 751 and *XRCC3* 241 did not change cancer risk. (W. Y. Huang et al., 2005).

Extension of a list of genes and their polymorphisms was done by De Ruyck et al. (2007) by an analysis (110 lung cancer v. 110 non-cancer controls) of 10 polymorphisms of genes involved in BER (*XRCC1*, *APE1*, *OGG1*, *XPA*, *XPC* and *XPD*). Primary significance was attributed to *APE1* Asp148Glu, and the secondary one to *XRCC1* ArgGln and *XPD* Lys751Gln concerning conversion of tobacco smoking effects into lung cancer. At this point it is necessary to admit the papers claiming no measurable effect of DNA repair genes polymorphism on cancer risk (London et al., 2001).

Because of a lack of convincing results concerning an impact of individual gene variants in cancer risk, recent years there is a tendency to study in parallel experiments a series of genes and multiple polymorphisms. Also a study groups tend to gain high numbers to get a reasonable statistic power. Within it a meta-analysis of previously published results plays an important role. An example of such situation is a paper Michiels et al. (Michiels et al., 2007) who studied polymorphism in 70 genes in lung cancer, head and neck cancer and healthy Caucasian individuals. None of the studied genes BER- or NER-associated genes was found to be associated individually with an influence of head and neck risk. Contrary, a few alleles of the genes attributed to DNA replication, translesion synthesis and transcription appeared to change a genetic risk. An international team anchored at International Agency for Research on Cancer, Lyon, France, presented an analysis of 28

SNPs in 18 DNA repair genes 9 SNPs in 7 cell cycle control genes on 811 cases with the upper aerodigestive tract v. 1083 individuals not related to tobacco and alcohol. In DNA repair genes only two variant alleles of *MGMT* and one allele of *OGG1* were found moderately more frequently in cases, whilst only three alleles including *XPA* variant were associated with a protective effect. The authors discuss a false positive results present in papers based on small study groups an postulate further extension of a number of individual include into study (Hall et al., 2007). Under the same auspices another broad analysis was done in connection with the upper aerodigestive tract (Canova et al., 2009). Studying the material derived from 10 European countries including 1511 cancer cases and 1457 controls the authors analyzed 115 SNPs from 62 genes already known to be associated with cancer. In 22 SNPs of DNA repair genes only three were found statistically significantly reducing the risk. The results are meaningful as that time it was the largest genetic epidemiologic study on the upper aerodigestive tract in Europe. Almost the same time there was published a large analysis of genetic polymorphism in breast cancer (Smith et al.,2010). Distribution of gene variants derived from 18 SNPs was estimated in 336 cases v. 416 controls (all Caucasians). An impact of individual genes only three cases reached a level of significance. The authors suggest (i) to perform combine SNPs analysis (polygenic model) and (ii) to increase the sample size.

Altogether, the hypothesis of a significant impact of polymorphism of DNA repair genes besides many research efforts was not sufficiently proven but it does not eliminate DNA repair from cancer risk estimation. Its moderate effect was shown and a necessity of gene-gene interaction was suggested.

4. Specific types of cancer

To unravel a link between DNA repair and risk of cancer an alternative way of studies explores sub-classification of cancer to eliminate potential differences connected with etiology, histology, progression and other factors.

Rodriguez et al. (2007) restricted their interest to the early oral squamous cell carcinoma on one site, and on *MGMT*, that protects against alkylating mutagens repairing DNA in BER pathway. Working on protein level they observed a loss of MGMT protein expression from leukoplakia to early oral cancer. MGMT expression was declining also undifferentiation, tumor thickness and grading. Hence, MGMT expression relates rather to cancer progression than to risk. It also seems to indicate a poor prognosis. Unfortunately the study was done on a small sample. An involvement of MLH1 gene, being a part of mismatch repair pathway early stage of oral cancer, was studied by Gonzales-Ramirez et al. (2010). It was shown that gene expression is inhibited by promoter methylation that also located an involvement of this gene rather in tumor progression than in risk to develop cancer.

For such a late stage of oncogenesis as entering metastasis, Sarassin and Kauffman (Sarasin & Kauffmann, 2008) put forward hypothesis on association of overexpression of DNA repair genes with metastasis. An assumption is that initial genetic instability need in time some genetic stabilization provided by over-expression specific DNA repair genes to invade and give rise to distant metastasis. To our knowledge the hypothesis has not been verified experimentally.

A risk of death for head and neck cancer is high for patients with second (multiple) primary tumors that encouraged clinical, molecular and genetic studies. Gal et al. (2005) were studying polymorphism of such DNA repair genes as *XRCC1*, *XRCC3*, *XPD* and *MGMT* in 279 subjects with already diagnosed and treated oral cancer who later on develop second primary tumors in upper aerodigestive tract. Polymorphism in *XRCC3* 241Met was found associated with an increased risk of second neoplasm. On the contrary *XRCC1* 399Gln gene was linked to a decreased risk of all-cause mortality in patients with oral cancer. In our studies we analyzed an impact of 11 polymorphisms of genes coding two activating enzymes, four detoxification enzymes and XPD, XRCC1 and XRCC3 DNA repair enzymes in 84 subjects with multiple primary tumors. The results were compared to that in 182 subjects with a single primary tumors and 143 cancer-free individuals. Looking at an impact of a single gene no correlation was found in case of DNA repair genes. The coexistence of some genotypes/alleles associated with higher cancer risk was established as an added factor for multiple primary tumor development. Our data indicate that the same group of low-penetration genes is involved in the development of single and multiple primary head and neck cancer, but their association with multiple primary tumor is significantly stronger (Rydzanicz, et al., 2005). Significance of NER core gene polymorphism was studied in the group of 1376 squamous cell carcinoma head and neck patients. Out of them 110 patients developed second primary tumors. None of seven studied genes had a pronounced effect for a risk to develop second primary tumors, that to some extent confirms our findings. However, the authors suggest that a profile of NER core gene polymorphisms might collectively contribute to the risk.

Nowadays the techniques exploring DNA microarrays technology became available and contribute well to the reviewed matter. An example of application of gene expression profiling of DNA repair genes is the paper of Rentoft et al. (2009) attempting to differentiate a pattern of DNA repair genes involved in development of head and neck cancer in young (<40 years) and elderly subjects. No genes were detected as significantly differentially expressed between young and elderly subjects.

5. Fanconi anemia pathway

Apart from previously described DNA repair systems present in human cells the Fanconi anemia pathway occupies equally important place. Fanconi anemia (FA) represents a specific and relatively rare syndrome, primarily described in 1927 by Guido Fanconi (Fanconi, 1927) (a Swiss pediatrician). He observed in 3 siblings hereditary form of aplastic anemia, panmyelopathy, short stature and hyper-pigmentation, nowadays syndrome known as Fanconi anemia. The FA is genetically and phenotypically highly heterogeneous condition, whereas patients display a wide variety of abnormalities. Some common features attributed to FA are multiple congenital malformations of skeleton and inner organs, radial ray defects, abnormal pigmentation and overall altered growth (Alter & Kupfer, 1993). However, the most important clinical feature are hematological abnormalities: bone marrow failure, aplastic anaemia, myelodysplastic syndrome (MDS), and high proneness to acute myeloid leukemia (AML). Besides AML FA patients also carry high risk of developing squamous cell carcinomas (SCC), especially of head and neck, gynecological and skin tumors (Alter, 1996; Lustig, et al., 1995, Rosenberg, et al., 2003). A considerable part of cancer biology knowledge was described thanks to rare genetic syndromes related with cancer proneness such as Fanconi anemia.

Physiologically, patients with Fanconi anemia demonstrate high susceptibility to cross-linking agents, which result in significantly increased number of DNA damage events (DNA cross-links are most common). As the consequence repair capacity is insufficient to maintain DNA integrity. Consequently, the FA pathway is frequently deregulated or inactivated.

An increased sensitivity of FA patient-derived cells to the lethal effects of numerous cross-linking agents was described already over three decades ago in mid 70s (Ahmed & Setlow, 1978; Fujiwara & Tatsumi, 1975). Cloning and cell fusion experiments have so far shown existence of fourteen FA complementation groups and corresponding genes *(FANCA, B, C, D1(BRCA2), D2, E, F, G, I, J(BACH1/BRIP1), L, M, N (PALB2), O(RAD51C), P (SLX4)* and combined functionally with FA repair pathway (Deakyne et al. 2011; Rego et al.,2009; Stoepker et al., 2011). However, their exact role have not yet been completely elucidated. The FA-associated genes are not clustered, but dispersed throughout the genome. Next to *BRCA2* (*FANCD1*) also *BRCA1* was corroborated to be involved in FA and comprises another FA associated factor (Garcia-Higuera et al., 2001; Zdzienicka & Arwert, 2002). Thus, FA pathway is often called Fanconi/BRCA pathway.

Complementation group A (mutation in *FANCA*) stands for majority of the Fanconi anemia cases (over 66%), C in 5-15% and G in 5-15% in most of the populations. Only some ethnic groups have founder mutation which accounts for most cases of disease (e.g. in Ashkenazi Jews mutation IVS4+4 A→T allele). The prevalence of other complementation groups is rather rare and many mutations are reported in different Fanconi genes with various frequency (Buchwald, 1995; Deakyne et al., 2011; Joenje et al., 1997). The open-access database of Fanconi genes mutations is available in the internet (*http://www.rockefeller.edu/fanconi/mutate*).

The hypothesis over the defect in the repair of damaged DNA is central to the etiology of Fanconi anemia. Moreover, recent studies have shown that FA is also clinically related to other hereditary chromosomal instability syndromes and the proteins mutated in Bloom Syndrome, Nijmegen Breakage Syndrome (NBS), Ataxia Telangiectasia (ATM) and Seckel Syndrome (ATR), which are also implicated and crosslink with FA pathway (Andreassen, D'Andrea, & Taniguchi, 2004; Nakanishi et al., 2002; Taniguchi et al., 2002). Therefore, an emerging body of evidence indicate Fanconi/BRCA DNA repair pathway proteins to operate in multiple DNA damage pathways, whereas FA-associated proteins have alternative roles. Disruption of any of the genes may lead to arrest of the DNA repair processes and accumulation of cancer-proneness events, which finally leads to non-FA associated cancer occurrence. Thus, Fanconi pathway appears to play remarkable role in the DNA repair capacity of a cell.

5.1 FA and head and neck cancer

Numerous clinical data reports, that FA patients demonstrate a high incidence of aggressive forms of squamous cell carcinoma, especially at young age, predominantly in head and neck sites (HNSCC). The estimated risk is increased over 700 times higher compared to non-FA population and rises much above the cumulative risk effect of environmental factors for this cancer. Average age of HNSCC patients is usually above 60 years who drink and smoke, in contrast to group so-called "young adults" of age below 40-45 years and not possessed by habits. Interestingly, FA patients are usually non-smokers and non-drinkers and demonstrate higher risk of HNSCCs with 40% cumulative incidence by the age of 40 years with 2-year survival rate much below 50% (Kutler et al., 2003). Seemingly, FA -associated squamous carcinoma of head and neck do not differ considerably from sporadic HNSCC, except hypersensitivity to crosslinking agents. FA/HNSCC patients are more vulnerable to the exposition of oral squamous mucosa as a first line absorbing carcinogens. Therefore, predominant site of cancer occur in oral cavity, oropharynx and tounge which is a major cause of high mortality in these patients. The repair of ICLs is mainly driven during cell arrest in late S/G2 phase. G2 phase is noticeable prolonged and, thus it rise the risk of viral infections, particularly Epstein–Barr virus (EBV) and oncogenic types of human papilloma virus (HPV). They integrate preferably to damaged sites of DNA. In previous study of FA/HNSCC over 80% have been infected with HPV (none of these showed mutation in *TP53*) in respect to 36% in non-FA HNSCC patients (Kutler et al., 2003). However, other studies could not demonstrate such high differences, but the disproportion was undisputed. Noteworthy is also that younger patients characterize with distinct sexual behavior, with higher preference to oral sex and thus high prediction of being HPV positive (Lustig et al., 1995; Rosenberg, Alter, & Ebell, 2008).

FA/HNSCC patients undergo strictly modified cancer therapy, eliminating ICLs inducers. Hematopoietic stem cell transplant (SCT) is nowadays the only efficient treatment for direct restoration of blood cells production in Fanconi anemia patients. There have been much of difficulties to optimize SCT protocols because of high toxicity of procedure to patients. From the other, side heavy SCT conditioning is frequently a cause of induction of squamous cell carcinomas, particularly head and neck cancers (Alter, 2005; Rosenberg et al., 2005).

It has been also suggested that single unrepaired ICLs in FA patients may be enough to promote the translocation of oncogenes or the deletion of tumour suppressor genes. Moreover, specific and well known oncogenic translocations such as loss of 1q, 3q or 9p and seems to be favored in FA (Sala-Trepat, et al., 1993; Tonnies et al., 2003).

5.2 DNA cross-linkers

As previously mentioned DNA in Fanconi anemia patients undergoes damage mostly by exposition to cross-linkers. Interstrand crosslinks (ICLs) are extremely toxic DNA damage type. Many drugs (mainly alkylating agents) producing interstrand cross-links in cellular DNA have been commonly used in clinical chemotherapy of solid and hematological malignancies. The idea of usage of crosslinkers to treat cancer was born out of horror of the Second World War. The autopsies of victims killed with chemical weapons (e.g. sulphur mustard) have shown selectively attacked blood white cells. The hypothesis has been established that those chemicals could have been useful for the treatment of leukemia (Deans & West, 2011) and further to other cancers. These include the nitrogen mustard class in use until now (e.g. melphalan, cyclophosphamide, chlorambucil etc), natural compounds: (mitomycin C, psoralen, aldehydes, formaldehydes), platinum drugs (cisplatin, carboplatin, oxaliplatin). Some physical agents such as UV light exposure or reactive oxygen species (ROS) are also capable to induce ICLs. Platinums and nitrogen mustard class require two active leaving groups, which are absorbed inside the cell by the sequential displacement of chloride ions by H_2O molecules. This active form predominantly crosslink DNA at *N*7-position of guanosine or adenosine on the opposite strands and forming ICLs. Mitomycin C and psoralens contain planar rings that must be activated by photon-mediated cycloaddition or cycloreduction, and attack DNA bases. The covalent bounds between two strands of DNA produced by cross-linkers leads to inhibition of fundamental processes such as replication and protein biosynthesis, preventing unwind for polymerase access. Clustering both DNA strands significantly reduces ability of DNA repair machinery to operate, and repair of cross-link involve a highly complexed networks. At the higher structural rank this cause high chromosomal instability (Bauer et al., 2008).

Noteworthy, major FA diagnostic method is still based on the cytogenetic analysis of lymphocytes that have been treated with ICL-inducing agents (MMC or DEB cross-linker) where chromosomal breaks are counted. As result, FA cells demonstrate highly increased levels of chromosome aberrations, such as: chromosome breakages and radical forms of chromosomes (Auerbach, 1988; Li et al., 1999).

5.3 DNA repair by FA/BRCA pathway

FA/BRCA pathway is currently conceived as the coordinator of several repair systems, including homologous recombination (HR), nucleotide excision repair (NER) and translesion synthesis (TLS). However, a major pathway for the repair of DNA interstrand cross-links (ICLs) is homologous recombination (also known as homology-directed repair, HDR). Postulated and partially elucidated model of FA processing with ICL repair begins when the replication forks are stalked and lesion recognition replication protein A (RPA) is recruited and responsible for stabilizing and coating of single DNA strands (L. C. Wang, Stone, Hoatlin, & Gautier, 2008). ICL invokes also FANCM with associated proteins (RMI 1 and RMI 2) which leads to the assemble of FA core complex (FANCA,B,C,E,F,G,L, M and N). FANCM also recruits the Bloom's syndrome complex (BTR), and cooperates with RPA protein. This activates checkpoint ataxia telangiectasia kinase ATR and its downstream effector kinase CHK1 and Rad3-related (ATR)-CHK1 signalling cascade. ATR and CHK1 phosphorylate several components of the core complex in order to activate them. UBE2T, the ubiquitin-conjugating enzyme (E2) binds to FANCL, the ubiquitin ligase subunit of the core complex. Activate core complex monoubiquitinate FANCD2 and FANCI (ID complex) a key event in FA pathway. BRCA1 and BRCA2 complex initiates homologous recombination and stabilizes the stalled replication fork. Monoubiquitinated FANCD2 forms DNA damage inducible foci together with core complex and several other downstream FA-associated DNA repair proteins such as: structure-specific nucleases and translesion polymerases, MRN complex (MRE11, NBN, RAD50), BRIP1, PALB2, FANCO and further participate and cooperate in ICL removal (Fig.2). Homologous recombination is performed on the basis of homologous sequence on sister chromatids and the mechanism in itself is similar to crossing-over during meiosis (Deakyne et al., 2011,; Guervilly et al 2008; Machida et al., 2006; Rego et al., 2009; Takata et al., 2009).

5.4 Disruption of FA/BRCA pathway in HNSCC

The DNA damage response pathway controlled by the Fanconi anemia/*BRCA* pathway genes can be disrupted by either genetic or epigenetic events.

Most FA-associated genes have a wide variety of mutations in FA/HNSCC patients and include deletions, frameshifts, stop codons, splice-site mutations and missense mutations.

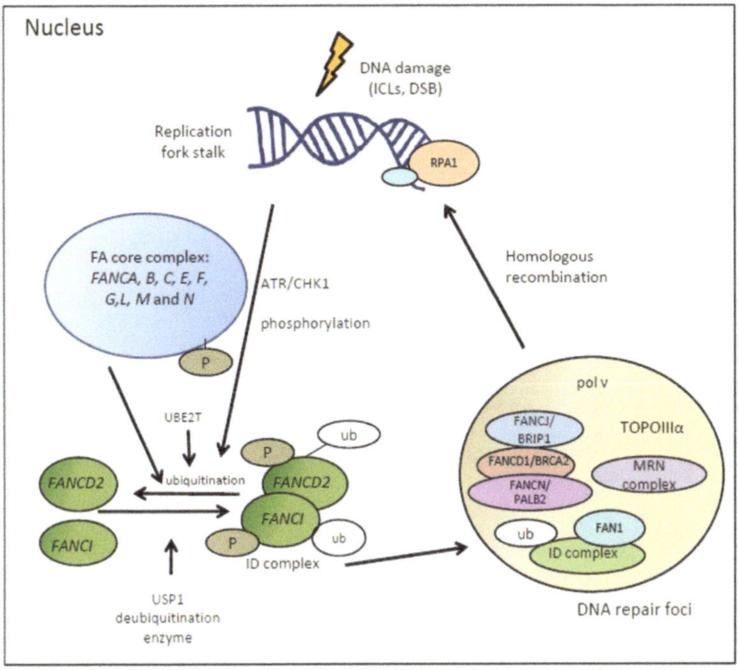

Fig. 2. Exemplary model of FA/BRCA pathway.

At this point of limited evidence, it seems that heterozygosity for any of FA gene mutation except *BRCA2* generates higher susceptibility to cancer, whereas biallelic mutation in single FA genes contribute to earlier cancer development and generally poorer prognosis. However, no specific mutations have been associated with head and neck cancer. Some array-based data (Sparano et al., 2006) demonstrates the copy number alterations (CNA) in regions covering FA genes *BRCA1, BRCA2, FANCD2*, and *FANCG* but no direct associations with the disease were found. In contrast, *FANCA* has been analyzed in arrayCGH-based study (Bauer et al., 2008), where the region 16q23–q24 (*FANCA locus)* showed a significant gain associated with lower survival rates in HNSCC patients.

Epigenetic mechanisms such as DNA methylation, a main posttranscriptional DNA regulation plays a predominant role in majority of developmental processes and regulates expression of most genes. Moreover, it maintains integrity of chromatin through stabilizing its structure. DNA methylation level is usually measured by methyl groups attached to position 5 in pyrimidine ring of cytosines.

Somatic inactivation of the FA pathway by epigenetic silencing has been observed in several different types of sporadic cancer (Lyakhovich & Surralles, 2006), such as bladder cancer (Neveling et al., 2007), ovarian cancer (Lim et al., 2008), breast cancer (Wu, Shin-ya, & Brosh, 2008) cervical cancer (Narayan et al., 2004) and of course in HNSCC (Marsit et al., 2004;

Szaumkessel et al., 2011 ; Wreesmann et al., 2007). Our own study has demonstrated the disruption of DNA methylation of promoter region in *FANCA, BRCA1* and *BRCA2* in squamous laryngeal carcinoma cell lines and primary tumors (Szaumkessel et al., 2011). *BRIP1* and *FANCB* have been shown to be higher and more frequently methylated compared to normal mucosa (Smith et al., 2010). *FANCB* is suggested to play important role in HNSCC pathogenesis as the hypermethylation was detected almost exclusively in cancerous samples. In other study (Wreesmann et al., 2007) *FANCB, FANCF, FANCJ* and *FANCM* were demonstrated to be affected by downregulation in HNSCC, however no methylation changes has been found comparing to non-tumor controls. *FANCF* promotoric DNA hypermethylation was demonstrated to be associated with smoking habit as the established risk factor in HNSCC (Marsit et al., 2004) but with no further reflection in other studies.

Recent years FA pathway is becoming of high interest because of versatile nature in respect to DNA repair. This would suggest that FA genes might be potentially widely used targets for future therapies of head and neck. Specific mutations or/and known deregulation mechanisms could provide a knowledge in order to design a targeted drugs to enhance existing anti-cancer therapies.

6. Summary

Despite the action upon improving the classical surgery and radio- and chemotherapy, a genetic background plays the supportive role and promise a significant enhancement in prevention and/or head and neck cancer curability. Last years has brought much of understanding in HNSCC biology, whereas many markers have been identified and utilized for genetic testing and therapies. Modern high-resolution techniques (e.g. CGH, aCGH, microarrays) has pointed relatively important DNA hotspots and greatly contributed to overall knowledge. However, the pathogenesis of HNSCC seems to be still elusive and ambiguous. The expectations always rise together with emerging new technologies and promise to develop brand new anti-cancer therapies.

7. References

Abou-Elhamd, K. E., Habib, T. N., Moussa, A. E., & Badawy, B. S. (2008). The role of genetic susceptibility in head and neck squamous cell carcinoma. *Eur Arch Otorhinolaryngol, 265*(2), 217-222.

Ahmed, F. E., & Setlow, R. B. (1978). Excision repair in ataxia telangiectasia, Fanconi's anemia, Cockayne syndrome, and Bloom's syndrome after treatment with ultraviolet radiation and N-acetoxy-2-acetylaminofluorene. *Biochim Biophys Acta, 521*(2), 805-817.

Alter, B. P. (1996). Fanconi's anemia and malignancies. *Am J Hematol, 53*(2), 99-110.

Alter, B. P. (2005). Fanconi's anemia, transplantation, and cancer. *Pediatr Transplant, 9 Suppl 7*, 81-86.

Alter, B. P., & Kupfer, G. (1993). Fanconi Anemia.

Andreassen, P. R., D'Andrea, A. D., & Taniguchi, T. (2004). ATR couples FANCD2 monoubiquitination to the DNA-damage response. *Genes Dev, 18*(16), 1958-1963.

Auerbach, A. D. (1988). A test for Fanconi's anemia. *Blood, 72*(1), 366-367.

Bauer, V. L., Braselmann, H., Henke, M., Mattern, D., Walch, A., Unger, K., et al. (2008). Chromosomal changes characterize head and neck cancer with poor prognosis. *J Mol Med, 86*(12), 1353-1365.

Becker, N., Nieters, A., & Rittgen, W. (2003). Single nucleotide polymorphism--disease relationships: statistical issues for the performance of association studies. *Mutat Res, 525*(1-2), 11-18.

Buchwald, M. (1995). Complementation groups: one or more per gene? *Nat Genet, 11*(3), 228-230.

Canova, C., Hashibe, M., Simonato, L., Nelis, M., Metspalu, A., Lagiou, P., et al. (2009). Genetic associations of 115 polymorphisms with cancers of the upper aerodigestive tract across 10 European countries: the ARCAGE project. *Cancer Res, 69*(7), 2956-2965.

Cheng, L., Eicher, S. A., Guo, Z., Hong, W. K., Spitz, M. R., & Wei, Q. (1998). Reduced DNA repair capacity in head and neck cancer patients. *Cancer Epidemiol Biomarkers Prev, 7*(6), 465-468.

David-Beabes, G. L., Lunn, R. M., & London, S. J. (2001). No association between the XPD (Lys751G1n) polymorphism or the XRCC3 (Thr241Met) polymorphism and lung cancer risk. *Cancer Epidemiol Biomarkers Prev, 10*(8), 911-912.

De Ruyck, K., Szaumkessel, M., De Rudder, I., Dehoorne, A., Vral, A., Claes, K., et al. (2007). Polymorphisms in base-excision repair and nucleotide-excision repair genes in relation to lung cancer risk. *Mutat Res, 631*(2), 101-110.

Deakyne, J. S., & Mazin, A. V. (2011) Fanconi anemia: at the crossroads of DNA repair. *Biochemistry (Mosc), 76*(1), 36-48.

Deans, A. J., & West, S. C. (2011) DNA interstrand crosslink repair and cancer. *Nat Rev Cancer, 11*(7), 467-480.

Denissenko, M. F., Pao, A., Tang, M., & Pfeifer, G. P. (1996). Preferential formation of benzo[a]pyrene adducts at lung cancer mutational hotspots in P53. *Science, 274*(5286), 430-432.

D'Errico, M., Parlanti, E., & Dogliotti, E. (2008). Mechanism of oxidative DNA damage repair and relevance to human pathology. *Mutat Res, 659*(1-2), 4-14.

Fanconi, G. (1927). Familiaere infantile perniziosaartige Anaemie (pernizioeses Blutbild und Konstitution). *Jahrbuch Kinderheild*(117), 257-280.

Fujiwara, Y., & Tatsumi, M. (1975). Repair of mitomycin C damage to DNA in mammalian cells and its impairment in Fanconi's anemia cells. *Biochem Biophys Res Commun, 66*(2), 592-598.

Gajecka, M., Rydzanicz, M., Jaskula-Sztul, R., Wierzbicka, M., Szyfter, W., & Szyfter, K. (2005). Reduced DNA repair capacity in laryngeal cancer subjects. A comparison of phenotypic and genotypic results. *Adv Otorhinolaryngol, 62*, 25-37.

Gal, T. J., Huang, W. Y., Chen, C., Hayes, R. B., & Schwartz, S. M. (2005). DNA repair gene polymorphisms and risk of second primary neoplasms and mortality in oral cancer patients. *Laryngoscope, 115*(12), 2221-2231.

Garcia-Higuera, I., Taniguchi, T., Ganesan, S., Meyn, M. S., Timmers, C., Hejna, J., et al. (2001). Interaction of the Fanconi anemia proteins and BRCA1 in a common pathway. *Mol Cell, 7*(2), 249-262.

Gonzalez-Ramirez, I., Ramirez-Amador, V., Irigoyen-Camacho, M. E., Sanchez-Perez, Y., Anaya-Saavedra, G., Granados-Garcia, M., et al. (2010) hMLH1 promoter methylation is an early event in oral cancer. *Oral Oncol, 47*(1), 22-26.

Guervilly, J. H., Mace-Aime, G., & Rosselli, F. (2008). Loss of CHK1 function impedes DNA damage-induced FANCD2 monoubiquitination but normalizes the abnormal G2 arrest in Fanconi anemia. *Hum Mol Genet, 17*(5), 679-689.

Hainaut, P., Olivier, M., & Pfeifer, G. P. (2001). TP53 mutation spectrum in lung cancers and mutagenic signature of components of tobacco smoke: lessons from the IARC TP53 mutation database. *Mutagenesis, 16*(6), 551-553; author reply 555-556.

Hall, J., Hashibe, M., Boffetta, P., Gaborieau, V., Moullan, N., Chabrier, A., et al. (2007). The association of sequence variants in DNA repair and cell cycle genes with cancers of the upper aerodigestive tract. *Carcinogenesis, 28*(3), 665-671.

Hao, B., Wang, H., Zhou, K., Li, Y., Chen, X., Zhou, G., et al. (2004). Identification of genetic variants in base excision repair pathway and their associations with risk of esophageal squamous cell carcinoma. *Cancer Res, 64*(12), 4378-4384.

Hecht, S. S. (2003). Tobacco carcinogens, their biomarkers and tobacco-induced cancer. *Nat Rev Cancer, 3*(10), 733-744.

Ho, T., Li, G., Lu, J., Zhao, C., Wei, Q., & Sturgis, E. M. (2007). X-ray repair cross-complementing group 1 (XRCC1) single-nucleotide polymorphisms and the risk of salivary gland carcinomas. *Cancer, 110*(2), 318-325.

Hou, S. M., Falt, S., Angelini, S., Yang, K., Nyberg, F., Lambert, B., et al. (2002). The XPD variant alleles are associated with increased aromatic DNA adduct level and lung cancer risk. *Carcinogenesis, 23*(4), 599-603.

Huang, W. Y., Olshan, A. F., Schwartz, S. M., Berndt, S. I., Chen, C., Llaca, V., et al. (2005). Selected genetic polymorphisms in MGMT, XRCC1, XPD, and XRCC3 and risk of head and neck cancer: a pooled analysis. *Cancer Epidemiol Biomarkers Prev, 14*(7), 1747-1753.

Huang, Y., Li, L., & Yu, L. (2009). XRCC1 Arg399Gln, Arg194Trp and Arg280His polymorphisms in breast cancer risk: a meta-analysis. *Mutagenesis, 24*(4), 331-339.

Husgafvel-Pursiainen, K. (2004). Genotoxicity of environmental tobacco smoke: a review. *Mutat Res, 567*(2-3), 427-445.

Jenkins, G. J., Zair, Z., Johnson, G. E., & Doak, S. H. (2010) Genotoxic thresholds, DNA repair, and susceptibility in human populations. *Toxicology, 278*(3), 305-310.

Joenje, H., Oostra, A. B., Wijker, M., di Summa, F. M., van Berkel, C. G., Rooimans, M. A., et al. (1997). Evidence for at least eight Fanconi anemia genes. *Am J Hum Genet, 61*(4), 940-944.

Kiyohara, C., & Yoshimasu, K. (2007). Genetic polymorphisms in the nucleotide excision repair pathway and lung cancer risk: a meta-analysis. *Int J Med Sci, 4*(2), 59-71.

Kumar, R., Angelini, S., & Hemminki, K. (2003). Simultaneous detection of the exon 10 polymorphism and a novel intronic single base insertion polymorphism in the XPD gene using single strand conformation polymorphism. *Mutagenesis, 18*(2), 207-209.

Kutler, D. I., Auerbach, A. D., Satagopan, J., Giampietro, P. F., Batish, S. D., Huvos, A. G., et al. (2003). High incidence of head and neck squamous cell carcinoma in patients with Fanconi anemia. *Arch Otolaryngol Head Neck Surg, 129*(1), 106-112.

Kutler, D. I., Wreesmann, V. B., Goberdhan, A., Ben-Porat, L., Satagopan, J., Ngai, I., et al. (2003). Human papillomavirus DNA and p53 polymorphisms in squamous cell carcinomas from Fanconi anemia patients. *J Natl Cancer Inst, 95*(22), 1718-1721.

Le Calvez, F., Mukeria, A., Hunt, J. D., Kelm, O., Hung, R. J., Taniere, P., et al. (2005). TP53 and KRAS mutation load and types in lung cancers in relation to tobacco smoke: distinct patterns in never, former, and current smokers. *Cancer Res, 65*(12), 5076-5083.

Le Marchand, L. (2005). The predominance of the environment over genes in cancer causation: implications for genetic epidemiology. *Cancer Epidemiol Biomarkers Prev, 14*(5), 1037-1039.

Li, L., Peterson, C. A., Lu, X., Wei, P., & Legerski, R. J. (1999). Interstrand cross-links induce DNA synthesis in damaged and undamaged plasmids in mammalian cell extracts. *Mol Cell Biol, 19*(8), 5619-5630.

Lim, S. L., Smith, P., Syed, N., Coens, C., Wong, H., van der Burg, M., et al. (2008). Promoter hypermethylation of FANCF and outcome in advanced ovarian cancer. *Br J Cancer, 98*(8), 1452-1456.

Loeb, L. A., & Harris, C. C. (2008). Advances in chemical carcinogenesis: a historical review and prospective. *Cancer Res, 68*(17), 6863-6872.

Lopez-Camarillo, C., Lopez-Casamichana, M., Weber, C., Guillen, N., Orozco, E., & Marchat, L. A. (2009). DNA repair mechanisms in eukaryotes: Special focus in Entamoeba histolytica and related protozoan parasites. *Infect Genet Evol, 9*(6), 1051-1056.

Lunn, R. M., Helzlsouer, K. J., Parshad, R., Umbach, D. M., Harris, E. L., Sanford, K. K., et al. (2000). XPD polymorphisms: effects on DNA repair proficiency. *Carcinogenesis, 21*(4), 551-555.

Lustig, J. P., Lugassy, G., Neder, A., & Sigler, E. (1995). Head and neck carcinoma in Fanconi's anaemia--report of a case and review of the literature. *Eur J Cancer B Oral Oncol, 31B*(1), 68-72.

Lyakhovich, A., & Surralles, J. (2006). Disruption of the Fanconi anemia/BRCA pathway in sporadic cancer. *Cancer Lett, 232*(1), 99-106.

Machida, Y. J., Machida, Y., Chen, Y., Gurtan, A. M., Kupfer, G. M., D'Andrea, A. D., et al. (2006). UBE2T is the E2 in the Fanconi anemia pathway and undergoes negative autoregulation. *Mol Cell, 23*(4), 589-596.

Marsit, C. J., Liu, M., Nelson, H. H., Posner, M., Suzuki, M., & Kelsey, K. T. (2004). Inactivation of the Fanconi anemia/BRCA pathway in lung and oral cancers: implications for treatment and survival. *Oncogene, 23*(4), 1000-1004.

Matullo, G., Peluso, M., Polidoro, S., Guarrera, S., Munnia, A., Krogh, V., et al. (2003). Combination of DNA repair gene single nucleotide polymorphisms and increased levels of DNA adducts in a population-based study. *Cancer Epidemiol Biomarkers Prev, 12*(7), 674-677.

Michiels, S., Danoy, P., Dessen, P., Bera, A., Boulet, T., Bouchardy, C., et al. (2007). Polymorphism discovery in 62 DNA repair genes and haplotype associations with risks for lung and head and neck cancers. *Carcinogenesis, 28*(8), 1731-1739.

Mohrenweiser, H. W., & Jones, I. M. (1998). Variation in DNA repair is a factor in cancer susceptibility: a paradigm for the promises and perils of individual and population risk estimation? *Mutat Res, 400*(1-2), 15-24.

Nakanishi, K., Taniguchi, T., Ranganathan, V., New, H. V., Moreau, L. A., Stotsky, M., et al. (2002). Interaction of FANCD2 and NBS1 in the DNA damage response. *Nat Cell Biol, 4*(12), 913-920.

Narayan, G., Arias-Pulido, H., Nandula, S. V., Basso, K., Sugirtharaj, D. D., Vargas, H., et al. (2004). Promoter hypermethylation of FANCF: disruption of Fanconi Anemia-BRCA pathway in cervical cancer. *Cancer Res, 64*(9), 2994-2997.

Neveling, K., Kalb, R., Florl, A. R., Herterich, S., Friedl, R., Hoehn, H., et al. (2007). Disruption of the FA/BRCA pathway in bladder cancer. *Cytogenet Genome Res, 118*(2-4), 166-176.

Paz-Elizur, T., Brenner, D. E., & Livneh, Z. (2005). Interrogating DNA repair in cancer risk assessment. *Cancer Epidemiol Biomarkers Prev, 14*(7), 1585-1587.

Phillips, D. H. (2002). Smoking-related DNA and protein adducts in human tissues. *Carcinogenesis, 23*(12), 1979-2004.

Phillips, DH. (2005). DNA adducts as markers of exposure and risk. *Mutation Research,* 577, 1-2, (Sept 2005), 284-292.

Radak, Z., Goto, S., Nakamoto, H., Udud, K., Papai, Z., & Horvath, I. (2005). Lung cancer in smoking patients inversely alters the activity of hOGG1 and hNTH1. *Cancer Lett, 219*(2), 191-195.

Rego, M. A., Kolling, F. W. t., & Howlett, N. G. (2009). The Fanconi anemia protein interaction network: casting a wide net. *Mutat Res, 668*(1-2), 27-41.

Reiter, M., Welz, C., Baumeister, P., Schwenk-Zieger, S., & Harreus, U. (2010) U. Mutagen sensitivity and DNA repair of the EGFR gene in oropharyngeal cancer. *Oral Oncol, 46*(7), 519-524.

Rentoft, M., Laurell, G., Coates, P. J., Sjostrom, B., & Nylander, K. (2009). Gene expression profiling of archival tongue squamous cell carcinomas provides sub-classification based on DNA repair genes. *Int J Oncol, 35*(6), 1321-1330.

Rodriguez, M. J., Acha, A., Ruesga, M. T., Rodriguez, C., Rivera, J. M., & Aguirre, J. M. (2007). Loss of expression of DNA repair enzyme MGMT in oral leukoplakia and early oral squamous cell carcinoma. A prognostic tool? *Cancer Lett, 245*(1-2), 263-268.

Rosenberg, P. S., Alter, B. P., & Ebell, W. (2008). Cancer risks in Fanconi anemia: findings from the German Fanconi Anemia Registry. *Haematologica, 93*(4), 511-517.

Rosenberg, P. S., Greene, M. H., & Alter, B. P. (2003). Cancer incidence in persons with Fanconi anemia. *Blood, 101*(3), 822-826.

Rosenberg, P. S., Socie, G., Alter, B. P., & Gluckman, E. (2005). Risk of head and neck squamous cell cancer and death in patients with Fanconi anemia who did and did not receive transplants. *Blood, 105*(1), 67-73.

Rossing, M. A. (1998). Genetic influences on smoking: candidate genes. *Environ Health Perspect, 106*(5), 231-238.

Rusin, P., Olszewski, J., Morawiec-Bajda, A., Przybylowska, K., Kaczmarczyk, D., Golinska, A., et al. (2009). Role of impaired DNA repair in genotoxic susceptibility of patients with head and neck cancer. *Cell Biol Toxicol, 25*(5), 489-497.

Rydzanicz, M., Wierzbicka, M., Gajecka, M., Szyfter, W., & Szyfter, K. (2005). The impact of genetic factors on the incidence of multiple primary tumors (MPT) of the head and neck. *Cancer Lett, 224*(2), 263-278.

Sala-Trepat, M., Boyse, J., Richard, P., Papadopoulo, D., & Moustacchi, E. (1993). Frequencies of HPRT- lymphocytes and glycophorin A variants erythrocytes in Fanconi anemia patients, their parents and control donors. *Mutat Res, 289*(1), 115-126.

Sales, K. M., Winslet, M. C., & Seifalian, A. M. (2007). Stem cells and cancer: an overview. *Stem Cell Rev, 3*(4), 249-255.

Sarasin, A., & Kauffmann, A. (2008). Overexpression of DNA repair genes is associated with metastasis: a new hypothesis. *Mutat Res, 659*(1-2), 49-55.

Schmezer, P., Rajaee-Behbahani, N., Risch, A., Thiel, S., Rittgen, W., Drings, P., et al. (2001). Rapid screening assay for mutagen sensitivity and DNA repair capacity in human peripheral blood lymphocytes. *Mutagenesis, 16*(1), 25-30.

Smith, I. M., Mithani, S. K., Mydlarz, W. K., Chang, S. S., & Califano, J. A. (2010) Inactivation of the Tumor Suppressor Genes Causing the Hereditary Syndromes Predisposing to Head and Neck Cancer via Promoter Hypermethylation in Sporadic Head and Neck Cancers. *ORL J Otorhinolaryngol Relat Spec, 72*(1), 44-50.

Sparano, A., Quesnelle, K. M., Kumar, M. S., Wang, Y., Sylvester, A. J., Feldman, M., et al. (2006). Genome-wide profiling of oral squamous cell carcinoma by array-based comparative genomic hybridization. *Laryngoscope, 116*(5), 735-741.

Stoepker, C., Hain, K., Schuster, B., Hilhorst-Hofstee, Y., Rooimans, M. A., Steltenpool, J., et al. (2011) SLX4, a coordinator of structure-specific endonucleases, is mutated in a new Fanconi anemia subtype. *Nat Genet, 43*(2), 138-141.

Sturgis, E. M., Castillo, E. J., Li, L., Zheng, R., Eicher, S. A., Clayman, G. L., et al. (1999). Polymorphisms of DNA repair gene XRCC1 in squamous cell carcinoma of the head and neck. *Carcinogenesis, 20*(11), 2125-2129.

Sturgis, E. M., Zheng, R., Li, L., Castillo, E. J., Eicher, S. A., Chen, M., et al. (2000). XPD/ERCC2 polymorphisms and risk of head and neck cancer: a case-control analysis. *Carcinogenesis, 21*(12), 2219-2223.

Szaumkessel, M., Richter, J., Giefing, M., Jarmuz, M., Kiwerska, K., Tonnies, H., et al. (2011) Pyrosequencing-based DNA methylation profiling of Fanconi anemia/BRCA pathway genes in laryngeal squamous cell carcinoma. *Int J Oncol, 39*(2), 505-514.

Taioli, E. (2008). Gene-environment interaction in tobacco-related cancers. *Carcinogenesis, 29*(8), 1467-1474.

Takata, M., Ishiai, M., & Kitao, H. (2009). The Fanconi anemia pathway: insights from somatic cell genetics using DT40 cell line. *Mutat Res, 668*(1-2), 92-102.

Talhout, R., Schulz, T., Florek, E., van Benthem, J., Wester, P., & Opperhuizen, A. (2011) Hazardous compounds in tobacco smoke. *Int J Environ Res Public Health, 8*(2), 613-628.

Taniguchi, T., Garcia-Higuera, I., Xu, B., Andreassen, P. R., Gregory, R. C., Kim, S. T., et al. (2002). Convergence of the fanconi anemia and ataxia telangiectasia signaling pathways. *Cell, 109*(4), 459-472.

Tonnies, H., Huber, S., Kuhl, J. S., Gerlach, A., Ebell, W., & Neitzel, H. (2003). Clonal chromosomal aberrations in bone marrow cells of Fanconi anemia patients: gains of the chromosomal segment 3q26q29 as an adverse risk factor. *Blood, 101*(10), 3872-3874.

Vineis, P., Alavanja, M., Buffler, P., Fontham, E., Franceschi, S., Gao, Y. T., et al. (2004). Tobacco and cancer: recent epidemiological evidence. *J Natl Cancer Inst, 96*(2), 99-106.

Vogelstein, B., Kinzler, KW. (2004). Cancer genes and the pathways they control. *Nature Medicine*, 10, 8, (August 2004), 789-799.

Wang, L. C., Stone, S., Hoatlin, M. E., & Gautier, J. (2008). Fanconi anemia proteins stabilize replication forks. *DNA Repair (Amst), 7*(12), 1973-1981.

Wang, L. E., Hu, Z., Sturgis, E. M., Spitz, M. R., Strom, S. S., Amos, C. I., et al. (2010) Reduced DNA repair capacity for removing tobacco carcinogen-induced DNA adducts contributes to risk of head and neck cancer but not tumor characteristics. *Clin Cancer Res, 16*(2), 764-774.

Wei, Q., Cheng, L., Hong, W. K., & Spitz, M. R. (1996). Reduced DNA repair capacity in lung cancer patients. *Cancer Res, 56*(18), 4103-4107.

Wreesmann, V. B., Estilo, C., Eisele, D. W., Singh, B., & Wang, S. J. (2007). Downregulation of Fanconi anemia genes in sporadic head and neck squamous cell carcinoma. *ORL J Otorhinolaryngol Relat Spec, 69*(4), 218-225.

Wu, Y., Shin-ya, K., & Brosh, R. M., Jr. (2008). FANCJ helicase defective in Fanconia anemia and breast cancer unwinds G-quadruplex DNA to defend genomic stability. *Mol Cell Biol, 28*(12), 4116-4128.

Yu, H. P., Wang, X. L., Sun, X., Su, Y. H., Wang, Y. J., Lu, B., et al. (2004). Polymorphisms in the DNA repair gene XPD and susceptibility to esophageal squamous cell carcinoma. *Cancer Genet Cytogenet, 154*(1), 10-15.

Zdzienicka, M. Z., & Arwert, F. (2002). Breast cancer and Fanconi anemia: what are the connections? *Trends Mol Med, 8*(10), 458-460.

Zhong, Q., Amin, S., Lazarus, P., & Spratt, T. E. (2010) Differential repair of polycyclic aromatic hydrocarbon DNA adducts from an actively transcribed gene. *DNA Repair (Amst), 9*(9), 1011-1016.

11

Tumour Repopulation During Treatment for Head and Neck Cancer: Clinical Evidence, Mechanisms and Minimizing Strategies

Loredana G. Marcu[1,2,3] and Eric Yeoh[4,5]
[1]*Department of Medical Physics, Royal Adelaide Hospital,*
[2]*School of Chemistry and Physics, University of Adelaide*
[3]*Faculty of Science, University of Oradea*
[4]*Department of Radiation Oncology, Royal Adelaide Hospital,*
[5]*School of Medicine, University of Adelaide*
[1,2,4,5]*Australia*
[3]*Romania*

1. Introduction

The poor clinical results reported when radiotherapy ± chemotherapy for the treatment of squamous cell carcinoma of the head and neck cancer and other sites such as the cervix is protracted has been attributed to accelerated repopulation of the tumour (Withers 1988, Fyles 1992).

Evidence from several pre-clinical studies indicates that the response of normal and cancerous squamous cells to cytotoxic injury regardless of the cause includes a greatly increased mitotic rate.

For example, experimental data have shown that the accelerated repopulation response of squamous epithelia (Dörr 1977) is analogous to the acute response of normal tissue after injury. It is suggested (Trott and Kummermehr 1991) that squamous cell carcinomas retain some of the homeostatic control mechanisms characteristic of their tissue of origin. Similarly, data from this and other studies support the evidence that normal and cancerous squamous epithelia share the same behaviour in response to injury (Trott and Kummermehr 1991, Denham 1996, Trott 1999). Therefore, the mechanisms responsible for normal tissue repopulation may be considered relevant for tumour repopulation.

Cell proliferation studies undertaken by Dörr *et al.* showed that accelerated repopulation of human squamous mucosa begins as early as 1 week after initiation of treatment (Dörr 2002). Histologic analysis of human mucosa from head and neck cancer patients during a course of radiotherapy indicated a considerable decrease in cellular density from approximately 1,000 cells/mm to 500 cells/mm by the end of the first week of treatment. The drop in cellular density radically slowed in subsequent weeks reaching around 400 cells/mm by the end of the treatment. This observation suggests that cell loss is overcome by an accelerated proliferation initiated within the first week of treatment.

Since the effect of both radiotherapy and chemotherapy results in damage to the DNA of malignant cells and eradication of irreparably damaged cells, it is likely that prolongation of treatment results in repopulation of clonogenic/stem cells surviving either treatment. This also provides a plausible explanation for the much better patient outcomes observed in the treatment of head and neck cancer when chemotherapy is given concurrently with radiotherapy than when chemotherapy is given in a neo-adjuvant setting i.e., before radiotherapy (Munro 1995, El-Sayed 1996). Surgery can also trigger repopulation in resectable head and neck tumours from undetected tumour foci inadvertently left behind (Peters 1997).

2. Mechanisms responsible for tumour repopulation

Head and neck cancers respond to the cytotoxic effect of radiation and chemotherapy by increasing the mitotic rate of surviving stem cells in order to regrow the tumour (figure 1).

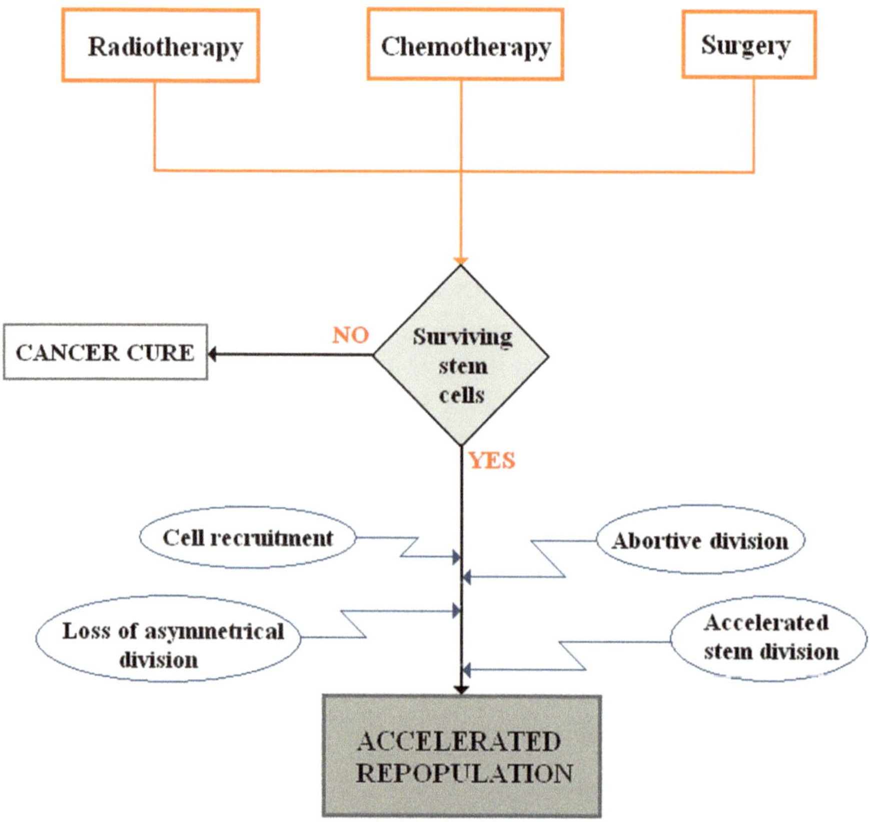

Fig. 1. Schematic diagram of the activation and the mechanisms responsible for accelerated repopulation.

Cell recruitment from the available pool of non-cycling (quiescent) cells is one plausible mechanism of tumour regrowth. In addition, other likely mechanisms, named by Dörr the three A's of repopulation, include acceleration of stem cell division, abortive division and asymmetrical loss in stem cell division. Accelerated stem cell division is a process whereby stem cells shorten the duration of the cell cycle thus resulting in a higher rate of mitosis. Abortive division is associated with loss of the limited number of cell divisions by stem cells destined to die, while asymmetrical loss in stem cell division results in stem cells dividing symmetrically into two stem cells instead of one stem cell and one differentiated cell.

While all of these repopulation processes contribute to accelerated tumour regrowth, the loss of asymmetrical division has been reported to be the most potent mechanism (Marcu 2004).

One of the latest studies looking at the mechanisms behind accelerated tumour repopulation showed that apoptotic tumour cells are the trigger for existing tumour cells to regrow (Huang 2011). The study showed, both *in vitro* and *in vivo,* that dying cells stimulate the re-growth of irradiated tumour cells more efficiently than non-irradiated cells. The mechanism of repopulation was found to be driven by the caspase 3 protease pathway. Head and neck cancer patient studies have confirmed the findings whereby high levels of caspase 3 expression are associated with a higher rate of tumour recurrence.

3. Strategies to overcome tumour repopulation

The first step to overcome tumour proliferation is to identify patients who are most likely to benefit from the strategy. Predictive assays of cell kinetic parameters and more recently, PET imaging using proliferation-specific radioisotopes can be used to identify patients with highly proliferative advanced head and neck tumours in order to tailor treatment individually (figure 2).

3.1 Pre-treatment approaches

3.1.1 Predictive assays

The ultimate aim of cancer treatment is towards its individualization because of the observed large inter-patient variability of tumour response to therapy even in patients with the same disease characteristics. Pre-treatment assessment of individual tumour parameters is a necessary first step towards this goal.

Predictive assays to evaluate the proliferative potential of individual tumours have been developed and applied with limited success in the treatment of patients. The purpose of assessing the tumour's proliferative potential is to distinguish between rapidly and slowly proliferating groups of cells within the tumour. Common methods to achieve this goal include measurements of cell kinetic parameters before treatment such as potential doubling time (Tpot) and the length of S phase (T_S) and to correlate these parameters with the treatment outcome. Measurement of kick-off time (T_K), which represents the time period from the start of radiotherapy until the initiation of accelerated repopulation, will provide a window of opportunity for adjustment of the conventional treatment schedule to that of any one of the 3 altered radiation dose fractionation schedules of (1) accelerated dose fractionation, (2) hyperfractionation or (3) hybrid hyperfractionated-accelerated radiotherapy schedules shown in randomised clinical trials to overcome accelerated tumour repopulation (discussed under Section III.2.1 below).

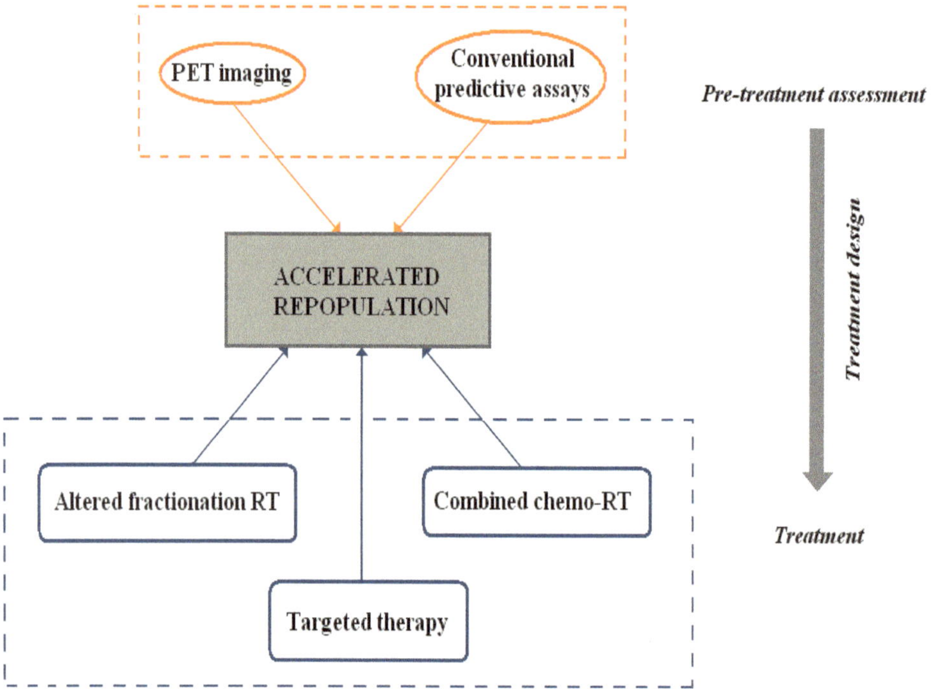

Fig. 2. Schematic diagram of pre-treatment and treatment approaches in overcoming accelerated repopulation.

Flow cytometric methods are common techniques used in the study of various pretreatment parameters of predictive value in treatment outcomes. Several studies have been undertaken to assess cell kinetic parameters and their relationships with treatment outcome (Corvo 1993, Bourhis 1996, Eschwege 1997, Begg 1999). The cytometry measurements have been based on tumour biopsies obtained after intravenous injection of bromodeoxyuridine, which is a thymidine analogue incorporated in DNA-synthesizing cells. Preliminary results obtained by Corvo *et al* (1993) have suggested that Tpot could be a prognostic factor influencing outcome of radiotherapy in head and neck cancer patients. Although the initial results were promising, very few further studies have confirmed the utility of Tpot as a predictor of treatment outcome. Tpot was not the only parameter reported to perform poorly in predicting treatment outcomes in subsequent studies, the majority of which show that other cell kinetic parameters such as the length of S phase, and the labelling index also had poor predictive power. On the other hand, the classic clinical prognostic factors of tumour stage and nodal status were strongly associated with treatment outcomes. Begg *et al* (1999) have established that the only pretreatment kinetic parameter with some association with local control in head and neck patients was the labelling index (LI), therefore concluding that pretreatment cell kinetic measurements determined by flow cytometry techniques provide a relatively weak overall prediction of radiotherapy outcome. Table 1 presents some of the most important cell kinetic parameters characteristic of head and neck squamous carcinomas.

The proliferation-associated nuclear antigen, p105, an antigen which identifies only proliferating cells has been reported to be a potentially useful predictor for loco-regional control and survival of treated head and neck cancer patients (Fu 1994). The method is also based on flow cytometry measurements, but instead of pretreatment injections with thymidine analogues, nuclei suspensions from paraffin blocks obtained from pretreatment biopsies are prepared and processed for p105 antibody and DNA staining. Subsequent flow cytometric quantification of p105 labelling indices and DNA content are undertaken and correlated with radiotherapy outcome. Later studies (Hammond 2003) however, showed no association between p105 labelling indices, DNA ploidy and treatment outcome.

Cell kinetic parameter	Mean value & range	Publication
Cell cycle time	43.5 hours (14 - 217)	Malaise 1973
Volume doubling time	57 days (43-75)	Steel 1977
Potential doubling time (T_{pot})	4.5 days (1.8 - 5.9)	Steel 2002
Kick-off time *(T_k)*	21-28 days	Withers 1993
Growth fraction determined by Ki67 LI (mean/median)	27.8%	Roland 1994
Labelling index *(LI)*	9.6% (5-17)	Steel 1977
Cell loss factor	91%	Steel 1977
Length of the DNA synthesis phase *(T_S)*	11.9 hours (8.8-16.1)	Begg & Steel 2002

Table 1. Cell kinetic parameters for head and neck carcinomas

The growth factor or proliferation rate within a tumour can also be given by the marker protein Ki-67, which is a nuclear antigen associated with cell proliferation due to its presence in the nuclei of cycling cells only. A recent study evaluating the prognostic value of Ki-67 in salivary gland tumours reported better survival rates for patients with lower Ki-67 values (< 15%) than for those with Ki-67 > 15% (Vacchi-Suzzi 2010). Nevertheless, a better prognostic indicator, REPP86 (restrictedly expressed proliferation-associated protein 86), a proliferation marker expressed in several phases of the cell cycle (S, G2 and M) has been reported in a recent clinical study (Cordes 2010). Retrospective analysis of REPP86 protein-level expression in patients with laryngeal squamous cell carcinoma, with a cut-off value between high and low tumour proliferation of 25% (i.e. percentage of proliferating cells of 25%) REPP86, showed a strong correlation between proliferation and long-term outcome. Patients with low proliferating activity tumours had a 95.8% overall survival rate after 5 years, whereas those with rapidly proliferating tumours only had a 23.3% survival rate.

A property of rapidly proliferating cells is to over-express sigma receptor proteins (Bem 1991). Sigma receptors are proteins with a very complex molecular physiology and they are involved in several aspects of cancer pathology yet to be elucidated. While the overexpression of sigma receptors in proliferating cells can be up to 10-times higher than in quiescent cells (Wheeler 2000), the usefulness of sigma-2 receptors in predicting treatment outcome in head and neck cancer patients has not been convincing so far. However, based on their molecular behaviour, these receptors are currently employed in the design of novel radiotracers. Radiolabelled ligands which bind to sigma-2 receptors are trialled for PET imaging to provide a quantitative assessment of proliferative versus quiescent cells in tumours.

To date, cell kinetic measurements have not conclusively established a correlation between pretreatment parameters and treatment outcomes. While some studies have shown a relationship between kinetic parameters and radiotherapy end points, the relationship is weak and worse in predicting treatment outcomes than the classic clinical prognostic factors (TNM staging classification) or tumour volume reported in other studies (Kurek 2003).

3.1.2 Positron Emission Tomography (PET) imaging with proliferation-specific radioisotopes

As previously mentioned, cell kinetic measurements have certain drawbacks including the need to establish a correlation between pretreatment parameters and treatment outcomes and inherent delays in obtaining results which have a potential for influencing treatment outcomes. There is, therefore, a great need for developing a more reliable tool which can accurately and expeditiously identify the proliferative potential of tumours. Functional imaging techniques employing proliferation kinetics-specific markers are being trialled with promising results (for a literature review see Marcu 2011).

The most common radiopharmaceutical used in Positron Emission Tomography for functional imaging is ^{18}F-FDG (fluorodeoxyglucose), a glucose analogue which is absorbed by cells with increased metabolism (reflected in high glucose consumption) such as malignant cells. There is strong evidence of the effectiveness, specificity and sensitivity of FDG in head and neck tumours. Based on a compilation of clinical studies Chiti et al (2010) reported a range of between 93-100% sensitivity and 90-100% specificity for the primary site, validating the use of this radioisotope for tumour staging, identification of the primary site of origin (if unknown) and for assessment of treatment response.

Despite its widespread use, ^{18}F-FDG has its limitations, particularly in quantifying tumour proliferation. Tumour proliferation-specific markers were used to develop new PET radiotracers in order to enable sub-volumes to be targeted for more aggressive treatment. To date, radiotracers employed for PET imaging of cellular proliferation in solid tumours can be divided into two categories: (1) thymidine kinase-1 based radiotracers which quantify the S-phase fraction, i.e. cells undergoing DNA synthesis during tracer uptake and (2) radiolabelled sigma-2 receptor ligands which quantify the ratio of proliferating versus non-proliferating tumour cells (Mach 2009).

Reactive lymph nodes are a common source for false-positive results in head and neck cancer patients. This factor confounds the interpretation of ^{18}F-FDG PET imaging as it does not distinguish between uptake in tumour and inflammatory cells (Abgral 2009, Corry

2008). To overcome this limitation of ^{18}F-FDG PET imaging, a new marker has been investigated which allows for uptake in actively proliferating tumour cells and inflammatory cells to be differentiated. The tumour proliferation marker, 3′-Deoxy-3′[18F]-fluorothymidine (FLT) is phosphorylated by **thymidine kinase 1 (TK-1)**, an enzyme with high activity in proliferating cells. Being a key enzyme in DNA synthesis, TK-1 presents with a peak activity during the S phase of the cell cycle, thus making the radiolabelled FLT a possible candidate for the imaging of cellular proliferation.

In a recent study conducted by Troost *et al* (2010) FLT was employed to evaluate sub-volumes of tumour with high proliferation in ten patients with oropharyngeal carcinoma. The patients underwent ^{18}F-FLT-PET scans before and during radiotherapy which helped in identifying sub-volumes of high proliferative activity within the gross tumour volume, enabling the radiation dose to be escalated in the highly proliferative tumour sub-volume in the treatment plan using intensity modulated radiotherapy.

The results of a kinetic analysis involving ^{18}F-FLT were reported by Menda *et al* (2009) in eight head and neck cancer patients before and 5 days after chemoradiotherapy (i.e. after 10Gy radiotherapy and one cycle of chemotherapy). The intense initial ^{18}F-FLT uptake by the tumour showed a significant reduction after 5 x 2 Gy of radiotherapy (mean SUV_{60} decreased from 2.53 ± 0.80 to 1.31 ± 0.67 between pre-treatment and mid-treatment scans), with the changes correlating with decrease in thymidine kinase activity after treatment. Though the number of patients involved in the study was small, the data are compelling particularly if confirmed by other studies.

One of the limitations when using thymidine analogues to assess tumour proliferation with PET imaging is dictated by the level of TK-1 activity of cells in the cell cycle. While in normal cells TK-1 is active in the S-phase, thus allowing quantification of cells undergoing DNA synthesis, regulation of TK-1 varies among tumours (Schwartz 2003). To characterize the proliferation activity of oral cancers, a recent study conducted by Troost (2010b) aimed to validate ^{18}F-FLT-PET against immunohistochemical expression of the TK-1. It was shown that despite the TK-1-positive staining in most tumours, the intensity of the staining was weak and no correlation was found between TK-1 activity and ^{18}F-FLT uptake. The lack of correlation was attributed to differences in biomarker characteristics, methods of quantification and also in the resolution of the imaging modalities used. Nevertheless, the high TK-1 labelling indices (50%-80%) obtained from other tumour sites (such as breast, and non-small cell lung) should stimulate further studies of immunohistochemical staining for TK-1 in head and neck carcinomas (He 2004, Mao 2005).

As mentioned above, another group of tumour proliferation-specific radiopharmaceuticals are **radiolabelled sigma-2 receptor ligands**. PET imaging with radiolabelled sigma-2 receptor ligands was shown to offer superior tumour specific information compared to thymidine kinase-1 based radiotracer imaging (Rowland 2006, Mach 2009). While their molecular function is still not fully understood, the evidence of sigma-2 receptor overexpression in proliferating cells offered the possibility of designing new agents for PET imaging.

Both ^{11}C- and ^{18}F-labelled sigma receptor ligands have been investigated with varying results (Mach 2009). While tumour uptake studies with ^{11}C-13 showed high uptake and good image contrast (Mach 2009b), ^{11}C-labelled compounds have the disadvantage of short half life of the radioisotope ^{11}C (20.38 min) as compared to ^{18}F (109.77 min). This drawback leads to a lower tumour to normal tissue ratio when ^{11}C agents are employed as image analysis after tracer injection is limited by the shorter half life of ^{11}C compared with ^{18}F. Tu *et al* (2007) investigated the effectiveness of fluorine-18-labelled benzamide analogues in imaging the sigma receptor status of solid tumours. Pre-clinical results demonstrated excellent tumour uptake at 5 min post-injection (2.5 – 3.7% ID/g percent injected dose per gram of tissue) which remained high 1 hour post-injection (1.2 - 2.7% ID/g) as compared to normal tissue uptake.

Another long-lived radioisotope evaluated *in vivo* is ^{76}Br, with a half life of 16.2 h and high affinity for sigma 2 receptors. A study conducted by Rowland (2006) compared the proliferation-specific imaging potential of ^{76}Br-labelled ligands with the more established ^{18}F-FLT. Although tumour uptake of the two compounds is driven by different mechanisms (^{76}Br-labelled sigma 2 receptors upregulation versus ^{18}F-FLT phosphorylation by TK-1 enzyme in proliferative tumours) a semi-quantitative comparison between their imaging characteristics allowed an assessment of their clinical utility in detecting tumours with high proliferative activity. It was found that 2 h after injection of the ^{76}Br labelled sigma 2 receptor-affinic agent, not only was tumour to normal tissue ratio (9x) higher resulting in better tumour visualization but also the metabolic clearance of non-specifically bound radioactive compounds was faster compared with ^{18}F-FLT. Although the clinical use of ^{76}Br-1 has been investigated in mammary adenocarcinoma cell lines, the relatively high tumour to normal tissue uptake ratio in head and neck cancer suggests the potential utility of ^{76}Br in tumour proliferation imaging of head and neck cancer.

A novel proliferation-specific radiotracer, ^{18}F-ISO-1, is trialled by Washington University School of Medicine in a study which is currently recruiting patients with one of the following three conditions: breast cancer, head and neck cancer and diffuse large B-cell lymphoma (ClinicalTrials.gov Identifier: NCT00968656). The primary goal of the trial is the "Assessment of Cellular Proliferation in Tumors by Positron Emission Tomography (PET) using [^{18}F]ISO-1 (FISO PET/CT)" and the evaluation of the diagnostic quality of [^{18}F]ISO-1-PET/CT images at the proposed 8 mCi dose. The trial also aims to quantify the relationship between tumour ^{18}F-ISO-1 uptake and various cellular proliferation markers and metabolic indicators such as: Ki-67, S-phase, mitotic index and sigma-2 receptors content of the tumour as secondary outcome measures.

Further studies are encouraged for the clinical validation of the existing radiotracers and for the development of new, tumour proliferation-specific PET markers for head and neck cancer.

3.2 Treatment approaches

As stated previously, an important outcome of pre-treatment assays is the identification of patients most likely to benefit from altered fractionation radiation therapy. While patients with highly proliferating head and neck tumours have been shown to gain from accelerated, hyperfractionated or combined accelerated and hyperfractionated radiotherapy alone or conventional radiation treatment schedules in combination with cytotoxic chemotherapy, patients who have tumours with low proliferation potential can be successfully treated with conventionally fractionated radiotherapy alone or in combination with cytotoxic chemotherapy.

3.2.1 Altered radiation fractionation schedules

In the treatment of head and neck cancer, three approaches to altering the schedule of conventional radiotherapy of 1.80 - 2.00 Gy week-daily dose increments have resulted in improved locoregional control without increasing late normal tissue complication rates based on randomised clinical trial data (as discussed and summarised in Table 2). These approaches are (i) accelerated fractionation dose schedules, (ii) hyperfractionated accelerated dose schedules and (iii) a hybrid of (i) and (ii) or hyperfractionated accelerated dose schedules.

An accelerated radiation dose schedule is one which is designed to shorten the duration of treatment without changing the fraction size or total dose. The ones successfully trialled have involved twice daily fractionation during some of the weekdays or once daily dose delivery six instead of the usual five days a week for conventional radiotherapy (Hlinak 2000, Overgaard 2000, see Table 2 for details).

Study	No of Patients	Experimental #	Standard #	Outcomes
(i) Hyperfractionation studies RTOG - Fu et al, 2000	1,073	81.6 Gy/68#/6.8 weeks, treating 2x/day	70 Gy/35#/7 weeks	Improved local control without increased late normal tissue complications although acute mucosal reaction enhanced.
Toronto - Cummings et al, 2000	331	58 Gy/40#/4 weeks, treating 2x/day	51 Gy/20#/4 Weeks	Improved local control without increased late normal tissue complications although acute mucosal reaction enhanced.
EORTC - Horiot et al, 1992	356	80.5 Gy/70#/7 weeks, treating 2x/day	70 Gy/35#/7 weeks	Improved local control without increased late normal tissue complications although acute mucosal reaction enhanced.
Pinto et al, 1991	98	70.4Gy/64#/6.5 weeks, treating 1x/day	66 Gy/33#/6.5 weeks	Improved local control without increased late normal tissue complications although acute mucosal reaction enhanced.
(ii) Accelerated fractionation studies Hliniak et al, 2000	395	66 Gy/33#/5.5 weeks treating 2x/day on one of 5 week days only	66 Gy/33#/6.5 weeks	Improved local control without increased late critical normal tissue complications although acute mucosal and skin reactions enhanced.
DAHANCA 6 & 7 - Overgaard et al, 2000	1,485	~ 66 Gy/33#/6 weeks, treating 6 days a week	~ 66 Gy/33#/7 weeks	Improved local control without increased late critical normal tissue complications although acute mucosal and skin reactions enhanced.

Study	No of Patients	Experimental #	Standard #	Outcomes
Skladowski et al, 2000	100	~ 70 Gy/35#/5 weeks, treating 7 days a week	~ 70 Gy/35#/7 weeks	Increased local control and overall survival but at expense of increased serious late normal tissue complications consequential to severe acute mucosal reactions.
Jackson et al, 1997	82	66 Gy/17#3-4 weeks, treating 2x/day on each of 5 week days	66 Gy/34#/6-8 weeks	Trial abandoned because of unacceptable severe mucosal toxicity preventing evaluation of treatment efficacy.
(iii) Hyperfractionated accelerated studies A. Continuous hyperfractionated accelerated studies TROG – Poulsen et al, 2001	350	59.4 Gy/36#/3.5 weeks treating 2x/day	66 Gy/33#/6.5 weeks	No difference in local control but reduced late normal tissue complications
GORTEC – Bourhis et al, 2000	268	63 Gy/35#/3.3 weeks treating 2x/day	70 Gy/35#/7 weeks	Improved local control without enhanced late normal tissue
UK – Dische et al, 1997	918	54 Gy/36#/2 weeks treating 3x/day	66 Gy/33#/6.5 weeks	No difference in local control but reduced late normal tissue complications
b. Split Course accelerated studies RTOG – Fu et al, 2000	1,073	67.2 Gy/42#/6.2 weeks treating 2x/day in 2 phases with 2 week break between	70 Gy/35#/7 weeks	No improvement in local control and no worsening of late normal tissue complications
EORTC - Horiot et al, 1997	500	72 Gy/45#/5 weeks treating 3x/day in 2 phases with 2 weeks break in between	70 Gy/35#/7 weeks	Increased local control but at expense of enhanced late critical normal tissue complications
c. Concomitant boost accelerated hyperfractionated studies MD Anderson – Ang et al, 2001	151	63 Gy/35#/5 weeks, treating 2x/day during last 2 weeks	63 Gy/35#/7 weeks	No statistically significant difference in local control or late normal tissue complications for whole patient group
RTOG – Fu et al, 2000	1,073	72 Gy/30#/6 weeks treating 2x/day duri8ng last 2.5 weeks	70 Gy/35#/7 weeks	Improved local control without enhancement of late normal tissue complications

Table 2. Phase III randomised trials of altered (experimental #) versus conventional (standard #) dose fractionation for radiotherapy of head and neck cancer

A hyperfractionated radiation dose schedule involves the use of lower dose fractions (typically 1.1 - 1.2 Gy) usually two times a day separated by at least 6 hrs between the dose fractions compared with the conventional 1.80 - 2.00 Gy once daily 5x/week. It is designed to enable higher total radiation doses to be delivered for improved local control without incurring increased normal tissue complication rates by exploiting the better ability of normal versus malignant cells to repair radiation damage between the multiple fractions provided a minimum time (of at least 6 hours) is allowed for the repair to occur (Fu 2000, Cummings 2000, Horiot 1992, Pinto 1991 as in Table 2). Strictly speaking the standard treatment arm of the Toronto hyperfractionation trial (Cummings 2000) does not fall within the definition of conventional dose fractionation because the treatment is delivered in 2.55 Gy once daily 5x/week and therefore incorporates a degree of acceleration but as the hyperfractionated treatment also involves the delivery of higher (1.45 Gy) than the typical 1.1 - 1.2 Gy twice daily fractions 5x/week, the study nevertheless provides data for a valid comparison of the hyperfractionation component.

By incorporating the radiobiological rationale of hyperfractionation and acceleration, hybrid hyperfractionated accelerated radiation schedules have been successfully trialled including treatment schedules of only two weeks duration albeit with up to an 18% reduction in total dose (Poulsen 2000, Bourhis 2000, Dische 1997, Fu 2000, Ang 2001 see Table 2 for details).

A dose reduction is necessary with hybrid schedules because for pure accelerated dose schedules, it has not proved possible to treat twice daily each week day nor to shorten the duration of treatment by two weeks treating daily, 7 days a week. This was because acute mucosal toxicity proved to be dose limiting which not only led to the abandonment of one of the pure accelerated dose fractionation trials but also resulted in increased rate of late normal tissue complications as a consequence of severe acute toxicity in another (Jackson 1997, Skladowski 2000, see Table 2 for details).

3.2.2 Combined chemotherapy and radiotherapy and the sequencing of the treatments

Whilst an optimal treatment regimen combining multiagent chemotherapy and radiotherapy is yet to be developed, clinical trials have established that platinum-based chemotherapy in combination with radiotherapy results in superior outcomes for locally advanced head and neck cancers compared with other cytotoxic agents in combination with radiotherapy or radiotherapy alone.

Cisplatin is among the most effective cytotoxic agents in head and neck cancer, with single agent response rates ranging from 25% to 30% (Schwachöfer 1991). Cisplatin interacts with cellular DNA to form interstrand and intrastrand crosslinks which then inhibit DNA replication and RNA transcription, leading to sublethal or lethal DNA breaks. Though inhibition of DNA synthesis implies S phase arrest, cells are blocked in the G2 phase of the cell cycle before dying (Sorenson 1990). The major mechanism of cisplatin-induced cell death is apoptosis.

In vivo studies examining the effects of combined cisplatin-radiotherapy concluded that the primary interaction between the two agents is the cisplatin-induced increased oxygenation of the hypoxic cells (Yan & Durand 1991). It was therefore suggested that cisplatin should be delivered before, rather than after irradiation. In addition, cisplatin administered daily with fractionated radiotherapy leads to improved tumour control compared with weekly cisplatin chemoradiotherapy. Trial designs have evolved together with better knowledge of the radiobiology and the implementation of novel treatment techniques. While in the 70s cisplatin was trialled as a single-agent, in the 80s and 90s the drug was combined with conventional radiotherapy. Later, radiobiological developments on the correlation between hypoxia, repopulation and treatment failure led to new radiotherapy schedule designs which altered the conventional fractionation pattern. Nowadays, for head and neck cancer patients, cisplatin is administered concurrently with either hyperfractionated or accelerated radiotherapy, employing intensity modulated techniques (IMRT) (see Table 3).

Clinical trial/study	Trial/study design	Treatment regimen	Observations
Phase III **trial** ***(SAKK 10/94)*** 224 patients Ghadjar **2011**	Concomitant cisplatin and hyperfractionated radiotherapy versus hyperfractionated radiotherapy alone	**RT:** median total dose, 74.4 Gy; 1.2 Gy twice daily; 5 days per week **Chemo:** two cycles of cisplatin (20 mg/m^2 for 5 consecutive days during weeks 1 and 5)	Locoregional failure-free survival at 10 years (40% vs 32%); metastasis-free survival (56% vs 41%); cancer-specific survival at 10 years (55% vs 43%) in the combined arm vs radiotherapy alone. No difference in late toxicity. *Significantly improved treatment outcome in the combined arm.*
Clinical study 43 patients Montejo **2010**	Accelerated radiotherapy with concurrent chemotherapy	**RT:** IMRT with simultaneous integrated boost (67.5, 60, and 54 Gy in 30 daily fractions of 2.25, 2, and 1.8 Gy) **Chemo:** cisplatin 40 mg/m^2 weekly or 100 mg/m^2 every 3 weeks during radiotherapy. + weekly cetuximab (3	Complete response: 74.4%; estimated 5-year locoregional control 82%; Tolerable acute and late toxicities. *IMRT with simultaneous integrated boost with concurrent chemotherapy improved local* and *regional control.*
Phase II trial (RTOG 99-14) 84 patients Garden **2008**	Concomitant boost-accelerated radiation regimen with cisplatin	**RT:** 72 Gy over 6 weeks **Chemo:**100 mg/m^2 on days 1 and 22	2- and 4-year locoregional failure rates: 33% and 36%; 2- and 4-year survival rates: 70% and 54%
			Worst overall late Grade 3 or 4 toxicity rate 42%. *A Phase III trial comparing AFX-C plus cisplatin against standard radiation plus cisplatin has completed accrual.*

Clinical trial/study	Trial/study design	Treatment regimen	Observations
Clinical study 31 patients (larynx and hypopharynx) Lee **2007**	Concurrent chemotherapy and Intensity Modulated Radiotherapy	**RT**: median prescribed dose 70 Gy at 2.12 Gy/fraction to the PTV_{GTV}; 59.4 Gy at 1.8 Gy/fraction to the PTV of high-risk subclinical disease **Chemo:** 2 to 3 cycles of cisplatin (100 mg/m^2 intravenously within 2 days every 3 weeks)	The 2-year local progression-free survival: 86%; regional progression-free survival: 94%; overall survival 63%. Grade 2 (and higher) mucositis occurred in 48% of patients; all had Grade 2 or higher pharyngitis during treatment.
Phase III ***trial*** 192 patients (oropharynx) Fallai **2006**	Conventional radiotherapy (arm A) *versus* Accelerated hyperfractionated radiotherapy (arm B) *versus* Concomitant radiotherapy and chemotherapy (arm C)	**RT:** ***Arms A and C:*** 66 to 70 Gy in 33 to 35 fractions ***Arm B:*** 64 to 67.2 Gy in two fractions of 1.6 Gy every day with a 2 weeks split after 38.4Gy **Chemo:** 3 cycles of carboplatin (75 mg/m^2 on days 1 to 4) and 5-FU (1000 mg/m^2 on days 1 to 4) every 28 days	Locoregional control: Arm A+B: 20% Arm C: 48% Toxicity: Arm C showed slightly more grade 3 side effects. *Patients with advanced oropharyngeal cancers should be treated with combined chemo-radiotherapy.*

Table 3. Concurrent chemo-radiotherapy regimens employing IMRT techniques

The general consensus regarding the concurrent administration of cisplatin-based chemotherapy with radiotherapy (usually IMRT) derived from the above-presented clinical studies is in favour of chemo-radiotherapy (as compared with radiotherapy alone). Phase II trials and small studies showed that further investigations employing novel treatment regimens are warranted. Therefore, as probably expected, phase III trials have proven the superiority of the combined chemo-altered fractionation radiotherapy as opposed to radiotherapy as single agent, particularly with respect to improved locoregional failure-free survival. Since locoregional failure is still a clinical challenge in the treatment of advanced head and neck cancer, more improvements in the rate of failure-free survival are desperately needed.

In order to reduce normal tissue toxicity, a recent phase II prospective trial has investigated the tumoricidal effect of standard dose weekly cisplatin (30 mg/m^2 once a week over 7-8 weeks) given concurrently with radiotherapy. Despite the low-dose drug regimen (the usual dose of cisplatin is 100 mg/m^2 per three weekly cycle) tumour control was high, with a locoregional control rate of 82% and a 5-year disease-free survival of 62% (Rampino 2011). Major acute toxicity (grade 3-4 mucositis) was observed in 35.2% of patients and mild late reactions occurred in 16% of patients. These results warrant further studies in a phase III randomised trial.

Beside concurrent chemo-radiotherapy, cisplatin and cisplatin-based chemotherapy have been trialled as neoadjuvant chemotherapy for definitive local treatment and for the management of distant metastases (Caponigro 2002, Posner 2005, Glynne-Jones 2007, Finnegan 2009). Induction chemotherapy has the potential to reduce the rate of distant metastases and to improve survival via the additional drug dose which targets both the systemic disease and the primary tumour (Paccagnella 2010). An overall response rate of 79% was achieved with induction chemotherapy consisting of two cycles of cisplatin on day 1, plus 5FU on days 2-5, with a 10-day interval between the two cycles (Zidan 1997). A similar result was obtained by Finnegan et al (2009), achieving an overall response rate of 75% with cisplatin- fluorouracil as induction therapy in patients with advanced head and neck cancers. A phase II randomized trial also employed a cisplatin-based neoadjuvant therapy, with cisplatin given on day 1 and 5FU-based chemotherapy on day 2, repeated every 2 weeks for four cycles (Caponigro 2002). Tumour response evaluation showed a complete response rate of 35%, which was deemed encouraging though unacceptable for further clinical implementation. Some trials have shown that the addition of 5-Fluorouracil and taxanes to neoadjuvant cisplatin further improves survival. The EORTC 24971/TAX 323 phase III trial employed cisplatin-based induction chemotherapy with and without taxanes in 358 advanced head and neck cancer patients, showing a 27% lower risk of death in the taxane arm (Vermorken 2007).

While all the abovementioned trials and studies employed injectable cisplatin, either intravenous or intra-arterial, with no significant differences in outcome between the two ways of administration (Ackerstaff 2011), physicians are striving to reduce normal tissue toxicities and unwanted side effects by trialling new ways of cisplatin administration. A recent dose-escalation trial administered oral cisplatin (CP Ethypharm®) in combination with radiotherapy to 18 head and neck cancer patients (Tao 2011). Four cisplatin dose levels were tested: 10 $mg/m^2/day$ in 4 patients; 15 $mg/m^2/day$ in 4 patients, 20 $mg/m^2/day$ in 5 patients and 25 $mg/m^2/day$ in 5 patients. Dose limiting toxicities were experienced at 25 mg/m^2 with the most frequent adverse events being gastrointestinal disorders. Therefore the dose recommended for phase II trial is 20 $mg/m^2/day$. Further clinical investigations are warranted to demonstrate the role of oral cisplatin in reducing the rate of adverse events.

Although chemo-radiotherapy has lately replaced radiotherapy for the management of advanced head and neck cancer, the optimal chemo-radiotherapy treatment regimen is yet to be established. While some trials showed promising results with concurrent chemo-radiotherapy, others suggest that loco-regional control can be improved with induction chemotherapy. However, meta-analyses of randomised trial data show that better treatment results are obtained when chemotherapy is administered concurrently with radiotherapy compared with chemotherapy given in a neoadjuvant setting (Munro 1995, El-Sayed 1996). Irrespective of the employed treatment, in order to overcome accelerated tumour repopulation, treatment gaps should be avoided and the timing of chemotherapy should be well designed. Cisplatin-based chemotherapy has the potential to partially synchronise cells in the cell cycle because of cisplatin's inherent characteristic of arresting cells in the G2 phase of the cell cycle. Given that cells in late G2 have high radiosensitivity, irradiation would be more effective if started before the next mitotic cycle. Furthermore, the effectiveness of induction chemotherapy could possibly be increased by starting radiotherapy as soon as tolerable to avoid tumour repopulation negating the gain in loco-regional control.

3.2.3 Targeted therapies

A major disadvantage of chemoradiotherapy in the treatment of locally advanced head and neck cancer is the increased normal tissue toxicity, particularly to the mucosa lining the upper aero-digestive tract. Whilst younger, fitter patients may be able to be medically supported during the treatment, older patients and particularly those with medical co-morbidities may be intolerant of the treatment regimen or refuse to continue it.

Fortunately, since the general acceptance of carcinogenesis as a multi-step event involving the deregulation of molecular pathways as a result of dysfunction of oncogenes and tumour suppressor genes (Hahn & Weinberg 2002), there has been a rapid increase in the number of therapeutic agents which target the "hallmarks of cancer" (Hahn & Weinberg 2011). These hallmarks include growth factor independence and insensitivity to growth suppressor signals leading to unrestricted proliferation, evasion of apoptosis, sustained angiogenesis, immortality and tissue invasiveness and metastasis.

Targeted therapies can be defined as the agent(s) which are designed to inhibit if not eliminate one or more the characteristics or hallmarks of cancer. These target specific agent(s) should spare normal tissues such as the mucosa of the entire digestive tract from the effects of chemotherapy and of the upper aero-digestive tract from the combined effects of chemo-radiotherapy although unexpected normal tissue effects have been reported (discussed below). Despite the absence of significant normal tissue toxicity, it is likely that a combination of agents will be needed as resistance to single agents is often inevitable as judged by later reports of the initially promising results of trastuzumab, a monoclonal antibody against one of the epidermal growth factor receptors, HER 2 in the treatment of metastatic breast cancer (Jones & Buzdar 2009) and imatinib, a tyrosine kinase inhibitor which targets the oncogenic protein BCR-ABL expressed at high levels in chronic myeloid leukaemia (Gorre 2001).

With respect to the treatment of locally advanced head and neck cancer, high dose radiotherapy combined with cetuximab, a monoclonal antibody against another epidermal growth factor receptor (EGFR) HER 1 associated with signalling pathways for cellular processes such as proliferation and differentiation has been shown to improve locoregional control and survival without increasing normal tissue toxicity compared with high dose radiotherapy alone (Bonner 2006). In this landmark clinical trial, 213 patients were randomised to radiotherapy alone and 211 patients to radiotherapy with cetuximab. The addition of cetuximab to radiotherapy significantly increased 3 year loco-regional control rates from 34% to 47% and overall survival rates from 45% to 55%. The main toxicity experienced by patients who received cetuximab was an acne-like rash and rather surprisingly sub-group analysis revealed that overall survival was better in patients with a moderate to severe (Grade ≥2) rash compared with patients who had no or a mild (Grade 0 or 1) rash. This finding opens up new possibilities for further minimizing the effects of tumour cell repopulation particularly as the improved treatment outcomes with Cetuximab in combination with high dose radiotherapy matches the best results of chemoradiotherapy without the increased normal tissue toxicity. For example, a randomized Phase III trial under the auspices of the Radiation Therapy Oncology Group (RTOG) comparing the addition of Cetuximab to accelerated radiotherapy and cisplatin chemotherapy versus accelerated radiotherapy and cisplatin chemotherapy for locally advanced head and neck cancer has been reported (RTOG 0552, 2007).

With advances in high throughput technology, gene microarray analysis is being used to predict tumour response to treatment thus heralding a future in personalised medicine (West 2007). Microarray technology used to derive a gene expression profile or signature from tumour samples has been shown to be a more powerful predictor of outcome of breast cancer in young patients than clinico-pathological staging systems (van de Vijver 2002). A small study of head and neck cancer patients treated by surgical excision reported that gene expression analysis of the tumour samples based on 205 genes discriminated between seven patients who recurred distally and eight patients who had no recurrence (Giri 2006). The implication of the study is that patients without the signature would be spared the toxicity of chemotherapy, particularly if the findings are confirmed in a larger study.

4. References

[1] Ackerstaff AH, Rasch CR, Balm AJ, de Boer JP, Wiggenraad R, Rietveld DH, et al, Five-year quality of life results of the randomized clinical phase III (RADPLAT) trial, comparing concomitant intra-arterial versus intravenous chemoradiotherapy in locally advanced head and neck cancer. Head Neck. 2011 doi: 10.1002/hed.21851.

[2] Ang K.K., Trotti A, Brown B.W., et al. Randomized trial addressing risk features and time factors of surgery plus radiotherapy in advanced head and neck cancer. Int J Radiat Oncol Biol Phys 2001; 51:571-578.

[3] Bonner J.A., Harari P.M., Giralt J et al. Radiotherapy plus cetuximab for squamous cell carcinoma of the head and neck. N Engl J Med 2006; 354: 567-578.

[4] Bourhis J, Lapeyre, Tortochaux J et al. Very accelerated versus conventional radiotherapy in HNSCC: results of the GORTEC 94-02 randomized trial. Int J Radiat Oncol Biol Phys 2000; 48:S111.

[5] Caponigro F, Rosati G, De Rosa P, Avallone A, De Rosa V, De Lucia L, et al, Cisplatin, raltitrexed, levofolinic acid and 5-fluorouracil in locally advanced or metastatic squamous cell carcinoma of the head and neck: a phase II randomized study, Oncology. 2002; 63(3):232-8.

[6] Cummings B, O'Sullivan B, Keane T et al. 5 Year results of a 4 week/twice daily radiation schedule: the Toronto trial. Radiother Oncol 2000; 56:S8.

[7] Denham J et al. Mucosal regeneration during radiotherapy. Radiother. Oncol. 1996; 41:109–18.

[8] Dische S, Saunders M, Barrett A et al. A randomized multicentre trial of CHART versus conventional radiotherapy in head and neck cancer. Radiother Oncol 1997; 44:123-126.

[9] Dörr W Three A's of repopulation during fractionated irradiation of squamous epithelia: asymmetry loss, acceleration of stem-cell divisions and abortive divisions Int. J. Radiat. Biol. 1977; 72:635–43.

[10] Dörr W, Hamilton CS, Boyd T, et al. Radiation-induced changes in cellularity and proliferation in human oral mucosa. Int J Radiat Oncol Biol Phys. 2002; 52:911–917.

[11] El-Sayed S & Nelson N. Adjuvant and adjunctive chemotherapy in the management of squamous cell carcinoma of the head and neck region. A meta-analysis of prospective and randomised trials. J Clin Oncol 1996; 14:838-847.

[12] Fallai C, Bolner A, Signor M, Gava A, Franchin G, Ponticelli P, et al, Long-term results of conventional radiotherapy versus accelerated hyperfractionated radiotherapy versus concomitant radiotherapy and chemotherapy in locoregionally advanced carcinoma of the oropharynx. Tumori. 2006; 92(1):41-54.

[13] Finnegan V, Parsons JT, Greene BD, Sharma V., Neoadjuvant chemotherapy followed by concurrent hyperfractionated radiation therapy and sensitizing chemotherapy for locally advanced (T3-T4) oropharyngeal squamous cell carcinoma, Head Neck 2009; 31(2):167-74.

[14] Fu K.K., Pajak T.F., Trotti A et al. A radiation therapy oncology group (RTOG) phase III randomized study to compare hyperfractionation and two variants of accelerated fractionation to standard fractionation radiotherapy for head and neck squamous cell carcinomas: first Report of RTOG 9003. Int. J Radiat Oncol Biol Phys 2000; 48:7-16.

[15] Fyles A, Keane TJ, Barton M et al. The effect of treatment duration in the local control of cervix cancer. Radiother Oncol 1992; 25:273-279.

[16] Garden AS, Harris J, Trotti A, Jones C, Carrascoza L, Cheng J, et al. Long-term results of concomitant boost radiation plus concurrent cisplatin for advanced head and neck carcinomas: A phase II trial of the Radiation Therapy Oncology Group (RTOG 99-14). Int J Radiat Oncol Biol Phys. 2008; 71:1351–1355.

[17] Ghadjar P, Simcock M, Studer G, Allal AS, Ozsahin M, Bernier J, et al, Concomitant Cisplatin and Hyperfractionated Radiotherapy in Locally Advanced Head and Neck Cancer: 10-Year Follow-up of a Randomized Phase III Trial (SAKK 10/94). Int J Radiat Oncol Biol Phys. 2011 (in press).

[18] Giri U, Ashorn CL, Ramdas L et al. Molecular signatures associated with clinical outcome in patients with high risk head and neck squamous cell carcinoma treated by surgery and radiation. Int J Radiat Oncol Biol Phys 2006; 64:670-677.

[19] Glynne-Jones R, Hoskin P, Neoadjuvant cisplatin chemotherapy before chemoradiation: a flawed paradigm? J Clin Oncol. 2007; 25(33):5281-6.

[20] Gorre ME, Mohammed M, Ellwood K, Hsu N, Paquette R, Rao PN and Sawyers CL. Clinical resistance to STI-571 cancer therapy caused by BCR-ABL gene mutation or amplification. Science 2001; 293:876-880.

[21] Hahn WC and Weinberg RA. Modelling the molecular circuitry of cancer. Nat Rev Cancer 2002; 2:331-341.

[22] Hahn WC and Weinberg RA. Hallmarks of cancer: the next generation. Cell 2011; 144:646-674.

[23] Hliniak A, Gwiazdowska B, Szutkowski Z. et al. Radiotherapy of the laryngeal cancer: the estimation of the therapeutic gain and the enhancement of toxicity by the one week shortening of the treatment time. Results of a randomized Phase III multicenter trial. Radiother Oncol 2000; 56:S5.

[24] Horiot J.C., Le Fur R.N, Guyen T et al. Hyperfractionation versus conventional fractionation in oropharyngeal carcinoma: final analysis of a randomized trial of the EORTC cooperative group of radiotherapy. Radiother Oncol 1992; 25:231-241.

[25] Huang Q, Li F, Liu X, Li W, Shi W, Liu FF, et al. Caspase 3–mediated stimulation of tumor cell repopulation during cancer radiotherapy. Nat. Med. 2011; 17:860–866.

[26] Jackson S.M., Weir L.M., Hay J.H., et al. A randomized trial of accelerated versus conventional radiotherapy in head and neck cancers. Radiother Oncol 1997; 43:39-46.

[27] Jones KL and Budzar AU. Evolving novel anti-HER 2 strategies. Lancet Oncol 2009; 10:1179-1187.

[28] Lee NY, O'Meara W, Chan K, Della-Bianca C, Mechalakos J, Zhung J, et al. Concurrent chemotherapy and intensity-modulated radiotherapy for locoregionally advanced laryngeal and hypopharyngeal cancers. Int J Radiat Oncol Biol Phys. 2007; 69:459–468.

[29] Marcu L, van Doorn T, Olver I, Modelling of post irradiation accelerated repopulation in squamous cell carcinomas, Physics in Medicine and Biology 2004; 49:3676-3779.

[30] Marcu L, Bezak E, Filip S, The role of PET imaging in overcoming radiobiological challenges in the treatment of advanced head and neck cancer, Cancer Treat Rev DOI: 10.1016/j.ctrv.2011.06.003, 2011 (in press).

[31] Munro AJ. An overview of randomised controlled trials of adjuvant chemotherapy in head and neck cancer. Br J Cancer 1995; 71:83-91.

[32] Overgaard J., Hansen H.S., Grau C, et al. The DAHANCA 6 & 7 trial: a randomized multicenter study of 5 versus 6 fractions per week of conventional radiotherapy of squamous cell carcinoma (scc) of the head and neck. Radiother Oncol 2000; 56:S4.

[33] Paccagnella A, Mastromauro C, D'Amanzo P, Ghi MG Induction chemotherapy before chemoradiotherapy in locally advanced head and neck cancer: the future? Oncologist 2010;15 Suppl 3:8-12.

[34] Peters LJ, Withers HR., Applying radiobiological principles to combined modality treatment of head and neck cancer--the time factor. Int J Radiat Oncol Biol Phys 1997; 39(4):831-6.

[35] Pinto L, Canary P, Araujo C et al. Prospective randomized trial comparing hyperfractionated versus conventional radiotherapy in stages II and IV oropharyngeal carcinoma. Int J Radiat Oncol Biol Phys 1991; 21:557-562.

[36] Posner MR, Paradigm shift in the treatment of head and neck cancer: the role of neoadjuvant chemotherapy, Oncologist. 2005; 10 Suppl 3:11-9.

[37] Poulsen M.G., Denham J.W., Peters L.J., et al. A randomized trial of accelerated and conventional radiotherapy for stage III and IV squamous carcinoma of the head and neck: a Trans-Tasman Radiaiton Oncology Group Study. Radiother Oncol 2001; 60:113-122.

[38] Rampino M, Ricardi U, Munoz F, Reali A, Barone C, Musu AR, et al, Concomitant adjuvant chemoradiotherapy with weekly low-dose cisplatin for high-risk squamous cell carcinoma of the head and neck: a phase II prospective trial. Clin Oncol (R Coll Radiol). 2011; 23(2):134-40.

[39] RTOG 0552: a randomised phase III trial of concurrent accelerated radiation and cisplatin versus concurrent accelerated radiation and cisplatin, and cetuximab [followed by surgery for selected patients] for Stage III and IV head and neck carcinomas. Clin Adv Hematol Oncol 2007; 5:79-81.

[40] Schwachöfer JHM, Crooijmans RP, Hoogenhout J, Kal HB, Theeuwes AGM Effectiveness in inhibition of recovery of cell survival by cisplatin and carboplatin: influence of treatment sequence. Int J Radiat Oncol Biol Phys 1991; 20:1235-1241

[41] Skladowski K., Macijewski J., Gohen M, et al. Randomized clinical trial on 7 day continuous accelerated irradiation (CAIR) of head and neck cancer: report on 3 year tumor control and normal tissue toxicity. Radiother Oncol 2000; 55:93-102.

[42] Sorenson CM, Barry MA, Eastman A Analysis of events associated with cell cycle arrest at G2 phase and cell death induced by cisplatin. J Natl Cancer Inst 1990; 82:749-755.

[43] Tao Y, Rezaï K, Brain E, Etessami A, Lusinchi A, Temam S, et al, A phase I trial combining oral cisplatin (CP Ethypharm) with radiotherapy in patients with locally advanced head and neck squamous cell carcinoma. Radiother Oncol. 2011; 98(1): 42-7.

[44] Trott K The mechanisms of acceleration of repopulation in squamous epithelia during daily irradiation Acta Oncol. 1999; 38:153–157.

[45] Trott K and Kummermehr J Accelerated repopulation in tumours and normal tissues Radiother. Oncol. 1991; 22:159–160.

[46] Van de Vijver MJ, He YD van't Veer LJ et al. A gene expression signature as a predictor of survival in breast cancer. N Engl J Med 2002; 347:1999-2009.

[47] Vermorken JB, Remenar E, van Herpen C, et al, Cisplatin, fluorouracil, and docetaxel in unresectable head and neck cancer. N Engl J Med 2007; 357:1695-1704.

[48] West CML, Elliott RM, Burnet NG. The genomics revolution and radiotherapy. Clinical Oncology 2007; 19:470-480.

[49] Withers H.R., Taylor J.M.G., Maciejewski B. The Hazard of Accelerated Tumor Clonogen Repopulation During Radiotherapy. Acta Oncologica 1988; 27(2):131-146.

[50] Yan R, Durand RE. The response of hypoxic cells in SCCVII murine tumors to treatment with cisplatin and x-rays. Int J Radiat Oncol Biol Phys 1991; 20: 271-4.

[51] Zidan J, Kuten A, Rosenblatt E, Robinson E, Intensive chemotherapy using cisplatin and fluorouracil followed by radiotherapy in advanced head and neck cancer, Oral Oncol. 1997; 33(2):129-35.

Part 5

Prosthesis and Reconstruction

12

Finesse in Aesthetic Facial Recontouring

Yueh-Bih Tang Chen[1], Shih-Heng Chen[1] and Hung-Chi Chen[2]
[1]*National Taiwan University Hospital, Taipei*
[2]*China Medical University Hospital, Taichung, Taiwan*

1. Introduction

Pursuing excellence in esthetically restoring a facial contour deformity is always a life-long endeavour for plastic surgeons. Significant facial defects, deformity or overt disfigurement, either soft tissue or skeletal or a combination of both, usually bring about aesthetic, functional and of course psychosocial impact. This situation is usually the formidable misery of the head and neck cancer patients with possible significant tissue loss. Strategy regarding the mode of reconstruction in order to obtain the most outstanding result is of utmost importance. Most reconstructions employing microvascular free tissue transfer often emphasize on tissue replacement and functional restoration. Based on 30 years experience in plastic surgery and free tissue transfers, the authors stressed on aesthetic refinement on each patient receiving either conventional methods or free tissue transfer for facial recontouring.

2. Material

The disease entity encompasses congenital anomalies, facial tumors (benign or malignant), or radionecrosis resulting in orbital, nasal, maxillary, mandibular or a combination of any of them, with functional defects amounting more than 1000 cases.

3. Methods

Minor defects might be reconstructed with various kinds of grafts, or miscellaneous implants. However, free tissue transfers should be selected for major reconstructions, which include groin flaps, radial forearm flaps, scapular flaps, anterolateral thigh flaps, latissimus dorsi, gracilis muscle, vascularized iliac bone, vascularized fibula or scapular bone, etc. Besides the success of the free tissue transfers, applications of various fundamental skills in plastic surgery will upgrade the result of the reconstruction to a higher hierarchy, which include Z-plasties, W-plasty, fat grafting, cartilage grafting, full-thickness skin grafting, specially designed sling surgery or even craniofacial skills--calvarial bone grafting, bilateral sagittal split osteotomy, sliding genioplasty, etc. Details of finesse in aesthetic facial recontouring using miscellaneous basic plastic surgery principles or microvascular free tissue transfers will be presented and discussed in the following selected representative cases.

As a plastic surgeon, pursuing excellence is always the gold standard. This involves technical mastery, enhancing experience, redeeming morality, development of accountability, eliciting ideas & innovations, emphasizing on humane solicitude, enriching artistic sense in order to get to the goal of pursuing excellence.

4. Considerations on facial recontouring

The basic fundamental principle of engaging in facial recontouring for the head and neck cancer patients is to aim at anatomical restoration as long as possible at the very beginning. If it's impossible, then tissue transfer with any measure should be employed—should it be a local flap, axial pattern flap, island flap or free tissue flap with any kind of tissue combinations. Certain percent of facial recontouring only requires volume reduction or volume replacement. Some patients with skeletal derangements need skeletal rearrangement—be it an osteotomy/ osteotomies with or without bone grafting or implant placement. Of course, proper anchorage of the facial interface is another important issue.

In patients with vascular malformations, skin problems should also be solved with intravascular embolization in collaboration with subtle use of appropriate selection of lasers in addition to sclerotherapy. Motor function disturbance at the face (facial paralysis or paresis) is another frequently encountered problem at the face, especially after trauma or tumor extirpation/ radical operation for malignant diseases. The facial expression/ symmetry should be deliberately restored with nerve transfers/ static sling operations/ regional functional muscle transfers/ free functional muscle transfers or combinations of any of the methods. The facial contours, not to mention, should be deliberately redefined and properly highlighted in order to get to a satisfactory result.

- Anatomy - restoration
- Volume - reduction, replacement
- Skeleton - rearrangement
- Interface - proper anchorage
- Skin - refinement, rejuvenation
- Motor Function - recreation; rehab.
- Contour - redefined, properly highlighted

Integration of craniofacial surgery, microsurgery and basic general plastic surgery principles is always indispensible in order to get to an esthetically satisfactory result.

Reconstruction may involve upper face, middle face, or lower face or combinations of any of them. It may also involve single layer reconstruction, double layers reconstruction, or triple layers reconstruction (sandwich reconstruction). Reconstruction can usually be finished in one operation by choosing the donor site with the least deformity and functional morbidity, and at the same time obtain the most benefit of the patient.

5. Table - Methods of facial recontouring

Aesthetic Facial Recontouring—Various Methods

- Replacement; Resurfacing
- Osteotomies– rearrangements; distraction
- Dynamic rehabilitation
- Reductions
- Augmentations
  - Autogenous tissue– bone, cartilage, fat, fascia
  - Alloplastic material-- silicone, PTFE, polyethylene, methylmethacrylate, hydroxyapatite, titanium implants, polyglycolic acids
  - Soft Tissue Fillers– HA, Alloderm, Gortex

6. Representative facial derangements

To esthetically recontour a face has been our main goal in daily encounters, here we select several interesting topics and representative instances to demonstrate the aforementioned methods used in treating facial derangements or enhancing facial esthetics.

6.1 The Fate of Different Reconstructive Modes for Mandibular Ameloblastomas.

6.2 Strategy of Reconstructing Combined Mandibular Defect and Facial Palsy.

6.3 Strategic Approaches to Revisions of Microvascular Oromandibular Reconstructions.

6.4 Upper Facial Recontouring after Facial Tumor Ablation.

6.5 Osteoradionecrosis of the mandible

6.1 The fate of different reconstructive modes for mandibular ameloblastomas

Mandibular ameloblastomas are not infrequently seen. However, most of the patients were primarily treated by oral surgeons, ENT surgeons or surgeons who were not comfortable with vascularized bone transfers. Therefore, many patients were left with formidable complications as malocclusion, deviation of chin, facial deformity, chronic intraoral/ extraoral drainage, extrusion and infection of dead bone, soft tissue wasting or even ultimate extrusion of the implant.

Material and methods

In 15 years, 57 patients were referred to us for management of the aforementioned problems, only 9 patients with mandibular ameloblastoma were treated primarily by the plastic surgeons. In 57 patients, 21 were reconstructed with nonvascularized bone, 10 of them were complicated with chronic drainage, and 11 of them were complicated with remarkable facial deformity. Thirty six out of the 57 patients were reconstructed with reconstruction plate without incorporation of bone. Ten patients were referred for progressive soft tissue wasting, 32 were referred for overt facial deformity, and 15 of them were referred for extrusion of the implant. The 9 patients treated primarily by the plastic surgeons all obtained satisfactory long term result.

The complicated cases were then reconstructed with vascularized iliac bone in 44 patients, vascularized fibula in 13 patients. The presenting symptoms were deformation and loosening of plates, soft tissue wasting, ended up with chronic drainage and ultimately extrusion of the plates.

6.1.1 Problems and difficulties of reconstructions with implant failures

1) Scarring and capsule formation around implants. 2) Difficulty in dissecting and approaching the glenoid fossa. 3) Lack of a clear plane to expand the pocket to accommodate a vascularized bone camouflaged ascending ramus. 4) Possibility of facial nerve injury or traction during dissection or expansion. 5) Placement of incision should be carefully designed since there had been soft tissue atrophy and thinning of skin.

Secondary mandibular reconstruction after implant failure may cause facial nerve injury or difficulty in approaching the glenoid fossa. Fascia lata sling operation is always required in hemimandibular reconstruction in patients with implant failures. Use of mandibular implants as a reconstruction tool should be limited. It is advised that vascularized bone is always the material of choice in major mandibular reconstructions.

6.2 Strategy of reconstructing combined mandibular defect and facial palsy

Either a significant mandibular bone defect or facial palsy presents a challenge to plastic surgeons. When these two conditions are present at the same time, the situation becomes even more complicated. The sequence of reconstruction should be thoroughly contemplated. The scars following a free osteocutaneous flap reconstructed mandibular defect will hamper further exploration of facial nerve lesion and vice versa. Here we report 5 patients with combined mandibular defects and facial palsy. The first case was a 28-year-old woman with an osteogenic sarcoma at left mandibular ramus. She underwent tumor resection, which was complicated with left complete facial palsy. Besides, left hemimandibulectomy was performed for osteoradionecrosis of the mandible as a complication of post-operative irradiation. The severely deformed face lasted for 6 years before she was referred for further reconstruction. An iliac osteocutaneous free flap was used for her mandibular defect followed by a temporalis muscle transfer in order to correct the deviated face. The second case was a 19-year-old young man who suffered from crush injury of the face resulting in right mandibular defect and right facial palsy. The patient received a fibular osteocutaneous free flap reconstruction and cross facial nerve grafting simultaneously. The 3rd patient was a lady with malignant parotid tumor, status post-tumor resection with subsequent radiotherapy. She was complicated with osteoradionecrosis of the mandible. Then, hemimandibulectomy and reconstruction with a plate was done by an oral surgeon which resulted in extrusion of the implant and significant facial deformity. The plate was removed and reconstructed with a vascularized scapular flap for the mandible and fascia sling operation for facial palsy. The last 2 cases were victims of oral cancer. Mandibular defect and lower facial palsy resulted after radical surgery. The bony defects were reconstructed with vascularized iliac bone and the lower facial palsy was reconstructed with masseter transfer and contralateral lower lip depressor myectomy. All the 5 patients demonstrated satisfactory functional and aesthetic results.

When mandibular reconstruction and facial nerve operations were carried out separately, it will be difficult to dissect out the facial nerve after mandibular reconstruction, and vice versa. For long-standing facial palsy as in the first case, static muscle transfer provides an alternative. There leaves much to be discussed about the reconstruction for patients with combined mandibular defect and facial palsy.

6.3 Strategic approaches to revisions of microvascular oromandibular reconstructions

Free tissue transfers have been employed for reconstructing oro-maxillo-mandibular defects in the past 30 years in our hands, amounting several thousands of patients.

Reconstruction of major oro-maxillo-mandibular defects employing microvascular free tissue transfers are always time-consuming task. In order to quarantee the survival of the flap, certain degree of swelling or tissue excess is usually inevitable. However, excellent result can always be obtained by virtue of proper selection of transferred tissue flap and post-operative refinement based on the basic plastic surgical and maxillofacial surgical principles. However, revisions are always the rule in order to reach an optimal result. The problems encountered can be summarized as:

6.3.1 Scar contractures - intra-oral/ extra-oral trapdoor scar contractures

Scar contracture at the oro-maxillo-facial area is inevitable in most of the reconstructed face. Mild forms may be released with Z-plasties, or W-plasty. Moderate contractures may be released with the addition of full-thickness skin grafts. Severe contractures should employ local flap or partial skin flap transposition with preformed free tissue flap (Revolving Door Switch-over Flap Technique).

6.3.2 Facial palsies - partial/ total

Complete facial palsy or paresis of branches of the facial nerve may be left with orofacial surgeries. For complete facial palsies, immediate bridging nerve grafting / hypoglossal nerve grafting/ cross facial nerve grafting can achieve satisfactory results. For facial paresis with incomplete recovery, cross facial nerve grafting with proper neurotization can significantly augment the facial reanimation. For weakness of the depressor anguli oris/

depressor labii inferioris, chemical denervation of the contralateral counterpart with botulinum toxin A can alleviate the asymmetry of the lower lip expressions.

6.3.3 Oral incompetence causing drooling

Oral incompetence often occurs after lip cancer/ buccal cancer/ gingival cancer operations. Therefore, it's advised that preservation of part of the orbicularis oris muscle and proper anatomical restoration is of utmost importance during tumor surgery, otherwise drooling will become a formidable and an unwelcome morbidity.

6.3.4 Loss of skeletal support

In mandibular tumors which resulted in insufficient skeletal height or even segmental bony defect, oral incompetence may also be noticeable with frequent sucking behavior during speaking.

6.3.5 Skin color mismatch

Partial skin resection and reconstruction at the face may result in skin color mismatch with possible trapdoor deformity, which necessitates further disposal.

6.3.6 Mandibular implant extrusions

Many of the mandibular reconstructions were done by ENT or dental-oral surgeons with bridging implant only without bony reconstruction or with conventional bone graft which ultimately resolved. In the long run, not only the implant extruded, but also the neighboring soft tissue would significantly shrink after daily friction which deemed to wasting with peri-implant capsular contracture.

6.3.7 Facial asymmetry / disfigurement

Facial asymmetry with different degree may be recontoured with addition of volume with fat grafting or injection with soft tissue fillers in order to minimize facial disfigurement.

Based on the experiences of doing more than 1500 oro-maxillo-mandibular reconstructions in our plastic surgery groups, we present our strategies in pursuing good results for our patients. There are a lot of amendment procedures to be carried out aiming at achieving not only functional recovery, but also aesthetic restoration. The procedures are as follows:

1. Release of trismus, deepening of buccogingival sulcus.
2. Debulking, Z plasties or W-plasty to alleviate trapdoor scarring.
3. Muscle transfers or tendon sling operation for facial palsies.
4. Skeletal recontouring.
5. Restoring oral competence/ oral commissuroplasty.
6. Fat grafting or using soft tissue fillers
7. Botulinum toxin A injection for dynamic asymmetry

With deliberate planning and proficient skills, optimal results can always be achieved ultimately. Details in dealing with miscellaneous problems in several representative patients will be presented and thoroughly discussed.

7. Case presentations

Case 1. Reconstruction for secondary mandibular deformity

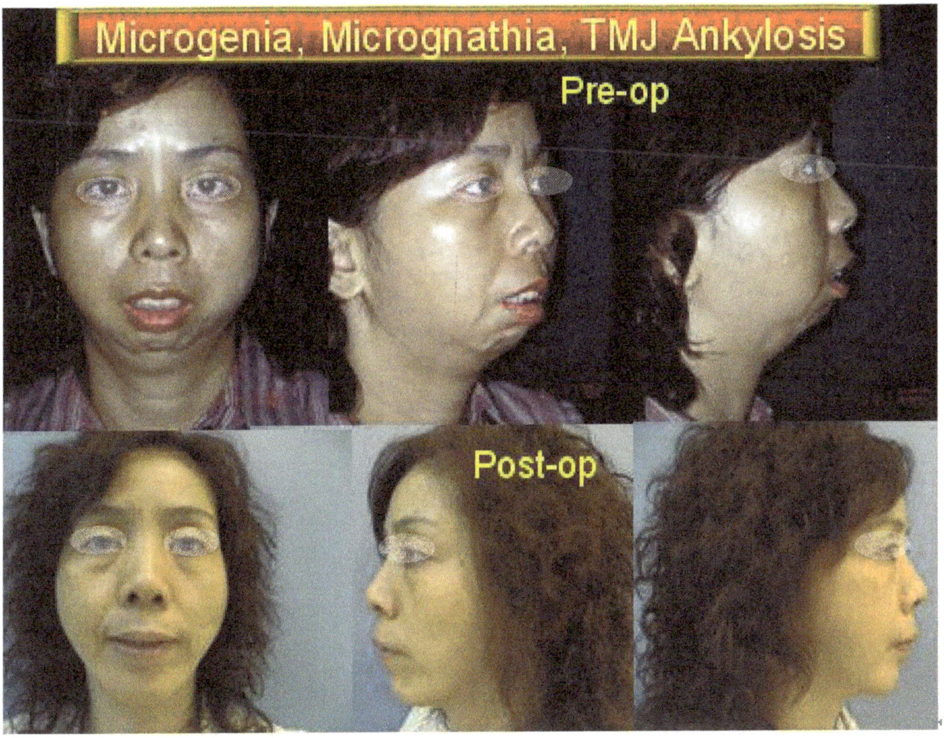

Fig. 1. Microgenia, Micrognathia, TMJ Ankylosis. This 42 year-old lady became microgenic and micrognathic with oral incompetence since she was very young due to some kind of ailment that she can not remember very well. She always shun herself from the public for not having a chin. Orthognathic surgery with bilateral sagittal split osteotomy, sliding genioplasty and Medpor chin implant placement were carried out after orthodontic treatment. She has been very satisfied with the operation.

Case 2. Reconstruction of combined major mandibular deficiency and facial palsy

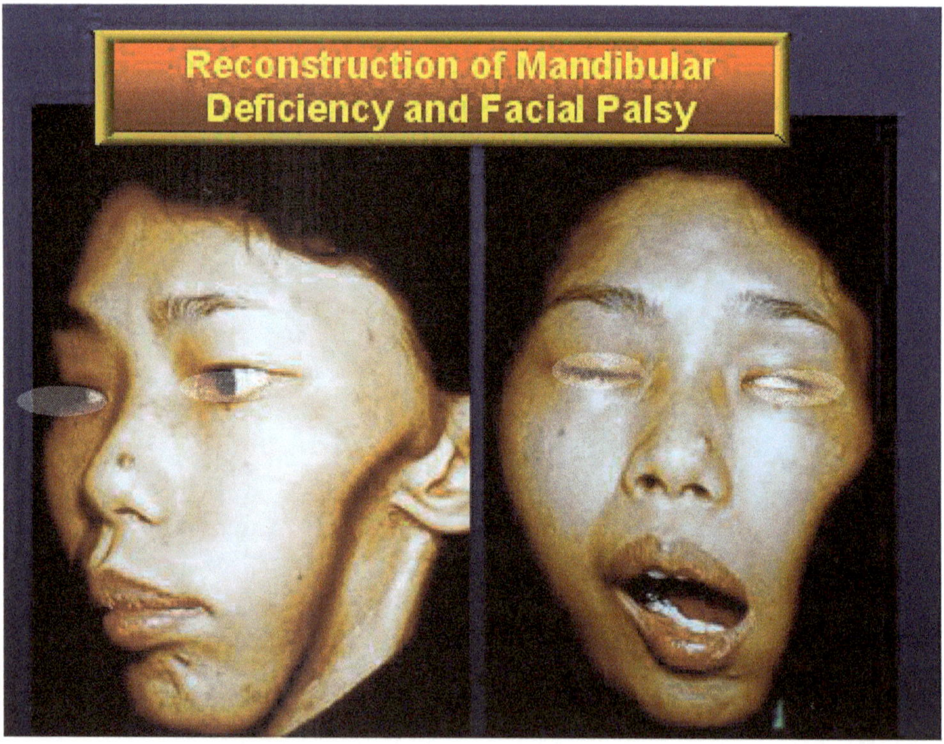

Combined Mandibular Deficiency and Facial Palsy. This 28 year-old lady suffered from osteogenic sarcoma at the left mandibular ramus at the age of 18.

Fig. 2.1. Reconstruction of Mandibular Deficiency and Facial Palsy.

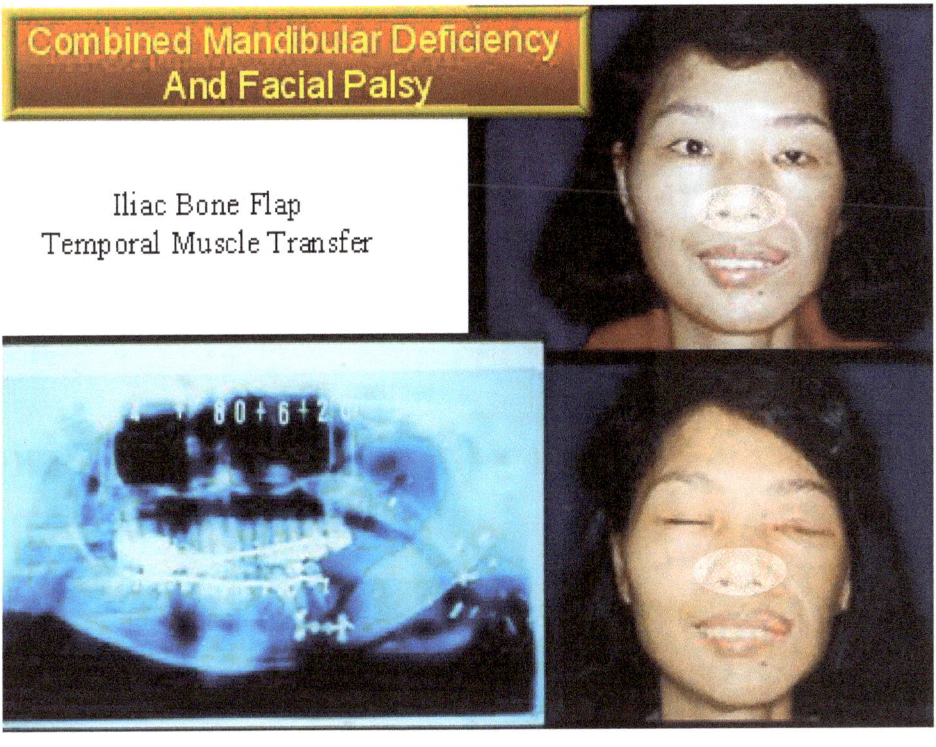

Fig. 2.2. Post-op. Combined Mandibular Deficiency and Facial Palsy. She received tumor excision by an ENT surgeon, and then was told to receive radiotherapy. She was then complicated with left facial palsy and osteoradionecrosis of the mandible and resulting in hemimandibulectomy. Since then, she suffered from a severely deformed face. Under her request, we reconstructed her left mandible with vascularized iliac bone flap which restored not only the hemimandibular defect but also soft tissue deficiency after previous extremely destructive surgery. After 6 months, we used left side temporalis muscle transfer and partial masseter muscle transfer to balance her left side face with that of the right side and also to treat left lagophthalmos.

Case 3. Reconstruction of upper facial deformity

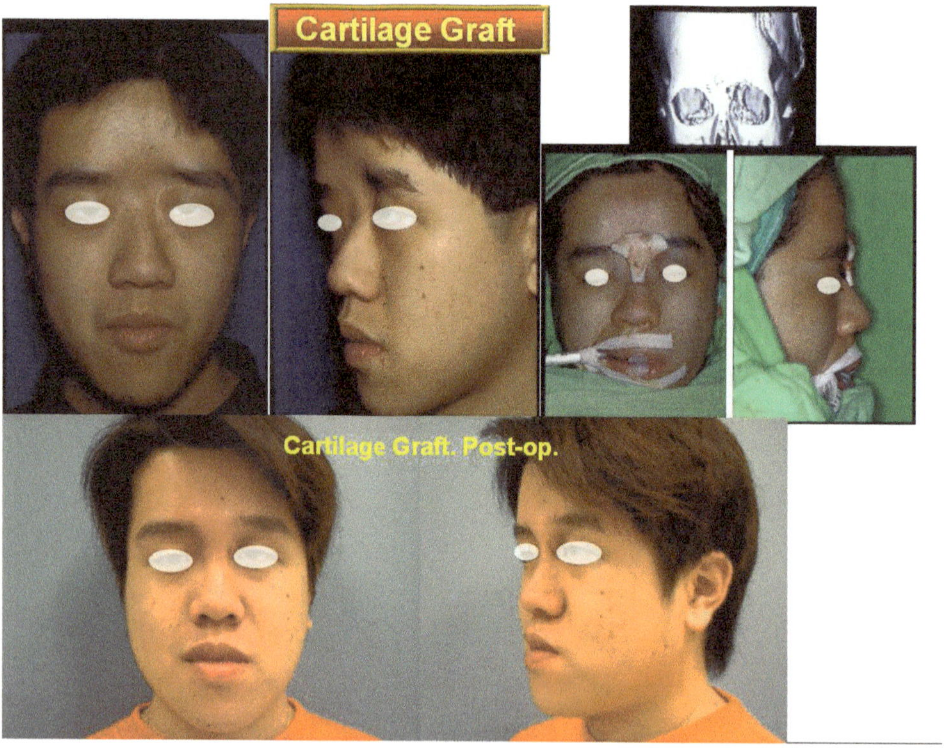

Fig. 3. Fronto-naso-orbital Defect
This 18 year-old boy was found to have a tumor at the left fronto-naso-orbital area when he was 6 year-old. Pathology after excision revealed an eiosinophilic granuloma, he then received chemotherapy afterwards. As he grew up, hypoplasia of the fronto-naso-orbital complex bothered him greatly. In order to recontour this area, we harvested a costal cartilage block which was carved to match the 3 dimensional configuration of the defect, and then wrapped with fascia graft, to be inserted into the defect through an incision at the frontal scalp. He then got a satisfactory facial contour.

Case 4. Reconstruction of mandibular implant extrusion

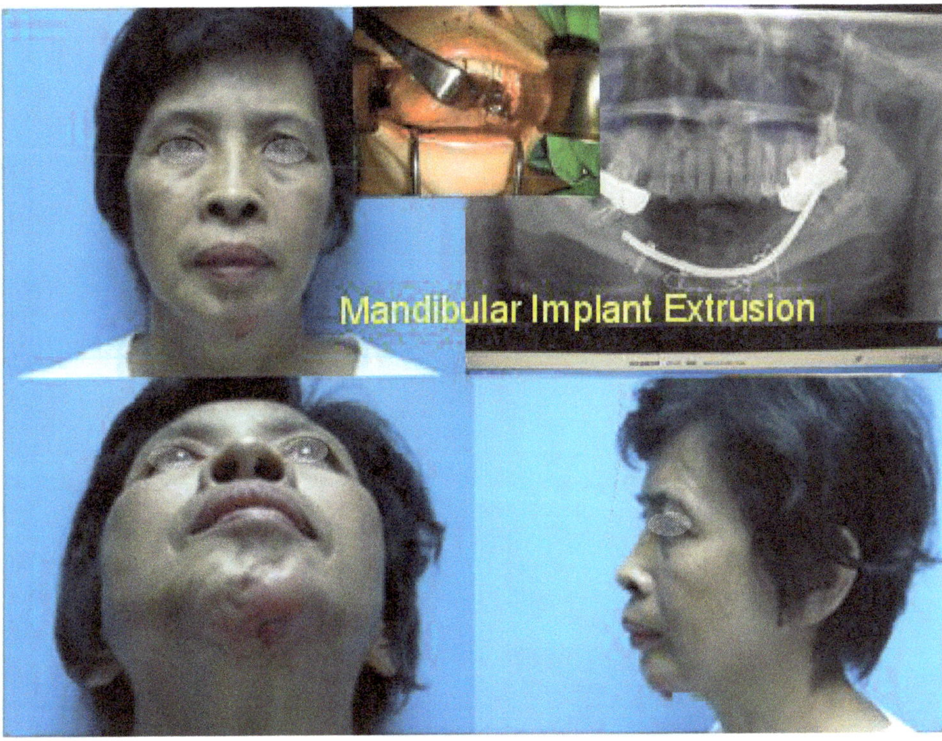

Fig. 4.1. Pre-op. This 56 year-old lady suffered from ameloblastoma of the mandibular symphysis 10 years previously. She received segmental mandibulectomy by an dental surgeon, and at the same time was reconstructed with a curved metallic implant. Several years later, she started to notice deformity of the chin, and then furtherly complicated with chronic drainage from the bottom of the chin with pointing out of the sharp tip of the implant piercing out the left side lower vestibular sulcus mucosa.

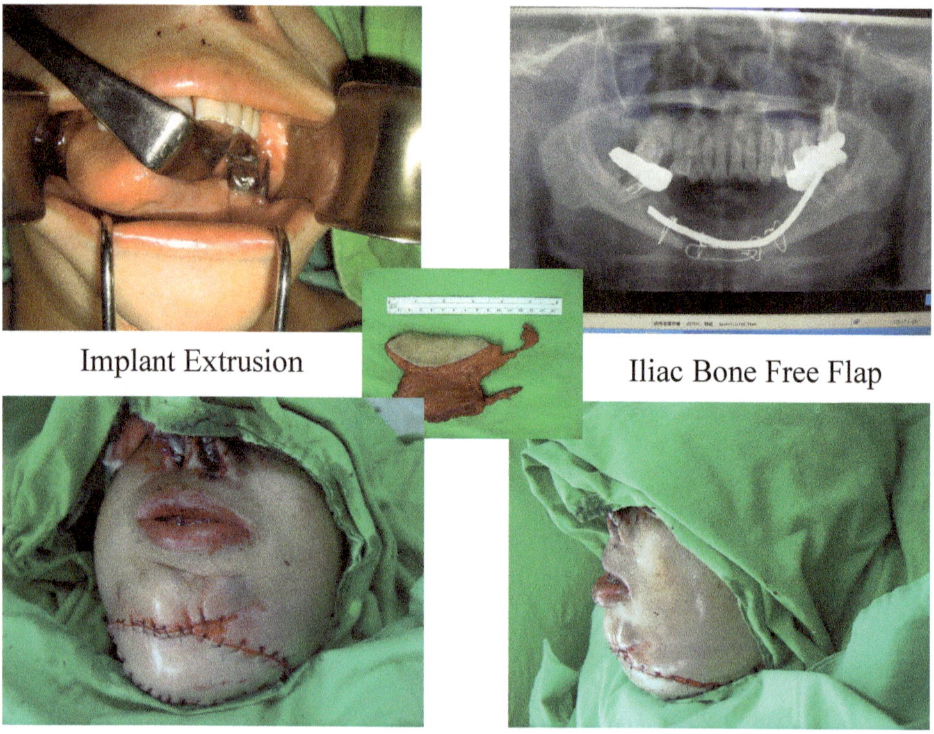

Fig. 4.2. At the first operation, the extruded and infected implant was removed and the wound was debrided thoroughly and the defect of the mandibular symphysis, skin and soft tissue was reconstructed with a vascularized iliac bone flap with complete success.

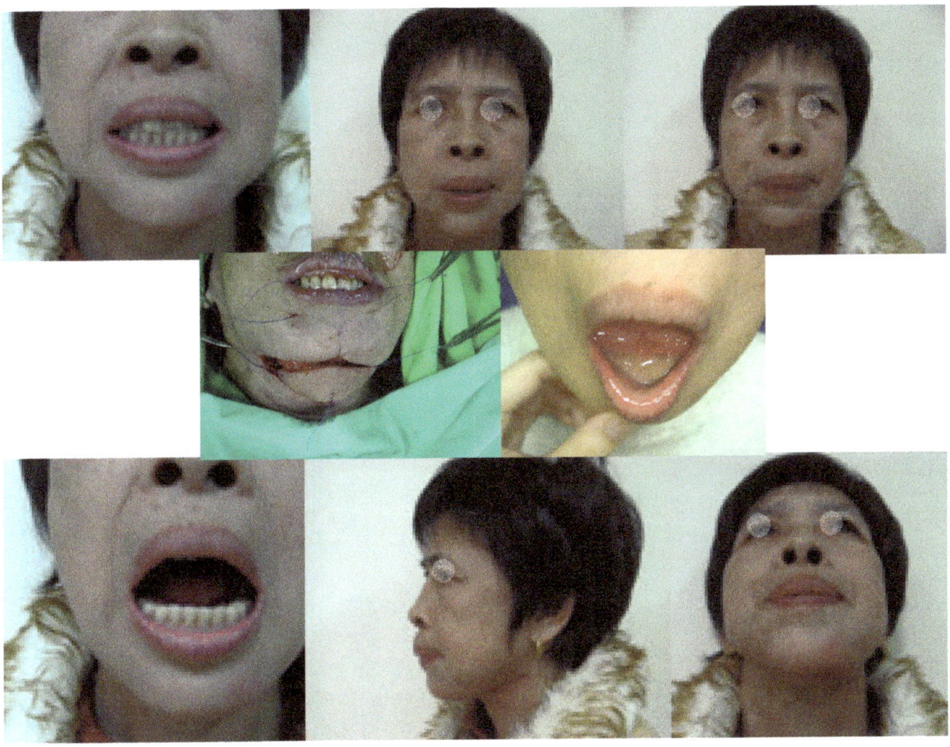

Fig. 4.3. Post-op. After 6 months, bone union had been secured and swelling of the reconstructed skin and soft t tissue bulk had subsided, the excess skin flap at the chin was used to deepen the insufficient lower sulcus by using the revolving door switch-over technique. In addition to deepen the sulcus to better accommodate dental implant placement, this measure also provided ample soft tissue for chin augmentation.

Case 5. Immediate anatomical restoration for mandibular ameloblastoma

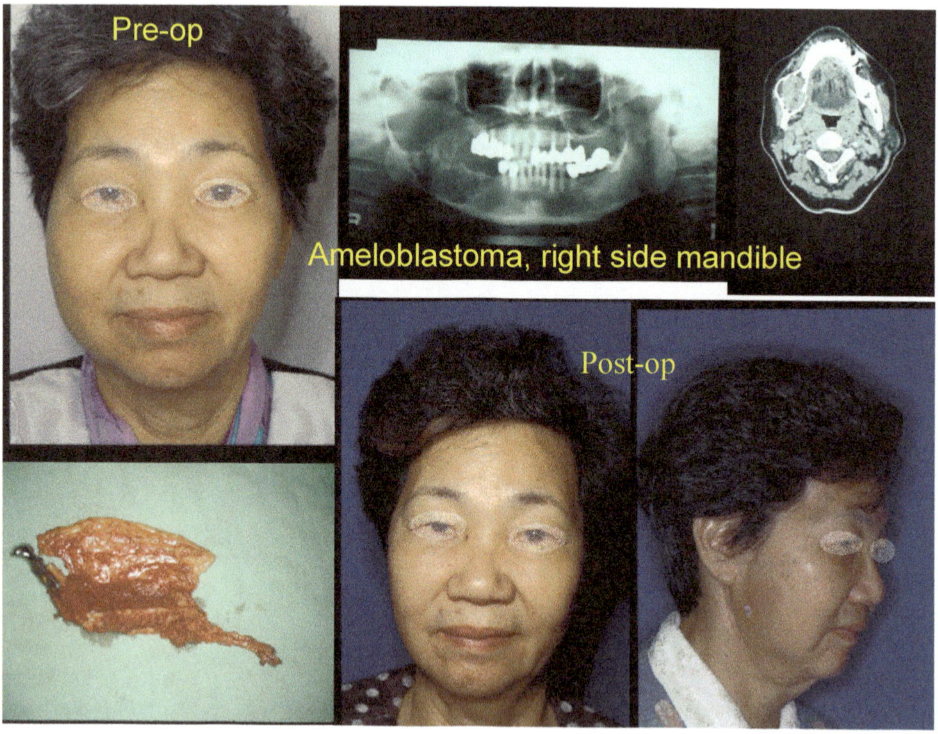

Fig. 5. This 63 year-old lady started to notice that she cannot open her mouth freely, and finally was found that she had a giant ameloblastoma at her right side mandibular body, extending to right mandibular ramus, condyle and coronoid process. She can hardly open her mouth as the tumor grew bigger and bigger. The tumor was resected en bloc, and at the same time replaced with a fibular osteocutaneous flap incorporating with a piece of titanium condyle to reconstruct her right side mandible and buccogingical lining. After 6 months, she received autogenous fat injection to further augment her right cheek for better facial contour and symmetry.

Case 6. Osteoradionecrosis of the mandible

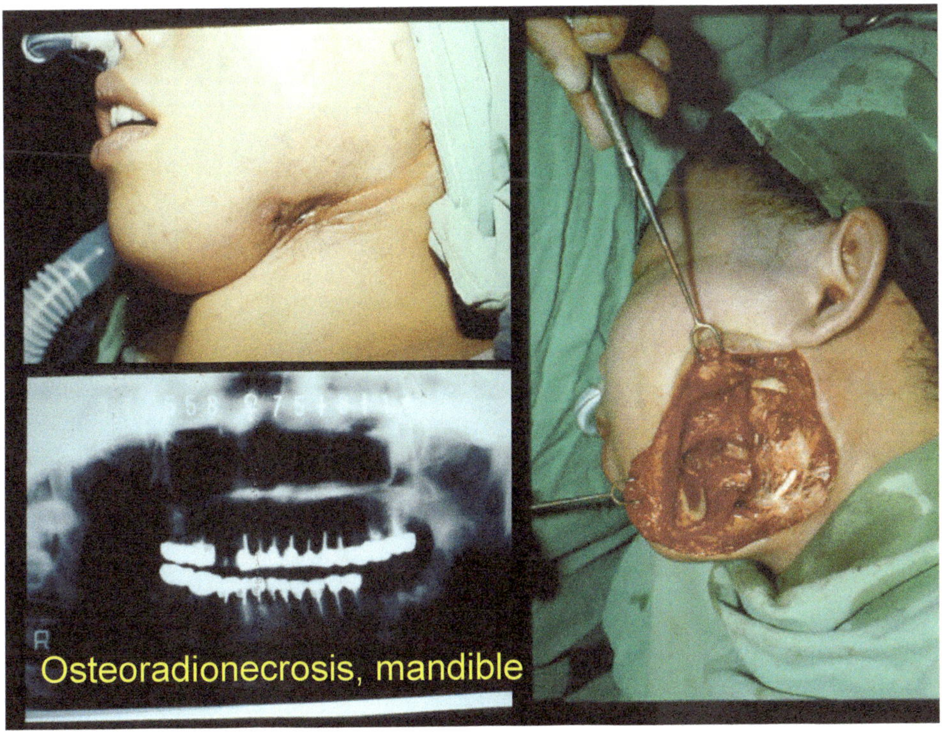

Fig. 6.1. This 42 year-old lady contracted a left submandibular tumor when she was 24 year-old. After resection, the pathology report revealed a mucoepidermoid carcinoma of the submandibular gland. She was arranged to receive radiotherapy. Eighteen years after the treatment, she suffered from left lower jaw teeth pain. Ever since teeth extraction by the dentist, the wound never healed and furthermore complicated with foul odor discharge from left side mandible, despite of 80 treatments of hyperbaric oxygen. Besides, she also suffered from intractable pain. Therefore, the osteonecrotic mandible was resected and the wound debrided thoroughly.

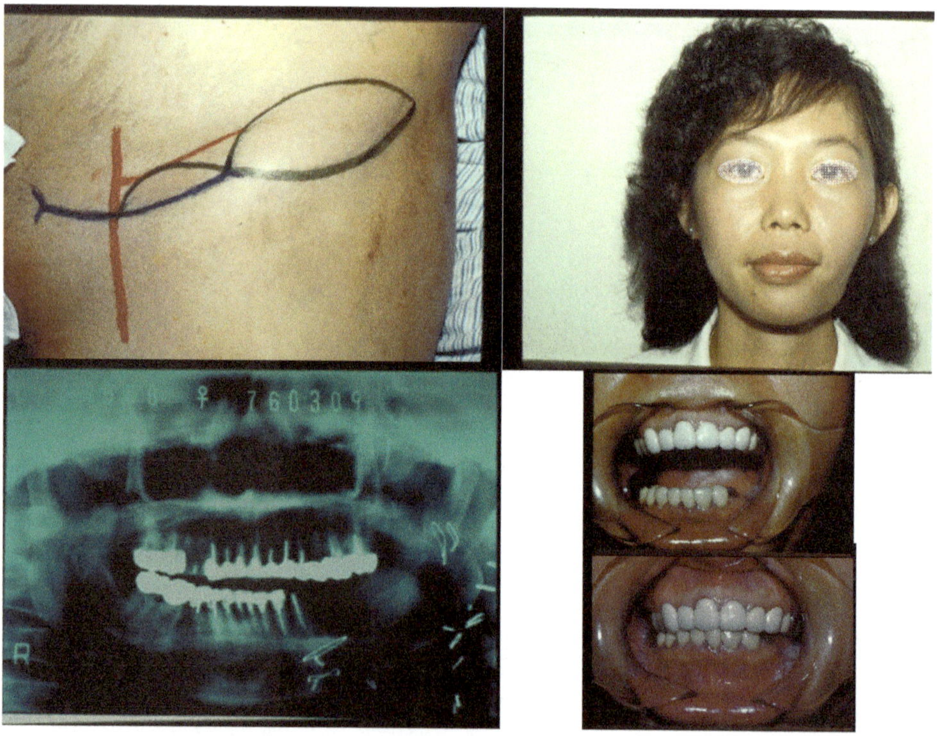

Fig. 6.2. The defect was reconstructed with a piece of vascularized iliac bone flap harvested from ipsilateral side with complete success. Besides maintaining satisfactory facial contour and symmetricity, the patient assumed good occlusion and can open her mouth freely without trismus.

Case 7. Reconstruction of secondary facial deformity

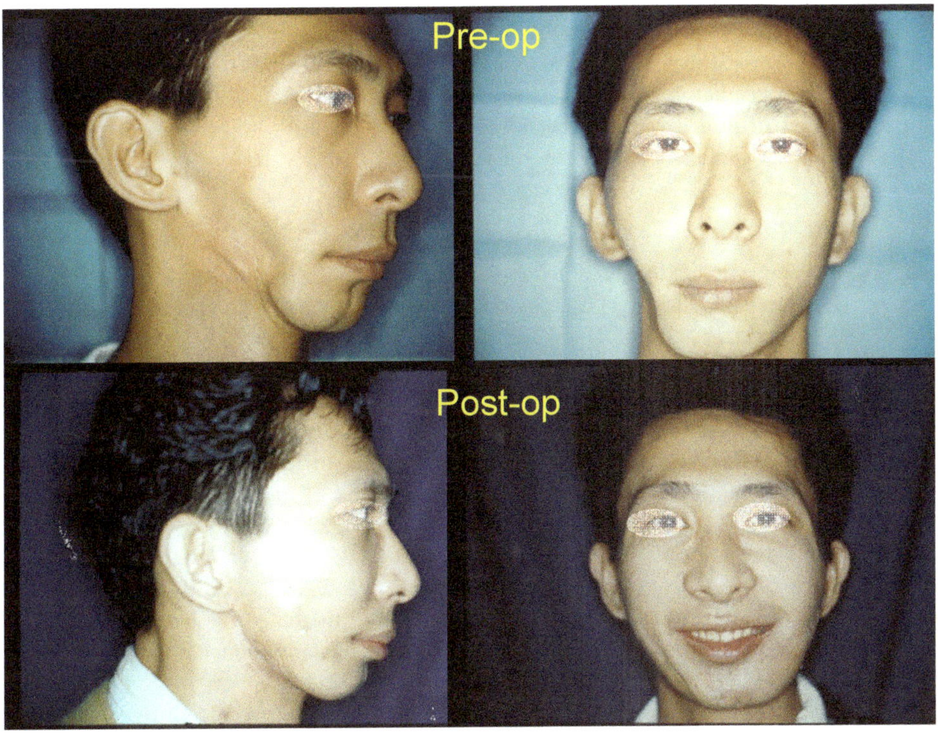

Fig. 7. This 25 year-old young man received resection of right side mandible by dental surgeons for ameloblastoma. He was left with a sunken cheek and deformed face, and became autistic and reluctant to go out. We reconstructed his right side mandible with a fibular osteocutaneous flap with 2 osteotomies and incorporating with a titanium mandibular condyle. After the operation, he regained facial symmetricity and normal facial contour, therefore resumed his bright smile again.

8. Conclusions

There are miscellaneous methods aiming at recontouring of the face for different purposes. Anatomical restoration is always the rule of thumb to achieve satisfactory aesthetic result. Overall, a comprehensive approach with integration of craniofacial surgery, microsurgery, aesthetic surgery and basic plastic surgical techniques will get to most outstanding results.

9. Acknowledgement

Reconstructions of facial derangements are usually time-consuming, and sometimes multi-stage tasks. Team approach is always a must. Here we would like to express our sincere thanks to whom ever joined the tedious works described in this text. Without their help, the difficult reconstructions can not be accomplished. The authors also have to give thanks to Mavis Kuo for her proficiency in editing this chapter.

10. References

Chao-Hsiang Lee, Ming Ting Chen, Yueh-Bih Tang*. (2008) Reappraisal of Using Platysma Myocutaneous Flap for Lower Facial Reconstruction. The Journal of Plastic surgical Association. ROC. Vol. 17, No.1, p.24-34.

Chen, CK. & Tang, YB. (2009). Myectomy and botulinum toxin for paralysis of the marginal mandibular branch of the facial nerve: a series of 76 cases. *Plast Reconstr Surg*. 2007 Dec; 120(7): 1859-64 SCI (27/167) Surgery. 2009

Chen, NC. ; Tai, HC. ; Chien, HF. & Tang, YB. (2002) Ancillary Procedures in Refining Microvascular Oromandibular Reconstructions. Proceedings of 18th Annual meeting of Taiwan Surgical Association. (2002/ 3/23-24). P173

Cheng NC, Ko JY, Tai HC, Horng SY, Tang YB*. (2008) Microvascular head and neck reconstruction in patients with liver cirrhosis. Head Neck. Vol.30, No.7, p.829-35.

Cheng, NC. ; Chen, MT. ; Tang, YB. & Tai, HC. (2005). Immediate Free Flap Reconstruction in the Management of Advanced Mandibular Osteoradionecrosis. *The Journal of Plastic surgical Association. ROC.* 2005 Vol. 14, No. 2, p.121-130.

Cheng, NC. ; Hsie, RH. ; Tai, HC. & Tang, YB. (2004). Ancillary Procedures for Refining Major Oromandibular Reconstructions. Proceedings of 19th Annual meeting of Taiwan Surgical Association. (2004 /3/27-28) P231

Colenan, JJ. & Woden, WA. (1990). Mandibular reconstruction with composite microvascular tissue transfer. *Am J Surg* 1990; 160 :390-5.

Hidalgo, DA. (1989). Fibula free flap: a new method of mandible reconstruction. *Plast Reconstr Surg* 1989 ;84 :71-9.

Hsieh, MH. ; Huang, CM. ; Peng, SF. ; Chen, CM. ; Wong, JM. & Tang, YB. (2003). Using Image Segmentation Technique in the Treatment of Craniofacial Soft Tissue Neoplasm. Proceedings of 18th Annual meeting of Taiwan Surgical Association. (2003/ 3/29-30). P220

Hung-Chi Chen, Ming-huei Cheng, Yueh-Bih Tang. (2003) Head and Neck Reconstruction in Trauma and Cancer. Seminars in Plastic Surgery, Vol. 17, No.1, p.23-37.

Hung-chi Chen, Yueh-bih Tang, Kuo-Lian Tseng. (2001) The Anatomical Variations of Posterior Interosseous Artery. Congress of the International Societies of the Hand (IFSSH) Turkey, Istanbul. (6/10-14) p.239-40.

Hung-chi Chen, Yueh-bih Tang, Kuo-Lian Tseng. (2001) Treatment for Avascular Necrosis of Scaphoid With Microvascular Free Cortico-periosteal Flap. Congress of the International Societies of the Hand (IFSSH). Turkey, Istanbul. (6/10-14) p.594-6.

Lei-Ming Sun, Han-Ming Tsung, Yuh-Yuan Shian, Shyh-Jye Chen, Ching-Shiow Tzeng, Yueh-Bih Tang *. (2002) Computer- Generated Simulation Template for Fronto-Naso- Orbtal Reconstruction. Formosan Journal of Surgery. Vol.35, No. 1. p.28-33.

Mark, RJ. ; Sercarz, JA. & Tran, L. et al (1991). Osteogenic sarcoma of the head and neck. The UCLA experience. *Arch Otolaryngol Head Neck Surg* 1991;117 :761-6.

Mon-Hsian Hsieh*, Shing-Guang Lai, Yueh-Bih Tang. (2005) Correction of the Webbed Neck Deformity in Noonan Syndrome. The Journal of Plastic surgical Association. ROC. Vol. 14, No. 4, p355-362.

Nai-Chen Cheng, M.D., Dar-Ming Lai, M.D., Mon-Hsian Hsie, M.D., Shu-Lang Liao, M.D., and Yueh-Bih Tang Chen*, M.D., Ph.D.(2006) Intraosseous Hemangiomas of the Facial Bone. Plastic and Reconstructive Surgery. Vol.117, No.7, p.2366-72.

Nai-Chen Cheng, Shyue-Yih Horng*, Shan-Chwen Chang, and Yueh-Bih Tang.(2004) Nosocomial Infection of Aeromonas Hydrophila Presenting as Necrotizing Fasciitis. J Formos Med Assoc. Vol.103, p.53-7.

Tang Chen, YB. (1999). Salvage mandibular Reconstructions after Implant Failures. Proceedings of 13th Symposium of the International Society of Reconstructive Microsurgery, (6/22-25) Los Angeles, USA.

Tang Chen, YB. & Chen, HC. (1995). Finesse in Microvascular Oromandibular Reconstruction. *Proceedings of Plastic, Reconstructive and Aesthetic Surgery*. p.531 San Francisco, USA.

Tang Chen, YB. ; Lai, SG. ; Chen, HC. (2003). Reconstruction of Combined Mandibular Defect and Facial Plasy. *Proceedings of the 8th Confederation of the International Society of Plastic, Reconstructive and Aesthetic Surgery*. Aug. Sydney, Australia.

Tang YB. & Hahn LJ. (1990). Major Mandibular Reconstruction with Vascularized Bone Graft. *J Formosan Med Assoc*, vol.89, No.1, p.34-40

Tang, YB. (1993). Long Term Survival of Mandibular Osteosarcoma. *British Journal of Plastic Surgery*. 1999; Apr; Vol.52, No.3, p.243-4

Tang, YB. (1997) Esthetic Considerations after Major Mandibular Reconstruction. The 90th Taiwan Medical Academic Lecture of Formosan Medical Association.(11/10) Taipei, Taiwan.

Tang, YB. (2008). Strategic Approaches to Revisions of Microvascular Oromandibular Reconstructions. Proceedings of American Society for Reconstructive Microsurgery 2008 Annual Meeting. Beverly Hills, USA.

Tang, YB. (2009). Long-term Outcome of Reconstructions for Mandibular Implant Failures. Proceedings of IPRASAP.(Oct) Tokyo, Japan

Tang, YB. (2009). Mandibular Reconstructions, Selection of Method according to the Ultimate Results. Proceedings of the 5th Congress of the World Society for Reconstructive Microsurgery.(1/10-13) Hawaii, USA

Tang, YB. (2009). The Fate of Different Reconstructive Modes for Mandibular Ameloblastomas. Proceedings of American Society for Reconstructive Microsurgery 2009 Annual Meeting. (1/10-13) Hawaii, USA.

Tang, YB. ; Chen, HC. & Hahn, LJ. (1994). Major Mandibular Reconstruction with Vascularized Bone Grafts-Indications and Selection of Donor Tissue, *Microsurgery*. Vol.15, p.227-237.

Taylor, GI. (1982). Reconstruction of the mandible with free composite iliac bone grafts. *Ann Plast Surg* Vol.9, p.361-76.

Taylor, GI. ; Townsend, P. & Corlett, R. (1979). Superiority of the deep circumflex iliac vessels as the supply for free groin flaps. *Plast Reconstr Surg* Vol.64, p.745-59.

Wang, CH. ; Horng, SY. & Tang, YB. (2002). Comparison of Vascularized Iliac and Fibular Bone Graft in Oromandibular Reconstruction. Proceedings of 18th Annual meeting of Taiwan Surgical Association.(3/23-24) p.174

Yoshimura, M. ; Shimarrura, K. & Yoshinobu, I. et al. (1983). Free vascularized fibular transplant, *J Bone Joint Surg Ser A.*. Vol., 65A, p.1295-301.

Yueh-Bih Tang*, C. H. Lee, and Y. M. Su. (2005) Aesthetic Facial Recontouring. Formosan Journal of Medicine Vol.2 No.9, p.214-222.

13

Functional and Aesthetic Reconstruction of the Defects Following the Hemiglossectomy in Patients with Oropharyngeal Cancer

Mutsumi Okazaki
Department of Plastic and Reconstructive Surgery, Graduate School, Tokyo Medical and Dental University, Tokyo
Japan

1. Introduction

In the patients who undergo the hemiglossectomy and reconstruction with free flap transfer, remaining oropharyngeal tissue and function is relatively large, and majority of patients recover speech and eating function, which allow them to live a normal life. Actually, many reports have described that the functional results are generally good after the reconstruction with flaps following hemiglossectomy [1-9]. However, it is rather difficult to perform the reconstruction that makes the best of remaining tissue and function. In this chapter, we describe our reconstructive concept and procedures from the plastic surgeon's standpoint, together with presenting the unfavorable results.

2. Concept of reconstruction and operative procedure

We itemize our concepts for the reconstruction of the defects following hemiglossectomy. The schematic of our reconstructive procedures is shown in Fig.1 and 2.

1. Employ long but not-voluminous flap because the short and voluminous flap spoil the tongue movement.

The length of flap corresponded to "epiglottic vallecula ~ lingual apex" requires 15~17 cm. The short flap less than 14 cm restricts thrust function of the tongue because the transferred flap has a tendency to shrink longitudinally after the operation. On the other hand, the volume of the flap should not be so large. Because the volume of remaining tongue is preserved enough for the eating function in the patients with hemiglossectomy, voluminous flap does not help but spoil eating and speech function.

2. Restore mobile tongue with long, narrow, and thin flap (Fig. 1 (A)).

After hemiglossectomy, restoration of mobile tongue with a voluminous flap tends to result in spoilage of speech function because a remaining tongue is "burdened with heavy flap". We recommend that the mobile tongue should be restored with long, narrow and thin flap. Namely, the mobile tongue is intentionally restored as long as and thinner than original tongue. We consider this is the best balance of aesthetic and functional restoration.

3. Apply several z-plasties at the back of tongue (Fig. 1 (B)), and oral floor (Fig. 1 (C)).

We often see a postoperative scar contracture along the suture line between flap and remaining tongue, which consequently reduces a range of lingual mobility. From the plastic surgeon's point of view, the occurrence of this scar contracture is inevitable, but it can be prevented to some extent by the application of several z-plasty (or insertion of triangle flap). We also see a contracture at the oral floor. To prevent this contracture, insertion of a triangle flap to the mucosa of oral floor at the ventral base of the tongue is effective (Fig. 1 (C)).

4. Filling dead space of oral floor not with muscle body but with adiposal tissue to avoid postoperative collapse of the oral floor and lingual root (Fig. 1 (D), Fig. 2)).

For the good eating function, appropriate reconstruction of the oral floor is mandatory. If the oral floor might be reconstructed with thin flap, the resultant oral floor would collapse, which occasionally causes the swallowing difficulty. Similarly, if the retro-mandibular dead space might be reconstructed with a muscle body, the muscle body would gradually become atrophic which causes collapse of oral floor. We recommend that the retro-mandibular space should be filled up with adiposal (deepithelized) flap (Fig. 2).

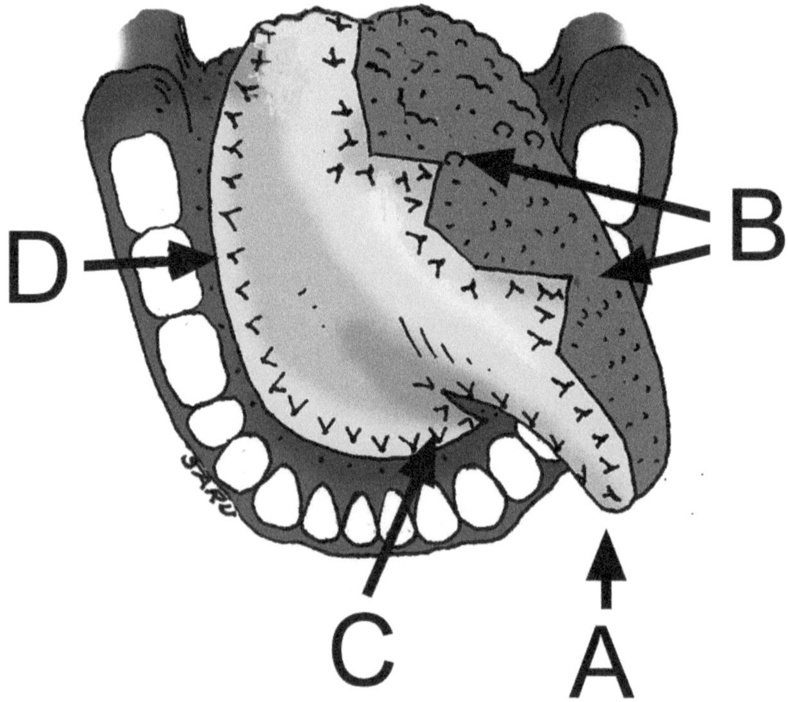

"A" indicates a long, narrow, and thin flap attached to the mobile tongue
"B" indicates the triangle flaps set to the back of tongue
"C" indicates the triangle flap set to to the oral floor
"D" indicates the part

Fig. 1. Schematic of the reconstruction of the defects after hemiglossectomy

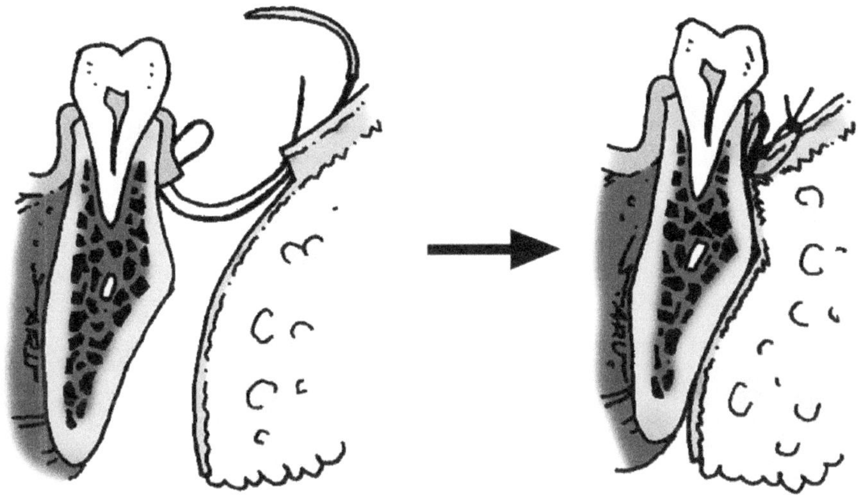

Fig. 2. Schematic of the reconstruction of the retro-mandibular space. A part of the flap is deepithelized and set at the retro-mandibular space attaching the dermis to the mandibular bone

5. Check whether residual tongue is in an appropriate position during flap transfer.

When a patient undergoes the operation under a general anesthesia, a tongue is placed in a glossoptotic position. So sewing of the flap on the tongue is performed pulling a remaining tongue out of a glossoptotic position.

6. Cover the great vessels (carotid artery and jugular vein) with the small muscle body if necessary.

In the patients with high risk of infection or leakage (due to chemo-radiation therapy, diabetes mellitus, and so on), small muscle body is harvested together with a flap during flap elevation, and set on the great vessels to prevent a rupture of them due to a leakage and/or infection.

7. Select appropriate flap depending upon the oral defects and thickness of the fat layer of a patient (whether a patient is obese or slender). We choose an appropriate flap chiefly among the radial forearm, anterolateral thigh, and deep inferior epigastric flap.
8. Choose the appropriate recipient artery among the branches of external carotid or subclavian arteries (referred to as "branch artery" hereafter). Anastomose two flap veins to the internal and external jugular venous system respectively.

When an appropriate branch artery to serve as the recipient is unavailable (ex. in patients with previous operation and/or irradiation therapy), end-to-side anastomosis directly to the external carotid artery (ECA) is a good option. For safer transfer, we recommend that two flap veins (a comitant and a cutaneous vein in the forearm flap, two comittant veins in the anterolateral thigh and inferior epigastric flap) should be anastomosed to the internal and external jugular venous system separately.

3. Representative case

A 57-year-old male patient with the lingual cancer underwent hemiglossectomy and modified radical neck dissection. A deep inferior epigastric flap (15 x 6 cm) with 3 triangle lobe was harvested including small amount of muscle body (Fig.3a). A part of the flap (2 x 7 cm:) was deepithelized to fill the retro-mandibular dead space (Fig. 3a (D)). The flap was sutured to the remaining tongue (Fig. 3b). The inferior epigastric artery was anastomosed to the superior thyroid artery, and two comitant inferior epigastric veins were anastomosed to the internal and external jugular vein respectively. The small muscle body was set on the great vessels. At this point, the reconstructed tongue protruded about 3 cm from incisor line (Fig.3c). Postoperative course was uneventful. The patient recovered good eating and speaking function with aesthetically-satisfactory tongue (Fig. 3d).

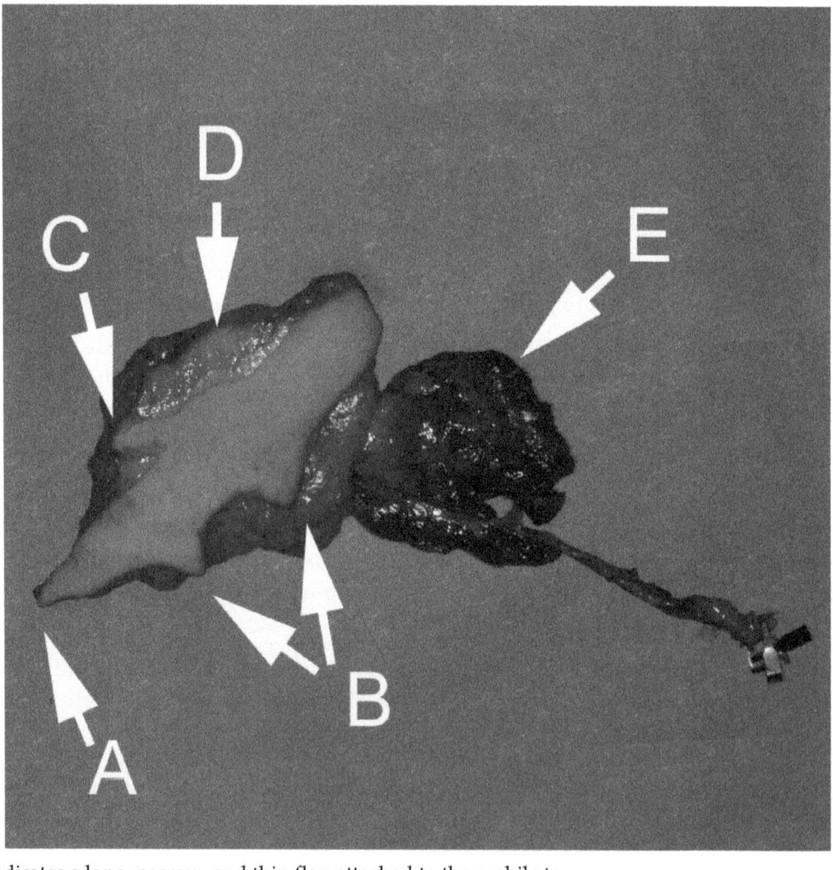

"A" indicates a long, narrow, and thin flap attached to the mobile tongue.
"B" indicates the triangle flaps to be inserted into the back of tongue.
"C" indicates the triangle flap to be inserted into the oral floor at the ventral base of tongue.
"D" indicates the deepithelized flap to be set at the retro-mandibular space.
"E" indicates the muscle body to be set on the great vessels.

Fig. 3a. Harvested flap.

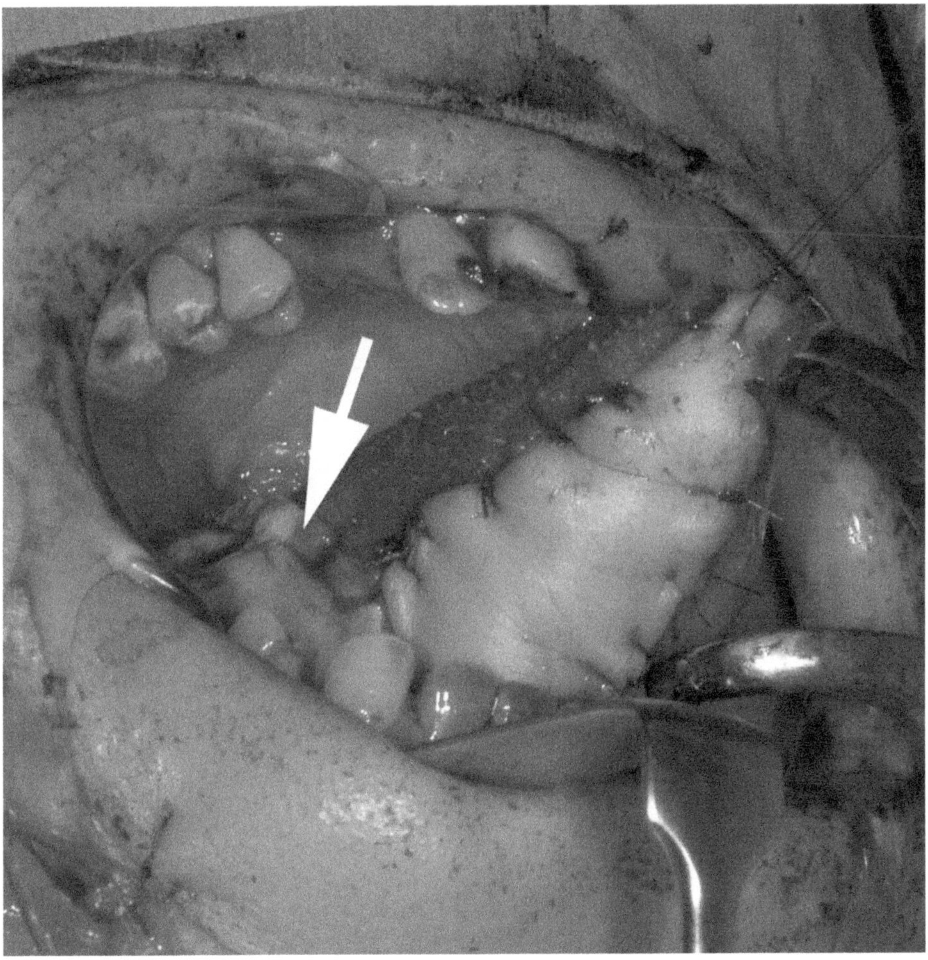

Fig. 3b. Reconstructed tongue. Arrow indicates a triangle flap inserted to the back of tongue.

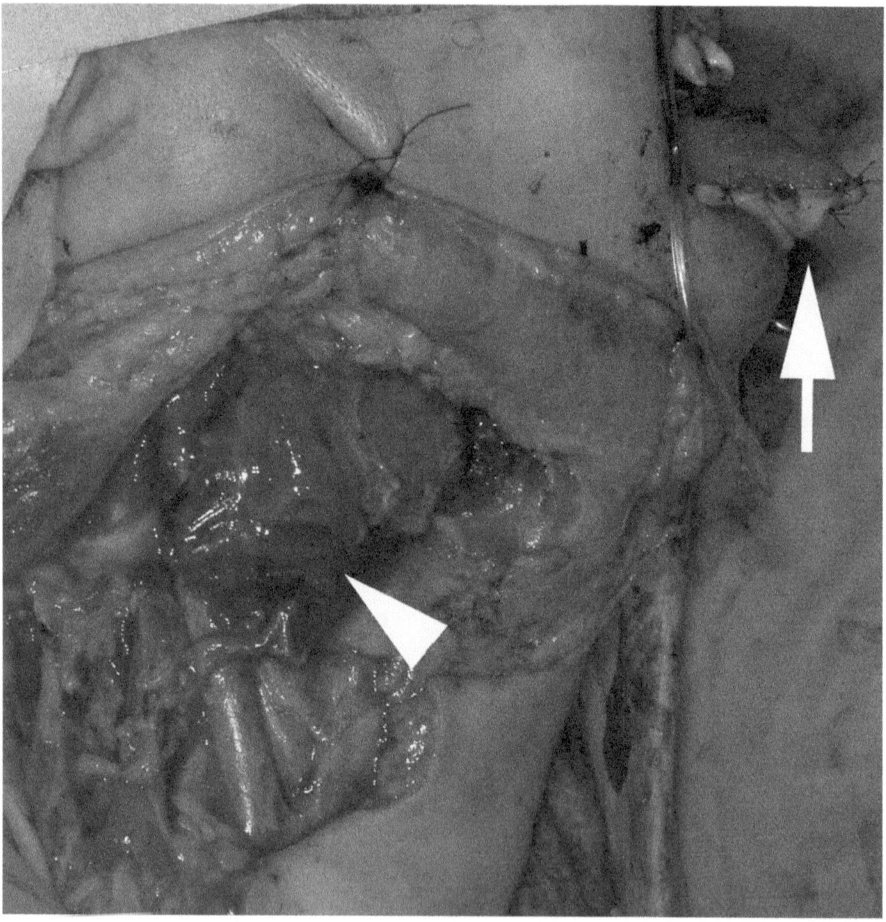

Fig. 3c. Findings of neck just after the vascular anastomosis. Muscle body covers the great vessels (arrowhead). Note the reconstructed tongue tip that protrudes beyond the incisors as it stands (arrow).

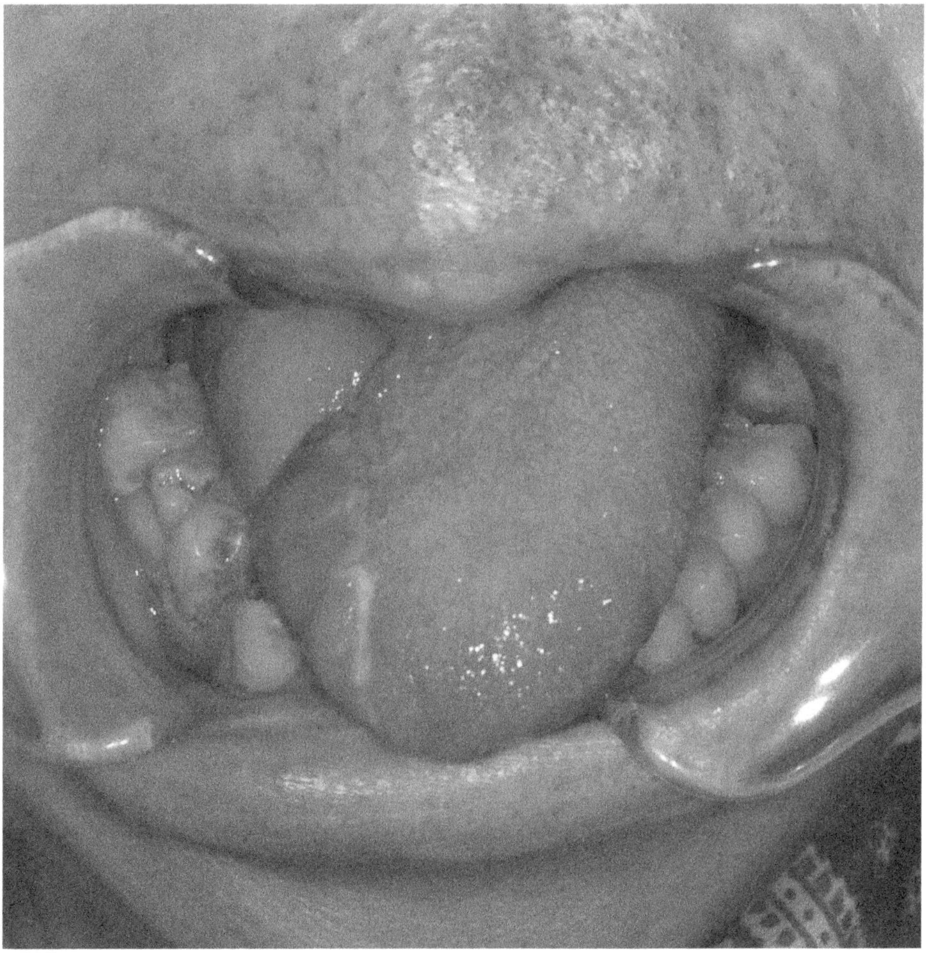

Fig. 3d. Postoperative findings. Although the size of reconstructed tongue is smaller than that of original tongue, the shape of tongue is natural. The eating and speaking function is excellent with wide range of mobility.

4. Discussion

Regarding the volume of the flap for the defects of hemiglossectomy, there was some reports that discuss whether the reconstruction with flap is necessary or not [10,11], but most papers describe that reconstruction with free flap provide good functional results [1-9]. The flaps seen in these papers are comparatively large, and the size of reconstructed tongues is as large as that of original tongue. However, the restoration of mobile tongue with a voluminous flap causes the spoilage of speech function because heavy flap hinders the motion of a remaining tongue (Fig.4a). We consider that the flap that restore the mobile part of the tongue (front half) should be long but thin and narrow.

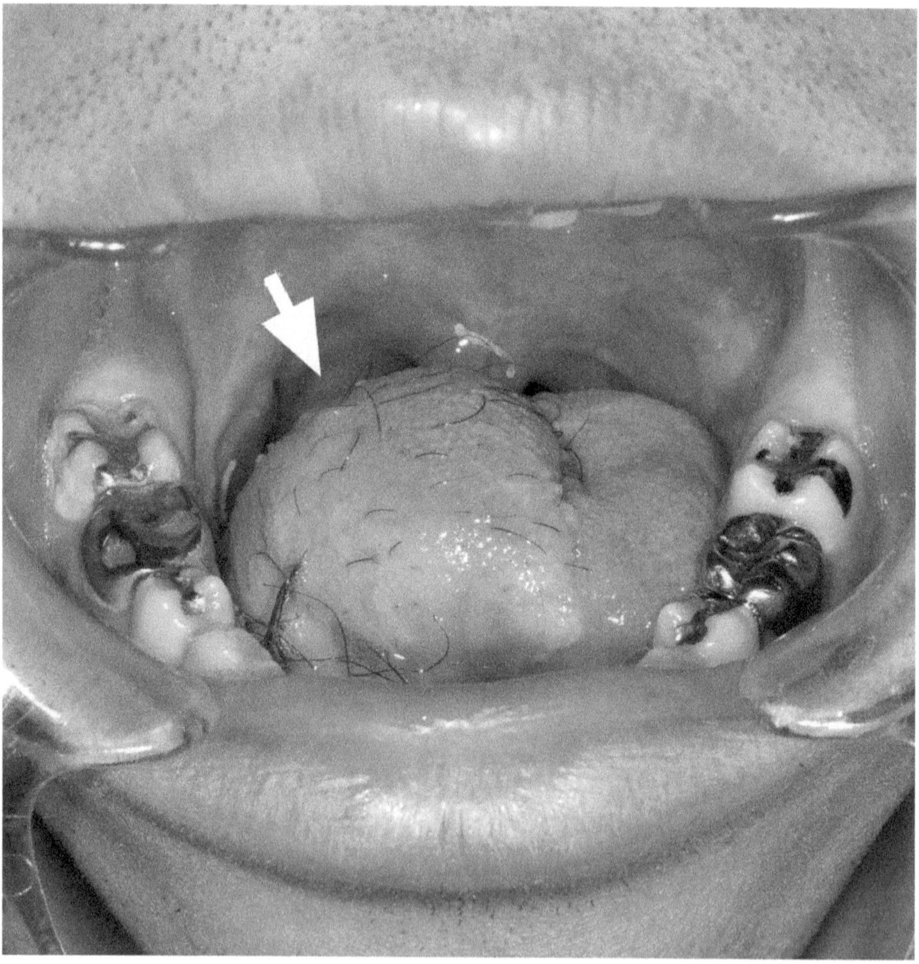

Fig. 4a. Examples of unfavorable results decreased mobility of tongue due to heavy voluminous flap (arrow) (Postoperative findings of a 32-year-old male with lingual cancer who underwent right hemiglossectomy and reconstruction with anterolateral thigh flap).

On the other hand, the lingual root requires some voluminous reconstruction to prevent miss-swallowing or dysphagia. It has been reported that the transferred muscle flap more decrease its volume postoperatively because of the interruption of muscle innervation compared with an adiposal flap [12,13]. So we recommend that lingual root and retro-mandibular space should be reconstructed with adipo-cutaneous tissue, not muscle. A part of the flap is deepithelized (Fig.3a (C)) and set at the retro-mandibular space attaching the dermis to the mandibular bone (Fig.2). We call this method "de-epithelialized flap overlapping method" which is useful also for the prevention of leakage in the flap-gingival suture [14].

Care should be taken whether residual tongue is in an appropriate position when the operators suture the flap to the tongue. Because the tongue is placed in a glossoptotic position under the general anesthesia, if the flap is sutured to the tongue as it stands, the tongue is fixed at the glossoptotic position. As a result, the patients have difficulty in deglutition and protrusion of their tongue. Chepeha and his colleagues [9] reported that tongue protrusion greater than 0.8 cm is associated with better swallowing results in the tongue reconstruction of the hemiglossectomy defect. So the operators should suture the flap to the tongue, pulling the tongue to the protruding position out of a glossoptotic position. By fixing a remaining tongue appropriately (protrusive position) to the mandible via flap, the larynx is consequently placed in an elevated position.

Insertion of a triangle flap to the oral floor at the ventral base of the tongue had been reported [8]. We observed that small triangle flap (less than 2 cm) shrunk postoperatively and was not so effective as was expected. So we recommend triangle flap with a size of more than 3 cm should be used. Applying several z-plasties at the back of tongue, to our knowledge, has not been reported up to now. In the majority of cases (not to say all cases), a postoperative scar contracture along the suture line between flap and remaining tongue occurs to a greater or lesser extent (Fig.4b). From the plastic surgeon's point of view, this inevitable contracture can be prevented by the application of several z-plasty (or insertion of triangle flap).

Concerning the question as to what is the best flap (radial forearm, anterolateral thigh, or deep inferior epigastric flap) for the reconstruction after hemiglossectomy, majority of recent papers suggest that the use of anterolateral thigh flap is the best option because the anterolateral thigh flap provide as good postoperative results as forearm flap whereas the former has less donor site morbidity than latter does [2-5]. We generally agree with them. The use of radial forearm flap may be the best in terms of not disturbing the movement of the tongue because the forearm flap is thin, soft and lithe compared with other two flaps. However, forearm flap is generally too thin for the adequate reconstruction of oral floor and its harvest leaves ugly scar on the forearm. So we recommend that the first choice is the anterolateral thigh flap while the deep inferior epigastric flap is indicated in patients with thin adiposal tissue in the thigh region.

We seldom have difficulties in the selection of appropriate recipient arteries for microvascular free flap transfer in the head and neck region because many sizable branches of the external carotid or subclavian artery are available. However, we occasionally encountered the lack of an appropriate recipient artery, especially in patients with recurrent cancer after previous surgery and / or irradiation therapy. For these cases, we have preferentially employed the ECA trunk as the recipient artery and anastomosed in an end-to-side fashion, with uneventful results [15]. Careful creation of a hole on ECA for anastomosis is an important key to successful anastomosis. In such difficult cases, the tunica intima of the ECA is as damaged as that of branch arteries, and careless operation may cause irrecoverable injury of the intima. The skin biopsy trepan is useful to create a hole without injuring the intima.

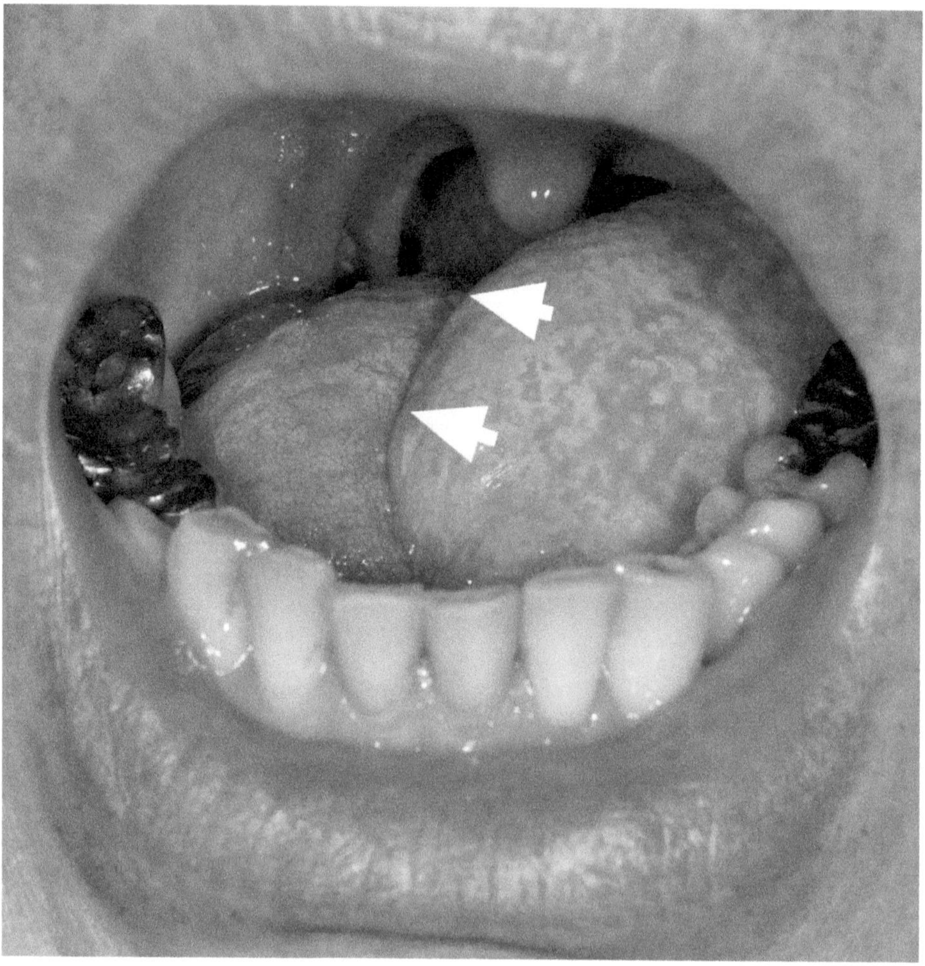

Fig. 4b. Examples of unfavorable results remarkable scar contracture along the straight suture line between the flap and remaining tongue (arrow) (Postoperative findings of a 51-year-old male with lingual cancer who underwent left hemiglossectomy and reconstruction with anterolateral thigh flap).

5. References

[1] Urken ML, Biller HF. A new bilobed design for the sensate radial forearm flap to preserve tongue mobility following significant glossectomy. Arch Otolaryngol Head Neck Surg 120: 26-31, 1994

[2] de Vicente JC, de Villalaín L, Torre A, Peña I. Microvascular free tissue transfer for tongue reconstruction after hemiglossectomy: a functional assessment of radial forearm versus anterolateral thigh flap. J Oral Maxillofac Surg 66: 2270-5, 2008

[3] Huang CH, Chen HC, Huang YL, et al. Comparison of the radial forearm flap and the thinned anterolateral thigh cutaneous flap for reconstruction of tongue defects: an evaluation of donor-site morbidity. Plast Reconstr Surg 114: 1704-10, 2004

[4] Hsiao HT, Leu YS, Liu CJ,et al. Radial forearm versus anterolateral thigh flap reconstruction after hemiglossectomy: functional assessment of swallowing and speech.J Reconstr Microsurg 24: 85-8, 2008

[5] Camaioni A, Loreti A, Damiani V, et al. Anterolateral thigh cutaneous flap vs. radial forearm free-flap in oral and oropharyngeal reconstruction: an analysis of 48 flaps. Acta Otorhinolaryngol 28: 7-12, 2008

[6] Haughey BH, Taylor SM, Fuller D. Fasciocutaneous flap reconstruction of the tongue and floor of mouth: outcomes and techniques. Arch Otolaryngol Head Neck Surg 128: 1388-95, 2002

[7] Engel H, Huang JJ, Lin CY, et al. A strategic approach for tongue reconstruction to achieve predictable and improved functional and aesthetic outcomes. Plast Reconstr Surg 126: 1967-77, 2010

[8] Koshima I, Hosoda M, Moriguchi T, et al: New multilobe "accordion" flaps for three-dimensional reconstruction of wide, full-thickness defects in the oral floor. Ann Plast Surg 45: 187-192, 2000

[9] Chepeha DB, Teknos TN, Shargorodsky J, et al: Rectangle tongue template for reconstruction of the hemiglossectomy defect. Arch Otolaryngol Head Neck Surg 134: 993-998, 2008

[10] McConnel FM, Pauloski BR, Logemann JA, et al: Functional results of primary closure vs flaps in oropharyngeal reconstruction: a prospective study of speech and swallowing. Arch Otolaryngol Head Neck Surg. 124: 625-30, 1998

[11] Hsiao HT, Leu YS, Chang SH, et al: Swallowing function in patients who underwent hemiglossectomy: comparison of primary closure and free radial forearm flap reconstruction with videofluoroscopy. Ann Plast Surg. 50: 450-5, 2003

[12] Wolff KD, Stiller D. Functional aspects of free muscle transplantation: Atrophy reinnervation, and metabolism. J Reconstr Microsurg 8: 137–14, 1992.

[13] Yla-Kotola TM, Kauhanen MS, Koskinen SK, et al: Magnetic resonance imaging of microvascular free muscle flaps in facial reanimation. Br J Plast Surg 58: 22–27, 2005.

[14] Okazaki M, Asato H, Takushima A, et al : Reconstruction with rectus abdominis myocutaneous flap for total glossectomy with laryngectomy. J Reconstr Microsurg. 23: 243-9, 2007

[15] Okazaki M, Asato H, Sarukawa S, et al: Availability of end-to-side arterial anastomosis to the external carotid artery using short-thread double-needle micro-suture in free-flap transfer for head and neck reconstruction. Ann Plast Surg, 2006; 56: 171-175.

14

Prosthodontic Rehabilitation of Acquired Maxillofacial Defects

Sneha Mantri[1] and Zafrulla Khan[2]
[1]*Hitkarini Dental College and Hospital, Jabalpur,*
[2]*James Graham Brown Cancer Center Louisville, Kentucky,*
[1]*India*
[2]*USA*

1. Introduction

In the last two decades treatment for head and neck cancers has evolved with multiple modality treatments, including radiation and chemotherapy in an effort to enhance local and regional disease control, reduce distant metastasis, preserve anatomic structures ,and improve overall survival and quality of life (QOL). Surgery is first choice for early cancers and for cancers that do not respond to radiation and chemotherapy in the form of salvage (Maureen, 2004).

Surgery can result in cosmetic, functional and psychological impairment greatly affecting the patient's quality of life (Roger, 2010). Presently the thrust in cancer care is not simply on survival but on rehabilitation, which aims to improve multiple impairments and QOL. Health related QOL refers to a multidimensional concept, which encompasses perception of both negative and positive aspects of at least four dimensions of physical, emotional, social and cognitive function (Moser et al., 2003).

Rehabilitation of such patients is quiet challenging and requires multidisciplinary team for comprehensive care and optimal post treatment functional outcomes. (Dingman, et al., 2008, Lemon et al., 2005, Logman, 1998, Hubalkowa, 2010). The team usually comprises of otorhinolaryngologist, radiation oncologist, medical oncologist, maxillofacial prosthodontist, speech therapist, psychologist, social workers, and nursing staff amongst the other disciplines for specific problems of the cancer patient. As a critical member of the team the maxillofacial prosthodontist co-ordinates the effort in many facets of patient care. Treatment is patient centered and patient directed, individualized to meet each patient's unique and specific needs.

Rehabilitation goals are focused on the restorative, supportive, palliative and preventive aspects of treatment (Moser, et al., 2003). Advanced cancers or trauma destroying structures, which may include soft and hard tissues of jaws, facial skeleton, oral tissues, lips, checks, nose and eyes, can affect the maxillofacial region. The defect may result in oroantral, oronasal, oronasal-orbital communication. The primary objective of rehabilitation is to preserve and restore the function of speech and swallow, preludes to the image restoration and boosts confidence of the patients so they can return to society; who have suffered the ravages of disfigurement.

2. Psychosocial intervention

The psychosocial effects of head and neck cancer are profound. Head and neck cancer strikes at some of the most basic human functions such as speech, taste, breathing, diet changes including facial disfigurement .This traumatic experiences poses great emotional threat to the patient and hinders their capacity to lead a normal life. The combination of exacerbated psychological distress and maladaptive coping strategies leads to impaired functioning and decreased rating of overall QOL (Haman 2008).

In specific reference to cancer, distress is defined as an unpleasant emotional experience of a psychological (cognitive, behavioral, emotional), social and / or spiritual nature that interferes with the ability to cope effectively with cancer, its physical symptoms and its treatment. Distress extend along a continuum, ranging from normal feelings of vulnerability, sadness and fears to problems that can become disabling, such as depression, anxiety, panic, social isolation and essential spiritual crisis (NCCN Practice Guidelines in Oncology 2005, as cited by Haman 2008).

An oncology social worker may help patients by providing access to valuable community resources and psychological assessment and intervention like head and neck support groups, which include other patients with similar cancers. Issues concerning treatment expectations, adjustment to diagnosis and coping strategies, during pretreatment counseling can reduce patient's uncertainty and help to restore their sense of control (Breitbart et al., 1988). The understanding of the psychological implications plays an important role in the management of patients with jaw defects (Rosenthal, 1964 as cited by Gillis, 1979). The primary goal should be to treat the person rather than just the defect (Lehman W.L. et.al. 1966 as cited by Gillis, 1979).

Rehabilitation is to help to readapt a disabled person to society, but ultimately it is the society that must be rehabilitated to reduce its prejudice, foster inclusiveness and increase acceptance of difference (Hearst, 2007).

3. Scope of prosthodontic services in rehabilitation of maxillofacial complex

Maxillofacial prosthetic services is to rehabilitate individuals who suffer anatomical compromise due to congenital disorders, trauma and oral/facial malignancies. Head and neck cancer patient presents a wide array of rehabilitative challenges associated with speech, mastication, deglutition and esthetics. Maxillofacial prosthetic treatment is not a substitute for plastic and reconstructive surgery, in certain circumstances it may be an alternative. Maxillofacial prosthesis provides a nonsurgical treatment for patients who are not good candidate for plastic surgery intervention because of advanced age, poor health, very large deformity or poor blood supply due to radiation. Moreover prosthetic treatment is indicated when anatomical structures of head and neck are not replaceable by living tissue, when recurrence is likely, when radiotherapy is administered or when fragment of fractured bones are severely displaced. (Chalian et al., 1972). Prosthodontic rehabilitation has specific advantages since it requires little or no additional surgery and the results are often more esthetically pleasing and less invasive than plastic surgery. The primary objectives of maxillofacial prosthetics and rehabilitation are to construct a prosthesis, which will restore the defect, improve function, enhance esthetics, return the patient back to society and thereby boost the morale of the patient contributing to the quality of life of the cancer patient.

4. Role of Maxillofacial prosthodontist as a member of multidisciplinary team

The role of maxillofacial prosthodontist varies depending on the modality of treatment. As a critical member of the multidisciplinary team, the maxillofacial prosthodontist co-ordinates the efforts in many facet of patient care. The prosthodontist must be acutely alert towards the medical health of the patient and be familiar with the various hospital protocols. He is best qualified to provide prosthetic support to the surgeon by preparing facial moulages and surgical stents to aid postoperative recovery. Communication with the surgeon as far as extent of disease, precise surgical technique, anticipated postoperative defects and healing time could help to plan the treatment. Recommendations can be made for the preservation of tissues or to improve the existing anatomical structures to improve the retention, stability and support for the prosthesis. (Zlotolow, 2001) Similarly, interaction with the radiation oncologist can render opinion regarding oral and dental condition, and recommended extraction of teeth, maintenance of teeth post radiation since the radiation might modify the care of teeth and mouth. Co-ordination with speech pathologist to gain knowledge about mechanics and physiology of speech can help to design the prosthesis, which can fulfill the requirements of resonance, phonation and articulation. (Chalian et al., 1972). Other specialists should be consulted as and when required. Primary concern of the treatment is to assure that the oral cavity is prepared to reduce the potential untoward effects of cancer treatment. The patients should be educated regarding the possible short term and long-term complications of chemotherapy and radiotherapy, trained in oral hygiene methods and therapeutics for oral health preservation and rehabilitate the post surgical defect utilizing prosthesis. Long term follow up and evaluation with an eye to the possibility of lesion recurrence is a part of the crucial contribution by the prosthodontist (Khan Et.al., 2006).

5. Presurgical prosthodontic intervention

A comprehensive oral and dental examination should be part of the presurgical intervention. The success of prosthetic treatment for a head and neck cancer patient may depend on the accuracy and adequacy of pre-surgical records. Presurgical records such as articulated diagnostic cast, jaw relation records, profile template of the midline of face, matching tooth shape and shade, radiographs, photographs of the mouth and face from strategic angles, facial moulage may be obtained for optimum post treatment outcome. Elimination of existing local infection, extraction of teeth with poor prognosis, restoration of teeth that has to be retained to support the prosthesis, modification of oral structures to anticipate the needs of subsequent treatment procedures such as alveoloplasty, gingivoplasty etc. may be required, as time permits. Existing dental prosthesis may be modified to serve as treatment prosthesis or preparation of surgical stents. Thus, an optimum oral environment should be maintained in order to provide freedom from infection and facilitate early recovery of tissues (Davenport, 1996, Jerbi, et al., 1968) Nutritional and psychological assessment and intervention should be included in the protocol.

Factors influencing the prognosis of prosthetic rehabilitation are size of the defect, availability of hard and soft tissues in the defect area to provide support for the prosthesis, proximity of vital structures, patient's attitude, temperament, systemic conditions and the patient's ability to adapt to the prosthesis. (Desjardins, 1978, Brown, 1970). Thus providing education, increasing awareness on possible changes, building of rapport and a working relationship with patients and their families are crucial during the pretreatment phase (Dingmam, et.al. 2008).These days CAD/CAM technology can be utilized in preprosthetic planning to prepare facial moulages and fabricate surgical stents for precise placement of implants when indicated.

6. Postsurgical prosthodontic rehabilitation of acquired defects

Head and neck cancer patients undergoing surgical resection as primary modality of treatment require prosthetic rehabilitation for restoration of speech deficits, control of oral secretions, mastication and swallowing dysfunction and possibly restoration of facial disfigurement. These defects can be divided into maxillary and mandibular defects.

6.1 Maxillary defects

Acquired defects of the palate may be due to surgery and or trauma. The defect may be in the form of a small opening resulting in communication from the oral cavity into the maxillary sinus, or it may include portion of the hard and soft palate, alveolar ridge and the floor of the nasal cavity (Chalian 1971).

Post surgical maxillary defects predispose the patient to hypernasal speech, fluid leakage through the nose including possibility of aspiration and impaired masticatory function (Keyf, 2001).The prosthesis constructed to repair the defect is termed as a maxillary obturator. An obturator (Latin; Obturare, to stop up) is a disc or plate used to close an unnatural opening or defect. The placement of an obturator restores oronasal separation to allow an increase in intraoral pressure and a decrease in nasal airflow rate. (Yoshida H., et.al. 2000). Obturators provide immediate improvement in speech articulation and intelligibility, voice quality and swallowing that approximates pre-surgical function enabling the patient to eat and drink immediately. Possible support is provided to the orbital content to prevent enopthalmous and diplopia, lips and cheeks are supported to restore the midfacial contour to improve the esthetics (Wang, 1997).Obturators are constructed in three phases, fulfilling different objectives in each phase.

6.1.1 Surgical obturator

It is constructed from pre operative cast after determining the approximate surgical boundaries of resection preoperatively by consulting the surgeon. At this point, it is an approximate guess relying on radiographic findings (Figure1a&b). The surgical obturator is inserted and sutured, screwed or wired at completion of resection. It separates the oral and nasal cavities, provides support for surgical packing, supporting the split thickness skin graft if used, minimizes wound contamination, enables the patient to speak and swallow immediately after surgery (Huryn, 1989).

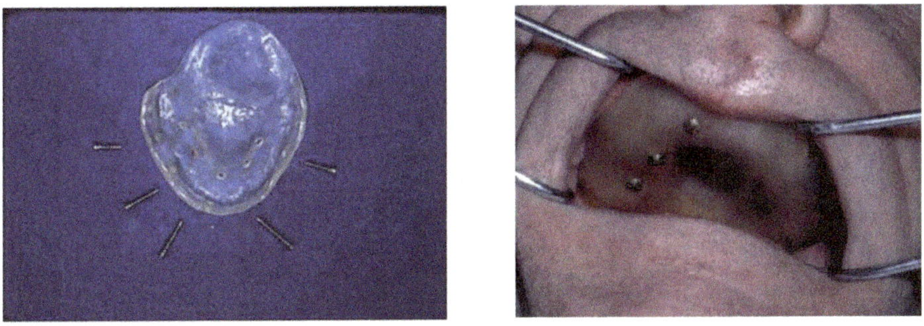

(a) (b)

Fig. 1. (a) Surgical Obturator with bone screws (b) Obturator screwed after resection

6.1.2 Interim/provisional obturator

The surgical obturator sometimes can be modified to compensate for tissue changes or surgical defect, which is different from the pre-surgical determination to form the provisional obturator. Usually it is constructed from post surgical impression to accurately reflect the defect. It replaces the surgical obturator and is worn in the postoperative healing period. The interim prosthesis in addition to clasps for retention can have anterior teeth for esthetics and a flange for lip and cheek support, which contributes to the patient's well being and social integration. Use of molar teeth is avoided to minimize occlusal pressure on the defect. The obturator is relined periodically for better adaptation as the healing progress. Good oral hygiene is encouraged during the healing phase. (Martin, 1993)

6.1.3 Definitive obturator

It is a more permanent prosthesis designed and fabricated when the surgical site is stable usually between six months to a year and local recurrence is ruled out. Precise impression of the defect is made for the fabrication of the prosthesis that allow maximum distribution of forces to all available teeth if present, remaining hard palate, lateral walls of the defect and remaining alveolus. In addition, occlusal relationship must be obtained to make the prosthesis cosmetic as well as functional (Fig.2a, b, c &d). Obturator bulbs for large defects can be made hollow to reduce the weight on the surgical side and improve retention of the prosthesis and comfort of the patient. (Payne,et al., 1965, Ampil, et al., 1967, Brown 1969, Chalian,et al., 1972, Buckner 1974, Benington,et al., 1982, Wiv ,et al., 1989, Wang,et al., 1999, McAndrews, et al., 1998 as cited by Keyf 2001).

6.1.4 Consideration for management of edentulous patients

Fabrication of an obturator for the edentulous patients provides major challenge because of the lack of support from teeth and lack of suction. In addition, excess resorption of the residual edentulous ridges may be encountered, demands equalization of stress distribution to available portions of the palate. In such conditions retention stability and support can be enhanced by maximum preservation of hard palate, skin grafting the cheek and maxillary sinus wall for better support and removal of inferior turbinates to provide a larger surface area for stress distribution (Jackob, et al., 2000).

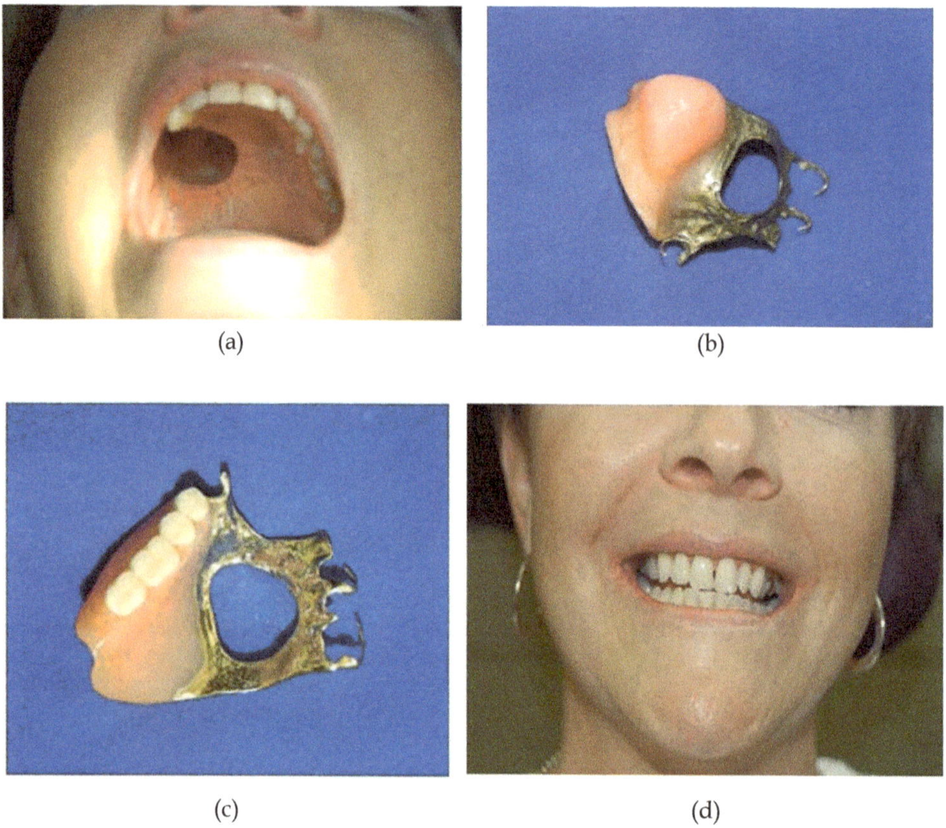

Fig. 2. (a) Hard Palate Defect (b) Partial denture definitive obturator
(c) Prosthesis replacing missing teeth (d) Prosthesis restoring esthetics and function

6.1.5 Hygiene considerations

Patients using an obturator must conduct meticulous daily cleaning of the defect and the prosthesis to prevent malodor and infection. As most patients remain with a resection, cavity, which allows the nasal and oral cavities to communicate, collection of mucous, and blood become encrusted and colonized by anaerobic bacteria in the area resulting in foul smell, nasal obstruction and discomfort. As the normal mucociliary, apparatus is no longer able to clear the secretions patients must be taught to clean and maintain the cavities themselves (Odell.et al., 2007). When teeth are present, high level of oral hygiene should be maintained especially for patients who exhibit xerostomia and have an increased risk of caries. Fluoride application and professional cleaning are mandatory (Fig.3).

6.2 Management of soft palate defects

Prosthesis for soft palate defects varies based on the extent and site to attain velopharyngeal closure during functions such as speaking and swallowing. Palatopharyngeal closure

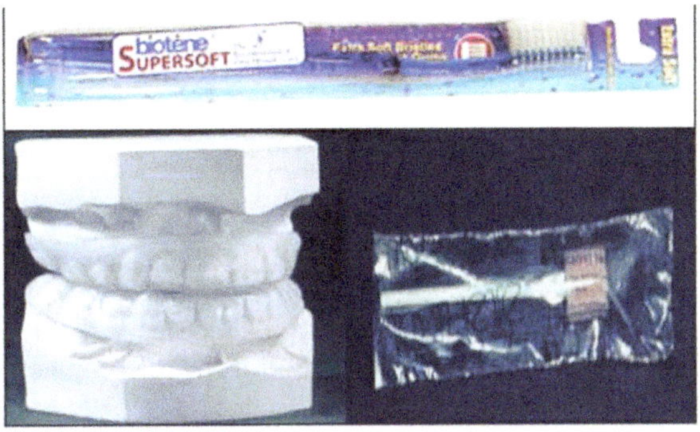

Fig. 3. Custom fluoride trays, soft toothbrush and toothette for cleaning teeth

normally occurs when the soft palate elevates and contacts the lateral and posterior pharyngeal walls of the nasopharynx. Acquired defects of soft palate results in insufficient tissues or altered function of the remaining structures to provide palatopharyngeal closure.

Prosthesis to aid in correcting palatopharyngeal insufficiency can be accomplished by providing pharyngeal obturator/speech bulb prosthesis. A portion of obturator extends into the pharynx to separate oropharynx and nasopharynx, restores the soft palate defect and allows adequate closure of palatopharyngeal sphincter (Abrew, et.al., 2007, Saunders, 1993, Beumer, et.al., 1996 as cited by Tuna, et al. 2010).

A meatus obturator is designed to close the posterior nasal chonchae through a vertical extension from the distant aspect of the maxillary prosthesis. (Eckert, et.al. 2000). This obturator design may be indicated when the entire soft palate has been lost in an edentulous patient.

Palatal lift prosthesis is provided for patients with speech disorders due to palatopharyngeal incompetency normally caused by closed head injuries. The purpose is to elevate the soft palate to the level of the palatine plane, enabling velopharyngeal closure by the actions of pharyngeal walls thus improving the quality of speech and reducing the effort required to speak (Gonzalez, 1970, Gibbons, et al., 1958).A speech pathologist is involved in training a patient to use the prosthesis to advantage. Palatal lift prosthesis cannot function by itself, but compliments a speech therapists training for the patient.

6.3 Defects of mandible, tongue and associated structures

Treatment of mandibular defects includes, defect from surgical resection of mandible, tongue, floor of mouth and associated structures. Disabilities resulting from such resection include impaired speech articulation, difficulty in swallowing, trismus, deviation of mandible during functional movement, poor control of salivary secretions and severe cosmetic disfigurement, (Beumer,etal.,2003). Based on the amount of resection or extent of bone loss, mandibular defects can be classified as continuity and discontinuity defects. Mandibular discontinuity can be managed by immediate on delayed surgical reconstruction to re-establish continuity. Loss of mandibular continuity if not re-established alters the symmetry of mandible, leading to altered mandibular movement and deviation of the residual mandible towards the affected side. Different methods used to reduce mandibular deviation are intermaxillary fixation, mandibular guidance appliances, sectional dentures or resection prosthesis. Resection prosthesis may require use of a guide flange or a maxillary occlusal platform incorporated in the prosthesis to guide the mandibular segment into optimal occlusal contact. This prosthesis is made four to six weeks after cancer surgery, after initial healing is complete and the patient is able to open and close the mouth adequately. Mandibular exercise regimen is advocated simultaneously.

According to Beumer and Curtis, intemaxillary fixation is most useful in patients with resection confined to the mandible with little soft tissue loss. The design of mandibular guidance prosthesis for partially edentulous mandible incorporates a rigid major connector, occlusal rest, guide planes and obtains major support from adjacent teeth and soft tissues. In edentulous patients, the dentures are extended into the soft tissue for added stability. An occlusal ramp is added to the palatal side of the maxillary denture to guide the mandible into proper occlusion. The severity of disabilities combined with composite resection of tongue, floor of the mouth and mandible is greatly reduced by the introduction of micro vascular free flap and possible osseointegrated implants depending on the amount and areas receiving radiation. A free tissue transfer with the fibula allows the possible placement of dental implants to support resection prosthesis. (Zlotolow, 2001)

6.3.1 Glossectomy defect

When a patient undergoes a partial on total glossectomy, the ability to masticate, swallow and formulate vowels and consonants for speech sounds is dramatically altered. The size, location and extent of the defect affect the degree of disability to swallow or speak. The areas of surgical resection that affects function of the tongue include removal of the anterior tip of the tongue, lateral (partial) glossectomy, removal of the base of the tongue and total glossectomy. Moore (1972) as cited by Zaki H.S., suggested tongue prosthesis as the treatment of choice in total glossectomy. This approach seldom restores the function of speech and swallow; it is mostly cosmesis. An artificial tongue of either hard or resilient acrylic is attached to the lower denture base, which covers the alveolar ridge as well as floor of the mouth. The artificial tongue is designed in such a way that the dorsum of the anterior two third of the tongue conforms to the anterior of the palate and comes almost in contact with the palate when the teeth are brought into occlusion. The posterior one third of the tongue is designed to act as a funnel, which directs the food and fluids into the oesophagus. Palatal augmentation (or drop) prosthesis is indicated when the tongue resection and reconstruction results in limited bulk and restricted movement of the reconstructed tongue resulting in reduced tongue palate contact. The palatal augmentation prosthesis allows reshaping of the hard and /or soft palate to improve tongue/palate contact during speech and swallowing. This could be a removable partial denture or complete denture prosthesis. (Laaksonen J.P. et al. 2009).

While rehabilitating a glossectomy patient the oral functions of the residual structures must be assessed. In addition to the extent of the defect factors such as mobility of the residual oral and paraoral structures, neuromuscular co-ordination and motivation will also determine the prognosis of the case.

7. Extraoral facial defects

The face is the most prominent visible part of the body and provides sense of identity to a person. Functionally, it animates emotion, communicate and intellect and provide the essential access routes to the respiratory and gastrointestinal system. Cognitively the region is the sole source of vision, hearing, taste and smell. Thus, facial disfigurement whether congenital or acquired has the potential to cause multiple problems and psychosocial dysfunction (Dropkin, 1999, Sarwer, Thompson, 2001 as cited by Wallace 2008). Such patients with facial disfigurement spend significant portions of their lives dealing with stigma. Stigma is a mark of disgrace attached to people who are considered different. When the actual social identity is perceived as departing from normality the individual is reduced in our minds from a whole and usual person to a tainted, discounted one "Such an attribute is stigma (Goffman 1963 as cited by Bonanno et.al., 2010). Stigmatized and socially excluded their ability to interact is often distorted and interaction is the source of problems including verbal and physical abuse, ridicule hostile behavior and isolation (Kish et.al. 2000, Furness et.al. 2006, Hagedoorm, t.al. 2006 as cited by Bonaeno, et.al. 2010).

Facial defects can be restored either surgically or prosthetically depending on the location and size of the defect, the surgeon is limited by the availability of tissues, changes due to radiation and the need for future visual evaluation for recurrent cancer.

Prosthetic restoration of facial defects is a combination of art and science requiring multidisciplinary approach focusing on the area involved for rehabilitation such as an eye, ear, nose or midface. A prosthetic replacement of an exterior part is termed as epithesis, which is described as early as seventh century (Van Doorne, 1994). There are definite limitations of both treatment modalities. The material available for facial restoration, movable tissue bed, limits the prosthodontist in retaining a large prosthesis and patient's willingness to accept the restoration (Beumer, et.al. 2003).

Prosthetic replacement of missing facial tissues has several advantages over surgical reconstruction. The process is relatively inexpensive, allows for periodic evaluation and cleaning of the site. It is a short process and the maxillofacial clinician has complete control of color, shape and position of the prosthesis. Disadvantages include possible irritation of he tissue site need for periodic remake and depending on adhesive on some other form of retention (Lemon, et.al. 2005). The goal of facial rehabilitation is to provide a natural, life like, integrated, esthetically pleasing, anatomically correct prosthesis, which blends with the body specially the surrounding structures. Knowledge of material science is the key to provide best care for patients.

7.1 Materials used for maxillofacial prosthesis

Desirable properties of a maxillofacial prosthetic material includes durability, biocompatibility flexibility light weight, color stability, hygiene, thermal conductivity, ease of fabrication and use, texture, availability and cost (Beumer, et al., 1996). Ambroise Pare who made varied contribution to standardize the indications for and material used in facial prosthetics. Amongst the large number of materials that have been tried out in the history of Anaplastology, example porcelain, natural rubber, gelatin and latex, two have established themselves, Methyl Methacrylates and Silicones (Andres, 1992). Methacrylates are relatively hard and more durable. Silicones are soft and flexible. Dr. Tsun Ma in a clinical overview of the materials stated that amongst the commercially available materials none of them is considered ideal. Different elastomers have their own physical and mechanical properties and share common clinical problem such as 1) discoloration over time (intrinsic and extrinsic discoloration due to environmental factors and loss of external pigments) and 2) degradation of physical and mechanical properties (tear) at the margin, lack of compatibility with medical adhesives, weakening of margins by colorants, adhesives, solvents and cleansers and deterioration of static and dynamic mechanical properties. Most discoloration and tear occurs when patients remove prosthesis or adhesives (Khan et al., 1992).Over the years there has been some improvement in facial biomaterials; but still there exists a clear need for new or improved facial materials in all clinical situations. (Lemon et.al. 2005).However studies have shown that chlorinated polyethylene may have advantage over conventional silicone rubber material in its ability to be repaired, relined or reconditioned, extending the life of the prosthesis. In addition, it can be used with any adhesive type. It has greater edge strength, does not support fungus growth and is cost effective as compared with silicone materials except processing of this material is complex and difficult (Gettleman et.al. 2004, Gettleman 1992, Gettleman et.al. 1989, Gettleman et.al. 1987, Gettleman et.al. 1985, as cited by Lemon et.al. 2005).

7.2 Types of extraoral prosthesis

These prostheses may include orbital/ocular, auricular, nasal or combination including midfacial prosthesis. The construction of facial prosthesis consists of four stages each equally important to the success of the rehabilitation effort and each requiring meticulous attention to detail (Andres,et al., 2000) Moulage impression and working cast fabrication, sculpting and formation of the pattern, including color match, mold fabrication and processing of the prosthesis with intrinsic and extrinsic coloration.

7.2.1 Auricular

Prosthetic replacement of the missing or altered ear can provide excellent cosmetic results. The advantage of an auricular prosthesis relates to the lateral face position and the effort to use hair to conceal the superior and posterior margin. When an auricular prosthesis is indicated, the entire ear should be removed except for the tragus. It provides a landmark for repeated placement since it is not easily displaced and helps to hide the anterior margin of the prosthesis (Carr, 1998). It also makes it easy for the patient in placement of the prosthesis especially if adhesives are used. Replacement of a complete ear is easy since it allows complete freedom of shape, size and location. The recipient areas should be flat or concave. Convexities from excessive bulk can hamper esthetic results (Parr et al. 1981 as cited by Lemon et al. 2005). Skin devoid of hair provides good adhesion base yet a split thickness graft is advantageous. Tissue pockets assist in the orientation and stability of the prosthesis and allow the margins to extend in a zero degree emergence profile. Craniofacial implants specifically designed to be placed in the mastoid temporal bone permit positive retention for auricular prosthesis and the ease of placement. (Fig.4a&b)

7.2.2 Nasal

Since nose is very prominent, centrally located and difficult to disguise on the face, making prosthesis with realistic effect is of vital significance. Presurgical photographs can aid for accurate replication of the patients original nose preservation of nasal bone to provide retention and support should be emphasized. Maintaining the anterior nasal spine helps to determine the final position of lip (Marunick, et al. 1985 as cited by Lemon, et al., 2005).

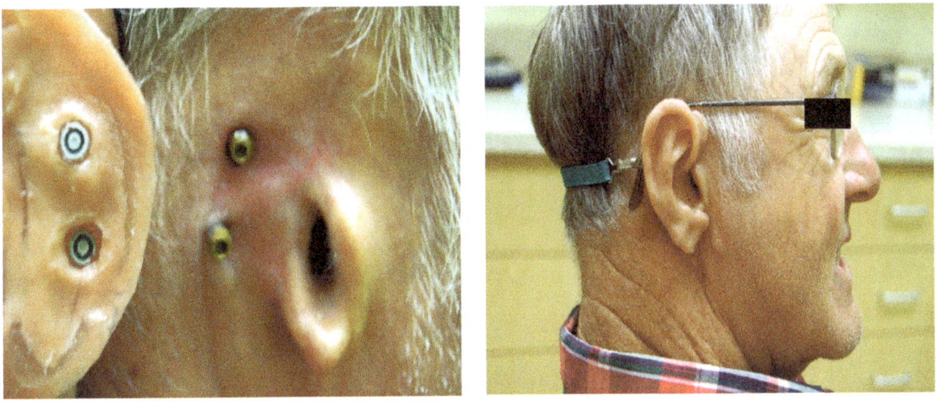

(a) (b)

Fig. 4. (a) Two Implants placed in mastoid/temporal region (b) Implant retained Silicone Auricular prosthesis

Attempts should be made to camouflage the margin with the surrounding anatomy and match the color, texture and translucency of skin. If cranio-facial implants are indicated-preferred site for implant placement is the anterior floor of the nose and maxilla region, which provides greatest bulk for the superstructure and retention mechanism (Carr, 1998).

7.2.3 Orbital/ocular

Different surgical procedures such as evisceration enucleation or an exenteration requires different prosthetic approach. Ocular prosthesis is simple as it replaces only the orbital contents, the eyelids are intact (Fig.5 a&b). Orbital excenteration defects are most challenging to restore. Facial expression around the margin makes it difficult to achieve an accurate fit without the margins being lifted. Skin grafting with split thickness graft, sufficient depth for placement of components, minimum margin tissue distortion, preserving eyebrow position and rounded orbital margin helps to enhance the prognosis of the prosthesis. Placement of craniofacial implants for larger defects is generally located in the supraorbital rim or lateral rim of the residual orbit. Medial placement of the implant is discouraged due to diminished bone quantity and quality (Nishimura et al., 1998). It is always recommended for the patient to wear glasses to protect the natural eye and to camouflage the non-blinking prosthetic eye.

7.2.4 Retention of extra oral facial prosthesis

Achieving adequate retention for maxillofacial prosthesis is quiet an uphill task. The surgical procedures often sacrifice a large part of retentive feature. A wide range of retention methods are available depending on the requirement of an individual case, consideration should be given to the location and size of the defect, tissue mobility, undercuts and the material weight of the prosthesis, (Chalian, et.al.)The retention action can be broadly classified as *Anatomical* factors such as already existing on created undercuts areas/concavities etc.Limitation with its use is irradiated tissues, which should be spared of undue stress. The prosthesis may abrade the tissues causing ulceration.

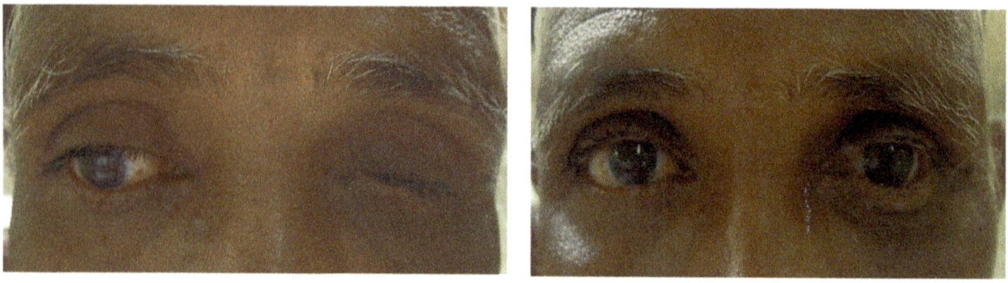

Ocular Defect Ocular Prosthesis

Fig. 5. Ocular Defect Ocular Prosthesis

Mechanical retention by means of attachment to external devices such as eyeglasses, headbands or straps, stud clips, snap buttons, magnets.

Adhesives are simple and commonly used form of the retaining extraoral prosthesis. They are available in two common form liquid (Silicone or acrylic based) or double sided medical grade tape. Adhesive choice will depend on the material it will bond. There are limitations to adhesive retention methods. Movement of the skin around the prosthesis, high humidity, oily skin or profuse sweating will loosen the marginal seal and border adaptation of the prosthesis. Meticulous cleaning is required to prevent moisture build up and infection. Some patients may be allergic to the adhesives used. Other, most reliable form of retention when indicated is craniofacial implants.

Retention is a significant challenge in rehabilitation of maxillofacial defects necessitating careful planning, meticulous surgical technique and skillful prosthetic planning.

8. Implants in maxillofacial prosthodontics

Osseointegrated implants forms a fixed bone anchored retention method providing a stable platform for retaining an extraoral or intraoral prosthesis. It is defined as a process whereby clinically asymptomatic rigid fixation of alloplastic materials is achieved and maintained in bone during functional loading (Zarb, et al., 1991). Since their introduction in 1977 to support, a bone conduction hearing processor (Tjellstrom 1990) osseointegrated implants have superseded their application in maxillofacial prosthetic rehabilitation than any other forms of retention. The improved retention enhances functional and esthetic advantages in facial prosthesis, greater accuracy and a better marginal fit enabling the thinner margins blend more effectively will adjacent tissues. This is dictated by the amount, type and area of radiation including proper placement of implants and remaining hard and soft tissues contours post surgically.

Most implants used in maxillofacial prosthesis are made of titanium and are cylindrical. They are anchored in the bone using threads. The placement of implant usually requires two minor surgeries, with high precision and aseptic conditions. The first surgery is the insertion of titanium fixtures/ implants into the bone and osseointegration is allowed to occur 4-6 month in accordance with the bone quality. In the second surgery, the implants are uncovered and the retentive element called as abutment is placed on the implant (Parr, et.al.

1981 as cited by Lemon, et al., 2005). The abutment can be used to hold a bar so that the prosthesis can be clipped into place or magnets can be used. Successful osseointegration depends on various factors. These include implant material biocompatibility, implant design and surface characteristics as well as surgical and loading conditions.

The introduction of advanced surgical procedures such as microvascular free tissue transfer has improved the treatment outcome. Free flap is an autogenous vascularized transplant, which involves the harvesting and detachment of bony and muscle tissue with its blood, and nerve supply and re-establishment by reanastomosis to suitable recipient site vessels (Mitchell, 2005 as cited by Fearraigh, 2009). Implants placed in the free flap reconstructed bone perform same as those placed in native bone. Use of implants in irradiated bone has been controversial. There is risk of developing Osteoradionecrosis of the mandible when carrying out surgical procedures such as implant placement. Certain factors needs consideration in placing implants in patients treated with radiation therapy for head and neck malignancies. The use of hyperbaric oxygen therapy (HBO) may help to revitalize the bone leading to improved success rate. It has been shown to prevent osteoradionecrosis in patients undergoing post radiation mandibular surgical procedures. The risk of ostcoradionecrosis is dependent on the radiation dose. Studies in the literature have suggested that an upper limit of 55 Gy should not be breached without the use of HBO. Disagreement as to when implants should be placed in irradiated bone remains. Zygomatic implants introduced by Branemark in 1988 are an alternative treatment modality to bone augmentation and sinus lift, where insufficient bone exists for maxillary implant placement (Kantas et al. 2002, Granstom, et al. 1992, Branemark 1998, Shaw, et al. 2005, as cited by Fearraigh P.O. et al. 2009).

9. Use of prosthodontic splints and stents in radiotherapy

Radiotherapy is increasingly being used in the management of head and neck cancer prior to or after surgery, either in combination with or without chemotherapy. Unfortunately, this treatment causes complications by increasing the morbidity of the surrounding tissues. This includes oral mucositis, infections, xerostomia, radiation caries, increased potential for osteoradionecrosis from infection (Fig.6a, b, c&d) or trauma to irradiated bone, trismus, altered taste sensation etc.

As a preventive measure, or to minimize the severity of the side effects, radiotherapy protective devices/stents can be fabricated and used during the treatment (Kaanders, et al., 1992, Chambers, et al., 1995, Schaaf, 1984 as cited by Mantri, et al., 2010). These stents are used to protect or displace vital structures, locate diseased tissues in repeatable position during treatment, position the beam, carry radioactive material or as a dosimetric device to the tumor site, recontour tissues to simplify dosimetry and shield tissues. (Figure 7, 8 &9) Before radiation treatment begins, flexible mouth trays can be fabricated which covers the teeth and are used to apply topical fluoride to prevent the onset of radiation induced tooth decay. Radiation of maxillary and hard palate tumors often includes the Temporomandibular joint and muscles of mastication, which causes stiffness of the joint, and fibrosis of the muscles followed by trismus, this can be minimized by oral exercises and use of appliances.

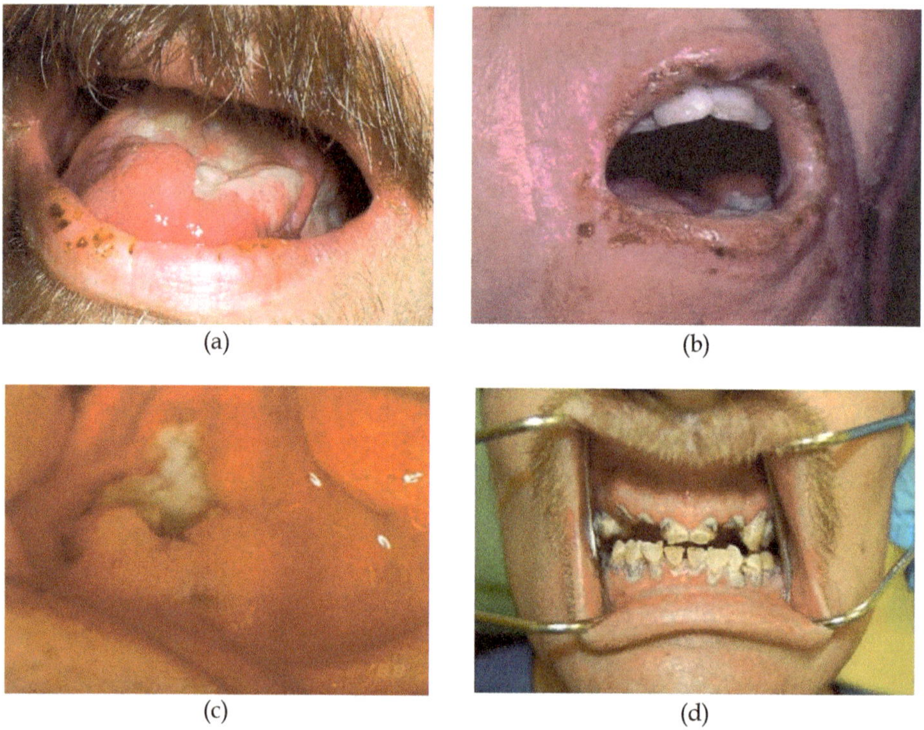

Fig. 6. a. Mucositis, post radiation showing desquamation of mucosa of dorsal surface of Tongue and Cheek. b. Keratitis of lips due to chemotherapy. c. Osteoradionecrosis showing ulceration, errythema of soft tissues, and bony sequestration. d. Radiation caries.

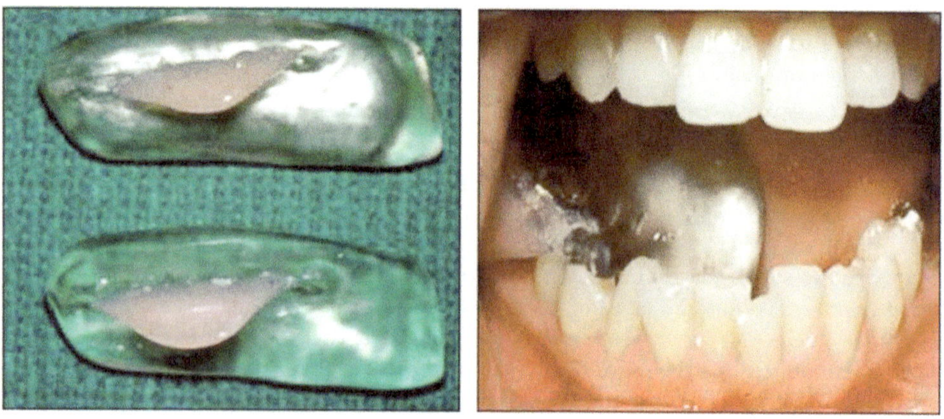

(a) (b)

Fig. 7. (a) Intraoral lead shield for unilateral radiation (b) Shield in position in mouth protecting tongue and opposite side of the jaw.

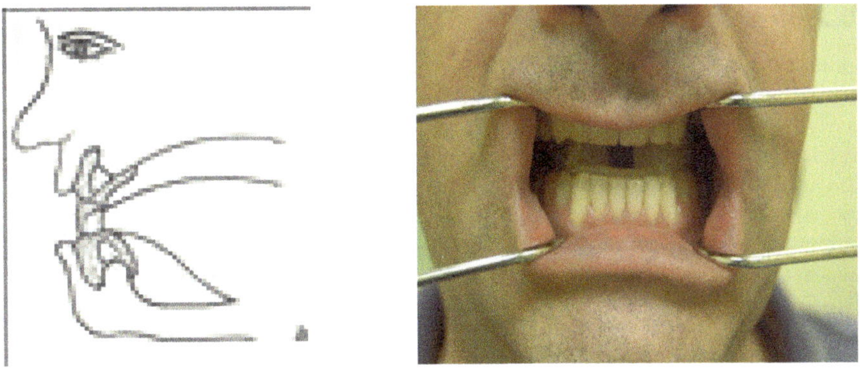

Fig. 8. Position maintaining stent

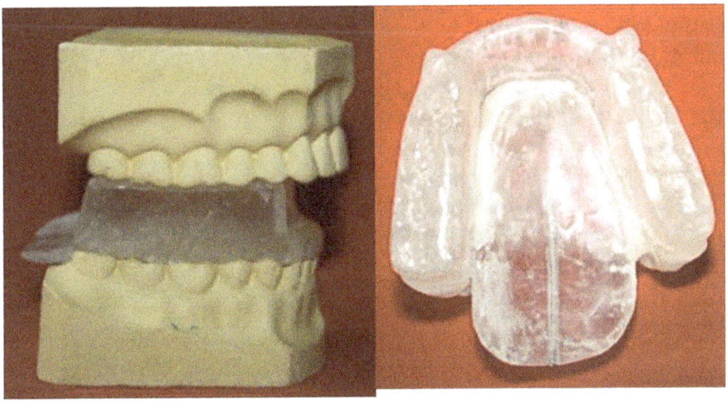

Fig. 9. Tongue depressing stent

Several prosthetic aids such as bite openers or exercises devices (Fig 10) can be used to help in the prevention of fibrosis of the muscles and to assist the patient in maintaining the mouth opening to eat and maintain oral hygiene.

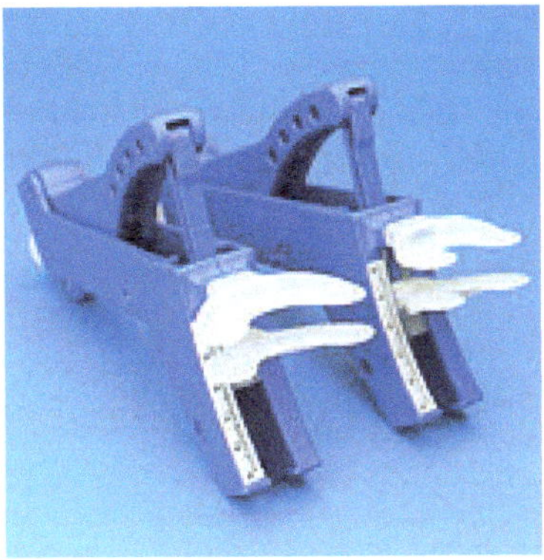

Fig. 10. Therabyte appliances for oral exercise

10. Patient education

Communication and education is the key for accepting the prosthesis. Successful use of prosthesis may depend on the patient's psychological acceptance. Rehabilitation is not a passive process. The patient must be an active participant. Patients participation in the decision making process with realistic expectations is of vital significance. They should be educated about the treatment choices and convinced of their personal responsibilities towards the use and care of the prosthesis. The need for professional re-evaluation on a frequent periodic schedule should be emphasized to determine its adaptability to soft tissues, stability, retention, tissue receptivity, occlusion function and esthetics.

11. Changing era in maxillofacial prosthetics

The field of maxillofacial prosthetics is embracing the rapid explosion of technology. The use of ossoeointegrated implants has broadened the treatment options. New technologies offer standardized quality, excellent precision of fit and outstanding biocompatibility, combined with adequate mechanical strength and provision for esthetic design. Success of implants is based on precise preoperative planning of the implant placement and the restoration. Modern three-dimensional (3D) imaging techniques such as digital volume tomography allow the acquisition of radiologic data with very low levels of radiation and excellent image accuracy and allow the processing of these data with various types of soft -ware application. It is possible to predetermine the precise 3-D position of the planned implant before the actual insertion of implant and thus enhance the placement process. Treatment planned in this way is fast, minimally invasive and predictable. This increases the quality of surgical procedure and restoration (Marquardt, et.al. 2009). The advent and increasing availability of 3-D cone beam computerized tomography (CT) and 3-D digital panoramic imaging machines makes it easier, timely and less costly to obtain images (Angelopoulos et.al. 2011 as cited by Serio F.G. 2011) C.T. images are extremely useful as a visualization and diagnostic tool. The use of CT also allows for the discovery of other lesions of head and neck not visible by older imaging technique. Magnetic Resonance Imaging (MRI) is another technology, which is more sensitive than CT at showing the difference between soft tissue types and is a useful tool for detecting the early stages of abnormalities in soft tissues.

The introduction of laser technology, 3-D computer aided designing (3-D-CAD) and computer aided manufacturing (CAM) also known as rapid prototyping (RP) or free form fabrication has revolutionalized the field of maxillofacial technology. CAD /CAM technologies are capable of alleviating most of the limitations of conventional techniques. With rapid prototyping, a life like prosthesis can be fabricated. CAD/CAM technology is changing the restorative quality and concepts of the future. Hopefully the cost for using these technologies in maxillofacial prostheses will drop with time for more wide utilization.

Biological improvements and the regenerative possibilities for regaining lost bone have shown continued advancement in the use of growth factor and bone proteins including recombinant bone morphogenetic protein and helping the clinician's ability to provide bone for accurate implant placement.

Color matching of facial prosthetic elastomers to skin color with portable spectrophotometer and computerized color formulation has been developed and has achieved clinical success (Seelaus R et.al. 2000, Troppmann R.J. et.al. 1996 as cited by Wolfaardtt J. et.al. 2003).

Relevant research on biomaterials advancement in surgical reconstruction such as microvascular free flap tissue transfers, bone-grafting methods have collectively helped to enhance rehabilitation outcomes.

12. Future vision

If the bridge between the existing chasm between oncology and rehabilitation has to be crossed several important challenges remains to be solved. Those challenges include 1) a paucity of outcome evaluation metrics 2) underdevelopment of the evidence base for cancer rehabilitation 3) the need for workforce development and 4) the absence of a health policy framework for cancer rehabilitation to support optimal service delivery, access to care and reimbursement (Mitchell S.A. 2010). Outcome is a major factor dictating treatment decisions and funding allocation. Quality of life outcome is equally important as survival rates. Those conducting research must ensure that evidence based research has its application to evidence based clinical practices. The reluctance to accept new treatment in clinical practice is a result of lack of adequate evidence. There is a need for transformation of educational programs. Core curriculum or competencies for cancer rehabilitation needs to be revised (Wolfaardtt et.al. 2003). The technological advancement as well as public demand for professionals accountability has increased the need for continuing and accessible education and specialized training for the professionals working with head and neck cancer patients. Interesting challenges are provided by robotics in the development of active prosthesis (Honda M. et.al. 1996, Klein M. et.al. 1999, as cited by Wolfaardt et.al. 2003) such as blinking and moving eye. Exciting developments in tissue engineering is likely to change the methods of reconstruction of tissue defects in the future. (Nusenbaum, et al., as cited by Kuriakose et al, 2007).Tissue engineering involves regeneration of new tissue with biologic mediators or scaffold. Success of tissue engineering depends on the effective participation of three components-scaffolds, signaling molecules and cells. Newer Scaffold materials with improved mechanical properties to provide tissue morphology and enhanced chemical properties to serve, as a bio-molecule carrier needs to be developed. Much research is being carried out in the field of muscular and neural tissue regeneration, which may have an impact in orofacial reconstruction in the future (Fearraigh, 2009).

Developing patient centered rehabilitation models, proposing evidence based guidelines through co-ordinated efforts of interdisciplinary teams should be on the agenda. Health policies to improve rehabilitation outcomes during and post surgical cancer treatment will be beneficial in rendering quality services to the cancer patient. Due to small number of newly diagnosed head and neck cancers in the United States, funding for research and development is limited. It is up to other countries where numbers are much greater to pursue this goal for helping these unfortunate patients. The economic impact of professional fees in maxillofacial prosthetics is difficult to summarize; since each case is unique and varies from region to region and country. It is also dictated by the treatment plan and the type of prosthesis. For example a nasal prosthesis retained by adhesive costs less than one retained by cranio-facial implants.

Restoration with a prosthesis is less expensive than plastic and reconstructive surgery.

Innovations in digital technology can be time saving and more precise but presently at significant cost for maxillofacial prosthesis. The investment in this technology should be based on subjective and objective assessment in terms of quantity and quality of outcome.

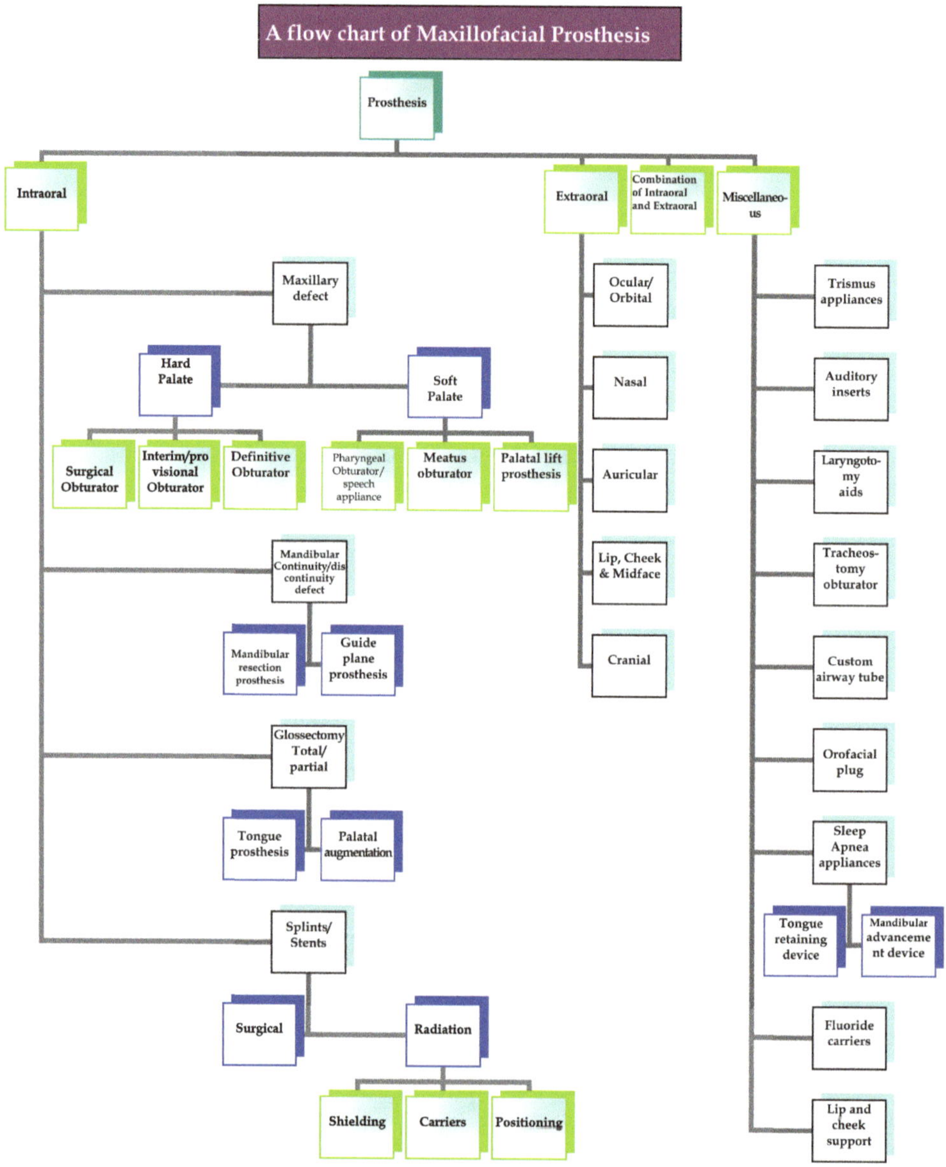

13. Conclusion

Rehabilitation of patients with acquired maxillofacial defects has always remained an enigma for the prosthodontist. The unpredictable nature of the defects and the uncertainty of recurrence have made the job of the prosthodontist more challenging. An attempt is made to discuss in brief the prosthetic aspects in rehabilitation of the patients with head and neck cancer. It stresses upon the need for multidisciplinary approach psychosocial consideration and the scope of prosthodontic services and the role of the maxillofacial prosthodontist in improving the QOL of such patients with different postsurgical defects. Although there are remarkable advances in technique and materials in past several years the full potential and utilization of maxillofacial prosthodontic services is yet not in sight. Today there is a need for dedicated and enthusiastic specialist coming forward and seeking specialized training for treating such patients. The integrated efforts, sound knowledge and practical implication in rehabilitating patients with acquired post surgical defects will help to bring smile and hope for patients with head and neck cancer now that longterm survival is achievable.

14. References

Andres. (1992) Survey of materials used in extraoral maxillofacial prosthetics. In Gettleman, L., Khan, Z. Eds. Proceedings of the conference on material research in maxillofacial prosthetics. Transactions of the Academy of Dental Materials. Vol. 5, pp. 25-40.

Andres, C.J. sss& Haugh, S.P. (2000) Facial prosthesis fabrication: Technical aspects. In Clinical Maxillofacial prosthetics, Taylor, T.D., Ed, ISBN 086715-391-1, Illions.

Beumer, J. III & Zlotolow, I. (1979) Restoration of facial defects, etiology, disability and rehabilitation. In Maxillofacial rehabilitation, Proshodontic and surgical considerations, Beumer, J., Curtis, T.A., Marunik, M.T., Eds. pp. 311-323, C.V. Mosby Company ISBN 0-8016-0676-4. USA.

Beumer, J., III, Zlotolow, I.M., & Sharma, A.B. (2003) Restoration of Palate, Tongue, Mandible and facial defect, in Oral Cancer. Silverman, S., Ed., B.C. Deker Inc., ISBN 1-55009-215-4, Ontario.

Bonanno, A and Choi, J.Y. (2010) Mapping out the social experience of cancer patients with facial disfigurement, Health , Vol. 2, No. 5, pp. 18-24.

Breitbart, W. & Holland, J. (1988) Psychological aspects of head and neck cancer. Semin Oncol, Vol. 15, pp 61-69.

Brown, K.E., (1970) Clinical Considerations in improving obturator treatment J. Prosthet Dent., Vol. 24, pp. 461-66.

Carr, A.B. (1998) Cosmetic and functional prosthetic rehabilitation of acquired defects. In OtolaryngologyHeadandNecksurgery, Vol.1, 3rdedition, Cummings, C.W., Fredrickson, J.M., Harker, L.A., et al Eds, Mosby Publication, pp. 1612-1634.

Chalian, V.A., Drane, J.B. & Standish, S.M. (1972) The Evolution and Scope of Maxillofacial prosthetics. In Maxillofacial prosthetics Multidisciplinary Practice. Chalian, V.A., Drane, J.B. and Standish, S.M. Eds., the Williams & Wilkins Company, ISBN 10:0683015125, Baltimore, USA.

Chalian, V.A., Bogan, R.L. and Snadlewick, J.W. (1972) Retention of Prosthesis. In Maxillofacial Prosthetics Multidisciplinary Practice. Chalian, V.A., Drane, J.B. & Standish, S.M., Eds., pp. 121-132, The Williams and Wilkins Company, ISBN 10:0683015125 Baltimore, USA.

Davenport, J. (1996) Managing the prosthetic rehabilitation of patient with head and neck cancer. Dent. News, Vol., 3, No.3, pp. 7-11.

Desjardins, R.P. (1978) Obturator prosthesis design for acquired maxillary defects. J. Prosthet Dent., Vol. 39, pp. 424-25.

Dingman, C., Hegedus, P.D., Likes, C., McDowell, P., McCarthy, E., & Zwilling, C. (2008) A Co-ordinated Multidisciplinary approach to caring for the patients will head and neck cancer. J. Support Oncol, Vol. 6, No.3, pp. 125-131.

Eckert, S.E., Desjardins, R.P. and Taylor, T.D. (2000) Clinical Management of the soft palate defect. In Clinical Maxillofacial Prosthetics, Taylor, T.D., Ed., pp. 121-132, Quintessence Publishing Co.Inc. ISBN 0-86715-391-1, Illinois.

Fearraigh, P.O. (2009) Review of Methods used in the reconstruction and rehabilitation of the maxillofacial region, J. of the Irish Dental Association. Vol. 56, No.1, 32-37.

Gibbons, P. & Bloomber, H. (1958) A supportive type prosthetic speech aid. J. prosthetic, Dent. Vol. 8, 362-374.

Gillis, R.E. (1979) Psychological Implications of patient care. In maxillofacial prosthetics, Laney, W.R. &, Gardner, A.F., Eds., pp. 21-40, P.S.G. Publication Company, ISBN 0884161609,Michigan.

Gonzalez, T.B. & Aranson, A.E. (1970) Palatal lift prosthesis for treatment of anatomic and neurologic palatal insufficiency. Cleft Palate Journal, Vol., 7, pp. 91-104.

Haman, K.L. (2008) Psychological distress, head, and neck cancer, Part 1- Review of the literature. J Support Oncol. Vol. 6, No.4, April 2008, pp. 155-163.

Hearst, D. (2007) Can't they like me as I am? Psychological intervention for children and young people with congenital disfigurement. Dev. Neurorehab., Vol. 10, No.2, pp. 105-12.

Hubalkowa, H., Holakovsky, J., Bradza, F. Diblik, P. & Mazenek, J. (2010) Team approach in the treatment of extensive maxillofacial defects. Five case report series. Prague Medical Report, Vol. 111, No.2, pp. 148-157.

Huryn, J.M. Piro, J.D. (1989) The maxillary immediate Surgical Obturator Prosthesis. J. Prosthet Dent, Vol. 61, pp. 343-47.

Jacob, R.F. (2000) Clinical Management of the Edentulous Maxillectomy patient. In Clinical Maxillofacial Prosthetics, Taylor, T.D. Ed., pp. 85-102. Quintessence Publishing Co., ISBN 0-86715-39-1 Illinois.

Jerbi, F.C., Ramey, W.O., Drane, J.B., Margetis, P., Lebley, J.P., & Goepp, R.A., et.al. (1968) Prostheses, stents and splints for the oral cancer patients. CA: A Cancer Journal Clinicians, Vol. 18, No. 6, pp 327-352.

Keyf, F. (2001) Obturator prosthesis for hemimaxillectomy patients. J.Oral Rehab. Vol. 28, pp. 821-29

Khan,Z.,Gettleman,L. & Jacbson,C (1992) Conference Report: Material Research in Maxillofacial Prosthetics Dent Res.,Vol.71,pp1541.

Khan, Z. & Farman, A.G. (2006) The prosthodontist role in head and neck cancer and introduction - Oncologic dentistry. J. Ind Prosthodont. Soc., Vol. 6, No.1, pp. 4-9.

Kuriakose, M.A., Sharma, M., &Ivyer, S. (2007) Recent advances and controversies in head and neck reconstructive surgery. Indian journal of Plastic Surgery.Vol.40, No.12, pp.3-12.

Laaksonen, J.P., Lowen, I.J., Wolfaardt, J., Rieger, J., Seikalay, H. & Harris, J. (2009) Speech after tongue reconstruction and use of a palatal Augmentation prosthesis. An acoustic case study. Canadian Journal of speech- language pathology and Audiology. Vol. 33, No. 4, pp. 196-202.

Lemon, J.C. Martin, J.W., & Jacob R.F. Prosthetic rehabilitation. In: Basal and squammous cell skin cancers of head and neck. Weber, R.S., Miller, M.J., Goepfert H., eds., pp. 305-312, Williams &Wilkins.

Lemon, J.C., Martin, J.W., Chambers, M.S., Kiat amnuay, S. Gettleman L. (2005) Facial prosthetic rehabilitation, preprosthetic surgical techniques and biomaterials. Curr. Opin. Otolaryngol head neck surg. Vol. 13, pp. 255-262, ISSN 1068-9508.

Logman, J.A. (1998) Rehabilitation for the head and neck cancer patient, oncology, vol. 10, No. 1,

Pascal, M., Siegbert, W. & Strub, J. (2007) Three-dimensional navigation in implant dentistry. Euro, J. Oral Implantology, Vol. 2, No.1

Mantri, S.S., Bhasin, A.S. (2010) Preventive Prosthodontics for Head and Neck Radiotherapy. Journal of Clinical and Diagnostic Research. 2010 August, Vol.4, pp.2958-62.

Maureen S. (2004). The expanding role of dental oncology in head and neck surgery.Surg Oncol Clin N Am.Vol.13, 37-46.

Mitchell, S.A. (2010) Framing the challenges of cancer Rehabilitation. Oncology Nurse Edition, Vol. 24, No.1, Suppl. pp. 33-4.

Moser, V.F., Crevenna, R., Korpan M. & Quiltan, M. (2003) Cancer Rehabilitation particularly with aspects of physical impairment J. Rehab Med. Vol. 35, pp. 153-162.

Nishimura, R.D., Roumanas, E., Moy, P.R., Suga, T., & Freymiller, E.G. (1998) Osseointegrated implants and orb ital defects: U.C.L.A. experience. J. Prosthet Dent., vol.79, no.3, pp.304-9.

Odell, M.J. and Gullane, P.J. (2007) Partial and total maxillectomy. In Lee, K.J. and Toh, E.H. Eds. Otolaryngology: A Surgical note book, pp 236-256. Thieme Medical Publishers ISSN 9783131383518 New York.

Roger, S.N. (2010) Quality of life perspective in patients with oral cancer. Oral Oncology, Vol. 46, pp. 445-47.

Tjellstrom, A. (1990) Osserintegrated implants for replacement of absent or defective ears. Clin. Plast. Surg. Vol. 17, pp 355-366.

Tuna, S.H., Pekkan, G., Gumus, H.O. & Aktas A. (2010) Prosthetic Rehabilitation of Velopharyngeal Insufficiency: Pharyngeal Obturator Prostheses with different retention Mechanisms. Eur J. Dent, Vol. 4, No.1, pp. 81-87.

Van Doorne, J.M. (1994) Extraoral Prosthetics: Past and Present. J Investigative Surg. Vol. 7, No. 4, 267-74.

Wallace, C.G. & Wei, F.C. (2008) The status, Evolution and future of facial Reconstruction. Chang Gung Med J. Vol. 31, No.5, 441-9.

Wang, R.R. (1997) Sectional prosthesis for total maxillectomy patient. A clinical report J. Prosthet Dent. Vol.78, No.3, pp. 241-244.

Wolfaardt, J. Gehl, G., Farmand, M. &Wilkes, G. (2003) Indication and methods of care for aspects of extraoral osseointegration 32:124-137.

Wolfaardt, J. et al. (2003) Advanced technology and the future of facial prosthetics in head and neck reconstruction. Int. J. Oral Maxillofacial Surg. Vol. 32, pp. 121-123.

Yoshida, H., Furuya, Y., Shimodaira, K., Kanazawa, T. & Kataoka, R. & Takahashi, K. (2000) Spectral characteristics of hypernasatity in maxillectomy patients. J. of Oral Rehab. Vol. 27, pp. 723-730.

Zarb, G.A. and Albrektsson, T. (1991) Osseointegration a requiem for the periodontal ligament. Int. J. Periodontics, Rest Dent., Vol. 11, pp. 88-91.

Zaki, H.S. (2000) Prosthodontic Rehabilitation following total and partial glossectomy. In: Clinical Maxillofacial Prosthetics. Taylor, T.D. Ed pp. 205-214, Quintessence Publication Co., ISBN 0-86715-39-1. Illinois.

Zlotolow, I.M. (2001) Dental Oncology and Maxillofacial Prosthetics. In Atlas of Clinical Oncology. Cancer of the Head and Neck pp. 376-373.,Shah, J.P. ed.,B C Decker Inc, ISBN 1-55oo9-084-4,Ontario.

Part 6

Health Outcomes

15

Health Related Quality of Life Questionnaires: Are They Fit for Purpose?

Kate Reid[1,2], Derek Farrell[2] and Carol Dealey[1,2]
[1]*University Hospital Birmingham NHS Foundation Trust*
[2]*University of Birmingham*
United Kingdom

1. Introduction

Patients frequently ask two poignant questions during their management: 'how will I be after my treatment?' and 'am I cured?' Focused or absolute answers are generally frustratingly absent and the multidisciplinary team are likely to be guarded in their response because at presentation the site of the tumour and the stage of the disease will influence treatment possibilities and outcome. Outcome from the varying treatment modalities have been reported in terms of survival-interval and more recently the patients' quality of life (QoL). The latter outcome is a multifaceted and dynamic concept which the World Health Organisation defined as a: "broad ranging concept affected in a complex way by a person's physical health, psychological state, level of independence and their relationships to salient features of their environment" (WHOQOL group, 1993). More specifically such data in the context of disease is described in terms of health-related QOL (HRQoL) the subjective experience of the impact of health status on QoL for the patient (Curtis, 1997;) and can in relation to H&NC patients be described as a patient's physical, emotional and social function at the pre and post-treatment stage(Hammerlid et al., 2001, Hammerlid and Taft, 2001).

The number of studies that routinely report on HRQoL has increased substantially over the last twenty years. In the literature it has been recommended that HRQoL tools should not only be used within the research arena but also within the clinical-setting (Velikova et al 2010). However the recommendation has not been put into practice and their use within the clinical setting remains limited. It would seem that clinicians have a poor understanding of what is available and are not able to link the findings with the clinical reality in which they work. This is despite patients reporting them both as a useful way of structuring their thoughts during outpatient appointments as well as a way of building a rapport with the teams involved in their care (Mehanna and Morton, 2006a, Velikova et al., 2010). Researchers have investigated why clinicians do not use QoL measures routinely within the clinical environment (Mehanna and Morton, 2006b, Kanatas et al., 2009). The results have suggested that clinicians do not view the findings as relevant to the clinical setting and that the logistical burden in the resultant collection and analysis of the data is too great. The volume of QoL questionnaires to choose from further complicates the situation. In a review of the head and neck cancer (H&NC) literature Kanatas and Rogers (2008) identified five broad categories of patient completed QoL questionnaires and as many as thirteen disease-specific questionnaires. Their conclusion was similar to a previous review by Ringash and Bezjak (2001) in which it was acknowledged that choice of questionnaire should be governed by the research questions being considered and the resources available.

The use of QoL data acknowledges that the patient aspect should be represented and that this information should be collected from the patient rather than from other sources such as health care professionals or carers, the former are likely to over estimate the physical symptoms (Reid et al., 2009) the latter under estimate the emotional aspects of the disease (Sollner et al., 2001). Complexity exists in all aspects of the field from the choice of questionnaire available to the possible influences on the results. Many and diverse variables would appear to impact on QoL scores and these include psycho-social factors: tumour characteristics,(Hammerlid et al., 2001) physical symptoms, (Campbell et al., 2004) treatments undergone,(Department of Health, 2011, Ronis et al., 2008) as well as psycho-social aspects of patients(Llewellyn et al., 2005, Howren et al., 2010).

The multi-dimensional and subjective nature of QoL makes it difficult to fit into the bio-medical model throughout the treatment management process. The link between QoL scores and survival for this group of patients has been noted to be neither strong nor proven (Mehanna et al., 2008). Over time the scores within categories or sub-categories might vary without an apparent change to the overall score, or the possibility that if scores do change they are often in relation to the patent's emotional response to a life-changing event and not as a consequence of a shift in physical symptoms. It is therefore very possible that scores are more a reflection of people's adjustment to their change of circumstances rather than a measure of their physical or emotional state. This notion has been demonstrated by a study by Logemann et al (Logemann et al., 2001) in which the impact of dry mouth on H&NC patients' function and perception of their swallow was investigated post radiotherapy. Logemann et al concluded that dry mouth did impact on sensory and comfort issues of swallowing but not on the actual function of the swallow. This would suggest that the patients are moderating or adjusting to the experience and that whilst objective measures are important there is value in collecting the diverse subjective aspects because this will influence patients' score to physical aspects of the disease or treatment. A systematic review of the HRQoL, for H&NC patients diagnosed and treated with reference to psychosocial variables Llewellyn et al (Llewellyn et al., 2005) suggested that personality, depressive symptoms, social support, satisfaction with consultation and information, consumption of alcohol and tobacco all influenced HRQoL scores. In the same year a study carried out by Scharloo et al (Scharloo et al., 2005) described how illness perceptions by patients -attention to symptoms, believing in a greater likelihood of recurrence, engaging in self-blame, and a strong emotional reaction to the illness- all contributed to lower QoL scores. There are therefore indications that the impact of the disease and treatment is moderated by subjective patient characteristics. A review of the QoL within the field of H&NC by Montazeri (Montazeri, 2009) identified eight papers that reviewed QoL and survival. Whilst four of the papers were not conclusive in their findings about the effect of QoL on survival a further four did show a clear relationship in areas such as cognitive function, (de Graeff et al., 2001) pain, appetite and eating scores (Karvonen-Gutierrez et al., 2008) and pre-treatment fatigue (Karvonen-Gutierrez et al., 2008, Fang et al., 2004) were reported as being linked to survival.

The conclusion of the review paper was that in order to really identify other variables more methodological and statistical rigor should be used in future studies. This recommendation is a recurring conclusion and perpetuates the concept that quantitative research is an adequate way of investigating the clinical complexity evident within the specialty H&NC. Such an approach holds with the belief that if homogeneity can be achieved between patient-groups eventually statistically significant variables can be identified. Perhaps this is currently an unrealistic goal with the instruments available and explains why different studies might appear to contradict one another. It is therefore possible that the actual variables that truly impact on outcome as measured by QoL remain both multiple, illusive and therefore uncertain.

It would be a limiting concept to suggest that H&NC impacts on the physical aspects of a patient with no influence on the emotional aspect. It would also be too simplistic to suggest that patients do not draw upon previous life events in order to help them mange the current diagnosis. From these two premises there is value in exploring the experience of H&NC at an individual level. The National Institute for Clinical Excellence estimates that 50% of all patients experience anxiety or depression at some point during their cancer assessment treatment and recovery (National Institue for Clinical Excellence, 2004). If the subjective aspect is left out in an attempt to follow a quantitative approach to study design the relevance of the results will remain, from the clinical perspective, poor representations of the patients. This will mean that clinicians fail to perceive a link between making clinical decisions and the research because it poorly depicts their caseload.

Being able to describe in a more representative way the disease and treatment is the preliminary stage of patient management. A United Kingdom government report has set out the outcomes which it would like to see developed and used within cancer care in England (Department of Health, 2011) The Department of Health cited research by Maddams within this document which predicted that by 2030 there will be more than three million people who will have been treated for cancer and survived, of which a third will be of a working age. The report emphasised the holistic nature of the patient experience acknowledging the financial and emotional aspect as well as the more frequently cited physical aspects. It is a real intention of the government's health care system that patients should achieve as much independence as possible from both the health care system as well as their own support network. Specific aims are set out within the report, one of which is that there should be a decrease in the proportion of people who report unmet physical and psychological needs post-cancer treatment. This is a significant challenge when considered in the context of a 2010 report that detailed patient experience and reported fewer cancer patients than in previous reports had understood the information they were given even at the point of diagnosis (Department of Health, 2010). Specifically within Britain therefore, despite more adherences to time-targets, a cultural shift needs to be achieved from a process-driven system towards a more personalised one. Part of this process has seen the development of Holistic Needs Assessment (HNA) for people with cancer (National Cancer Action Team, 2011). The publication suggested that if the holistic needs of patients were identified patients would be more likely to be engaged with their care, and identify the possible resources or services available during later stages of their treatment. Another government publication published in the same year, Improving Outcomes-A strategy for Cancer Care (Department of Health, 2011) has also recommended outcomes derived directly from patients should form the basis of outcome measures. It would seem therefore that there are two influences that might recommend more qualitative methodologies for the ongoing care of H&NC patients (i) the lack of clear and consistent QoL results (ii) a political expectation, which encourages the description of care at an individual level. It is within this context that the current study was devised. The purpose of which was to establish whether H&NC QoL measures adequately reflect a) the literature on patient experience b) the reported experience of H&NC patients undergoing curative treatment.

2. Methods

2.1 Research design

A qualitative methodology was used in order to identify the themes associated with the experience of H&NC. Three different sources of information were systematically explored using a previously described method of analysing information (Attride-Stirling, 2001). The sources were:

1. The three most commonly used HRQoL questionnaires in the H&NC literature; These had been identified by previous research carried out by Rogers et al (Rogers et al., 2007) who had reviewed a five year period (2000-2005) and reported on the range and most frequently used questionnaires.
2. A review of the literature that describes the H&NC patient's experience of the condition, its treatment and sequelae;
3. Semi-structured interviews recorded and transcribed from six H&NC patients. The interview questions were informed by the themes developed from the literature, in source 2.

For each of the three sources the themes were derived using a thematic analysis protocol as described by Attride-Stirling (2001). The application of thematic networks is a way of organising qualitative data in a systematic way. The thematic-analysis entailed development of a coding-framework that could be used to analyse and categorise each of the three sources of data: The themes were generated independently for the HRQoL questionnaires; but the literature review was used as a way of forming the semi-structured interview structure. This meant the process was sequential and relied upon the literature generating the initial interview structure. In effect the third source was dependent on the themes described in the second. Following categorisation, basic themes that evolved from each source were grouped, re-read and re-framed. The intention was to identify underlying patterns that might not be apparent on reading each in isolation. Finally, a review process took place in order to decide which organising themes were discrete or broad enough, to represent a group of ideas. The themes that were identified were organised in relation to one another such that they could be classified as either super-ordinate, or sub-ordinate to one another. Using the Attride-Stirling (2001) thematic analysis this meant that the themes were classified as basic, organising or global thematic networks. Independent assessment was provided to confirm the validity of the themes. Diagrams which represent and summarise visually the global themes between each of the three sources are presented within the section marked findings.

2.2 Data gathering

Source 1: Thematic analysis of HRQoL questionnaires

Rogers et al (2007) had previously carried out a structured review of the H&NC QoL literature in order to determine what questionnaires were used within the research. Three HRQoL questionnaires had been identified as the most commonly used within the research over a five year period (2000-2005). These were: The University of Washington (Hassan and Weymuller, 1993); the EORTC C30 and H&N C35 (Bjordal et al., 1994, Bjordal and Kaasa, 1992); which are used in conjunction to one another and the Functional Assessment of Cancer Treatment -Head and Neck Subscale FACT (List et al., 1990). Thematic analysis was carried out on these questionnaires.

The areas represented by each questionnaire require patients to describe in the past week which statement is most representative of their current situation. The University of Washington (UoW) reviews: pain, appearance, activity, recreation, swallowing, chewing, speech, shoulder function, taste, saliva, mood and anxiety. Patients also represent these aspects of their health or function by one of five statements, which grade their abilities from 'no' to 'severe change' in function. Patients also have to identify three domains that are most affected, rate their health to prior to the cancer diagnosis, during the past week and their overall quality of life during the past week from outstanding through to very poor. The Functional Assessment of Cancer Treatment -Head and Neck Subscale (FACT H&N) has a five point scale ranging from a description of "not at all" to "very much" examining specific areas and which include: seven questions re physical well being, seven questions regarding social well being six questions regarding emotional well being and seven questions regarding functional well being one of these questions asks the patient to rate their current satisfaction with their QoL. There are also twelve H&NC specific questions that investigate eating, communication, appearance, smoking, and drinking behaviours and pain. The EORTC reviews via a four-point likert scale with descriptors ranging from "very much" to "not at all" the presence of the quality a range of issues. The general questionnaire EORTC C30 is composed of 30 multi-item scales and single items assessing areas of functioning (physical, role, emotional, cognitive, and social), as well as general symptoms -fatigue, pain, emesis, dyspnea, insomnia, appetite loss, constipation, and diarrhea. The patients are also asked to rate on a seven-point scale their attitude to their own health and quality of life status over the past week. The disease specific module EORTC H&N35 consists of 35 questions including seven symptom scales: pain, swallowing, senses, speech, social eating, social contact, and sexuality. There are 11 additional, single items covering problems with teeth, mouth-opening, dry mouth, sticky saliva, cough, feeling ill, weight loss, weight gain, use of nutritional supplements, feeding tubes, and painkillers. The patient can complete all three questionnaires independently.

Source 2: Thematic review of the literature

A literature search was carried out in July 2009 using MEDLINE, EMBASE, the Science Citation Index (ISI), the Cumulative Index to Nursing and Allied Health Literature (CINAHL), the PsycINFO, the Allied and Complementary Medicine (AMED) and Global Health databases to review the literature surrounding H&NC patients' experience and or coping with the disease The search terms used were "head and neck cancer" and "experience"; and "head and neck cancer" and "coping". There was also a manual review of topic areas specific to experience and H&NC.

Source 3: Thematic analysis of patients' perspectives.

A purposive sample of six H&NC patients was recruited for the study from a UK cancer centre. The bio-clinical details and treatment undergone for each participant are presented in Table 1a and Table 1b.

	Sex	Age	Smoker	*Alcohol	Job	Tumour site	**Pathology
n							
1	f	68	X	none	Secretary	Mandibular alveolus	PT4N0
2	m	45	√	≤ 21	Craftsman	Floor of mouth	PT2NO
3	m	68	ex	≤7	Health wk	Laryngeal	PT1N0
4	m	62	√	≤ 21	Hairdresser	Laryngeal	PT4N1
5	m	66	√	≤ 21	Accountant	Laryngeal	PT4N2b
6	f	82	ex	≤7	Linguist	Buccal	PT4N1

*number of units of alcohol consumed in a week
**pathological classification UICC 6th edition

Table 1a. Bio-Social Statistics of participants n=6

	Surgery	Neck dissection	RT	Chemo RT	Complications
n					
1	Scapula-flap (failed) Pec major	Unilateral	√		flap failure salvage surgery pec major
2	Radial fore arm free flap	Bilateral	X	X	Paralysed tongue due to neuro praxis of tongue
3	Laser excision	None	X	X	None
4	Pharyngo-Laryngectomy Free flap (ALT) Tracheal oesophageal puncture	Bilateral	X	√	Infected donor site skin grafts
5	Pharyngo-Laryngectomy Tracheal oesophageal puncture	Bilateral	X	√	Trachy pre surg at time of biopsy
6	Fibula flap	Unilateral	√	X	None

Table 1b. Treatment and complications for participants

The participants were eligible if it was a year since the definitive treatment date of a squamous cell carcinoma, were judged to be cognitively intact and able to speak English. Thirty questions acted as the structure of the interview and are reproduced in Table 2. A year post-treatment was judged an appropriate time-interval so that participants would

Pre diagnosis
What made you go to the doctor in the first place? Did you suspect you had cancer when you first went to your doctor? If so, what made you suspect this?
At the time of diagnosis
How do you feel about the care you've been given? How do you feel about all the people that you have had to meet directly so your care could take place? How did having a diagnosis of H&NC impact on your life before you were treated? How do you feel about the information you've been given? Can you explain the effect the amount of information had on you? What has been the best thing about the information? Can you explain how the information written or verbal impacted on your ability to cope with the situation? Who did you feel the key people were? What helped you to cope with the pre treatment phase?
Post treatment What are your main concerns now? Has the H&NC affected the way you see yourself What was the lowest point for you over the past year? Has anything been particularly difficult to cope with? Are there particular symptoms that you continue to experience? How comfortable have you felt when discussing your situation with the team and why? What has been the most difficult time or thing to deal with? Are you still smoking or drinking -why? Is there anything particular that the team can do to help you cope? What enables you to cope with all that has happened? How do you feel about being reviewed in outpatients? Do you think that the team managing you have any idea how the treatment and disease has impacted on you? Do you feel the team understands your problems and concerns? Is there anything you wish you could tell the team that would make a difference to your care or others? What have been your feelings about undergoing the treatment? Since the treatment how do you think the disease and the treatment has impacted upon you psychologically What were the expectations you had of the disease and treatment and how did the reality compare? How has your disease and treatment impacted on those around you at home and socially?

Table 2. Questions used to generate interviews of the H&NC patients.

have recovered from the acute phase of treatment and not be overwhelmed by some of the pervasive physical symptoms that have been well documented (Rogers, 2010). Each interview was digitally recorded and independently transcribed before being analysed by the primary researcher. The length of interview ranged from 40-70 minutes.

3. Findings

3.1 Findings from questionnaires, literature and semi-structured interviews

Six global themes were evident; four from all three sources: day to day physical comfort, emotional well being, place in society and own mortality; one from the literature and semi-structured interviews; quality of care; and one from the semi-structured interviews: reality.

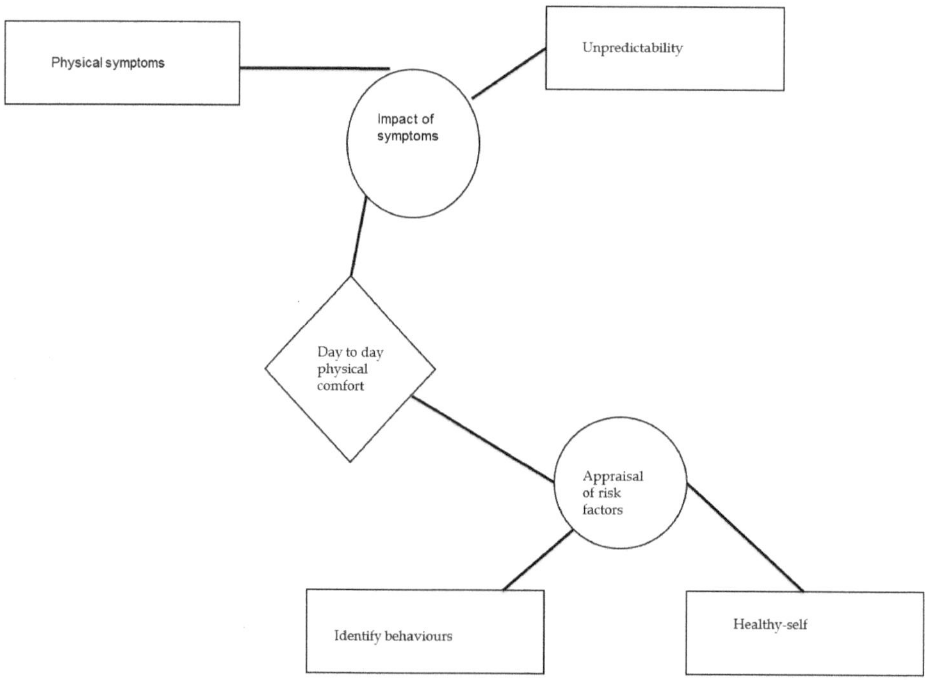

Diagram 1. Thematic network: Day to day physical comfort

The global themes that were evident from all three sources however differ in the detail covered. The questionnaires were at a basic theme level and remained at the identification and quantification of symptoms function and role. The literature and semi-structured interviews revealed a wider range of physical and emotional symptoms and demonstrated increased subtleties. This meant that there was more explanation into how participants coped with physical and emotional symptoms, as well as place in society.

Participant 1: "We have an away day in October. I said I don't think I can go because I think it would bother me. They said "oh no we would ask for something special for you at mealtimes" I said "no I don't want to eat around a table with people, if I could just bring my drinks and be somewhere separate where no one would bother me or say "come and eat with us" then I'll come."

Participant 2: "People don't know how much you rely on your tongue. There are a lot of things I can't do. I can't touch the top of my lip. If I get a piece of meat stuck in the back of my tooth, before I'd use my tongue..... But now I can't. I have to use the toothbrush to get it out..... There's no point in getting irritated because I can't change it. I might do it one day but I just get on with it."

Participant 3: You try not to let it get to you, how bad you are and the pain you're in(pointing at anterior lateral thigh donor site) so you cope with it more because if you're not showing it you can cope."

All three of the above semi-structured interview excerpts describe symptoms and function - eating in public, reduced tongue mobility and the ongoing issue of pain- but also describe what strategies the participants use to over come them.

Whilst as a basic theme identification of primary risk behaviours such as tobacco and alcohol use were evident within one of the three questionnaires-the FACT (I smoke Cigarettes; I drink alcohol); the semi-structured interviews were able to develop the theme into a personal appraisal of such behaviours being renewed.

Participant 2:"I was diagnosed on the Wednesday, I went outside and lit up; I had half a cigarette and went home, had a cup of tea and a sandwich and smoked half a cigarette. About five o'clock, I lit up another cigarette up and had half. I finished the other half about eight o'clock and I said when I go to bed tonight I'll have a cigarette in the morning. I woke up and never touched one.

I used to smoke thirty or forty per day. I don't know how I just stopped and I'd been trying to pack up for ten years as my New Year resolution"

Participant: 3 More than ever, I still crave a cigarette I've actually banned it from the house now. If it's raining I'll let them smoke in the kitchen with the door closed and the windows open but it's not for me."

Within the global theme place in society the HRQoL questionnaires revealed the basic theme of personal roles identified at work, -"my work is fulfilling" and within social and family circles " I get emotional support from my family", " I feel close to my partner" (FACT H&N). Within the interviews the global theme was expressed more in terms of the alienation from society and the purpose of some roles that participants had. Participants were very specific and actively chose who would or would not know about the diagnosis and the treatment, a way of maintaining a particular role but which within the FACT might still be labelled as having family support and so overlook certain choices made to protect other members of the family.

Participant 1:"I couldn't tell my brother and sister, or my children. One of my sons had a first child on the way and he was born three days after I left the hospital so I couldn't possibly worry him. ....My younger son had had a terrible accident when he was ten months old, he poured a kettle over himself, so knowing that I had mouth cancer, I didn't even want him to come and see me, I thought it would bring it all back to him, so I shut them out of life whilst I was in the hospital."

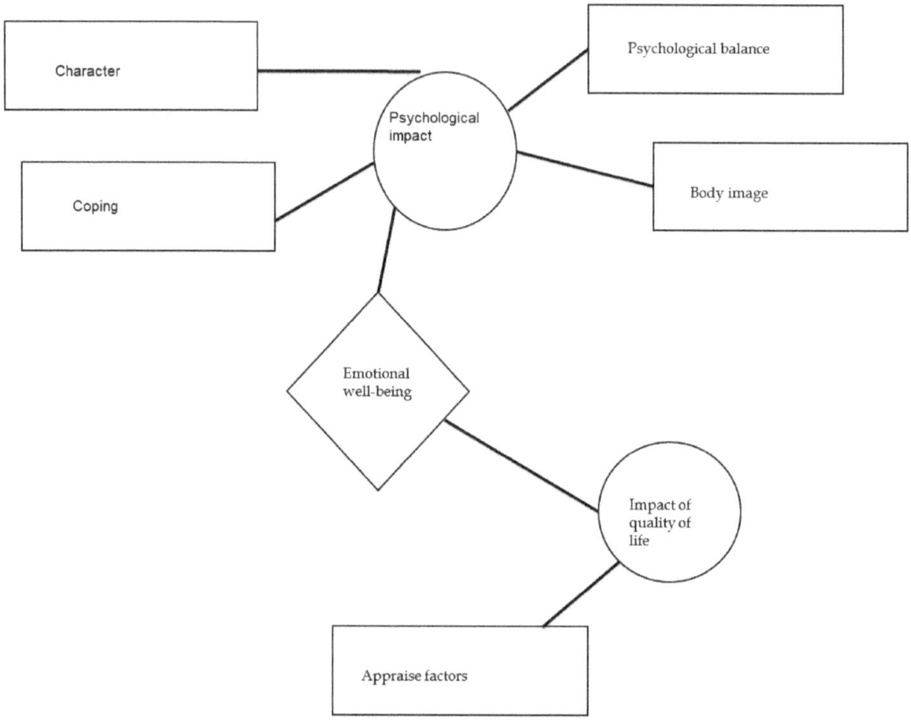

Diagram 2. Thematic network: Emotional well-being

The semi-structured interviews also revealed the detail of explicit secondary gain that predominantly focussed around enhanced relationships. This included the adjustment of values and priorities such that more time was spent with family members. Situations were also reappraised in the context of health and survival.

Participant 4: "I allow a lot of trivialities to go out the window, which I wouldn't have done before........domestic situations at home, I'll break something it would have bothered me before, and I would have fixed it quickly but it can wait. I'll get it done when I feel like it when it's convenient.......... I can't wait to see my grandkids. It makes you more appreciative of your family."

The final common theme between all three sources "Own Mortality" was again explored to different depths by each source. Within the HRQoL questionnaires it was evident with the FACT questionnaire "I worry about dying" In the literature it was explored through the theme of disease recurrence- a substantial part of the H&NC survivor literature (Llewellyn et al., 2008, Humphris et al., 2003)and an acceptance that death is a possibility (Chaturvedi et al., 1996). Fear of recurrence within the semi-structured interviews was openly expressed.

Participant 5 "Now and then I worry it might come back."

Participant 1 "Now and then the worry comes over you. I don't worry if it will come back; I wonder if I would have the courage to meet new people with that diagnosis again, I'm ok where I am."

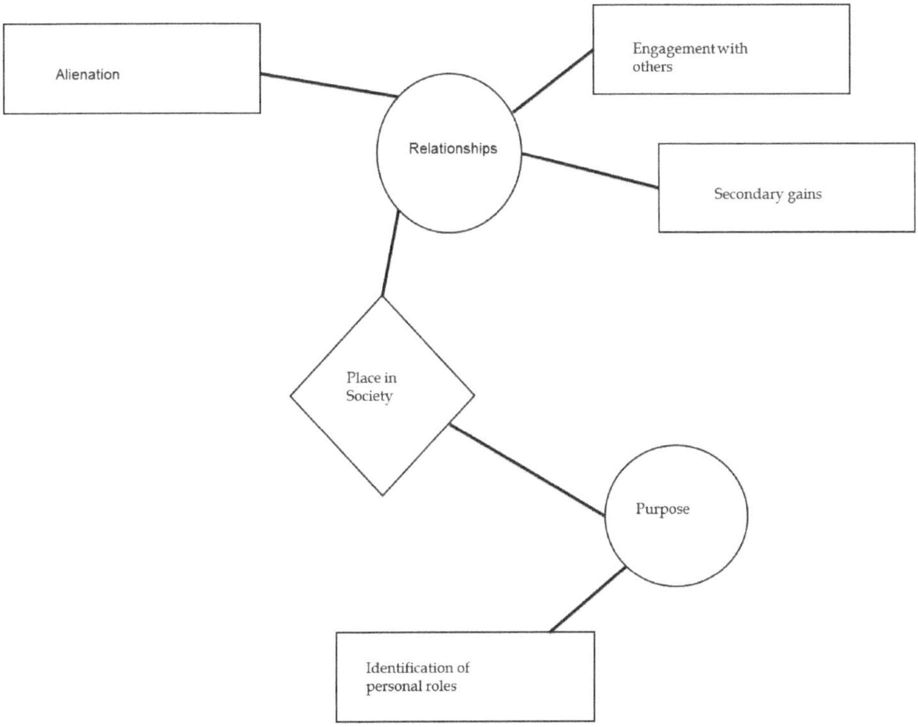

Diagram 3. Thematic network: Place in society

There was acknowledgement that participants had actively prepared for the possibility of dying soon after treatment. Five of the six participants had made personal preparations in the event of not recovering enough to adequately deal with personal effects.

Participant 1: "All day for a couple of weeks I didn't think I would survive the operation and I knew the house would have to be cleared so I just spent day after day clearing books. One day I had eight bags for the charity shop."

Two participants within the global theme of mortality expressed regret at having the treatment. There was a sense of reappraisal in the context of having the treatment and an admission that the current existence was hard to reconcile because of the change in function.

Participant 3: "I wish to God now that I had not had it done and I would have just carried on for twelve months with a bottle in one hand, well not for twelve months I most probably would have had three. I'm not used to being ill for longer than a couple of weeks."

One of the participants commented on the difference for them between the questionnaires and an interview discussion.

Participant 4 : "if you do the normal surveys when you've come round and asked me questions, I tick and cross the response but I don't think I give out that much information,............ but some people like me when you start talking never stop and then you find out so much in twenty minutes, -all in one go."

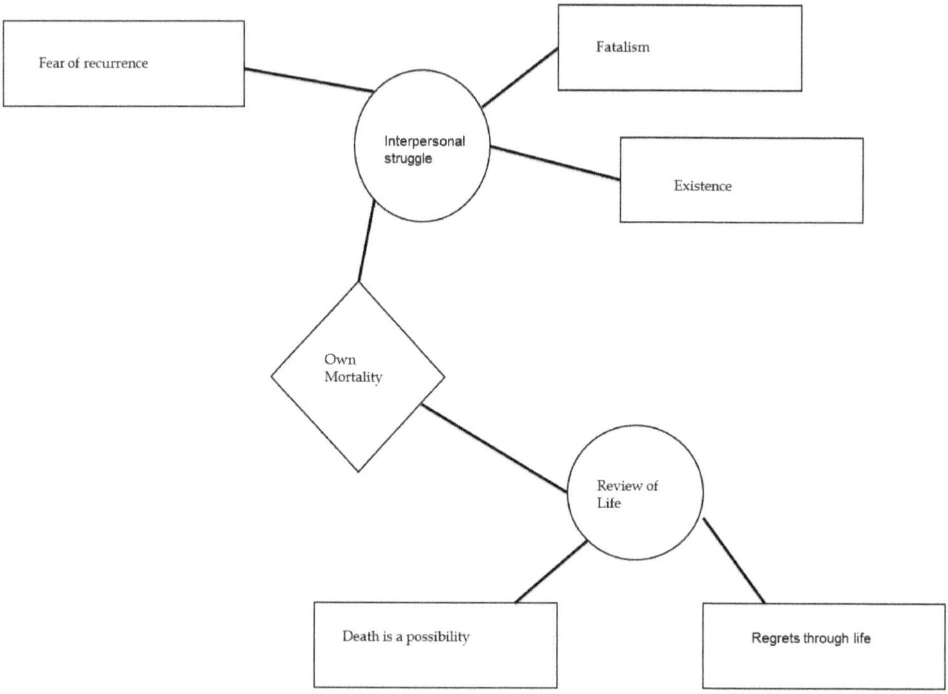

Diagram 4. Thematic network : Own mortality

3.2 Findings from literature and interviews

The literature and interviews added a further global theme: quality of care.

The quality of care theme was able to illustrate patient vulnerabilities and assumptions that might be present during the treatment process. There was a sense from participants interviewed that it was not possible to really appreciate how long it would take to begin to recover from the treatment. The semi-structured interviews gave evidence of the difficulty participants had in the assimilation of written and verbal information, and more specifically the implications of not understanding information. One participant explicitly described how it was difficult to appreciate what the real meaning was of a neck dissection until it had happened, relating it then to physical changes.

Participant 2: "The surgeon was saying what he was going to do, he said he would cut me from here to here and he would take my glands out. I understood but I suppose I didn't understand the extent of what the operation involved. Does that make sense? They are alien words; when you say you are going to make a line from here to here and take away glands I don't really know what that means. I didn't know the glands were as big as they were. It was obvious what was happening but I didn't understand what it would mean."

Another described how despite needing three operations within the space of three weeks it was not possible to be prepared any more comprehensively because of it being so difficult to predict the course of recovery. Research has concluded that the timeliness, individuality and amount of written and verbal information given to patients are vital if trying to reduce evident mismatch between patient expectations and experiences (Llewellyn et al., 2008, Llewellyn et al., 2006).

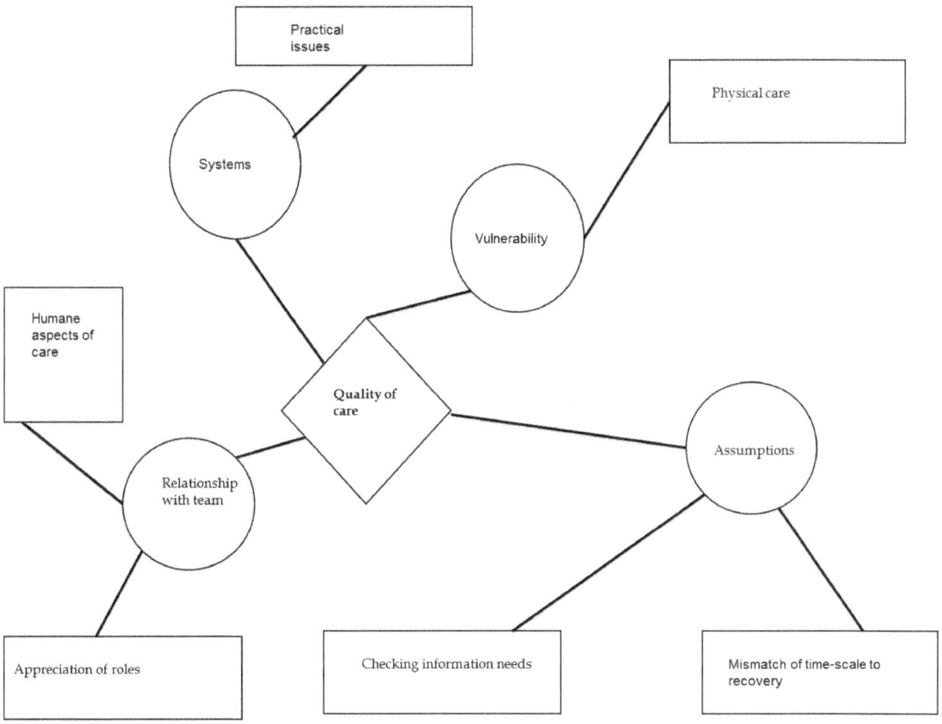

Diagram 5. Thematic network: Quality of care

A substantial organising theme was the relationship with the team. Examples were given within the literature of individual and patient orientated care and although the teams judged this as time consuming,(McLane et al., 2003) it was seen to have value and focus to the team and patient interactions. H&NC patients undergoing treatment have been described as resilient and resistant to offers of help (Wells, 1998), an issue echoed within the semi-structured interviews when a participant described not wanting to bother busy ward staff unless there was a real need. For example it might also be that there is some difficulty in patient compliance and adherence to treatment programmes that needs to be identified and addressed (Edmonds and MaGuire, 2007). Specific to the semi-structured interviews there was evidence of institution organisation difficulties. These included logistical and practical issues relating to appointments. Both the literature and semi-structured interviews disclosed information relating to the humane judgments in patient care. There was evidence to suggest that it was expected that there would be good advanced communication skills used, which would result in a consistent and understood message from the teams (Moore et al., 2004, Llewellyn et al., 2006). Specifically the semi-structured interviews highlighted the utter trust, vulnerability and belief in key members of the clinical team that the participants had.

Participant 1 "Well you couldn't be in better hands anywhere in the world, from first meeting my surgeon I had no fear and trusted him. I always felt better when I left the appointment he was just so down to earth and gave me so much confidence."

Participant 2 "And the surgeon's reputation is important, because you're thinking if you are going to do this to me, and you are telling me its going to work, I have to believe you are the best to do it, because if I don't then you are completely lost...They don't make you feel like a number. If I've got a problem I can raise it with somebody. It's not as though you go to the bottom of the pile and have to repeat it all the next time you visit they remember the conversation and what was on your mind at the last appointment."

3.3 Findings from the semi-structured interviews

The semi-structured interviews revealed a specific global theme, reality that reflects some of the stoical aspects of the participants in dealing with the situation. In this context participants described unremitting symptoms, the acceptance of being reactive rather than in control, the need for an inner strength and the stark choices that had been faced during the assessment and treatment phase of their disease. Participants did not perceive choice at the time of treatment because in reality little choice existed in deciding whether to have treatment.

Participant 5: You've got no option, it's that or nothing, so you have to have it done you don't have to think about it at all-there is no choice."

The perceived choice by others was not in reality available to the participants. This aspect of stark choices linked to the basic theme of alienation that participants felt in the global theme "place in society". The inner strength that became an organising theme was made up of examples of physical and emotional loneliness and a sense of if the participants did not deal with the issues then no one else would.

Participant 3 "I just worried that I'm not going to feel much better and I'm finding it difficult to cope."

Participant 5 "The days pass and you go to sleep and you relax and you don't think about it even with the tube in your neck (tracheostomy) you have to learn to switch off and let the nurses do the worrying."

There was also evidence of unremitting symptoms, both physical and emotional that were continually present and difficult to ignore. This in part explained the reactive state that participants expressed in which they were not able to take control of certain symptoms. There was a sense of needing to wait to heal; knowing that to be too active would lead to frustration, fatigue and deterioration in function.

Participant 6: "For me it is a very ongoing thing and also to the point where you can have what are called one of my 'good days' and you think this is great only to feel the next two days are horrid and you think I'm back to where I was. I count my good days and enjoy and do what I can .... You have to let time pass, you can't hurry (the recovery) and you have to let it go at it's own pace."

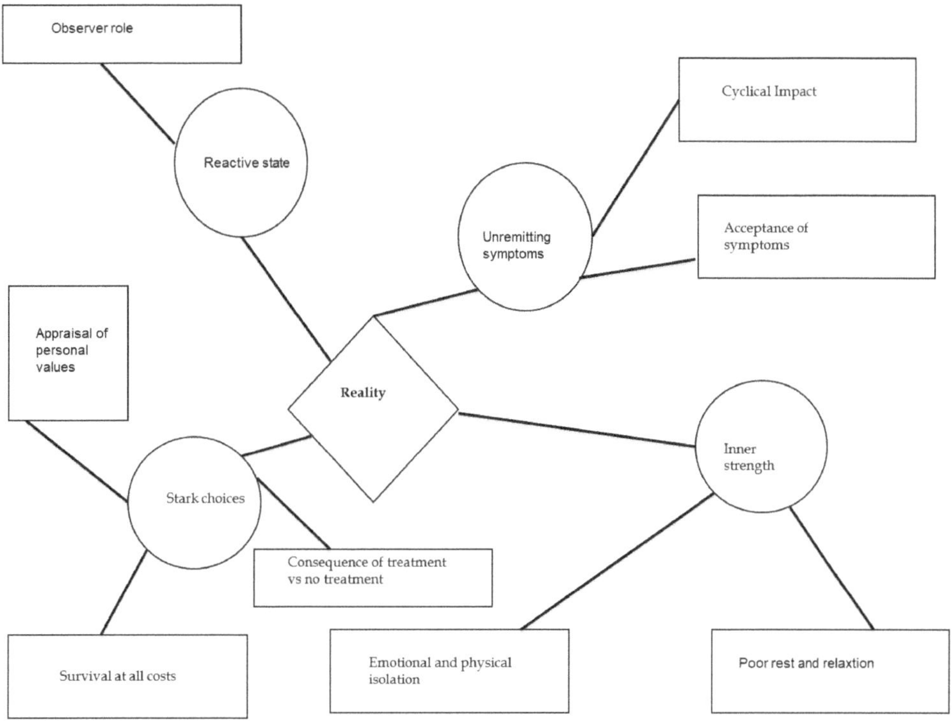

Diagram 6. Thematic analysis: Reality

The evident stoicism and depiction that participants presented that they were emotionally coping hid the reality of the gruelling impact that participants dealt with.

Participant 3 "Once you let your defences down that's when you start to crumble, so it's as though I'm standing on the outside of the building, but I've crumbled inside, ...there are times in the last few weeks I've felt 'oh hell what's the point, I'm not bothered but I don't let on."

From the semi-structured interviews it was possible to represent the global themes from statements made by the patients such that statements could be categorised under the global themes and perhaps give some real salience to the experience of the disease and treatment of H&NC. Diagram seven represents the 45 statements under one of the six global themes.

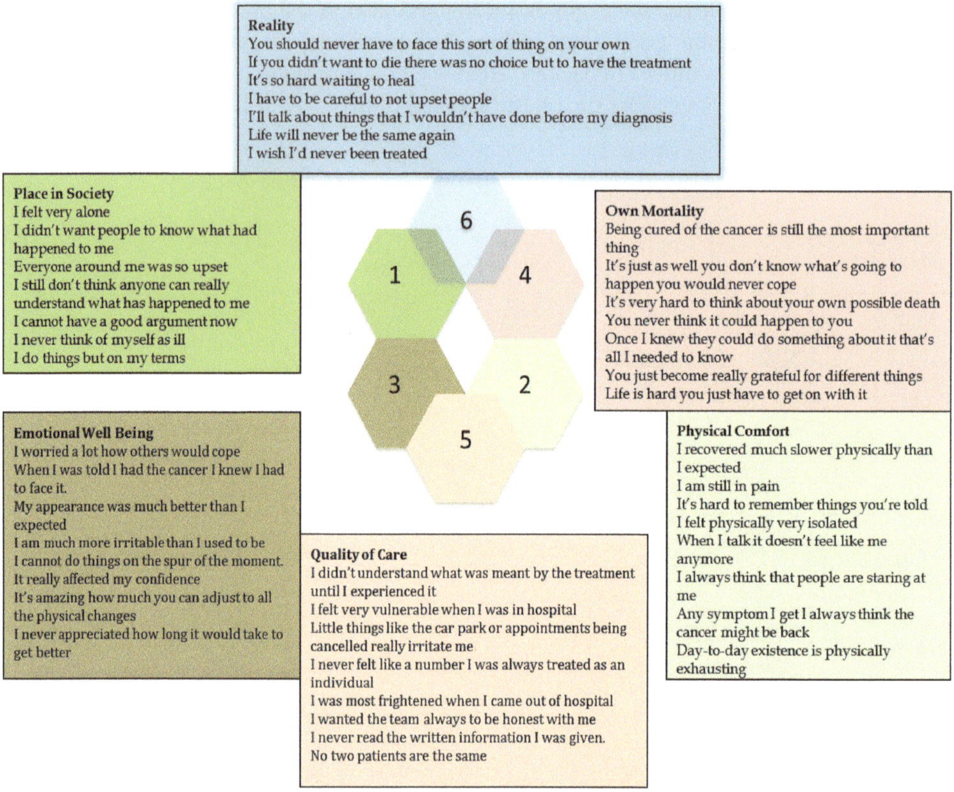

Diagram 7. Statements from participants that represent six themes.

4. Discussion

Three sources of information relating to the experience of H&NC have been thematically analysed using a previously described approach (Attride-Stirling 2001). HRQoL questionnaires focus on symptoms and function, which mean they remain at the level of basic themes. They do not allow the influences or the connections between scores to be understood so that patient adjustment and reappraisal when undergoing treatment is poorly represented. Whilst there might be changes identified by HRQoL questionnaires when they are repeated, there is limited explanation as to how the patient might have achieved this or the relevance of the symptom or change in function for the patient. This perspective is verified further in the context of the literature which has suggested that H&NC patients will under-report symptoms, due in part to a sense of hopelessness and loss of meaning to life following treatment for the disease (Moore et al., 2004). It might be therefore that the use of HRQoL questionnaires under-represents patients' real experience both in terms of intensity and scope.

This investigation of the experience of H&NC enables one to conclude that there are perhaps complex and interactive patient characteristics that will impact on the H&NC patients' QoL scores. The semi-structured interviews identify in participants a reappraisal of values, numerous coping strategies, and adaptation. It might therefore be that HRQoL questionnaires are measuring other effects, that modify patients' scores which are not directly related to the treatment and disease and which might, if better understood, give insight to the patient, carers and health care team which might secure a more successful management of the patient. A specific example of this can be seen within health behaviours. If a patient is still smoking or drinking alcohol the behaviour should not only be identified but have a patient specific commentary so that the health care professional might become more informed of the context for the continuing behaviour. If this could happen cessation programmes if appropriate might be more successful. Assessment of the existence of risky behaviours is only evident within one of the three most regularly used HRQoL questionnaires the FACT. It would seem therefore discussion of health behaviours is poorly represented within HRQoL questionnaires.

The current study demonstrates that the focus of HRQoL questionnaires is narrow and that it is important to build a context in which the HRQoL variables are a part rather than the whole. Whilst physical, emotional symptoms and personal relationships are a substantial part of a patient's description of their well-being they are not the complete picture. In order to achieve this, patients' needs and possible current limitations, quality of care and the reality of the situation for them as individuals should be discussed. If this aspect of the whole person can be better understood then personalised care can be described and care plans created which meets UK government policy (National Cancer Action Team, 2011). It might also be that the process of semi-structured discussion allows a patient to review their concerns and have them recognised as important aspects of their care. Through this method of investigation the health care team might begin to truly understand, in the context of the patient's own previous life-experiences why they might have reacted in a particular way during their treatment and recovery. Such understanding and reflection might allow patients to recognise at an earlier stage their needs, which might avert a crisis; a further intention of the Holistic Needs Assessment set out by the National Cancer Action Team (2011). It might also mean that patients are able to discuss and understand dissatisfactions in life without having feelings labelled as either anxiety or depression.

It has been suggested by Salander (Salander, 2011) that the added burden of the cancer diagnosis and treatment prompts patients to seek support in order to lessen the total psychological burden. He went onto suggest that whilst patients need medical input to cure them of the cancer they are capable of lessoning some of the emotions associated with the situation. As part of this process they may respond well to the opportunity to reappraise their life. Within a treatment paradigm patient data should not only act as a descriptor but also as a way of formulating a treatment plan. If this could be achieved, studies would move beyond recognising the presence of the impact towards aiming to describe more specifically how treatment has affected patients. Discussion via semi-structured interview enables much more explanation of the patient's situation and allows for the true context of the symptom or feeling to be described. This approach is more holistic and might allow for the medical team to make judgements with the patients, which relate to their tolerance of the situation. This method of enquiry is less likely to be open to misinterpretation and might add more satisfactorily detail so that care-plans might be formulated. It might be that HRQoL questionnaires can act as a screen of needs assessment for some of the more obvious physical and emotional impacts of the disease and treatment, but they should not take the place of detailed discussion between the team and patient, and in no way can they be said to be representative of the whole experience.

5. Conclusion

Outcome should be represented in more meaningful terms than length of survival or clinical process targets. HRQoL measures might identify some of the more superficial aspects of outcome but a more rounded understanding of the covert aspects may positively support both the patient and their carers through such life-changing experiences. HRQoL questionnaires cannot be said to adequately reflect either the available literature on patient experience or the reported experiences of H&NC patients themselves. Review of all three sources would suggest that when used HRQoL questionnaires are used there is a narrow, symptoms biased collection of information. The questionnaires cannot capture the wealth of the data that is potentially available or offer an explanation to some of the measures that are taken.

Health care teams, patients and their families should understand the impact of H&NC and its management from a holistic perspective so that the care can be achieved successfully for each individual. HRQoL measures by necessity have a narrow focus on symptom and function and these can be mistakenly seen as representing a patient's QoL rather than as some of the constituent parts. Within a clinical setting it would seem valuable to routinely invite patients who have undergone treatment to discuss, in a semi-structured way, the individual impact of the disease and the treatment. The purpose of this would be to facilitate a deeper understanding through explanation of the individual experience and to enable specialist teams to support patients more appropriately in outpatient settings. If this were to happen it would enable teams to move away from the quantifying process, in which a change in score has limited real meaning towards more a detailed explanation. Moving towards a more holistic needs assessment should enable patients to explain what has happened to them and to appreciate a more complete picture of the impact. If this could be achieved one might expect that a patient is less dependent on others for their well-being and that they could seek help earlier. There should be a recognition that patients' minds are intrinsically linked to their physical status and are not well represented because they are hard to describe in a meaningful way.

This study only examined the experience of six H&NC patients' experience of their treatment within a UK cancer centre. The statements gathered from them can be used in a more formal way to investigate the experiences of other H&NC patients. A future study will use the list of statements generated from the six identified themes with other H&NC patients and invite them to rank them according to how like or unlike their experience of the disease the statements are. The current study has therefore acted as a way of creating a set of statements from three sources, and is part of the a method called Q Methodology, which has been described as a way of looking for patterns in the way people think (Webler, 2009). There is perhaps a role for more qualitative methodologies to be used alongside quantitative methods in order to discover what factors affect people who survive the disease, which to date has been poorly identified. This may allow a structured approach that is replicable with more groups of patients and this might be said to be an influential method of gathering key factors that are important for patients at an individual level. The ultimate goal will remain to collect information that can inform the management of patients who live with the consequences of a life changing event so that they can live as independently as possible from health care systems and carers.

6. Ackowlegement

The first author would like to thank Professor Carolyn Hicks, Mr Sat Parmar, and Mr Andrew Brown for their significant and most insightful professional support that they have provided over many years.

7. References

Attride-Stirling, J. 2001. Thematic-networks: an analytic tool for qualitative research. Qualitative Research, 1, 385-405.

Bjordal, K., Ahlner-Elmqvist, M., Tollesson, E., Jensen, A. B., Razavi, D., Maher, E. J. & Kaasa, S. 1994. Development of a European Organization for Research and Treatment of Cancer (EORTC) questionnaire module to be used in quality of life assessments in head and neck cancer patients. EORTC Quality of Life Study Group. Acta Oncol, 33, 879-85.

Bjordal, K. & Kaasa, S. 1992. Psychometric validation of the EORTC Core Quality of Life Questionnaire, 30-item version and a diagnosis-specific module for head and neck cancer patients. Acta Oncol, 31, 311-21.

Campbell, B. H., Spinelli, K., Marbella, A. M., Myers, K. B., Kuhn, J. C. & Layde, P. M. 2004. Aspiration, weight loss, and quality of life in head and neck cancer survivors. Arch Otolaryngol Head Neck Surg, 130, 1100-3.

Chaturvedi, S. K., Shenoy, A., Prasad, K. M., Senthilnathan, S. M. & Premlatha, B. S. 1996. Concerns, coping and quality of life in head and neck cancer patients. Support Care Cancer, 4, 186-90.

Curtis, J. R., Martin, D.P, Martin, T.R. . 1997;. Patient-assessed health outcomes in chronic lung disease: what are they, how do they help us, and where do we go from here? Am J Respir Crit Care Med 156, 1032–1039.

De Graeff, A., De Leeuw, J. R., Ros, W. J., Hordijk, G. J., Blijham, G. H. & Winnubst, J. A. 2001. Sociodemographic factors and quality of life as prognostic indicators in head and neck cancer. Eur J Cancer, 37, 332-9.

Department Of Health 2010. National Cancer Patient Experience Survey Programme - 2010 National Survey Report.

Department Of Health. 2011. Improving Outcomes: A Stratedgy for Cancer [Online]. Available: http://www.dh.gov.uk/prod_consum_dh/groups/dh_digitalassets/documents/digitalasset/dh_123394.pdf.

Edmonds, M. & Maguire, D. 2007. Treatment adherence in head and neck cancer patients undergoing radiation therapy: challenges for nursing.

Journal of Radiology Nursing, 26, 87-92.

Fang, F. M., Liu, Y. T., Tang, Y., Wang, C. J. & Ko, S. F. 2004. Quality of life as a survival predictor for patients with advanced head and neck carcinoma treated with radiotherapy. Cancer, 100, 425-32.

Hammerlid, E., Bjordal, K., Ahlner-Elmqvist, M., Boysen, M., Evensen, J. F., Biorklund, A., Jannert, M., Kaasa, S., Sullivan, M. & Westin, T. 2001. A prospective study of quality of life in head and neck cancer patients. Part I: at diagnosis. Laryngoscope, 111, 669-80.

Hammerlid, E. & Taft, C. 2001. Health-related quality of life in long-term head and neck cancer survivors: a comparison with general population norms. Br J Cancer, 84, 149-56.

Hassan, S. J. & Weymuller, E. A., Jr. 1993. Assessment of quality of life in head and neck cancer patients. Head Neck, 15, 485-96.

Howren, M. B., Christensen, A. J., Karnell, L. H. & Funk, G. F. 2010. Health-related quality of life in head and neck cancer survivors: impact of pretreatment depressive symptoms. Health Psychol, 29, 65-71.

Humphris, G. M., Rogers, S., Mcnally, D., Lee-Jones, C., Brown, J. & Vaughan, D. 2003. Fear of recurrence and possible cases of anxiety and depression in orofacial cancer patients. Int J Oral Maxillofac Surg, 32, 486-91.

Kanatas, A. N., Mehanna, H. M., Lowe, D. & Rogers, S. N. 2009. A second national survey of health-related quality of life questionnaires in head and neck oncology. Ann R Coll Surg Engl, 91, 420-5.

Karvonen-Gutierrez, C. A., Ronis, D. L., Fowler, K. E., Terrell, J. E., Gruber, S. B. & Duffy, S. A. 2008. Quality of life scores predict survival among patients with head and neck cancer. J Clin Oncol, 26, 2754-60.

List, M. A., Ritter-Sterr, C. & Lansky, S. B. 1990. A performance status scale for head and neck cancer patients. Cancer, 66, 564-9.

Llewellyn, C. D., Mcgurk, M. & Weinman, J. 2005. Are psycho-social and behavioural factors related to health related-quality of life in patients with head and neck cancer? A systematic review. Oral Oncol, 41, 440-54.

Llewellyn, C. D., Mcgurk, M. & Weinman, J. 2006. How satisfied are head and neck cancer (HNC) patients with the information they receive pre-treatment? Results from the satisfaction with cancer information profile (SCIP). Oral Oncol, 42, 726-34.

Llewellyn, C. D., Weinman, J., Mcgurk, M. & Humphris, G. 2008. Can we predict which head and neck cancer survivors develop fears of recurrence? J Psychosom Res, 65, 525-32.

Logemann, J. A., Smith, C. H., Pauloski, B. R., Rademaker, A. W., Lazarus, C. L., Colangelo, L. A., Mittal, B., Maccracken, E., Gaziano, J., Stachowiak, L. & Newman, L. A. 2001. Effects of xerostomia on perception and performance of swallow function. Head Neck, 23, 317-21.

Mclane, L., Jones, K., Lydiatt, W., Lydiatt, D. & Richards, A. 2003. Taking away the fear: a grounded theory study of cooperative care in the treatment of head and neck cancer. Psychooncology, 12, 474-90.

Mehanna, H. M., De Boer, M. F. & Morton, R. P. 2008. The association of psycho-social factors and survival in head and neck cancer. Clin Otolaryngol, 33, 83-9.

Mehanna, H. M. & Morton, R. P. 2006a. Patients' views on the utility of quality of life questionnaires in head and neck cancer: a randomised trial. Clin Otolaryngol, 31, 310-6.

Mehanna, H. M. & Morton, R. P. 2006b. Why are head and neck cancer clinicians not measuring quality of life? J Laryngol Otol, 120, 861-4.

Montazeri, A. 2009. Quality of life data as prognostic indicators of survival in cancer patients: an overview of the literature from 1982 to 2008. Health Qual Life Outcomes, 7, 102.

Moore, R. J., Chamberlain, R. M. & Khuri, F. R. 2004. Communicating suffering in primary stage head and neck cancer. Eur J Cancer Care (Engl), 13, 53-64.

National Cancer Action Team. 2011. Holistic needs assessment for people with cancer [Online]. Available: http://www.ncat.nhs.uk/our-work/living-with-beyond-cancer/holistic-needs-assessment.

National Institue for Clinical Excellence 2004. Improving supportive and palliative care for adults with cancer:the manual The Stationary Office London.

Reid, K., Hicks, C., Herron-Marx, S. & Parmar, S. 2009. Effect of oral tumour size on quality of life judgements by health care professionals working with head and neck cancer patients: a pilot study. J Laryngol Otol, 123, 1352-7.

Rogers, S. L., D. Yueh, Bevan, A. Weymuller, E, A., JR 2010. The Physical Function and Social-Emotional Function Subscales of the University of Washington Quality of Life Questionnaire. J Arch Otolaryngol Head Neck Surg, 136, 352-357.

Rogers, S. N., Ahad, S. A. & Murphy, A. P. 2007. A structured review and theme analysis of papers published on 'quality of life' in head and neck cancer: 2000-2005. Oral Oncol, 43, 843-68.

Ronis, D. L., Duffy, S. A., Fowler, K. E., Khan, M. J. & Terrell, J. E. 2008. Changes in quality of life over 1 year in patients with head and neck cancer. Arch Otolaryngol Head Neck Surg, 134, 241-8.

Salander, P. 2011. Why doesn't mind matter when we are to find out what is helpful? Psychooncology, 20, 441-2.

Scharloo, M., Baatenburg De Jong, R. J., Langeveld, T. P., Van Velzen-Verkaik, E., Doorn-Op Den Akker, M. M. & Kaptein, A. A. 2005. Quality of life and illness perceptions in patients with recently diagnosed head and neck cancer. Head Neck, 27, 857-63.

Sollner, W., Devries, A., Steixner, E., Lukas, P., Sprinzl, G., Rumpold, G. & MAISLINGER, S. 2001. How successful are oncologists in identifying patient distress, perceived social support, and need for psychosocial counselling? Br J Cancer, 84, 179-85.

Velikova, G., Keding, A., Harley, C., Cocks, K., Booth, L., Smith, A. B., Wright, P., Selby, P. J. & Brown, J. M. 2010. Patients report improvements in continuity of care when quality of life assessments are used routinely in oncology practice: secondary outcomes of a randomised controlled trial. Eur J Cancer, 46, 2381-8.

Webler, T. D., S. and Tuler, S. 2009. Using Q Method to Reveal Social Perspectives in Environmental Research. Available: www.seri- us.org/pubs/Qprimer.pdf [Accessed January 20th 2011].

Wells, M. 1998. The hidden experience of radiotherapy to the head and neck: a qualitative study of patients after completion of treatment. J Adv Nurs, 28, 840-8.
Whoqol Group 1993. Whoqol Study Protocol, Geneva, WHO.

16

Pain Control in Head and Neck Cancer

Ping-Yi Kuo and John E Williams
Royal Marsden Hospital Foundation NHS Trust
United Kingdom

1. Introduction

"An unpleasant sensory and emotional experience associated with actual or potential tissue damage"(Merskey & Bogduk, 1994), pain is one of the most common symptoms in cancer (Lorenz et al., 2006). Pain associated with head and neck cancer could result from the following causes (Williams & Broadley, 2009):

- Local or metastatic disease causing infiltration, pressure or ulceration
- Side effects from anti-cancer treatment: medication, chemotherapy, radiotherapy, surgery
- Incidental causes such as infection or coexisting morbidity

The assessment of pain should be thorough, the treatment prompt and carefully considered. The current international consensus is that "...the unreasonable failure to treat pain is poor medicine, unethical practice, and is an abrogation of a fundamental human right" (Brennan et al., 2007).

Undertreatment of pain may result in patients having increased morbidity (Carr et al., 1992; MacIntyre 2005), increased prevalence of depression and anxiety (Brennan et al., 2005; Gureje et al., 1998), poor sleep (Thorpe 1993; Cleeland et al., 1996), poor concentration and poor personal interactions (Ferrell, 1995). It also has massive socioeconomic costs including loss in productivity (Steward et al., 2003; van Leeuwen et al., 2006), work days (Brennan et al., 2005) and litigations (Blyth et al., 2003).

Management options should be kept as simple and easy to follow as possible to ensure compliance to treatment. Patients may prefer medication in liquid form as mouth opening may be difficult. However it has been noted that some oral elixirs may contain alcohol, which cause local irritation in a patient with oral mucositis, and tablets which are crushed may feel gritty and unpleasant (Weissman, 1989). Also in patients with dysphagia, the tablets may be difficult to swallow. Suffice to say that it is extremely important to keep re-assessing the patient to make sure that the treatment prescribed is not more unpleasant than the symptom itself! The clinician may need to be flexible and imaginative in finding ways for the patient to comply with treatment. Other routes of administration may need to be considered, including the use of suppositories, subcutaneous infusion pumps, nasogastric feeding tubes, percutaneous enteric gastric tubes and transdermal patches.

2. Prevalence of pain

Despite guidelines for treatment of cancer pain available from agencies such as the WHO (1996, 2008) and the Expert Working Group of the European Association for Palliative Care (2001), it has been shown in a recent meta-analysis involving 26 studies that nearly half of patients with cancer have pain that is undertreated (Deandrea et al., 2008). Another meta-analysis showed that cancer pain prevalence is around 53%, irrespective of staging - in particular for patients with head and neck cancer, the prevalence is the highest of all cancers at 70% (Van den Beuken-van Everdingen et al., 2007). In a pan-European survey screening over 5000 cancer patients, 56% had moderate-to-severe pain at least monthly (Breivik et al., 2009). Patients with brain cancer and squamous cell cancer of the head and neck were amongst those with the highest prevalence of pain – 90% and 86% respectively.

The prevalence of pain at diagnosis of head and neck cancers vary from 40% to 84% (Keefe et al., 1986; Chaplin, 1999; Epstein, 1993; Saxena et al., 1995). A higher incidence of pain was noted in more advanced disease i.e. stages III or IV (Keefe et al., 1986). A recent study showed that a third of patients who attend head and neck cancer outpatients had pain from any cause within the previous seven days, with over two-thirds of those having severe pain (Williams et al., 2010). No specific risk factors for pain were found in this population.

3. Aetiology of pain

The cornerstone of effective pain management is to determine the aetiology of the pain (Miaskowski et al., 2005). Pain can be due to the cancer itself, as a result of anti-cancer treatment such as surgery, radiotherapy or chemotherapy, or pain which is wholly unrelated to cancer – for example, incidental arthritic pain (Table 1). The type of pain suffered by patients could be nociceptive, neuropathic or mixed nociceptive and neuropathic.

Nociceptive pain often results from tissue damage - for example tumour pressure, the recurrence of tumour, bony infiltration, deafferentiation or neuroma formation secondary to nerve damage during neck dissection, mucositis, related or unrelated infection and inflammation (e.g. sinusitis), osteoradionecrosis, lesions in the cervical spine causing head and neck pain, to name but a few causes (Chua et al., 1999; Williams & Broadley 2009).

Some authors also distinguished myofascial pain from nociceptive *per se*. Talmi et al. (2000) in particular discussed a type of pain resulting from a musculoskeletal imbalance, and associated changes occuring in the shoulder as a result of surgical neck dissection and removal of neck muscles. They cited Fialka and Vinzenz (1988) who noted that 77% patients had shoulder dysfunction and strong to severe pain after radical neck dissection, and Krause (1992) who noted that 31% of patients develop shoulder-arm syndrome after radical neck dissection. Pain resulting from anti-cancer treatment is important as it may be long-lasting and may also adversely affect compliance to continued anti-cancer treatment.

Reference	Pain due to cancer	Pain due to anti-cancer treatment	Pain associated with cancer disease	Non-cancer sources of pain
Grond et al., 1996	81%	31%	19%	7%
Williams et al., 2010	37%	42%	-	25%

Table 1. Presumed aetiology of pain in patients with head and neck cancer

Neuropathic pain is pain associated with injury or disease of the peripheral or central nervous systems, which may result in pathophysiological changes such as ectopic (spontaneous or evoked) discharge by nerves, microneuroanatomical changes, central sensitization, and many others beyond the scope of this review (Macintyre & Schug, 2007). Neuropathic pain for patients with head and neck cancer may involve all sensory nerves in the face, skull, neck and shoulders (Vecht et al., 1992). Some common symptoms of neuropathic pain experienced by the patients include spontaneous continuous burning (81%), shooting pain (69%) and allodynia (88%) - which describes abnormal pain elicited by light touch (Sist et al., 1999; Merskey & Bogduk, 1994). The percentage of patients with head and neck cancer in various studies who were assessed to have neuropathic pain is shown in Table 2.

Reference	Neuropathic (Mixed neuropathic /nociceptive)	Comments
Grond et al., 1993*	28%	From surgical treatment
Grond et al., 1996	47%	377 patients
Forbes, 1997	26%	
Vecht et al, 1992	23%	25 patients, from surgical treatment
Sist et al., 1999	100%	25 patients, post radical-neck dissection
Chua et al., 1999	7.5% (37.5%)	40 outpatients
Williams et al., 2010	10%	70 outpatients

Table 2. Numbers of patients with head and neck cancer and neuropathic or mixed neuropathic/nociceptive pain. * Cited by Talmi et al., 2000

4. Assessment of pain

Prior to commencing analgesic therapy, a detailed history and careful examination is required in the patient with head and neck cancer to determine the cause of the pain, and the potential role of anti-cancer therapy in treating the cancer and thus decreasing or relieving the pain. The relative impact of analgesic drugs and techniques should also be explored. Investigations such as radiological examinations may be required to accurately determine the cause of the pain.

The assessment of pain in any patient requires attention not only to the physical and physiological aspects, but also to psychological, including how the pain and disease may impact on their quality of life (Portenoy et al., 1999). The emotional and cognitive components of pain may be more significant in cancer compared with non-cancer pain (Huber et al., 2007). In patients with head and neck cancer additional functional problems including ability to swallow, speech, hearing, sight etc also may need to be assessed. All of which will have an additional impact on their quality of life. The expertise of specialties such as psychological medicine, psychiatry, neurology, allied health staff and others are required to provide a multi-disciplinary approach to pain. Palliative care medicine encompasses many of these facets of cancer management, and as such is an invaluable source of information and assistance.

Patients with cancer often have more than one distinct pain syndrome (Grond et al., 1996), or more than one location (Valeberg et al., 2008). In 377 patients with primary head and neck cancer, they described their regions of pain as in Table 3. Assessment and treatment of these patients must then be thorough so as to not miss symptoms and potential problems.

Pain region	
Head/face/mouth	78%
Cervical region	45%
Upper shoulder/limbs	9%
Thoracic	7%
Lower back, lumbar spine, sacrum, coccyx	7%
Pelvic region	1%

Table 3. Pain regions in patients with head and neck cancer (Grond et al., 1996)

5. Application of pain pharmacology and physiology in the clinical setting

Pain as a subject is still under research and much is yet not understood about the mechanisms of chronic pain. Treatment methods of pain, particularly those of chronic and neuropathic pain, are still being refined. Table 4 shows some aspects of pain pharmacology and physiology linked to clinical relevance.

Pain Pharmacology and Physiology	Clinical Relevance
Peripheral nerve injury leads to ectopic discharge, microneuroanatomical and phenotypical changes*	Chronic, neuropathic pain is not easily treatable by conventional analgesics
Central sensitization as a result of neuroplasticity*	Treat early before persistent changes to CNS synaptic processing take place due to neuronal damage
Acute severe pain post-operatively is an important predictor of persistent pain*	Acute post-operative pain need to be aggressively treated to prevent long term problems with persistent pain
Evidence for pre-emptive analgesia is inconclusive*	No good evidence in humans for analgesics given pre-painful stimulus versus post-stimulus
Preventive analgesia to reduce chronic pain syndromes* †	"Preventative analgesia" is a description of when the effects of the analgesics administered exceed the expected duration of effect of the analgesic strategy. There is some evidence in the effective use of ketamine and early use of calcitonin in preventive analgesia.
NMDA receptor activation in central sensitization*‡	NMDA receptor antagonists, particularly ketamine, is of special interest, having been shown to have preventive analgesic effects in some circumstances
Role of reorganisation in the somatosensory cortex*	May contribute to neuropathic pain states such as phantom limb pain and complex regional pain syndrome (CRPS)
Multimodal analgesia to combat central and peripheral plasticity†	Use of more than one type of analgesic to treat pain
Evidence for effectiveness of the multidisciplinary approach to pain treatment‡	A holistic view of the patient situation should be employed, involving other practitioners in pain management

Table 4. Clinical relevance of pain pharmacology and physiology. (Brennan & Kehlet, 2005†; Macintyre & Schug, 2008*; Williams & Broadley, 2009‡)

6. Acute pain

Patients with head and neck cancer may suffer from acute cancer-related, or acute anti-cancer treatment related pain. Acute cancer-related pain may occur as a result of inflammatory and tumourigenic pain mechanisms such as local tumour pressure, or infiltration of tissues or bone, which may cause subsequent obstruction or compression of visceral structures or nerves and also paraneoplastic effects at distant sites (Portenoy & Lesage, 1999; Delaney et al., 2008). Anti-cancer treatments such as surgery, chemotherapy or radiotherapy can be a means of alleviating pain as the tumour is debulked, but they may also have side-effects causing acute pain after the treatment.

6.1 Acute post-surgical pain

In the patient with head and neck cancer, surgical procedures such as radical neck dissection or other major head and neck surgery will cause acute post-surgical pain - this is not unexpected by most people. The treatment of this acute post-surgical pain commences peri-operatively by the anaesthetist administering analgesics or local anaesthetic techniques such as local infiltration to the wound or nerve blocks. Some patients may be given analgesics as a pre-medication pre-operatively. Treatment of post-surgical pain continues into the recovery area and onto the wards and eventually home ideally using multi-modal analgesia via all routes of administration, as will be discussed later in the chapter.

Acute post-surgical pain is usually easily amenable to treatment and as such should be promptly and adequately treated to prevent development of chronic post-surgical pain (CPSP). Patients reporting high levels of acute post-operative pain and at 4 days post-operation are at high risk of increased pain, poor global recovery with functional limitations and lower quality of life at 6 months post-operatively (Peters et al., 2007). This is concordant with review articles by Perkins & Kehlet (2000) and Kehlet et al. (2006) citing numerous studies to show that acute moderate to severe post-operative pain is a predictive factor for CPSP. Occasionally acute post-surgical pain is difficult to treat as nerve damage occurs peri-operatively from direct resection, bruising or stretching, particularly patients undergoing radical neck dissection (Talmi et al., 2000). Referred shoulder and arm pain may also occur (Chaplin, 1999; Talmi et al., 2000).

6.2 Acute pain following radiotherapy and chemotherapy

Pain following radio- and chemo-therapy in patients with head and neck cancer normally manifests itself as oral mucositis. However, other problems such as radiation fibrosis syndrome, infection and chemotherapy-induced peripheral neuropathy can also cause acute or chronic pain.

6.2.1 Oral mucositis

Radiation-induced mucositis is common in head and neck cancer patients, with increasing frequency due to the use of more intensive altered radiation and concurrent chemotherapy regimes (Rosenthal & Trotti, 2009). The incidence however will significantly vary amongst different treatment regimens and modalities. Oral mucositis normally becomes symptomatic between the second and fourth week of treatment of radio- or chemotherapy. In many patients, oral mucositis is associated with considerable pain, which may lead to dose reductions, delays and abandonment of further anti-cancer treatments, to increases in healthcare costs, and impairment in the patient's quality of life. Details of the pathophysiology of oral mucositis is beyond the scope of this chapter. As an outline, the available evidence supports the view that oral mucositis is a complex, interactive process involving all the tissues and cellular elements of the mucosa, with suggestions of genetic risks of developing mucositis (Sonis et al., 2004). Further detailed work is required to clarify the process.

Pain is only one symptom of oral mucositis. Dysphagia, another common complaint, leads to a dependency on feeding tubes and its associated complications or parenteral nutrition, dehydration, micronutrient deficiencies, weight loss, and aspiration (Rosenthal & Trotti, 2009, Sonis et al., 2004). Mucositis also leads to ulceration and subsequent infection, which are both additional causes of pain. In children with mucositis, it should be remembered that their smaller airways may prove problematic with airway compromise. Hospitalisation is sometimes necessary both for initial control of pain and treatment of the other complications already mentioned.

Treatment of oral mucositis was recently the subject of a Cochrane Collaboration Review (Clarkson et al., 2008). They concluded that the evidence for allopurinol mouthwash, granulocytemacrophage-colony stimulating factor, immunoglobulin and human placental extract to improve or eradicate mucositis is weak and unreliable and requires further research.

Symptomatic control of oral mucositis pain by using analgesics may be via many different routes. Many patients with head and neck cancer are still able to take oral analgesics, so the oral route should not be disregarded altogether. One must bear in mind however the other routes of administration, including the transdermal patch, intravenous, intramuscular or subcutaneous routes. Although there is no evidence that patient controlled analgesia (PCA) is more beneficial than a continuous infusion method for controlling pain, patients using PCA used less opiate per hour, and had shorter durations of pain (Clarkson et al., 2008), and thus may suffer less from the side-effects of opiate medication. Multi-modal analgesia should also be considered. In particular, there is evidence that concomitant administration of adjuncts such as gabapentin is useful in radiation-induced mucositis (Bar et al., 2010a, 2010b).

6.2.2 Other complications of radio- and chemotherapy

Radio- and chemotherapy can also cause other pain syndromes in patients with head and neck cancer, such as radiation fibrosis syndrome, chemotherapy-induced peripheral neuropathy and infection.

With fibrosis from radiation pain may occur when the skin and underlying structures contract. An example is "dropped head syndrome", described by Rowin et al. in 2006 as one potential complication of radiation of the mantle field (neck, axillary and mediastinal lymph nodes). This is a late complication of radiotherapy, characterised by fibrosis and contractures of the anterior cervical muscles and atrophy of the posterior neck and shoulder girdle.

Chemotherapy-induced peripheral neuropathy (CIPN) is frequently a complication of common anti-cancer treatments, but is often under recognised and undertreated, with additional difficulties of it being difficult to diagnose, with no universally accepted assessment tools and a lack of interobserver agreement (Stephens et al., 1997 and Postma et al., 1998, as cited in Farquhar-Smith, 2011). As an example, docetaxel causes less CIPN than pacitaxel, carboplatin can also cause CIPN, but less than ciplatin (personal communication, Farquhar-Smith, 2011). Being neuropathic in nature, it is not easy to treat and is commonly a problem in the cancer survivor. There is conflicting, inconclusive evidence that anti-neuropathic agents such as gabapentin may be effective for CIPN (Farquhar-Smith, 2011, quoting Tsavaris et al., 2008; Rao et al., 2007). The heterogeneous nature of CIPN with different anticancer therapies, resulting in distinct neuropathies adds another layer of complexity to its management.

As with other complications of anti-cancer treatment, the discomfort of CIPN may impact on the willingness of patients to enter into future anti-cancer treatments. Additional clinician and patient education is required to highlight the potential problems with this syndrome and further research is necessary to improve current treatment options and potential preventative measures.

Infections, both local and systemic, may also play a role in exacerbating pain in the patient with head and neck cancer. This can occur at any stage of treatment and may often present as a worsening pain problem. Local infections are common with patients who have head and neck cancer. Celluitis, localised tumour infections and orocutaneous fistulae contribute to more than 20% of febrile episodes in patients with head and neck cancer. Infections may or may not be accompanied by clinical signs such as local inflammation or systemic involvement with fever and leucocytosis (Bruera & MacDonald, 1986 and Hussain et al., 1991, as cited by Williams and Broadley, 2009), particularly due to their already immunosuppressed state from the disease itself or the treatment already undergone. Treatment of the pain will be symptomatic as well as treating the infection itself.

7. Chronic pain

The definition of chronic pain as according to the International Association for the Study of Pain (IASP) is "pain which has persisted beyond normal tissue healing time", which, in the absence of other criteria, is taken to be 3 months (IASP, 1986). Chronic pain may be accompanied by severe psychological and social disturbances. Whilst acute pain management focuses on the cause of the pain, the aim of chronic pain treatment is about managing the effects of the pain, including the physical and psychological aspects, to maximise the function of the patient with chronic pain (Clinical Standards Advisory Group, 2000).

Chronic pain in cancer often occurs as a consequence of cancer treatment. With survival being the primary goal of cancer treatment, side-effects or risks to treatments such as pain are frequently being brushed aside as inconsequential (List et al., 2004), although it is essential to bear in mind - a survey of chronic pain patients in the UK revealed that the second most common aetiology of chronic pain was surgery (Crombie et al., 1998).

Figure 1 shows 3 different pain transmission states:

1. Normal physiological pain transmission – the pain stimulus causes action potentials to travel from the periphery to the brain, with no neuroplasticity ("wind-up" mechanism).
2. Nociceptive pain transmission, with both peripheral stimulation and some central sensitization. Pain may be persistent, but should resolve once the stimulus is removed/resolved.
3. Neuropathic pain transmission. Abnormal transmission of action potentials as a result of "wind-up", causing altered sensations to both noxious and normally non-noxious stimuli, leading to symptoms such as allodynia and other descriptions of "nerve pain" such as "shooting", "burning", "pins and needles" etc.

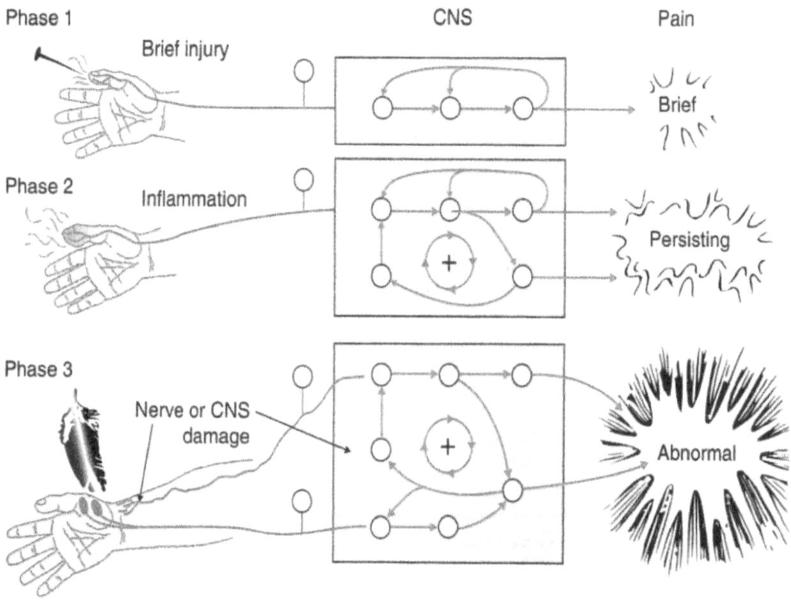

Fig. 1. Three pain transmission states: Phase 1 - normal physiological pain transmission; Phase 2 - nociceptive pain transmission, with peripheral stimulation and central sensitization; Phase 3 - neuropathic pain transmission. Reproduced with permission, Williams & Broadley, 2009.

8. Treatment of pain

The mainstay of the management of pain in the patient with head and neck cancer is to target the source of the pain. According to the WHO (2008), up to 90% of cancer pain can be effectively managed. Pain can often be controlled with anti-cancer treatments such as radiotherapy, chemotherapy and surgery. Analgesic drugs and techniques are used concurrently to alleviate pain.

8.1 Drug therapy

The WHO guidelines for the treatment of cancer pain advocate a stepwise increase in drug dosages and drug type. The recommendation is summed up as in Table 6.

Head and Neck Tumour/Treatment	Neuropathic Pain Syndrome
Intraorbital	Sharp, lancinating pains in the distribution of the ophthalmic nerve
Maxillary antrum	Sharp, lancinating pains in the maxillary nerve distribution
Infratemporal fossa	Mandibular nerve distribution neuralgia, trismus, temporal pain
Nasopharynx, oropharynx, tonsillar region, oral cancers	Glossopharyngeal and vagal nerve distribution neuralgia and palsies, occipital pain radiating to vertex, referred pain causing otalgia, tinnitus, dental pain
Postherpetic neuralgia	Commonly affects trigeminal nerve with stabbing pains and hyperaesthesia
Post-radical neck dissection	Diffuse burning sensation neck and shoulders, sensation deficits, allodynia, shooting pain, severe shoulder pain and dysfunction, superficial cervical plexus neuralgia
Chemotherapy	Chemotherapy-induced neuropathic pain, causing distal "stocking and glove distributions", usually symmetrical, predominantly sensory symptoms

Table 5. Neuropathic pain syndromes in head and neck cancer, adapted with permission from Willams & Broadley, 2009 (Talmi et al., 1997; Chua et al., 1999; Sist et al., 1999; Farquhar-Smith 2011)

WHO recommendation	Comments
By mouth	Use the oral route unless contra-indicated. In the patient with head and neck cancer, drugs can still be taken enterally by nasogastric or gastrostomy tubes or rectal administration. Patients unable to use the enteral route could try different preparations such as subcutaneous, intravenously or transdermal patches.
By the clock	Regular administration to be given before the previous dose wears off. Breakthrough analgesia is not a substitute but is given in addition to regular.
By the ladder	Follow the WHO 3-step ladder
For the individual	There are no standard doses - the correct dose is one that relieves pain. Titrate dose and add adjuvant therapy as necessary.
Attention to detail	Individualised details such as timing, side effects, response, follow-up, weaning etc. Regular reviews to ensure a personalised treatment plan.

Table 6. WHO guidelines for the treatment of cancer pain. (WHO, 1996)

The WHO 3-step ladder was developed for the treatment of cancer pain (WHO, 1996). It encourages the clinician to assess the severity of pain, administer the appropriate medication, and then re-assess. The patient may then be moved up or down the ladder depending on the clinical assessment of his/her pain. An additional step 4 is now often advocated for some patients (Figure 2). Patients often are prescribed analgesia from more than one step, as part of the concept of "multi-modal analgesia". Drugs from Step 1 in particular have been shown to work synergistically with opioids and can often be opioid-sparing, which helps to decrease the side-effect profile of the opioids used (Macintyre & Schug, 2007).

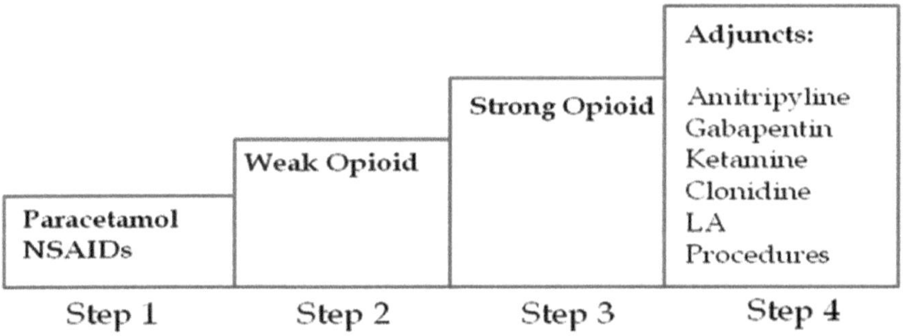

Fig. 2. The WHO 3-step ladder, with step 4 modification

8.1.1 WHO Step 1 – Non-opioid drugs

Step 1 drugs on the WHO ladder consist of paracetamol (acetaminophen) and non-steroidal anti-inflammatory (NSAIDs) drugs only. Paracetamol is used widely for mild-to-moderate pain with a well-established safety profile. Its mechanism of action is surprisingly not well defined, for such a prevalent drug, but it is thought that paracetamol acts as a centrally-acting cyclooxygenase enzyme inhibitor, with suggested modulations of the serotoninergic system and interference with peripheral delivery of β-endorphins (Remy et al., 2006). Paracetamol is known to act synergistically with NSAIDs and is opiate-sparing. Intravenous paracetamol is particularly useful for those patients who are unable to use the oral route due to clinical or symptomatic reasons.

The class of NSAIDs include both non-selective cyclooxygenase enzyme inhibitors (COX-I and II), such as aspirin, ibuprofen, naproxen, diclofenc, and also selective cyclooxygenase II (COX-II) inhibitors such as celecoxib and paracoxib. Cyclooxygenase produces prostaglandins, which is one contributor to the peripheral inflammatory response, as well as playing a part in thrombosis, body salt and water homeostasis, blood pressure, and gastric protection (Gislason, 2009, citing Grosser et al., 2006). There are many well known potential complications with NSAIDs, including renal impairment, gastrointestinal (GI) irritation, leading to ulceration and haemorrhage, haematologic (anti-platelet effects) and aspirin-exacerbated respiratory disease (Risser et al., 2009). The COX-II selective NSAIDs are shown to have a lower incidence of problems with GI irritation compared to non-selective NSAIDs, however risk varies depending on the individual NSAID. An additional GI risk is a long plasma half-life and also the slow-release formulation (Massó González et al., 2010). The cardiovascular system is also affected, increasing the risk of fluid retention, oedema and destabilise existing heart failure. COX-II selective NSAIDs are particularly known to have effects on the cardiovascular system, but the rates of these events in general are so low, that probably the estimates are imprecise and it is difficult to design a trial which would investigate this ethically and be financially viable (Trelle et al, 2011).

8.1.2 WHO Step 2 – Weak opioid drugs

In the UK the weak opioid drugs currently available are codeine, dihydrocodeine and tramadol. Weak opioids are used for mild-to-moderate pain, often in combination with Step 1 analgesics.

CYP2D6, an isoenzyme of the cytochrome P450 family, is important for the metabolism of codeine and tramadol. There are many variants of the CYP2D6 enzyme, which impact upon the metabolism of weak opioids (Leppert, 2011). This polymorphism results in some people being "poor metabolisers", whereas some people are "extensive metabolisers". The effects can be unpredictable. One metabolite of codeine is morphine, but the analgesic effect of codeine is approximately $1/10^{th}$ of morphine analgesia. Tramadol is centrally-acting, on opioid receptors, but also on other mechanisms such as noradrenaline and serotoninergic reuptake mechanisms (Macintyre & Schug, 2007). Both mechanisms are implicated in neuropathic pain pathways. The metabolism of dihydrocodeine is not affected by CYP2D6 (Leppert, 2011).

Some clinicians prefer to go directly from Step 1 to Step 3, to avoid the potential for uncertainty with CYP2D6 polymorphism. Instead, strong opioids are titrated carefully to the patients' needs.

8.1.3 WHO Step 3 – Strong opioid drugs

Strong opioid drugs include morphine, diamorphine, oxycodone, fentanyl, which are mu-opioid receptor agonists, and also partial agonists such as buprenorphine. These Step 3 analgesic drugs are used for moderate-to-severe pain.

The most commonly used drug is morphine, of which there are several preparations. For patients with head and neck cancer who find tablets difficult to swallow, there are elixirs which can be taken orally or passed down a feeding tube. Both immediate release preparations and sustained-release preparations are available in elixir form.

Other forms of strong opioid drugs include the transdermal patch for fentanyl or buprenorphine. Buccal preparations of fentanyl are also available - as a lozenge or lollipop to be sucked, or a tablet which slowly dissolves. The type of preparation most suitable for the patient depends on their particular circumstances - for example, a head a neck cancer patient who has painful oral mucositis, with a persistently dry mouth may find it uncomfortable to use lozenges or buccal tablets, and may prefer transdermal patches, or intravenous or subcutaneous patient controlled analgesic devices (PCAs).

Some patients become resistant or tolerant to strong opioids, particularly if they have required Step 3 medication for a prolonged period of time. In this case it may be necessary to change to a different drug. Any other strong opioid may be chosen - methadone is good option which is often forgotten. It is particularly convenient as a once daily administration due to its long half life.

The potential adverse effects of opioid medication, both weak and strong, must not be overlooked. The most common problems are constipation, nausea and vomiting, and sedation. For constipation, the patient should be advised to keep well hydrated, mobilise, and if prescribed opioid for more than a few days, all patients should also be prescribed laxatives - a stool softener and a bowel stimulant. Dose reduction of the opioid does not help with constipation. Newer agents such as the combined oxycodone/naloxone, and opioid antagonists such as methylnaltrexone have been shown to be effective in this regard (Clemens et al., 2011; Candy et al., 2011). Nausea and vomiting is perhaps the most unpleasant side-effect for the patient. Numerous classes of anti-emetics are available, and as with analgesic drugs, a combination of anti-emetics acting at a combination of sites may be a more effective method than single treatment (Macintyre & Schug, 2007). Mild sedation and cognitive impairment are common side effects of opioid therapy, however tolerance develops quickly. Sedation can be a warning sign of excessive opioid therapy, and will almost always precede respiratory depression. A decrease in respiratory rate is actually a late and unreliable sign of opioid-induced respiratory depression. Both sedation score and respiratory rate should be monitored, particularly when starting patients on new medications, in the acute setting.

8.1.4 WHO additional Step 4 – Adjuvant drugs and interventions

Step 4 is a modification commonly proposed to the original 3-step WHO analgesic ladder (Vargas-Shaffer, 2010). Consisting of both drug and interventional therapy, step 4 adjuncts may be added at any point, with any combination of other steps. The adjuvant drugs proposed are those that are now commonly used for chronic or neuropathic pain, including anti-depressants (amitriptylline, nortriptylline), anti-convulsants (gabapentin, pregabalin), NMDA-receptor antagonists (ketamine), steroids, capsaicin and so forth. Local anaesthetics are also included in this group - either as part of an intervention such as local anaesthetic infiltration/nerve blocks, or as a transdermal patch (lidocaine patch). As we have already seen, patients with head and neck cancer will often have neuropathic pain, and chronic pain. The addition of a step 4 adjunct may help in the treatment of their pain, and may also decrease the amount of opioids necessary to help control pain.

8.2 Interventional therapy

In the patient with head and neck cancer, interventional therapy for pain caused by cancer or cancer treatment is now not longer at the forefront of pain management. It was not possible to use single nerve blocks to relieve pain, as sensory innervations in the head and neck region typically arises from multiple cranial or cervical nerves. Numerous other methods have been tried with reasonable success. Examples include cervical plexus block (Dwyer 1972), lumbar CSF morphine injections (Sullivan 1987), long-term intraventricular infusion of morphine (Dennis & DeWitty, 1990) and intrathecal administration of analgesics (Crul et al., 1994). However, these interventions described are not without potentially very serious complications. The modern analgesics and their methods of delivery are now so well established such that these interventions are largely no longer performed.

8.3 Characteristics of studies investigating pain in patients with head and neck cancer

Study (Number of patients)	Cancer type	Duration of follow-up	Prevalence of head and neck pain
Bjordal (N = 126) 1992	Head and neck cancer	None	18% ("quite a bit" or "very much" pain)
Chaplin and Morton (N = 93) 1998	Newly diagnosed, curable head and neck cancer	2 years	48% at diagnosis (8% severe) 25% at 12 months (3% severe) 26% at 24 months (4% severe)
Forbes (N = 38) 1997	End-stage head and neck cancer	None	79% (26% neuropathic)
Keefe (N = 30) 1986	Head and neck cancer (100% squamous cell carcinoma)	3-6 weeks after initial evaluation 2-3 months after initial evaluation	40% at initial evaluation 50% at final evaluation
Olson (N = 51) 1978	Head and neck cancer, undergone surgical treatment previously	Unknown	32-39% mild to moderate (8% moderate) No patients reported severe pain
Robertson and Hornibrook (N = 522)	Head and neck cancer (~90% squamous cell carcinoma)		8% to 66%, depending on cancer type
Saxena 1995 (N = 117)	Head and neck cancer (90% clinical stage III or IV)		84% (55% moderate to severe, 50% of whom had unrelieved pain)
Talmi (N = 62) 1997	Terminal head and neck cancer (87% squamous cell carcinoma)	None	77%
Epstein (N = 34) 1993	Head and neck cancer pre-/post-radiotherapy (91% squamous cell carcinoma)	6-12 months	82% at diagnosis 100% at midpoint of treatment 46% 6-12 months after treatment
Weissman (N = 14) 1989	Newly diagnosed head and neck cancer patients undergoing radiotherapy	Unknown	29% before treatment 100% during treatment (moderate to severe pain on 37% of treatment days)

Talmi (N = 88) 2000	Head and neck cancer	1-8 months (prospective)	85% after neck dissection; 3% after 2 months
		>2 years (retrospective)	0%
		6-24 months (retrospective)	15%
Terrel (N = 175) 1999	Head and neck cancer	None	Unknown
Chua (N = 40) 1999	Head and neck cancer (83% squamous cell carcinoma; 60% T3 or T4)		100% at presentation (severe in 52%)
Grond (N = 167) 1993	Head and neck cancer	Unknown	100% at referral

9. Holistic care

Aside from direct treatment of the cancer itself by surgery, radiotherapy or chemotherapy, one must remember that treatment of the patient with head and neck cancer should always be undertaken in a holistic manner. As cancer treatments are improving, so too are the rates of cure and length of remission. `Cancer survivorship' issues such as quality of life, good pain and symptom control are important aspects of holistic care that should be prioritised (World Health Organisation [WHO], 1996) - the patient may debilitated for a long time with pain.

Holistic care in patients with head and neck cancer involves not only being concerned about the practical aspect of physical problems, but also the less `medical' problems of psychological distress and social aspect of cancer as a disease, in particular the aesthetic appearance of head and neck cancer or anticancer treatment causing disfigurement. The functional aspect of having cancer in this region also requires particular care - speech and swallow may well be affected, as well as the possibility of requiring medical adjuncts such as the tracheostomy. This in turn will clearly have an effect on the psychosocial state of the patient with head and neck cancer. These symptoms may or may not be directly mentioned by the patient, and it may take a clinician who pays attention to detail to elicit this information. By identifying and resolving issues quickly, holistic needs assessment and care allows the opportunity for clinicians to make a huge difference to the overall experience of cancer, and the potential to improve outcome. Patients are also allowed to be fully engaged in their own care, thus feel empowered to support self-management of their condition (National Cancer Action Team, 2010).

Symptomatic control is relevant during all stages of the cancer, be it at diagnosis, during treatment for cure or palliation, after anti-cancer treatment, at palliation, or even once `cured'. Commonly pain with head and neck cancer will occur as a result of anti-cancer treatment, as well as due to disease progression. Sometimes the most effective method of symptom management or palliation may be further anticancer treatment. The potential adverse effects must then be weighed up when considering the expected benefit to undergoing therapy for pain. The patient and family members should be well informed before making a joint decision with the clinician to undergo any further treatment.

Treatment of pain in the patient with head and neck cancer may well be adequately managed by an experienced clinician. However many studies quoted by Brennan et al (2007) showed that many clinicians are not comfortable in prescribing opioids, having a lack of knowledge of pharmacology of the relevant drugs and experience of pain management. The Pain Management or Palliative Care Teams are experts in the hospital in this regard and timely advice should be sought when problems arise to prevent complications developing further down the line. Quite as importantly, bearing in mind the subjective nature of the pain as a whole, the clinician needs to believe in patients in their descriptions of their pain, and take action to help alleviate the pain.

10. Conclusion

Patients with head and neck cancer will often suffer from pain, resulting from the cancer itself, anti-cancer treatment, or wholly unrelated causes. A high percentage of patients will suffer from neuropathic pain, or mixed nociceptive and neuropathic pain, which may be difficult to treat. Many patients with head and neck cancer will also have pain in more than one location. When treating these patients, it is vital to carefully assess and determine the aetiology of their pain in order to effectively treat their symptoms. Early treatment is advised to help avoid progression into chronic pain and will further complicate treatment strategies. A multi-modal, multidisciplinary approach to pain management encapsulates the concept of holistic care and may make a huge difference to the experience of cancer for the patient. We should aim to empower our patients and encourage them to take ownership of their pain issues. By doing so, we will be positively contributing to the quality of the patient journey with cancer.

11. References

Bar Ad, V., Weinstein, G., Dutta, P.R., Chalian, A., Both, S., & Quon, H. (2010a).Gabapentin for the treatment of pain related to radiation-induced mucositis in patients with head and neck tumors treated with intensity-modulated radiation therapy. Head and Neck. Vol. 32, No. 2, February 2010, pp.173-177, Online ISSN 1097-0347

Bar Ad, V., Weinstein, G., Dutta, P.R., Dosoretz, A., Chalian, A., Both, S., & Quon, H. (2010b). Gabapentin for the Treatment of Pain Syndrome Related to Radiation-Induced Mucositis in Patients With Head and Neck Cancer Treated With Concurrent Chemoradiotherapy. Cancer, Vol. 116, pp.4206-4213, ISSN: 1097-0142

Bjordal K, Kaasa S. Psychometric validation of the EORTC Core Quality of Life Questionnaire, 30-item version and a diagnosis-specific module for head and neck cancer patients. *Acta Oncol.* 1992;31(3):311–321.

Blyth, F.M., March, L.M., Nicholas, M.K., & Cousins, M.J. (2003). Chronic pain, work performance and litigation. Pain, Vol. 103, pp.41-47, ISSN: 0304-3959

Brennan, F., Carr, D.B., & Cousins, M. (2007) Pain Management: a fundamental human right. Anesthesia Analgesia, Vol. 105, No. 1, pp. 205-221, ISSN 0003-2999

Brennan, F., Carr, D.B., & Cousins, M. (2007). Pain Management: a fundamental human right. Anesthesia and Analgesia, Vol. 105, No. 1, pp.205-221, ISSN 0003-2999

Brennan, T.J., & Kehlet, H. (2005). Preventive Analgesia to Reduce Wound Hyperalgesia and Persistent Postsurgical Pain: Not an Easy Path. Anesthesiology, Vol. 103, pp. 681-683, ISSN: 0003-3022

Candy, B., Jones, L., Goodman, M.L., Drake, R., Tookman. A. (2011). Laxatives or methylnaltrexone for the management of constipation in palliative care patients. Vol.1, January 2011, CD003448. Cochrane Database Systems Review, The Cochrane Library, John Wiley & Sons, Ltd, ISSN: 1465-1858

Carr, D.B., Jacox, A.K., Chapman, C.R., Ferrell, B., Fields, H.L., Heidrich, G (III)., Hester, N.K., Hills, C.S. Jr., Lipman, A.G., McGarvey, C.L., Miaskowski, C.A., Mulder, D.S., Payne, R., Schechter, N., Shapiro, B.S., Smith, R.S., Tsou, C.V. & Vecchiarelli, L. (1992) Acute Pain Management: Operative or Medical Procedures and Trauma. Clinical Practice Guideline. Agency for Health Care Policy and Research, Public Health Service, US Department of Health and Human Services, AHCPR Pub. No. 92-0032, ISBN-13: 978-0788146114, Rockville, MD

Chaplin J.M. & Morton R.P. (1999). A Prospective, Longitudinal Study of Pain in Head and Neck Cancer Patients. Head and Neck, September 1999, pp. 531-537, Online ISSN 1097-0347

Chua, K.S.G., Reddy, S.K., Lee, M.C., & Patt, R.B. (1999). Pain and loss of function in head and neck cancer survivors. Journal of pain and symptom management, Vol.18, No.3, September 1999, pp.193-202, ISSN: 0885-3924

Chua, K.S.G., Reddy, S.K., Lee, M.C., & Patt, R.B. (1999). Pain and loss of function in head and neck cancer survivors. Journal of pain and symptom management, Vol.18, No.3, September 1999, pp.193-202, ISSN: 0885-3924

Clarkson, J.E., Worthington, H.V., & Eden, T.O.B. (2008). Interventions for treating oral mucositis for patients with cancer receiving treatment. The Cochrane Collaboration, The Cochrane Library, John Wiley & Sons, Ltd, ISSN: 1465-1858

Cleeland, C.S., Nakamura, Y., Mendoza, T.R., Edwards, K.R., Douglas, J., & Serlin, R.C. (1996) Dimensions of the impact of cancer pain in a four country sample: new information from multidimensional scaling. Pain, Vol. 67, pp. 267-273, ISSN: 0304-3959

Clemens, K.E., Quednau, I., & Klaschik, E. (2011). Bowel function during pain therapy with oxycodone/naloxone prolonged-release tablets in patients with advanced cancer. International Journal of Clinical Practice, Vol. 65, No. 4, April 2011, pp. 472-478, Online ISSN 1742-1241

Clinical Standards Advisory Group. (2000). Services for Patients with Pain. National Pain Audit, CSAG, Retrieved from http://www.nationalpainaudit.org/media/files/services forpatientswithpain.pdf

Crombie, I.K., Davies, H.T. & Macrae, W.A. (1998). Cut and Thrust: antecedent surgery and trauma among patients attending a chronic pain clinic. Pain, Vol. 76, pp.167-171, ISSN: 0304-3959

Crul, B.J., van Dongen, R.T., Snijdelaar, D.G., & Rutten, E.H. (1994) Long-term continuous intrathecal administration of morphine and bupivacaine at the upper cervical level: access by a lateral C1-C2 approach. Anesthesia and Analgesia, Vol.79, pp.594-597, ISSN 0003-2999

Deandrea, S., Montanari, M., Moja, L., & Apolone, G. (2008) Prevalence of undertreatment in cancer pain. A review of published literature. Annals of Oncology, Vol.19, pp.1985-1991, ISSN 0923-7534

Delaney, A., Fleetwood-Walker, S.M., Colvin, L.A., & Fallon M. (2008). Translational medicine: cancer pain mechanisms and management. British Journal of Anaesthesia, Vol.101, pp.87-94, ISSN 0007-0912

Dennis, G.C., & DeWitty, R.L. (1990) Long-term intraventricular infusion of morphine for intractable pain in cancer of the head and neck. Neurosurgery, Vol. 26, No. 3, pp.404-408, Online ISSN 1524-4040

Dwyer, B. (1972). Treatment of pain of carcinoma of the tongue and floor of the mouth. Anaesthesia and Intensive Care, Vol. 1, No. 1, pp.59-61, Electronic 1448-0271

Epstein J.B. & Stewart K.H. (1993) Radiation Therapy and Pain in Patients with Head and Neck Cancer. European Journal of Cancer with Oral Oncology, Vol. 29B, No. 3, pp.191-199, ISSN 1359-6349

Farquhar-Smith, P. (2011). Chemotherapy-induced neuropathic pain. Current Opinion in Supportive and Palliative Care, Vol. 5, No. 1, March 201, pp.1-7, ISSN: 1751-4258

Ferrell, B.R. (1995). The impact of pain on quality of life. A decade of research. Nursing Clinics of North America, Vol. 30, pp.609-624, ISSN 0029-6465

Forbes, K. (1997). Palliative Care in Patients with Cancer of the Head and Neck. Clinical Otolarngology, Vol. 22, pp. 117-122, Online ISSN 1749-4486

Gislason, G.N. (2009). Editorials: NSAIDs and Cardiovascular Risk. American Family Physician. December 2009, Vol.80, No.12, pp.1366-1368, ISSN 0002-838X

Grond, S., Zech, D., Diefenback, C., Radbruch, L. & Lehmann, K.A. (1996). Assessment of Cancer Pain: A Prospective Evaluation in 2266 Cancer Patients Referred to a Pain Service. Pain, No. 64, pp.107-114, ISSN: 0304-3959

Gureje, O., von Korff, M., Simon, G.E., & Gater, R. (1998). Persistent pain and well-being: a World Health Organization study in primary care. Journal of the American Medical Association, Vol. 280, pp. 147-151, ISSN 0098-7484

Hanks, G.W., de Conno, F., Cherny, N., Hanna, M., Kalso, E., McQuay, H.J., Mercadante, S., Meynadier, J., Poulain, P., Ripamonti, C., Radbruch, L., Roca, i Casas, J., Sawe, J., Twycross, R.G., & Ventafridda ,V. (2001). Morphine and alternative opioids in cancer pain: the EAPC recommendations, British Journal of Cancer, Vol. 84, pp.587–593, ISSN 0007-0920

Huber, A., Suman, A.L., Rendo, C.A., Biasi, G., Marcolongo, R. & Carli, G. (1995). Dimensions of "Unidimensional" Ratings of Pain and Emotions in Patients with Chronic Musculoskeletal Pain. Pain, Vol. 130, pp. 216-24, ISSN: 0304-3959

International Association for the Study of Pain. (1986). Classification of chronic pain. Pain, Supplment 3: S1-S226, ISSN 0167-6482

Keefe, F .J., Manuel, G., Brantley, A. & Crisson, J. (1986). Pain in the head and neck cancer patient: Changes over treatment. Head and Neck Surgery, Vol. 8, pp.169-176

Kehlet, H., Jensen, T.S. & Woolf, C.J. (2006). Persistent postsurgical pain: risk factors and prevention. Lancet, Vol.367, pp.1618–1625, ISSN 0140-6736

Leppert, W. (2011). CYP2D6 in the Metabolism of Opioids for Mild to Moderate Pain. Pharmacology, Vol. 87, pp.274–285, ISSN 0031–7012

Lorenz, K., Lynn, K., Dy, S., Hughes, R., Mularski, R.A., Shugarman, L.R., & Wilkinson, A.M. (2006). Cancer Care Quality Measures: Symptoms and End-of-Life Care.

Evidence Report/ Technology Assessment No. 137. Southern California Evidence-based Practice Center AHRQ Publication No. 06-E001, Agency for Healthcare Research and Quality, Rockville, MD.

MacIntyre, P. (2005) Acute pain management: scientific evidence, on behalf of the Working Party of the Australian and New Zealand College of Anaesthetists. 2nd ed, Melbourne, Australia: Australian and New Zealand College of Anaesthetists, Retrieved from http://www.nhmrc.gov.au/publications/synopses/ cp104syn.htm

Macintyre, P.E. & Schug, S.A. (2007). Acute Pain Management: A Practical Guide (3rd edition), Elsevier limited, ISBN 978 0 7020 2770 3, Edinburgh

Massó González , E.L., Patrignani, P., Tacconelli, S.,& García Rodríguez, L.A. (2010). Variability Among Nonsteroidal Antiinflammatory Drugs in Risk of Upper Gastrointestinal Bleeding. Arthritis & Rheumatism, Vol. 62, No. 6, June 2010, pp 1592–1601, ISSN 0004-3591

Merskey, H., & Bogduk N. (1994). Part III: Pain Terms, A Current List with Definitions and Notes on Usage, In: Classification of Chronic Pain, Second Edition, pp. 209-214, IASP Task Force on Taxonomy, IASP Press, Seattle. IASP Subcommittee on Taxonomy Pain Terms: A list with definitions and notes on usage, Retrieved from <http://www.iasp-pain.org/Content/NavigationMenu/GeneralResourceLinks/PainDefinitions/default.htm ISBN-13: 978-0-931092-05-3

Miaskowski, C., Cleary, J., Burney, R., Coyne, P., Finley, R., Foster, R., Grossman, S., Janjan, N.A., Ray, J., Syrjala, K., Weisman, S.J., & Zarbock, C. (2005). Guideline for the management of cancer pain in adults and children. APS clinical practice guidelines series, Vol 3. American Pain Society, Glenview, IL

National Cancer Action Team. 2010. Holistic Needs Assessment for people with cancer. A practical guide for healthcare professionals, Cancer Action Teams, London

Olson , MS, Donald P. Shedd. Disability and rehabilitation in head and neck cancer patients after treatment Mrs. & Neck Surgery Volume 1, Issue 1, pages 52–58, September/October 1978

Perkins, F.M. & Kehlet, H. (2000). Chronic Pain as an Outcome of Surgery. A Review of Predictive Factors. Anesthesiology, Vol. 93, pp.1123–1133, ISSN: 0003-3022

Peters, M.L., Sommer, M., de Rijke, J.M., Kessels, F., Heineman, E., Patijn, J., Marcus, M.A.E., Vlaeyen, J.W.S., & van Kleef, M. (2007). Somatic and Psychologic Predictors of Long-term Unfavorable Outcome After Surgical Intervention. Annals of Surgery, Vol. 245, No. 3, March 2007, pp.487- 494, ISSN 0003-4932

Portenoy, R.K, & Lesage, P. (1999). Management of Cancer Pain. Lancet, Vol. 353, pp. 1659-1700, ISSN 0140-6736

Remy, C., Marret, E. & Bonnet, F. (2006). State of the art of paracetamol in acute pain therapy. Current Opinion in Anaesthesiology, Vol. 19, pp.562–565. ISSN 0952-7907

Risser, A., Donovan, D., Heintzman, J. & Page, T. (2009). NSAID Prescribing Precautions. American Family Physician, Vol. 80, No. 12, December 2009, pp 1371-1378, ISSN 0002-838X

Rosenthal, D.I. & Trotti, A. (2009). Strategies for managing radiation-induced mucositis in head and neck cancer. Seminars in Radiation Oncology, Vol. 19, No.1, January 2009, pp.29-34, ISSN 1053-4296

Rowin, J.; Cheng, G.; Lewis, S.L. & Meriggioli, M.N. (2006). Late appearance of dropped head syndrome after radiotherapy for Hodgkin's disease. Muscle & Nerve, Vol.34, No. 5, November 2006, pp.666-669, Electronic ISSN 1097-4598

Saxena, A., Gnanasekara, N. & Andley M. (1995). An epidemiological study of prevalence of pain in head and neck cancer. Indian Journal of Medical Research, Vol. 12, July 1995, pp.28-33, ISSN 0971-5916

Sist, T., Miner, M. & Lema, M. (1999). Characteristics of Postradical Neck Pain Syndrome: A Report of 25 Cases. Journal of Pain and Symptom Management, Vol. 18, No. 2, pp.95-102, ISSN: 0885-3924

Sonis, S.T., Elting, L.S., Keefe, D., Peterson, D.E., Schubert, M., Hauer-Jensen, M., Bekele, B.N., Raber-Durlacher, J., Donnelly, J.P. & Rubenstein , E.B. (2004). Perspectives on Cancer Therapy-Induced Mucosal Injury. Pathogenesis, Measurement, Epidemiology, and Consequences for Patients. Cancer, Supplement, Vol. 100, No. 9, May 2004, pp.1995-2025, ISSN: 1097-0142

Steward, W.F., Ricci, J.A., Chee, E., Morganstein, D., & Lipton, R. (2003). Lost productive time and cost due to common pain conditions in the US workforce. Journal of the American Medical Association , Vol. 290, pp.2443-2454, ISSN 0098-7484

Sullivan, S.P. & Cherry, D.A. (1987). Pain from an Invasive Facial Tumor Relieved by Lumbar Epidural Morphine. Anesthesia and Analgesia, No. 66, pp.777-779, ISSN 0003-2999

Talmi, YP; Horowitz, Z; Peffer, MR; Stolik-Dollberg, OC; Shoshani, Y; Peleg, M; Kronenberg, J (2000). Pain in the neck after neck dissection. Otolaryngology - Head and neck surgery, Vol.123, No. 3, pp.302-306, September 2000. ISSN: 0194-5998

Terrell JE, Nanavati K, Esclamado A prospective, longitudinal study of pain in head and neck cancer patients. Head Neck. 1999 Sep;21(6):531–537.

Thorpe, D.M. (1993). The incidence of sleep disturbance in cancer patients with pain. Proceedings of the 7th World Congress on Pain: Abstracts 451, IASP Publications, ISBN 978-0-931092-07-7, Seattle, WA, August 1993

Trelle, S., Reichenbach, S., Wandel, S., Hildebrand, P., Tschannen, P., Villiger, P.M., Egger, M., & Jüni, P. (2011). Cardiovascular safety of non-steroidal anti-inflammatory drugs: network meta-analysis. British Medical Journal, Vol. 324, c7086, ISSN 0959 8138

Valeberg, B.T., Rustoen, T., Bjordal, K., Hanestad, B.R., Paul, S., & Miaskowski, C. (2008). Self-reported prevalence, etiology, and characteristics of pain in oncology outpatients. European Journal of Pain, Vol. 12, pp. 582-590, ISSN 1090-3801

Van den Beuken-van Everdingen, M.H., de Rijke J.M., Kessels, A.G., Schouten, H.C., van Kleef, M., & Patijin, J. (2004). Prevalence of pain in patients with cancer: a systematic review of the past 40 years. Annals of Oncology, Vol. 18, pp.1437-1449, ISSN 0923-7534

Van Leeuwen, M.T., Blyth, F.M., March, L.M., Nicholas, M.K., & Cousins, M.J. (2006). Chronic pain and reduced work effectiveness: the hidden cost to Australian employers. European Journal of Pain, Vol. 2, pp.161-166, ISSN1090-3801

Vargas-Schaffer, G. (2010). Is the WHO analgesic ladder still valid? Twenty-four years of experience. Canadian Family Physician, Vol. 56, pp.514-7, Online ISSN 1715-5258

Vecht, C.J., Hoff, A.M., Kansen, P.J., de Boer, M.G., & Bosch, D.A. (1992) Types and Causes of Pain in Cancer of the Head and Neck. Cancer Vol. 70, No. 1, July 1992, pp. 178-184, ISSN: 1097-0142

Weissman, D.E., Janjan, N., & Byhardt, R.W. (1989). Assessment of pain during head and neck irradiation. Journal of Pain and Symptom Management, Vol. 4, No. 2, pp.90-95, ISSN: 0885-3924

Williams, J.E., & Broadley K.E. (2009). Palliation of advanced head and neck cancer, In: Principles and practice of head and neck surgery and oncology, Ed: Montgomery, P.Q., Rhys Evans P.H., & Gullane, P. J., pp.151-159, Informa Healthcare, ISBN-10: 0415444128, ISBN-13: 978-0415444125, London

Williams, J.E., Yen, J.T., Parker, G.M., Chapman, S., Kandikattu, S., & Barbachano Y. (2010). Prevalence of pain in head and neck cancer out-patients. Journal of Laryngology and Otology, Vol.124, No. 7, pp.. 767-773, ISSN 0022-2151

World Health Organisation (2008) Pallative care, WHO, Retrieved from http://www.who.int/cancer/palliative/en/

World Health Organisation. (1996). Cancer pain relief. World Health Organisation, 2nd edition, ISBN 92-4-1544-82-1, Geneva

17

A Health Promotion Perspective of Living with Head and Neck Cancer

Margereth Björklund
Kristianstad University
Sweden

1. Introduction

1.1 Public health and head and neck cancer

All definitions of public health share a mutual aim, i.e. to decrease disease and preserve health (Beaglehole & Bonita, 2001). In the nineteenth century public health (i.e. the old public health approach), search for changes in the physical environment and point at e.g. education of personal hygiene, and development of social standard of living satisfactory for maintenance of health, further infection control, medical and nursing services for early diagnosis and preventive treatment of disease. In the mid-1970s, the movement towards a new public health approach sought changes in, social, political, economic and environmental conditions believed to enhance health. The topics are fundamental, socioeconomic determinants of health and disease, in addition to more proximal risk factors. These determinants of health- i.e. our life circumstances linked not only to living with illness, genetic disorders, or other disease, are linked to income, educational status, and not least to social relationship to others. All these factors seem to prompt linking public health research to individuals and groups living with Head and Neck Cancer [HNC]. Additional, it is not uncommon that the location of the tumour and the side effects of treatment (surgery and radiation) often result in everlasting, visible disfigurement, and those affected could experience this as a social disability (Vickery et al., 2003). Visible disfigurement is known to be associated with extensive psychosocial worries, considering the face is the initial focus in encounters and central to verbal and non-verbal communication (Rumsey et al., 2004). Even a brief glimpse of the affected person informs the observer of a dissimilarity of ordinary look. Furthermore, these persons often have poor speech and might avoid social contact, often restricting them to a close circle of friends and relatives (ibid).

When a person contracts an HNC disease he/she always carries the primary concern for individual health. If he/she is too sick, the responsibility shifts to the next of kin. As a final point, the responsibility shifts to society. On the individual level, public health aims to promote health and enhance comfort to those groups and individuals that are most vulnerable to ill health (Beaglehole & Bonita, 2001). Patients with HNC search for relief and health resources when they experience lifelong feelings of ill health (cf. Aarstad, 2008). Nevertheless, it seems to be challenging for them to achieve better health and well-being since they live constantly with chronic problems, e.g. swallowing and eating disorders that go with their increasing age.

1.2 Head and neck cancer

HNC is comprised mainly of squamous cell and adenocarcinoma and includes cancer of the lip, mouth, sinuses, ear, nose, salivary gland, thyroid, larynx, tongue, pharynx and oropharynx, nasopharynx, and hypopharynx (cf. Feber, 2000). HNC is most common in people in aged >50 years, and the percentage of aged patients is rising due to the increasing lifespan. HNC presents diverse aetiologies and pathology, but tobacco and alcohol use, particularly in combination, are known risk factors (cf. Langius, 1995). The pattern of HNC is not same for both sexes, e.g. women have three to four time greater chance for thyroid cancer than men have (cf. Feber, 2000). In contrast, cancer incidence in the tonsils has increased threefold in men since 1970s and this could be an indication of an epidemic of virus-induced carcinoma, since nearly all tonsils cancer originates from a human papilloma virus infection of the mucosa (Näsman et al., 2009). HNC is the fifth most common cancer in the Nordic countries and the annual incidence of this cancer is increasing, and its prevalence reflects a long term survival rate. The survival rate has increased in recent decades due to the many advances in surgery and development in combining radiation therapy and chemotherapy. These findings correspond to other cancer research showing that advancements in cancer research have reduced the risk of cancer death across lifespan. Consequently, cancer should be recognised as a chronic illness (cf. Carnevali & Reiner, 1990).

Traditionally, Western medicine that follows oncology guidelines is used in treating HNC in Denmark, Finland, Island, Norway and Sweden. Treatment is based on clinical factors, i.e. histological diagnosis, primary site, tumour size and spread, likelihood for total surgical resection, and potential to save speech and swallowing functions. Additional factors are patients´ wishes, cooperation, physical function, social status, and education, experience, and physician qualifications (cf. Feber, 2000).

Radiotherapy is standardised with 60 to 68 Grey given once or twice a day, five days a week, for 35 to 50 days. Unceasing improvement in radiotherapy are allowing clinicians to target only the diseased tissues, thus resulting of fewer side effects compared to previous therapy (Sharp, 2006). Likewise, chemotherapy has also advanced and can be used as both curative and palliative treatment, or as an integral part of radiotherapy, with drugs given five days on three or more occasions (cf. Aarstad, 2008).

These treatment offer cure and/or palliation for patients but have also side effects such as acute breathing and bleeding problems. In addition to long-term changes with swallowing and/or communication, this could cause psychological and existential problems for patients (cf. Björklund, 2010). In recent decades, services for patients´ emotional and practical needs related to support, care, and knowledge have been available at ear, nose, and throat clinic (cf. Larsson, 2006). However these clinics are not easily accessible for everyone with HNC, since the patients often need acute support when experiencing harsh side effects of treatment. Access to health care can be difficult and frequently patients try to find additional treatment known to be health promoting in people with cancer (cf. Hök, 2009). This treatment is often referred as complementary and alternative medicine, but this and traditional medicine is context-dependent (World Health Organisation [WHO], 2002). The term complementary and alternative medicine speaks of a set of health care practices that are not part of a country´s own traditions, or not integrated into a dominant health care system. Hence, a particular practice such as acupuncture might be referred as complementary and alternative medicine or treatment in Western (developed) countries, while it is classified as traditional medicine in China. Traditional medicine includes diverse health practices, approaches, knowledge, and beliefs to treat, diagnose, or prevent illness. Additionally, it can incorporate plant-, animal-, and/or mineral-based medicines, spiritual therapies, manual techniques, and exercises applied singularly or in combination to maintain well-being (ibid).

Complementary and alternative therapies such as Yoga and human touch are shown to be effective and valuable for patients' with different cancer forms (Leddy, 2003). Both therapies integrate awareness of breathing, improved muscle relaxation, exercise and social support, and their documented positive effects on fatigue, sleep, mood, and sense of well-being. Since the patients have specific problems, e.g. living with deformity, perhaps complementary and alternative medicine could be used as self-care to help these patients be capable of daring to present and touch their deformed face after surgery (Dropkin, 2001). Siegel (1990) stresses that an individual´s attitude towards self and the power of positive thinking could be the most important factor in healing a cancer and promoting health, and this has always been an integral part of Eastern healthcare culture (cf. Dossey et al., 2000).

1.3 Everyday life with head and neck cancer

It is known that the experience of living with an illness is based on the context of the individual's reality i.e. at home, at work or in health care, and is related to subjective discomfort and practical implications of life (Carnevali & Reiner, 1990). The personal uneasiness of having HNC often begins with insidious symptoms that could be similar to experiences from minor ailments, e.g. blocked nose, sore throat, hoarseness, earache, mouth ulcers and swollen lymph glands (Feber, 2000). But the patient's symptoms progress to become a struggle of daily problems with breathing, bleeding, odour from nose or mouth, eating, swallowing, fatigue, speaking, and pain in addition to changes in appearance. Larsson (2006) revealed the patients' eating and swallowing problems as a very specific contextual phenomenon, and highlight the need to focus on the patients' needs on the whole. Patients' nutritional problems often lead to extreme weight loss, in addition to fatigue. Fatigue is a subjective, unpleasant symptom, especially during and after radiotherapy and can range from tiredness to exhaustion. Together with pain in the shoulder and arm, due to neck dissection, it affects with the patient's ability to perform domestic tasks (cf. Björklund, 2010). Also, patients' complex communication problems, with limited speech or no voice at all, complicates life and their contact with health professionals. Also, patients must often learn to live, and Semple et al. (2008) suggest that patients' with disfigurement could be more vulnerable since appearance affects a person's identity, self-image, ability to converse, and success in interpersonal relationships. These physical problems could lead to psychosocial consequences, e.g. changed mood, social anxiety, and behavioural avoidance that could minimize patients' sense of health and well-being in life (Björklund, 2010). Living with HNC is challenging because of its acute and long- term health consequences for those affected, and since health is such an important resource in everyday life it is important to focus on how the patients can experience better health (WHO, 1986).

HNC cancer corresponds to the chronic illness definition; an illness that is prolonged, does not resolve spontaneously, and is rarely cured completely (National Center for Chronic

Disease Prevention and Health Promotion [NCCDPHP], 2010). Despite the long-term problems, patients' with HNC seemed to adjust to their new situation; to live with the disease and maintain their well-being (cf. Björklund, 2010). These thoughts and behaviour of maintaining well-being can be understood through the Shifting Perspectives Model of Chronic Illness (Thorne & Paterson, 1998; Paterson, 2001). This model suggested that people with chronic illness has element of both illness and wellness that effect their life and outlook on living. This determines how people respond to the disease, themselves, caregivers and situations, and it represents their beliefs, perceptions, expectations, attitudes and experiences of what it means to live with a chronic illness within a specific context (Paterson, 2003). They either putting the illness itself in the foreground, or they live their life in essence as a well person. The wellness-in- the-foreground perspective focuses on one's self as a person and allows patients to distance themselves from the disease and to find meaning and hope when focusing on emotional, social and spiritual wellness (Paterson, 2001). It permits people to rate their overall health as good even when their physical function is significantly impaired, and could provide opportunities for personal growth and change. However, keeping wellness in the foreground could prevent individuals from getting the service or attention they need since patients are forced to focus on their limitations and weakness to receive help, and this could threaten their integrity and sense of self (ibid.). The illness-in-the-foreground perspective focuses on the sickness, the suffering, and the loss, and patients are absorbed and overwhelmed by the illness. The model illustrate that the perspective is not static and suggest that understanding the individual's perspective at any given time enables health professionals to provide appropriate care and support for people with either perspective (Paterson, 2003).

1.4 Health

Health is formed, lived and promoted by people in the settings of their everyday life; where they learn, work, play and love (WHO, 1986). The word *health* has its roots in the word *heal*, which originally meant *whole*, and implies considering a person in his/her entirety as a social being. Hippocrates (about 400 BC) described health as a condition in which the functions of the body and soul are in harmony with the outside world. Health is valued through each individual's personal experience and can be known only through personal description (Hover-Kramer, 2002). Antonovsky (1996) defines health as a continuum between the extremes of health and disease, implying that health is present for the entire lifetime. When individuals move towards the healthier or positive end of the continuum it is called salutogenic as opposed to pathogenic. This focuses on patient's personal strength and health resources, i.e. salutogenic factors, and supposedly contributes directly to health and predicts favourable health outcomes. This perspective of viewing health, referred to as holistic health, is represented by Nordenfelt (1995; 2007) who describes health as being related to the extent to which the individuals can realise their vital goals under standard or reasonable circumstances. Furthermore, he stresses that all individuals have the right to determine and to decide what health signifies to them specifically, i.e. health relates to the affected and their situation and goal in life (Nordenfelt, 1995). However, some patients have cognitive disorders, or no strength, and then their next of kin or health professionals need to act as spokespersons, look after the patient's needs, and find out what could improve their health (Björklund et al., 2010). However it is known that patients living with HNC may experience ill health from the acute and long-term side effects of tumour growth and treatment, and this could impact on their entire life situation. But every human being has his/her motives for health and the experience of health, and this relates to the person's attentiveness to their own potentials, i.e. their own health resources. If the person feels well and can function in his/her social context, then that is their experience of health and feelings of well-being irrespective of illness or health condition (Nordenfelt, 1995).

1.5 Health promotion

The concept of health promotion is a theoretical concept and has been interpreted in many ways. Expressions such as equality, partnership, collaboration, participation, self-determination and mutual responsibility, and empowerment are used in the Ottawa Charter when describing health promotion (WHO, 1986). Health promotion is a positive concept emphasising personal, social, political, and institutional resources, as well as physical capacities. As such, not a responsibility for health services alone, since subjective feeling of health and well-being are a necessity and require participation from the individual self.

Leddy (2003) highlight to look at the patients as active individuals with strength to decide for themselves what they think promotes their health. The human being's power lies in his/her inner strength, i.e. the ability to be free to act, which also implies ability to refrain from actions. Some describe health promotion as being consistent with the disease perspective, which is based on risk factors that cause disease, i.e. a pathogenic perspective (Tones & Tilford, 1994). In this context, the patients in focus are recipients of information and education from health professionals who inform about risk factors, e.g. smoking that could cause biological changes resulting in disease, and encourage health activities that could prevent ill-health or promote health. Though, health promotion in relations to patients with HNC could mean that an individuals' viewpoint defines what counts as healthful. This is a transformation from expert- driven care to patient- centred care (Young & Hayes, 2002). Although this perspective involves education and information, it emanates from the patient's own questions and overall life situation (ibid.). For instance giving up smoking or alcohol is a reliable way to prevent and lessen the recurrence of some HNC (cf. Feber, 2000. Yet, giving up these habits will not directly lead to achieving vital goals in life; nor will it spontaneously reinforce patient's ability to act (Aarstad, 2008). Further, Allison's (2002) research shows that using wine during recovery can lead to decreased sense of illness. It is also known that intake of citrus fruits could be protective and reduce risk of developing a secondary primary tumour in the lung, but often the patients' anatomical problems make it impossible to eat the recommended food (Larsson, 2006). Pender (1996) stresses that health promotion aims to, and includes, advocating health wishes and intensifies patients' positive potentials for health. Berg et al. (2006) assert that patients (hospitalised elderly) perceived health as being able to be the person they were, to do what they want, and feel well and have strength. They view health promotion as being enabled- through the person they were, through information and knowledge, and through hope and motivation. Health professionals ought to work in partnership with their patients as relational beings, i.e. health promotion is a matter of power distribution and joint responsibility (Young & Hayes, 2002). Effective communication, understanding and insight were experienced as enhancing health and well-being for patients in HNC care (Richardson, 2002). Wells (1998) research reveals that some patients with HNC have resilience and profound reluctance to ask for help despite extensive physical and emotional trauma. Perhaps this is not necessarily attributed to characteristics of the patient. Research shows health professionals' behaviours e.g. rejection, annoyance, and being stressed could discourage patients from expressing their needs (cf. Halldórsdóttir & Hamrin, 1997). To experience feelings of positive human encounter when receiving care, patients need respect and balance in every care contact with health professionals (National Institute of Public Health [NIPH], 2005). Consequently, perhaps patient- centred care (Institute of Medicine [IOM], 2000) and accessible information could strengthen hope and motivation and help these patients build the strength to decide to act and ask for help if and when they need it. This corresponds to The Ottawa Charter, which underlines the individuals' own activities in the health promotion definition- a process of enabling people to increase control over and to improve their health, i.e. empowerment (WHO, 1986). Empowerment is a multi-dimensional social process. At the core is the idea that we could accept that power can change and expand and make empowerment possible. Empowerment is part in health promotion and as such is said to be essential, implying a mobilisation of individuals (and groups) by corroboration of their basic life skills, and enhancing their decisions and actions affecting their health (Nutbeam, 1998).

Empowerment is strongly connected to the idea of holistic health (Dossey et al., 2000), in particular when defined as the ability to act to realise vital goals (Nordenfelt, 1995). It may be understood to promote health if it implies the growing capability of patients to succeed in their self-formulate goals, with an outcome of better health. This concept encompasses the idea that people can form relationships with others, and that the empowerment process could be similar to a journey that develops as we work through it (Leddy, 2003). Mok et al. (2004) revealed that empowerment leads to increased self-determination, self-worth, creating of autonomous decision making and ultimately a mastery over and acceptance over the illness and the meaning in everyday life.

1.6 Rationale of the studies

The intent of the studies is to describe 35 participants' experiences from a health promotion and salutogenic perspective. There is a value in focusing on patients' personal strength and other health resources, though possessing a sense of better health and well-being could be of significance for patients as they endure their vulnerable situation. An increasing number of people are contracting HNC and patients face both acute and long- term chronic problems from the illness and side-effects from treatment. These factors reflect the illness burden for patients and their next of kin, and need for continuing and long-lasting access and support from healthcare and society. HNC often causes visible disfigurement combined with speech and eating disorders that could lead to psychosocial problems. Such features underline that this fairly large group in society could be a concern of public health services. In view of this, it was important to reach understanding of how patients could find a balance between ability, demands, and actions for realising their vital goals, under realistic conditions, during this long-term illness. This goes far beyond a superficial knowledge of the situation- it means trying to understand and enter into the affected individual's experiences and sphere of thinking, trying to gain insight and share feelings of another individual and understand the meaning that he or she attaches to a phenomenon.

2. Aims

The studies aims to reach a deeper understanding of living with head and neck cancer and to identify the experiences that patients felt promoted their health and well-being.

2.1 Specific aims

- to describe cancer patients' experiences of nurses' behaviour in terms of critical incidents after nurses had given them health promotion care (Bjorklund & Fridlund, 1999; paper **I**).
- to describe the characteristics of health promoting contacts with health professionals as encountered by individuals with head and neck cancer (Björklund et al., 2009; paper **II**).
- to shed light on health promotion from the perspective of individuals living with head and neck cancer (Björklund et al., 2008; paper **III**).
- to illuminate what it means to live with head and neck cancer (Björklund et al., 2010; paper **IV**).

3. Methods

3.1 Design

A qualitative research design was chosen since this type of design generates an awareness of human experiences, as expressed by the individuals themselves in their natural context (Polit & Beck, 2008). The design is flexible, and the researcher is the tool for data collection and analysis while engaging in on-going reflection and decision-making throughout the studies' progression. The studies employ different qualitative methods. The first study was conducted in Denmark, Finland, Island, Norway and Sweden, with one individual from each of the four participating Nordic countries and 17 from Sweden (paper **I**). Since costs, logistics, and time would have been prohibitive in conducting a qualitative follow-up study in five countries, the remaining studies (papers **II**, **III**, **IV**) focused on the Swedish HNC care context. Furthermore, it was not the intention to conduct comparative research between the countries.

3.2 Study context

The first study was conducted from 1997 through 1998 in the Nordic countries (paper **I**), and the second study during 2005 in Sweden (paper **II** and **III**), and the last study was conducted from 2005 through 2007 in Sweden (paper **IV**). All participants had received or were receiving treatment for HNC i.e. surgery, radiotherapy or chemotherapy at their regional oncology centre or local ear, nose, and throat clinic. During these treatment periods the patients had contact with numerous health professionals, i.e. different surgical, radiation and medical oncology experts, dentists, pathologists, physiotherapists, speech therapists, social workers, dental hygienists, dieticians and nurses. Healthcare policies concerning the treatment of HNC in the Nordic countries have changed during the past decade, from inpatients care in general to short hospital visits and outpatient care. Adding, policymakers have stipulate sharper guiding principles towards more health promoting care (cf. NIPH, 2005).

3.3 Participants

All patients' (n= 35) interviewed were purposively selected in consultation with medical and nursing staff involved in their care. The selection criteria were:

- Men and women above age of 18 years
- Willingness and interest to verbalise and communicate their own experiences
- Diagnosed and treated for different forms and stages of HNC
- Curative or palliative treatment of HNC

Nine of the patients (six men and three women) originated from seven other countries outside of Sweden (Southern Europe, Middle East and other Nordic countries).

Of the 21 men (aged 38- 83 years; median 62.6 years) 15 were married or cohabited, two lived apart, and the rest were divorced, widowed, or single. Of the 14 women (aged 59-81 years; median 65.4 years) nine were married or cohabited, one lived apart, and the rest were divorced, widowed, or single. All but two men and two women had children, and several had grand-children. One participant was unemployed, and 14 were employed, one was a student, five had disability pension, three had early retirement pension and eleven were retired. Of the patients who chose not to participate 12 were men (aged 35-65; median 48.6 years) and seven were women (aged 32-80; median 55.7 years). Six men and four women of those initially asked chose not to participate in the first study (paper **I**), and six men and three women chose not to participate in the second study (papers **II** and **III**). All agreed to participate in the last study (paper **IV**). In nearly half of the participants (n= 15), seven men and eight women) the cancer had not spread, but nearly all patients had large tumours. Eighteen participants had lymphatic gland metastases and eleven had recurrence near the first tumour. Seven had both metastases and recurrence. The severity of the HNC sickness could have impacted on both the unique patient's everyday life and on the next of kin who shared his/her experiences.

Some of the patients' problems, symptoms and changes could be particularly unpleasant, for instance:

- 33 participants experienced eating and swallowing difficulties
- 31 participants had visible tumours or skin defects in the face or neck after surgery or radiation
- 20 participants had hoarseness
- 18 participants had increased phlegm with coughing or spitting, or no saliva and dry mouth
- 16 participants had articulation problems
- 5 participants who had undergone laryngectomy had pseudo voice
- 4 participants had nasal voice

3.4 Interviews

All studies were based on individual open-ended semi-structured, qualitative interviews (Kvale, 1996). A semi-structured guide with written topics for all studies was developed in advance, reflecting the author's interest in everyday life, especially in what promotes better health and well-being for patients' with HNC. In the first study, a semi-structured interview

Diagnosis	No. of participants	Male/female	
Cheek cancer	3	3/0	
Epipharynx cancer	1	0/1	
Gingival cancer	2	0/2	
Laryngeal cancer	6	4/2	
Lip cancer	1	1/0	
Mandible cancer	1	1/0	
Maxilla cancer	2	1/1	
Mouth bottom cancer	2	1/1	(2/2) [1)]
Nasal cancer	1	1/0	
Oro-pharyngeal cancer	1	0/1	
Unspecified head and neck cancer	2	1/1	
Oesophagus cancer	0	0/0	(0/1) [1)]
Salivary gland cancer	1	0/1	
Tongue cancer	4	2/2	
Tonsil cancer	7	6/1	
Thyroidal cancer	1	0/1	
Other solitary cancer in the body	5	2/3 [2)]	

Table 1. Presents an overview of the 35 participants' diagnosis and was designed to include the specific diagnoses while ensuring the confidentiality and integrity of all participants when grouped together. [1)] Side diagnoses are indicated in brackets, [2)] Prostate, stomach, breast, lymphoma, and melanoma.

guide was constructed by following Flanagan's (1954) advices, i.e. questions were derived from the aim of the study (Bjorklund & Fridlund, 1999). After one test interview, both the technique and the questions proved to be satisfactory and were included in the study. In the second study, a semi-constructed interview guide was constructed and used, and three test interviews were conducted. Since these were unsatisfactory, the guide was divided into two areas, one to cover topic for paper **II** (Björklund et al., 2009) and one for paper **III** (Björklund et al., 2008). After revision, all participants were re-interviewed using the two-part guide. The first three test interviews were included into the respectively participant's interview. A semi-structured guide was further constructed for the last study. One test interview was conducted and showed the guide to be useful. Hence, the interview was included in the study (paper **IV**). In this last study, the interviews were repeated and extended over 1-year illness experiences, dissimilar in points in time for each participant (Björklund et al., 2010).

3.5 Interview process

All patients' (n=35) gave their written consent before the interviews and chose the time and place for their interview. Some patients were interviewed once (Bjorklund & Fridlund, 1999, Björklund et al., 2008, 2009) while others were interviewed up to four times (Björklund et al., 2010).The patients were interviewed at their homes (n=30), at hospitals (n= 21), or at their place of work (n=2). Since it could be problematic to interview patients with impaired speech, sufficient time was allowed to reach an understanding. The interviewer focused on topics, however the participants were allowed to talk freely about topics and narrate in their own words. Problems could arise because Swedish was not every patient's native language. Hence, parts of some interviews were performed in English. Neither the participant nor the interviewer had English as their native language, but all were familiar with the language. Body language was also used frequently, e.g. facial expressions and lip movement or pointing at the body to describe surgery, pain, disgust or cheerfulness. Some participants clarified their answers in writing or had next of kin nearby during the interview, but comments from next of kin were included only if the participant asked them to fill in words and gave a nod of approval. Several of the participants glanced through private diaries or at photographs or brochures during the interviews to trigger memories of their illness experiences. All discussions during the interviews were tape recorded. The interviews lasted 30-120 minutes, but contact time with the patients was substantially longer. The researcher transcribed the tapes verbatim in the days following the recorded interviews. At that time she could recall her experiences of the interview situation and if necessary add small notes to the transcripts of what happened, e.g. when participants experienced episodes of coughing or crying. This helped capture the illness impact on the participant's entire body. The transcriptions yielded 1083 pages (1.5 spacing).

3.6 Text analyses

Owing to the richness of the text and the ability to interpret the data on different levels, different qualitative analyses were used for interpret the collected information. Qualitative content analysis is an interpretation process that focuses on similarities in and differences between different parts of text that lead into categories and/or themes (Polit & Beck, 2008). A category contains several codes with similar content that answers the *what* question and relates to the content on a descriptive level. A theme answers the *how* question i.e. the 'read thread' throughout the condensed meanings units, codes or sub-categories A meaning unit is a constellation of statements or words that relate to the same meaning, and codes are a process of identifying recurring words, themes, or concepts within these meanings units. There are different levels or dimensions of interpretations ranging from the concrete surface level of words down to deeper level of meaning. The researcher's pre-understanding was treated as a part of the interpretation process as well as a tool to guide it, thus, the text analysis was open to several possible interpretations. The first study (Bjorklund & Fridlund, 1999) was analysed with the critical incident technique (Flanagan, 1954). The second study (Bjöklund et al., 2008; 2009) with a qualitative content analysis i.e. thematic and latent (Berg, 2004). The last study (Björklund et al., 2010) was analysed with an interpretative descriptive analysis (Thorne et al., 1997; Thorne et al., 2004).

3.6.1 Critical incident technique

In 1954, Flanagan described the critical incident technique and this method obtains data from participants by in-depth exploration of critical incidents and human behaviours related to the topic under study. The technique differs from self-reported approaches as it focused on something specific that the participants can likely give evidence on as an expert (Polit & Beck, 2008). It includes a detailed description of the situation that led to the incident, acting or behaviour, and the result. This study (Bjorklund & Fridlund, 1999) aimed to describe cancer patients' experiences of nurses' behaviour in terms of critical incidents after nurses had given them health promoting care. A critical incident was defined as an event of great importance to the patient, which had either positive or negative impact on the patients' experience of feeling better health and well-being. All the incidents were classified into groups and reformulated into different types of actions i.e. sub-categories. These sub-categories were allocated into the nurses' behaviour i.e. categories. Then the categories were placed into one of the main areas (ibid).

3.6.2 Qualitative content analysis

The content analysis of narrative data aims to identify prominent themes and patterns among the themes (Polit & Beck, 2008). It involves breaking down text into smaller units, and coding and naming these units according to the content they represent. Thereafter, the coded material is grouped by focusing on similarities and differences. The thematic (Baxter, 1991) and latent (Berg, 2004) qualitative content offers alternatives for analysis when researcher use wording to develop qualitative descriptions when analysing different qualitative content of text. The questions to the patients were asked in positive sentences, but throughout the process of identifying meaning units the analysis revealed both positive and negative experiences and even the desire for health promoting contacts. For that reason the text was divided into two parts and named *health promoting contacts*, and *not health promoting contacts*. The latter holds participants' wishes for health promoting contacts, since these were not experienced contacts, but they might broaden the findings on the meaning of the concept. Then the meaning units were grouped according to which period in the participants' illness trajectory they belonged, and were then condensed and labeled with a code. All coded data were grouped together based on their similarities and difference, and ultimately three themes were named (Björklund et al., 2009). Latent qualitative content analysis seemed to be appropriate to use since it involves an interpretative reading of the representation of what is essential in the text to reveal the deep structural meaning conveyed by the message. The first reading revealed that health could be promoted in three ways; by means of oneself, family and others, and various actives (Björklund et al., 2008). The meanings unit were marked condensed and label with a code, and the codes were sorted into sub-themes. A search was conducted for a pattern in the sub-themes, and the themes were named. Every theme was further analysed, and one main theme could be formulated (ibid.).

3.6.3 Interpretative descriptive analysis

Before the final study began (Björklund et al., 2010), the findings and methods used in the other studies were discussed in attempting to form a critical review and basis for a preliminary analytic framework (Thorne et al., 2004). The pre-analytic understanding was that the findings had in some way captured the experiences of 35 patients as regards contact and care involving health professionals, and the patients had reported when these contacts had promoted health and well-being. Some patients, however, reported negative experiences, e.g. being exposed and vulnerable in contacts with health professionals. The findings also mirrored the patients' process of empowerment by being enabled to act and take control over everyday life with help from internal and external resources. Although patients were obviously troubled by tumour location and the side effects of treatment, which placed a heavy burden on everyday life, none of the studies revealed this profoundly.

This pre-analytic understanding revealed a need for deeper understanding of what it meant to live with HNC. It was decided to repeat the interviews with a small sample of patients and follow, for one year, the unique experiences of individuals living with the illness.

Already during the interviews the narrated stories revealed the individuality of what it meant to live with HNC, and therefore each patient's text was analysed and coded separately. The interview text was rich and deep in structure, and the researcher moved in and out of the text, critically examining the initial codes by asking questions such as: What was said here? What, where and when did it happen? What does/ could it mean for this person? By changing between the codes and the exclusive patient's complete text, the progression of understanding evolved from the surface to a deeper level of interpretation. From this investigation of uncover patterns in the text grew an interpretation of sub-themes from each interview, and these were further analysed when locking for changes over time. After that, one theme was interpreted for the complete transcripts of each unique patient. In the final stage, a main theme was interpreted, i.e. an association that could mirror living with HNC for all the patients (Björklund et al., 2010).

3.6.4 The author's pre- understanding

I am a registered nurse with over 25 years of experience in working in an ear, nose, and throat clinic that treats patients with different stages of HNC. Additional, for the past decade I have been a lecturer, teaching e.g. health sciences, nursing and oncology proficiency. The pre-understanding was a requirement for performing the interview studies, given the practical knowledge of the care context and the communication problems that these patients can encounter. I was also aware that individuals in this group of patients are vulnerable when meeting strangers, due to their changed appearance or other issues, e.g. coughing and spitting necessitated by increased phlegm. I have grown proficient in shaping a dialogue and participating in and providing equality in the interview situation. I know the importance of being an attentive listener, respecting the patients' life situation, and paying attention to their will to communicate. I recognise the need to probe and to prolong the waiting time for answers, not necessary verbal but also responses expressed in body language or in writing.

The pre-understanding about living with HNC and the concept of health promotion has changed during the research work. As a consequence, the concept of health promotion is not equivalent in the four studies. I realise that as a health professional you can perceive, but not experience, the inner feelings and needs associated with having an illness. This awareness can grow and be used as part of caring or the interpretative research process. Since the pre-understanding could interfere with the findings, this should be taken into consideration especially regarding the concept of health promotion.

4. Ethical considerations

The Lund University Ethics Committee (LU, 348/1997, LU 772/2004) approved the studies in Sweden. In the other Nordic countries, chief physicians at the regional ear, nose, and throat hospitals where the patients had been treated were informed about the studies and agreed to its implementation. All studies compiled with ethical principles, i.e. the principles of respect for autonothe, non-maleficence, and beneficence (Northern Nurses Federation

[NNF], 2003, World Medical Association [WMA], 2004). The data collected were coded and kept in strictest confidence, and the participants were guaranteed confidentiality in the presentation of study findings. The first study revealed no unique details, e.g. diagnosis together with country, age and gender (Bjorklund & Fridlund, 1999). Participants in the next two studies were treated in a specific area in the southern Sweden, and it was important to act with strict confidentiality (Björklund et al., 2008; 2009; 2010). The researcher was careful not to reveal the specific diagnosis, age, gender and exact day when the interviews were performed, or other such details. Participants who originated from other countries, but were living in Sweden, were not referenced in terms of mother country or language. Confidentiality was also explained to next of kin if they were present during the interviews.

4.1 The principles of respect for autonomy

In all the studies, patients were presented with a written form asking if they would be willing to participate and be interviewed. In the first study, the written form was written in their native language, but the open interview questions were posed in Swedish, English and occasionally in the participants' native Nordic language (Bjorklund & Fridlund., 1999). The researcher provided verbal information about the study and obtained the patients' written, informed consent before they enrolled. The participants also gave oral informed consent before the repeat interviews in the final longitudinal study. All the patients' were informed that their participation was voluntary and that they could withdraw at any time during the research process without explaining the reason, and with no consequences to usual care. The patients' physical and psychological conditions received special attention, and added value was shown to severely ill individuals. Since many of the participants had difficulty speaking, an attachment to the written form encouraged them to use the interviewer's telephone number, address or e-mail if they wanted to raise some questions or leave the study, but no participant made such request. On occasion participants asked to postpone the interview, and death precluded some interviews (Björklund et al., 2010).

4.2 The principles of beneficence and the principle of non-maleficence

When conducting qualitative research with patents who are in vulnerable life situation the principles to do no harm and to do good are highly important and were applied in this research, e.g. when taking the individual's very specific speech impairment into consideration. Hence, the same interviewer with extensive working experience as a nurse in this care context conducted all the interviews. Potentially, problems concerning physical ability, language or culture could have arisen, but none did. The interviewer made a concerted effort to respect and intuitively perceive the needs of the individual participants.

5. Findings

The deep understanding of living with HNC, and the experiences of what the patients felt promoted health and well-being, was interpreted as *having strong beliefs in a future in face of living on a rollercoaster.* This interpretation was built on the patients' experiences of the unique impact of HNC, its threat against their identity, and an existence with swiftly changeable feelings oscillating between hopelessness and hopefulness. Inherent in these feelings were the patients' struggle and orientation towards the health, power, and control that offered them belief in the future. Yet the findings also revealed the opposite - that some patients showed less energy and a sense of facing insurmountable barriers against achieving feelings of health. Hence, they felt less command over life and less belief in the future.

All participants' experiences were of course based on specific everyday situations. Hench, their capacities, difficulties, needs, and access to support differed substantially. Many of the patients felt vulnerable, exposed, and even disempowered in their contact with health professionals. Especially before and after treatment they experienced feelings of being alone, abandoned, and insecure. Nevertheless, inherent in the interpretations was their search for ways to promote health and well-being, although they experienced this as a means to find ways of thinking about a future life. The success of this work was interpreted as depend on their connection with enabling, which could involve internal motivation to act i.e. internal strength, and external resources, i.e. when others stimulate him/her to engage in processes to look forward.

The researcher's pre-understanding of the health promotion concept is not equivalent in the studies. The first study revealed her traditional biomedical and pathogenic standpoint; dependent, of course, on the aim of the study (Bjorklund & Fridlund, 1999). The nurses engaged in monitoring, caring, inspecting, observing, informing, and educating patients about risk factors in the context of health promotion activities, helping patients cope with the environment to reach well-being. In the subsequent studies, the affected individuals' perspective on living every day with HNC dominated. These findings are rooted in the affected individuals' activities and experiences of what they thought promoted their own health and well-being (Björklund et al., 2008; 2009; 2010).

The most important findings will be presented under the following headings: living with head and neck cancer; experiences of what promotes health and feelings of well-being; and experiences of what hinders health and feelings of well-being.

5.1 Living with head and neck cancer

Some of the patients' experiences of living with HNC meant an existential loneliness, and was interpreted as a unique and complex feeling, not unlike that of living in captivity. This imprisonment was a result of the participants' illness-related experiences of living alone in existential insecurity and encapsulation, reliant day and night on how the illness impacted their vital needs for survival. Although the physical impact could reveal similarities, it always involved unique experiences that were *(1) physically, (2) emotionally, (3) socially,* and *(4) existentially* confining for the patient.

(1) Patients experienced physical confinement when choking sensations and extreme swelling in the throat forced them to exhibit ungraceful behaviour, e.g. massive phlegm stagnation resulted in constant hawking, clearing of throat, and spitting, and they felt trapped in an alien body. These feelings were intensified and interwoven with their changed appearance and dependence on technical and medical devices, e.g. feeding tube and/or tracheal tube. Further, it was understood that feeling breathless made patients extremely anxious, and they were afraid of choking during sleep, and this discomfort mirrors confinement in a rouge body.

(2) Experiences of emotional confinement were revealed when hovering between despair and hope, where patients first had a sense of uncertainty, anxiety, and depression, and then experienced a swing in the opposite direction. It was as if they were living on a virtual rollercoaster. Their feelings of despair intensified when needing an alter ego to deal with the complexities of speaking, and the findings revealed living in a compromised state. The experiences of hope were most noticeable in comforting meetings with next of kin, good friends, and sometimes with health professionals that gave them emotional support.

(3) Experiences of social confinement were revealed when eating difficulties and disfigurement altered the patients' interactions and encounters with others. In social encounters it was understood that the patients were met by stares or avoidance in addition to changed attitudes and reactions, and they felt an altered sense of affiliation. It was not uncommon that they preferred to be alone and limited their social life to conserve energy, and the findings revealed this self-induced isolation. Some patients felt that the social circumstances that forced them into dependency on others also made them vulnerable, and they felt as if they were trapped in a social net. The distribution of domestic work changed, affecting everyday life for both the patients and their next of kin. Further, their life could be affected by financial problems because both the patients and their next of kin experienced increases in the cost of living, e.g. medicine, treatment, special diet, travel expenses, or inability to work. The patients often shouldered the responsibility for protecting their total family's economic situation and the findings revealed that they looked ahead to prepare for their own departure and their next of kin's future economic security. The findings showed that the patients' working life changed and feelings of harassment from employers when being on sick-leave, no consideration given to their new life situation, and feeling threatened by legal proceedings.

(4) Experiences of existential confinement were revealed when unemployment seemed to affect the patients with feelings of existential disequilibrium, and they presented spiritual beliefs that their total life situation had brought forth the latent cancer in their body. Patients developed an existential loneliness and feelings of living in the land of the sick; an experience amplified by the patients' perceived rejection by next of kin and changed sexual relationship.

5.2 Experiences of what promotes health and feelings of well-being

The findings revealed the patients' unique willpower to fight for something that could enhance their feelings of better health. The patients' focus could be understood as an endeavour to improve health and to find hope, i.e. to achieve the best possible well-being to fulfil new life goals of health. The ability to reach goals for better health was connected to the patients' *internal* and *external enabling* to regain control and empower oneself.

5.2.1 Ability to reach internal enabling

Factors that impacted on the patients' internal or intra-personal ability to enable and use inner strength could be observed in the dialogue with the inner self when the patient practised mental training and praying. They learned to use their inner potential and adeptness to discover and take charge of solving their own problems by their transformed and improved self-esteem. Internal enabling was connected to thoughts and persona of how they looked at their existence and self, i.e. their self-confidence and self-image, and this seemed to impact on their ability of self-determination. As a result, the findings revealed an intention not to act as a victim of circumstance, but to somehow reconcile with the illness. They actively took action to explore new life conditions and felt a need, and were relieved, to meet soul mates having similar experiences. The patients seemed to recognise and embrace existentiality and to be totally focused on being present in the here and now as a grateful survivor. The findings revealed patients' free spirit and spiritual confidence and faith with no fear of dying and the conviction of re-incarnation and death as a transition.

5.2.2 Ability to reach external enabling

Factors that impacted on the patients' external or inter-personnel enabling of ability were revealed in support from **(a)** social networks **(b)** contact with environment, **(c)** and health care. Helped by these external enablers, the patients could reach their own strength and form and enhance their health.

(a) Being enabled by means of contact with a social network was revealed as *emotional* and *practical support* from the patients' next of kin and close friends. *Emotional support* 24 hours a day was particularly precious - to have one important person to talk to, someone who dared to listen and contained their fears when the patients' thoughts were in turmoil from their sickness and existence. The patients revealed cheerful, humorous, and amusing interactions that gave them strength and motivation to live, and they revealed that having HNC was a family affair. They also revealed the *practical support* they received, e.g. assistance with household work, personal hygiene, and phone calls.

(b) The patients' external enabling of ability was revealed by means of contact with and appreciation for the environment, categorised as *nature, hobbies, and activities. Nature* was understood to have a healing power, and when being outdoors in any weather conditions the patients enjoyed nature's colour and peacefulness. Outdoor activities seemed to increase the patients' physical strength and reduce their psychological stress. Although appreciation for the environment offered external enabling of ability, the findings also revealed that nature helped them acknowledge their own existence, and they found it easier to connect with and find transpersonal relatedness to a supernatural power. The findings revealed that if patients experienced something that suited their capability, something they found pleasurable and motivating, this *hobby and activity* created flow and positive feelings and joy, and they practiced it over and over again.

(c) Other factors that impacted on the patients' external enabling of ability were revealed in their contact with health care, categorised into *health care organisation, health professionals' knowledge and experiences,* and *health professionals' attitudes.* The findings revealed that patients had a better feeling of health when the *health care organisation* successfully provided long-term, continuing access with individualised, tailored care from, e.g. physicians, dieticians, dentists, dental hygienists, and nurses. This corresponded to the findings revealed when patients experienced confidence in health care and turned over the medically responsibility to health professionals because of their own lack of medical knowledge. *Health professionals' knowledge and experience* was an expectation, and the patients always assumed that health professionals were skilled, knowledgeable, effective, and updated on medical and technical issues. The patient needed to be respected as a unique person and needed to be believed when telling their illness story. Contacts with health professionals could then facilitate improved health and these contacts were named *health promoting contacts* and were mainly experienced during the treatment phase when patients had daily contact with specific, qualified health professionals. Kind and considerate treatment was invaluable in contacts with health professionals and enhanced a patient's sense of autonomy. It was obvious that patients wanted to remain as independent as possible. However, during acute life-threatening situations they had a sense of well-being despite their dependence, i.e. when health professionals cared for, checked, examined, and observed them. The findings revealed that *health professionals' attitudes* or behaviours, e.g. silent body language or outspoken views on mankind, were especially important for the patients' learning and confidence in performing self-care. Further, in dealing with the patients' speech impairments it was important for health professionals to be attentive and have a humble attitude, then patients felt that co-operation and a practical working relationship were achievable. The patients wanted to be seen and respected as active persons and meet health professionals that supported their health objectives and positive potential for health rather than focusing on the disease and related problems. The findings revealed that the patients' strengths, competencies, and health resources grew in the course of participating and co-operating with health professionals through mutual or individual initiatives. Also, the patients revealed that they were surprised to meet health professionals that showed solicitude and were available, engaged, respectful, confirming, and did more than expected.

5.3 Experiences of hindrances to health and feelings of well-being

In the face of the patients' vulnerability and new life circumstances, accompanied by distressing illness experiences, the findings revealed how complicated it could be to set and attain goals for better health. In addition, it was understood that in human encounters, and especially in the dependant position of being a patient and seeking health care, people could feel that they had lost their power and self-control. Consequently, the patients' could experience hindrances to health as a lack of ability to connect to his/her *(1) internal* and *(2) external enabling.*

5.3.1 Lack of ability to reach internal enabling

Some patients revealed a lack of ability to reach goals for health, due to their inability to connect to inner strength, and the findings revealed feelings of diminished strength of mind. The changed self-image seemed to burden the patients with feelings of low self-esteem and decreased self-confidence, and these shortcomings in self-directed support could result in a self-depreciated sense of how other people viewed them, and they felt as if they were living in a compromised state. The feeling of self-imposed incarceration was obstructed, giving rise to feelings of being taken hostage by health care. The findings also revealed that the patients' weakened self-worth interfered with their autonomy and performance, and they felt left out of treatment decisions, like a guinea pig.

5.3.2 Lack of ability to reach external enabling

Hindrances in reaching external enabling were connected to the same factors and revealed a lack of support from **(a)** social networks, **(b)** contact with environment, **(c)** and health care.

a) Patients' diminished inner feeling of self could influence their social contacts and change their relationship to next of kin, thereby increasing isolation. In addition to the adverse physical and communicative impact of their illness, patients felt discomfort from being in situation that forced them to depend on others day and night.

b) However, the findings also revealed feelings of insecurity caused by the gravity of illness that forced the patients to stay home alone, having little contact with nature. Patients revealed that they felt a necessity for restrictive living. Hence, in addition to the fatigue that diminished or stopped their involvement in hobbies and other activities, this created feelings of ill-health and powerlessness.

(c) The same external factors could also be experienced as hindrances in enabling patients' contact with health care, and could also be categorised into *health care organisation, health professionals' knowledge and experiences,* and *health professionals' attitudes.* The findings revealed that *health care organisation* could be experienced as a barrier to patients' feelings of well-being, and the patients frequently revealed feelings of abandonment and lack of confidence in health care. When problems arose, the patients were often uncertain who to contact amongst the numerous health professionals and they felt lost and, due to their vulnerability, dared not ask questions. Moreover, they felt exhausted by the massive, impersonal, one-way information and other limitations in human encounters. It was understood that at times *health professionals* did not comprehend patients' feelings of vulnerability resulting from dependency on health care, and this insensitivity increased the patients' suffering and contradicted their feelings of health. The findings revealed deficiencies in accessibility and continuity of health care. This, added to a sense of being caught in a permanent illness trajectory, compounded the patients' vulnerability and stress in life. Contacts with health professionals that revealed hindrances against improving health were named *not-health-promoting contacts,* and were experienced predominantly before and after treatment. Still it was understood that the most important factor to patients was to be believed when expressing their illness story. If the patients were met by *attitudes* from *health professionals* of not being respected, or even listen to, it led them to search for attentive health professionals. Patients revealed being put off balance, i.e. less capacity to grasp health goals, when encountering unengaged or incompetent health professionals with paternalistic or superficial attitudes who seemed to lack respect for the individual behind the patient role. When patients worried about the imperfections in their body such encounters were often accompanied by feelings of not having their opinions valued.

6. Discussion

The findings concerned 35 individuals diagnosed with HNC, revealing their experiences of and connection with *enabling,* i.e. providing somebody with the ability or means to do something was important to their success in experiencing health and well-being and the process of taking control over of new life situation. This process of empowerment, i.e. the goal of health promotion (WHO, 1986), was an on-going process of contacting and using their inner strength; their internal ability or skill to motivate action. Further, enabling was associated with external connection to environmental factors e.g. relationship to family/ friends, health professionals, nature, hobbies, and activities that stimulated patients to engage in processes to move forward, belief in a future, and take command over everyday life.

Living with HNC was like living on a virtual rollercoaster, on one hand, fighting day and night with HNC's life-threatening impact and the side-effects of the treatment or tumour growth, e.g. breathlessness, and bleeding. On the other hand, making it through the 'downs' helped the patients believed in the future, since it gave them an enhanced feeling of confidence in their ability to orient themselves towards health and self-empowerment. This correspond to Antonovsky's (1987) research when he put forward that as long as there is breath of life in us, we are all to some degree healthy and we are always moving between two extremes of ease and dis-ease on the health continuum. This interpretation of *life in a symbolic roller coaster* is not exceptional and could be experienced by many people, with or without a sickness. Many people struggle with life- threatening diseases combined with treatment complications and an insecure future, e.g. people with diverse cancer forms or other chronic diseases.

An important factor could be the researchers' perspective (pathogenic or salutogenic) in interpreting the findings. Although the participants in the studies had numerous physical symptoms and experienced many 'ups and downs', they tried (and often succeeded) to repress negative feelings to make life bearable. Being positive might be part of a process where patients actively seek meaningful and therapeutic interactions with health professionals, thereby gaining important knowledge. Positive thinking could be a way to take responsibility for prevention of and recovery from cancer, i.e. one strategy to cope with cancer and its treatment (McCreaddie et al., 2010). However, it could place another burden on the already afflicted person, i.e. if you think positive enough the cancer can be cured.

For some of the patients living with HNC, the disease was understood as be on a permanent illness trajectory that changed their life into a state of physical, emotional, social and existential captivity. This translated into a difficult everyday life, especially highlighted by the findings showing their aloneness, even when cohabiting or having close relationships to next of kin and/or friends. Trillin (1981) emphasized that having cancer signifies entering the land of the sick, where those from the land of the well could visit, but always leave. This corresponds to other research showing that patients on a cancer trajectory often experienced uncertainties, vulnerability, and isolation (Halldórsdóttir & Hamrin, 1997). Also, HNC causes potentially life threatening problems, e.g. involving respiration, nose bleeding, choking while eating and swallowing, and it also causes lifelong physically problems with, e.g. altered appearance and communication (cf. Rumsey et al. 2004). No research was found that addressed the findings on patients' feelings on an altered relation to their body, which confronting them with embarrassing behaviours, e.g. phlegm stagnation resulted in a need to repeatedly clear the throat and spit. Problems seemed to have a huge impact on patients' entire everyday life and correspond to other research on HNC's bodily impact that seemed to confront patients' both a psychosocial and existential struggle (cf. Mok et al, 2010).

The findings stress the importance of meeting soul mates, since the patients experienced a substantial difference in talking to and receiving information and support from someone that had life experiences with this illness. Research has shown that active memberships in patient organisation improved patients' well-being and perhaps these meetings could alleviate some of their loneliness, and help regain power and control over everyday life (Aarstad, 2008). Still, as Mok et al. (2010) point out, there is no medication for alienation, loneliness, despair, meaninglessness, and fear or death. Hench, findings on patients' endeavours to find meaning in life through love, hope, confidence and belief in the future, i.e. to reach the best possible well-being to achieve new life goals, were important. Mok et al. (2010) also stressed that it was essential for the patients' emotional and spiritual well-being to meet health professionals that showed caring attitudes and delivered expert information with a cheerfulness and kindness.

HNC can cause discomfort and suffering since it is located in the body's most visible area and this could either enhance personal growth or damage or destroy self-esteem (Rumsey et al. 2004). Lindenfield (1996) suggested that if a person believes that he/she is worthless or ugly it could generate negative feelings and depression. Mok et al. (2004) asserted that if health professionals focus on resources rather than health deficits this could more effectively influence the individuals' thoughts and attitudes in a positive way. Feber (2000) highlighted coaching in intrapersonal skills as a means of promoting optimum health and well-being for the individual with HNC. Dropkin (1999) showed that self-care could be beneficial and reduce anxiety in disfigured persons, since it helps patients find their true self and adapt to their new body image. This corresponds to research by Turpin et al. (2008) showing that patients with HNC went through an active process to retain a positive sense of self when the illness impact altered their relationship to their own body.

It was the individuals improved sense of self-worth when they took control over their new life situation, and this helped them break many years of lifestyle habits, e.g. smoking and alcohol consumption. Adopting new lifestyle habits required inner strength and will, and it could be valuable for health professionals to draw on these findings when following public health advice (NIPH, 2005), and start smoking cessation programmes in HNC care (Sharp, 2006), and begin to find out if patients are motivated to make lifestyle changes. The findings also correspond to the research of Mok et al. (2004) regarding patients' motivational process, process of seeking mastery, and transformation of thoughts.

The patients' often used their power of mind when meditating or praying i.e. self-transcendence are shown to be helpful in drawing on one's own strength and health resources (cf. Dossey et al., 2000). Some patients expressed high self-confidence in spirituality and being present in the here and now, with no fear of dying - hence, finding meaning in life by thinking that death was a transition to another state of being. Acceptance of death as a process in life, and letting go, corresponds to the research of Mok et al. (2010) claiming that inner spiritual well-being is attained from having faith and being aware of possibilities in life and after death. The findings revealed that integration of spiritual and personal beliefs lead to peacefulness, harmony, and spiritual growth. In addition, it is known that patients with HNC often use complementary and alternative methods, such as spiritual therapies, herbs and vitamins, physical therapies, and body/mind therapies (Molassiotis et al. 2006). Frenkel et al. (2008) advocate integrating these methods into health care and advise health professionals to engage with, support, and give appropriate advice to patients wanting to complement their medical treatment with such alternatives.

The findings revealed that some patients found a glass of wine or beer to be beneficial and relaxing and this correspond to Allison's (2002) research showing that using (as opposed to abusing) wine during recovery can lead to better physical and role functioning, less fatigue, and fewer feelings of illness. This way of caring for and encountering patients with HNC requires health professionals to be attentive, listen to and respect patients - and to relinquish some of their own power to trust in, and dare to support, patients' actions and wishes.

Good interpersonal relationships and emotional support 24 hours a day, i.e. external enablers such as next of kin or friends, were essential. It was vital to have someone to talk to, and perhaps particularly when patients experienced new illness and acute, life- threatening problems. Again, this corresponds to the research of Mok et al. (2010) on the necessity for patients to have well-functioning relationships and connection with next of kin and friends. However, research also shows that the relationship between two individuals could be experienced as difficult, due to a dependency on support that one might need from the other (cf. Carnevali & Reiner, 1990). The findings also support this, revealing strained relationships and changed life situations for the family as an entity. It could be altered role function at home, and some participants felt rejection from next of kin. Vickery et al. (2003) highlight that partners could report greater distress than the sick person they care for. Additionally, the findings revealed transformed emotional and sexual relationships, particularly amongst the women interviewed in the studies. For example Carnevali & Reiner (1990) confirm that relationships and intimacy seem to be more important for women to discuss. These problems might relate to the patients' problems with phlegm production or mouth odour, which both parties could experience as unpleasant. It is known that this cancer could be experienced as more traumatic than other cancers because of the visible disfigurement involved (cf. Vickery et al., 2003). The findings revealed high psychological stress and vulnerability in the patients, partly because of how they viewed the life situation of their next of kin. It was essential for them to take an active role, to be responsible for their own self-care, and seek support from next of kin or good friends when needed. The findings also presented various confirmations on the importance of long-term support for next of kin. Co-operative care seems to alleviate fear by providing self-care education in a home setting, and has been shown to conserve health resources and improve and facilitate communication amongst the family and health professionals involved in care (McLane et al., 2003). Interest has been growing in psycho-oncology and emotional well-being for patients and their next of kin (Hodges & Humphris, 2009). Training courses for patients and next of kin, e.g. on learning to live with cancer, seemed to be valuable and these courses were based on a teaching-learning process with an interactive and systematic bottom- up approach (Grahn et al., 1999) that could help patients and their next of kin choose topics they wanted to discuss, ultimately empowering and supporting them in achieving defined health goals. The findings also revealed the patients' eagerness to learn and preserve independence and autonothe and to practice self-care. This corresponds to research by Mok et al. (2004) suggesting that when patients owned knowledge and skills and practice self-care, they could accept the illness and could lead to feelings of better health and well-being.

All the patients narrate that they received strength and felt good when being outdoors and following the changes in nature, i.e. also an external enabler. Nurturing plants to survive and blossom also gave patients a sense of hope for the future; to be alive despite their sickness. The link between nature, health, and healing are well-known and nature can be viewed as an unused public health resource since it has the potential to increase people's sense of well-being. Hence, it appears that parks and natural areas are potential 'gold mines' for a population's health promotion (cf. Björklund, 2010). This means a responsibility for health care to creating an atmosphere that is pleasing for the eyes, and combining this with easy access or views to parks and green spaces, since it enhances everyone's wellbeing (patients, next of kin, and health professionals).

Hobbies and cultural activities suited to the situation are other external enablers, and by practising these activities over and over again the patients experienced control and power over everyday life. This corresponds to other research showing, e.g. that art therapy could decrease anxiety and facilitate recovery and the use of music enhance effects of analgesics, and decrease pain, anxiety, and depression (cf. Leddy, 2003).

Working relationships with respectful and competent health professionals could encourage a patient's activity, participation, co-operation, and self-care. It was also understood that positive human encounters could contribute towards counterbalancing the often unequal position that patients sometimes felt in health care. This was named *health promoting activity* (Bjorklund & Fridlund, 1999) or *health promoting contact* (Björklund et al., 2009). In this context, the patients experienced health professionals to be available, engaged, respectful, and validating and to express knowledge, competence, solicitude, and understanding. Good interpersonal relationship between the patient and health professionals can be seen as both 'means and end' in an interaction/contact (cf. Halldórsdóttir & Hamrin, 1997). These health promoting contacts could, to a certain extent, correspond to research on supportive clinics that could help patients with emotional and practical needs (Larsson, 2006). Nevertheless, the findings showed that, especially before and after treatment, the patients felt abandoned and lost amongst all the members in the multidisciplinary team that were involved in their care. These findings suggest that the current healthcare organisation is characterised by large-scale production that is function oriented - not a patient-process-oriented organisation. It seems that a health-care organisation with supportive clinics must be developed and be accessible 24 hours a day. Care needs to focus on the unique patient and be designed as individually tailored, patient-centred care, throughout the lengthy trajectory of illness (IOM, 2000).

To improve the organisation of HNC care, it should develop in teamwork with patient organisations, health professionals, and policy makers (cf. NIPH, 2005). Patient organisations are vital because of their potential influence as the voice for an entire group of patients. It can raise demands on behalf of their members, who have less opportunity to speak up in society due to the impact of the illness on their ability to communicate (Aarstad, 2008).

It is, however, known that these patients often have long-lasting and slowly progressing health problems. In addition the findings showed lack of individual, tailored care outgoing from a salutogenic perspective. It was also understood that some patients experienced discouraging obstacles against better health and feelings of well-being, and these vulnerabilities seemed to cause low self-esteem and low self-performance. This highlights a) the need for easy access to care with a salutogenic focus to long-term psychological rehabilitation and b) the need for good contact with health professionals who follow patients throughout the entire course of their illness trajectory (cf. Larsson, 2006). Rehabilitation services should also involve any next of kin engaged in a patient's everyday life and care.

The findings also indicated that the patients experienced many *not health promoting contacts* (Björklund et al., 2009) and a *lack of health promoting activities* (Bjorklund & Fridlund, 1999). Such encounters could lead to feelings of ill-health and powerlessness. Some health professionals seemed to be insensitive to the patients' vulnerabilities and did not listen to or respect patients' opinions, reflecting a superficial and paternalistic view of mankind. These findings correspond to the research by Halldórsdóttir & Hamrin (1997) about caring versus uncaring. When patients perceived that nurses were incompetent in some way; nonchalant or uninterested in the patient's competence, this created an obstacle in the patients' well-being and recovery. Professionals working in health care, especially in cancer care, must have special skills such as being an attentive listener, i.e. open for patients' questions and narratives.

One challenge could involve being responsive to behaviour and psychosocial responses to bad news, and delivering information in a series of processes along with the cancer trajectory (cf. Thorne, 2006). Patients want health professionals to openly share bad and uncertain information, however to do it sensitivity. A recommend approach was to follow up uncertain or bad news with slightly better information to avoid of diminishing opportunities for hope or future optimism (ibid.).

Patients experienced many hindrances in accessing health services, particularly the first contact with health professionals in the front line of care was problematic, and often the patients felt they were not believed when telling their illness history. Feber (2000) highlight the dynamic and context-specific nature of communication, and research shows the complex communication problems that patients with HNC can experience. It is of importance for health professionals to check that the information supplied has been understood and to be ready to provide further information if necessary. Patients' experienced also being in a disadvantaged position due to their vulnerability and dependence when seeking care. Research confirms the inequity of power in health care, due to the patient's dependency, and this could be an obstacle in interpersonal relationship between patients' and health professionals (cf. Halldórsdóttir & Hamrin, 1997). Ineffective communication can lead to delay in seeking care, failure to access appropriate care, and early withdrawal from treatment (cf. Thorne, 2006). Research has shown that some resilient HNC patients exhibited a profound reluctance to ask for help, despite extensive physical and emotional trauma (Wells, 1998). This could correspond to the patients that choose the wellness-in-the-foreground perspective, as described in the Shifting Perspectives Model of Chronic Illness, where some patients have trouble receiving the services or the attention they need (Thorne & Paterson, 1998; Paterson, 2001). Then patients struggle to maintain a positive attitude, keep active and independent, and try to live everyday life as normally as possible, strategies aim to maintain hope and to distance one's self from certain aspects of authenticity. Health professionals are accustomed to working with the-illness-in-foreground perspective and are skilled in supporting patients with information and teaching them how to manage their illness. HNC patients undergoing treatment wanted as much information as achievable, both good and bad, especially about the treatment and its side-effects (cf. Björklund, 2010). On the other hand, patients had express being overloaded with information that they do not understand. Research revealed that health professionals at times provide patients with 'hard core' information as part of their professional duty and not as a result of a sensitive dialogue (cf. Thorne, 2006). The-illness-in-foreground perspective was understood to be good in HNC context of the studies, if patients had the strength and motivation to learn. However, some health professionals could find it puzzling when a patient talks of well-being while having a multitude of problems. The Shifting Perspectives Models of Chronic Illness represents the patients' viewpoints, perceptions, hope, attitudes, and life experiences and appears to be a valuable tool in this care context. It enables health professionals to understand the patients' perspective at any given time and make suitable care and support available to patients with either perspective (Paterson, 2001).

It was understood that some patients experienced unemployment as distressing while others, in contrast, felt threatened by their employer and felt forced to continue working. It is well known that loss of occupational identity can be a source of significant anxiety and depression in everyday life. Further, HNC patients frequently experienced becoming employed because of their unique problems regarding, e.g. eating, speaking, pain, fatigue, and appearance (cf. Feber, 2000). Thoughtfulness must be exercised when supporting patients to continue working, and they need rehabilitation that is comprehensive and takes into account their contextual situation and burden of everyday life (cf. Hodges & Humphris, 2009). The findings highlight the need for health professionals to deepen their understanding of the patients' everyday life with HNC in relation to health, illness, and suffering. Hench, a vital factor for patients with chronic diseases is to have a well-functioning everyday life (cf. Carnevali & Reiner, 1990).

The patients experienced social and economic strains and Semple et al. (2008) addressed the increased cost of living with HNC, e.g. medicine, special diets, and lengthy treatment periods with related travel expenses, and inability to work. The findings also revealed long lasting side effects of treatment, e.g. jaw- and tooth-related pain. Adell et al. (2008) confirmed that some of the former HNC patients could never be rehabilitated to overcome the inconveniences in the jaw and teeth, and in those who could, it took years to restore dentition. The findings in the studies mirror the long-term struggle with distress, pain, and social and economic hardship in the patients' everyday life, and reflect a demand for public health and psychosocial interest for this group of patients. There is a need for society and health services to support cancer patients and their next of kin with psychosocial care and rehabilitation of good and equal quality at all stages of disease and survivorship (Björklund, 2010).

6.1 Methodological considerations

A qualitative design was chosen and was judged to be the most accurate means to describe and explore the patients' subjective truth and reality of their own life experiences. The four studies were based partly on different concepts related to health promotion. This could be viewed as a threat to the internal conceptual validity of the research as a whole. On the other hand, however, this conceptual variety reveals the versatility of health promotion strategies and points of departure. It reveals how the own way of thinking about health promotion developed during the research. The transformed view of the concept could be attributed in part to the many years that elapsed between conducting the first study and conducting the later studies. Another possible factor could be that society changed during this period, as did the concept of health promotion. Nevertheless, the approach towards the central concept of health promotion remained consistent with several of the basic principles, e.g. participation, partnership, equity, and inter-sector cooperation, but not always with others, e.g. holism and empowerment.

During the first study the view towards the patients were quite objectified, i.e. a person 'within' a specific form and stage of HNC (e.g. patient with stage 4 oropharynx cancer). This was accompanied by the 'mental image' as a nurse of these patients' common problems and needs. The standpoint on the concept of health promotion came from this traditional biomedical and pathogenic view, i.e. nurses should inform and educate patients about risk factors for acquiring diseases and should advise patients to change lifestyle (Bjorklund & Fridlund, 1999). However, the understanding about everyday life with HNC and persons' inherent capacity grew and in the later studies, the view on the concept health promotion changed. As a result, the concept shifted towards a more subjective-oriented understanding of the need to focus on the affected individuals' own experience of what promoted health and well-being. This represent a shift from the traditional 'top-down' approach to 'bottom-up' approach integrating the individual's own capacity to take control and become empowered. When health professionals view the patient as a person- an expert on his/her situation and co-producer of his/her health- it strengthens the patient's confidence in drawing on their own resources to improve their personal health and well-being.

In focus for the studies are 35 patients with HNC. Data were collected via individual, audio-taped, semi-structured, qualitative interviews. This semi-structured interview approach seemed appropriate since the aims were to identify areas that each participant would cover e.g. what promotes health in everyday life or what promotes health in contact with health professionals. The questions were open-ended so the participants could speak restrictions about these topics and could also initiate new topics. Different methods and analyses, all sensitive to human experiences, were used to interpret the data. Despite some differences between the four analysis methods used, they have followed basically the same approach throughout the studies. First, the researcher(s) read the full text of each interview to determine the most important aspects of the phenomenon under investigation. Second, the researcher (s) developed a more structured thematic analysis of every interview searching for meaning units/codes in sub theme. Finally, the researcher(s) examined the sub themes in the context of more superior theme, all at different levels of interpretations.

To ensure the quality of the findings, methodological considerations have been considered in terms of the five criteria for trustworthiness: credibility, dependability, transferability, confirmability, and authenticity (Polit & Beck, 2008). The central aspect is to confirm that the findings truthfully mirror the experiences and viewpoints of the participants, rather than perceptions of the researchers. The aspects undertaken to guarantee creditability also serve to guarantee dependability.

Credibility refers to confidence in the data and their interpretation. The strength lies in the process of purposively selecting the patients - in consultation with medical and nursing staff involved in their care - and following the criteria, i.e. patients' with diverse HNC diagnoses, stages, and treatment. Although variation in socio-demographics was not the most important criterion, it was important to find patients with the willingness and interest to communicate and verbalise their lived experiences. The first study (Bjorklund & Fridlund, 1999) makes reference to strategically chosen patients, but it also conveys a purposive selection since the interviewer worked in one hospital and therefore could ask some patients if they would participate. A limitation could be the unbalanced sample in this article (i.e. 17 individuals from Sweden and one from each of the other four Nordic countries). Although the purpose was not to generalised or compare the findings between the countries, more participants from the same country might have given more contextual data. In view of the research design, the data are not sufficient to make generalisations of the findings.

The patients' gender and age differences are in line with data showing that HNC is two to three times more frequent in men and most common in the group >50 years of age (cf. Feber, 2000). A weakness could be that although 54 persons were invited, 19 did not agree to participate. The non-participants were mainly men and younger people. Hench, a weakness could be that the findings may not reveal the experiences of younger people and people that did not match the selection criteria, e.g. confused or cognitive disable patients that could not communicate their experiences. Those who did participate were eager to contribute information about their experiences, and they provided rich descriptions. It should be noted that three of the participants heard of the studies and asked to participate and contacted a nurse at the ward on their own initiative. These participants had severe speech difficulties because of surgery and tumour growth, yet they gave concise information and lengthy interviews.

Communication between the interviewer and the interviewee during the interview situation may have influenced the quality of the data; since it is the researchers themselves that serve as data gathering and analytic instruments in qualitative studies. However, the participants could talk freely about the topic, and the interviewer thoughtfully went back and forth between the questions in the guide. Every interview were rich in content, quality, and meaning i.e. they were experienced as open, profound, and emotionally charged, and no problems were observed regarding the request to audio tape the interviews. The patients' showed an eagerness to contribute to the research, and together with the relaxed atmosphere during the interviews this fulfilled the criterion of a trusting and confidential relationship (Polit & Beck, 2008). The interviewer was familiar with the care context, and her interviewing skills progressively expanded as she conducted more interviews. This was evident from the interview transcripts. In the first study, she spoke and asked questions frequently, but in the latter studies the patient's voice dominated, and the patient was often first to break the silence. Since patients' speech problems could potentially jeopardise understanding, at times the questions were reformulated to achieve a shared understanding of the core response to these questions and avoid misinterpretation or the possibility that patients' answered in a way they thought might please the interviewer. The patients always chose the interview site, and most interviews were performed in the home. In-hospital interviews with inpatients were often shorter. On the whole, interviews conducted in hospital were shorter, but more convenient for outpatients who wanted to combine the interview with their hospital appointment.

Nine of the patients did not have Swedish as their native language. These patients received a written inquiry in their own language (Nordic language), and their interviews could include English words, notes of non-verbal interaction, body language, and help from next of kin. The small contributions from next of kin seemed to benefit; they not only elucidated and endorsed information, they also confronted the patient to talk, often about things not mentioned previously.

Although the interview questions were asked in positive sentences, e.g. what they felt promoted their health, the patients' answers occasionally revealed negative experience. It seemed, if we wanted to understand or know that something was good then we needed to confront it with the opposite, and thereby reach a deeper understanding of the subject under study (cf. Halldórsdóttir & Hamrin, 1997). Other researchers have used this approach when obtaining both positive and negative findings and looking at the findings (Bjorklund &

Fridlund, 1999) and the category *the nurse showed personal consideration* and the subcategory *the nurse showed empathy*. The positive form conveyed that the patients experienced the nurse as attentive, and she respected him: *the nurse was so calm and collected and sympathetic.* The negative form conveyed that the patients experienced that the nurses lower his self-esteem by trespassing his integrity; *the nurse was too good-nature, she felt sorry for me, I didn't like it.* In Björklund at al., 2009 p. 266 the positive form in the theme *receiving individualised, tailored care,* conveys experiences of being confirmed and feeling secure; *she called the dentist to prescribe medication for thrush ... I felt that I was well taken care of.* The negative form conveys the patient's experiences of being abandoned because no health professional wanted to take responsibility of their care; *they just remit patients from one place to another.*

The purposeful sampling with participants that had eagerness and interest to verbalise their lived experiences yielded rich interviews, and the participants acted safe and comfortable in revealing their often negative experiences. When researchers have a sense of what they need to know the use of purposive sampling could strengthen a comprehensive understanding of a phenomenon. By searching for disconfirming evidence and competing explanations the researcher could challenge a categorisation or explanation (Polit & Beck, 2008).

The value of repeating the interviews after a time was immense since the interviewer's understanding of the patients' everyday life grew with this extended relationship. Further, a longitudinal approach gives you an idea about the participants' experiences over time and what it could mean for them in process of healing, learning and continued empowerment. It allows the researcher to revisit issues and discuss new areas that have emerged from the data, and also allows the participants to discuss areas they may have forgotten or decided to withhold during previous interview (Polit & Beck, 2008).

Dependability concerns the stability of data over time and conditions, and was assured by using semi-structured guides and the same interviewer to conduct and transcribe all interviews verbatim. The verbatim transcripts allowed the researcher to remain close to the content of the interviews, and thereby ensure trustworthy and dependable interpretation. Different qualitative analyses were chosen because of the richness and profoundness of the text, making it possible to interpret the data on different levels. Interpretation was an on-going process that began already when the patients described their everyday life during the interview, and during the process they began to see and narrate new connections, free of interpretation by the researcher. In a way, the interviewer condensed and interpreted what the patient said and then transmitted the meaning back, especially during probing. This also took place during transcription when a new cognitive interpretation emerged.

Confirmability refers to objectivity and was assured when analyses and interpretations were checked and discussed on a repeated basis with supervisors and in seminar groups with researchers. Confirmability implies that procedures were followed to ensure that the findings are rooted in the data and are not resting on insufficient analysis or preconceived assumptions. A potential limitation in the first study is the considerable overlap between the categories, and the analysis could be done more rigorous (Bjorklund & Fridlund, 1999).

All over the studies transparency and credibility enable readers to be 'co-examiners' in gaining insight from analysing the patients' quotations and arriving at different interpretations. In the studies, the patients' quotations have been translated into English, but presented as their own choice of wording. A few minor revisions in grammar and vocabulary improved readability.

Transferability refers to the extent to which qualitative findings can be transferred or applied to other settings or groups. It could be successful if patients, and health professionals working in this care context, recognise the descriptions and interpretations as credible. Reasonably, transferability could be considered successful if people with cancer or neurological diseases, and who have similar severe communication and swallowing difficulties, could recognise the descriptions and interpretations as their own. However, the core question in transferability is whether it is logic to carrying out the innovation in a new practice setting. If some aspects of the settings contrast with the innovation, e.g. regarding philosophy, clients, personnel, or administrative structure, then it might not be sensible to try to apply the innovation (Polit & Beck, 2008). An important factor in promoting transferability is the quantity of information the researcher present about the context on their studies. Kvale (1996) stated that a post-modern shift towards the search for general knowledge, and the individually unique, is being replaced by the importance on the heterogeneity and contextuality of knowledge. 'Thick description' refers to a rich and thorough description of the research settings, performance, and approach (Polit & Beck, 2008). Perhaps the contextual descriptions are thick enough for the purpose of the studies, and consequently could contribute to the reader's capability to assess whether findings would be applicable to other groups or contexts. Transferability is analogous to generalisability. Naturalistic generalisation rest on personal experiences and derives from tacit knowledge of how things are and leads to expectations rather than formal predictions (Kvale, 1996). The findings show the participants' experiences and many quotations and interpretations of the findings are generally applicable to everyone, regardless of having HNC, e.g. the importance of emotional support from family and friends, and the importance of nature and culture in health. Analytic generalisation involves a reasoned judgement about the extent to which the findings from a study can be used as a guide to what might occur in another situation, and is based on similarities and differences of the two situations. However, how much should the researcher formalise and argue generalisations, or could this be left to the reader? Kvale (1996) put forward Freud's therapeutic case stories as examples for reader generalisation, since his descriptions and analyses are so colourful and persuasive that readers today still generalise many of the findings to modern cases.

Authenticity refers to the extent to which qualitative researchers honestly and truly show a variety of diverse realities in analysing and interpreting their data (Polit & Beck, 2008). This was assured since many of the findings and interpretations convey diverse shades of feeling in reference to patients' experiences and what it means to live with HNC. In many ways, the text invites readers into a vicarious experience of the lives being described, and enables readers to expand their sensitivity to the issues being depicted. Thereby, perhaps the reader can reach a deeper understanding of the patient's life, e.g. when reading quotations that contain non-verbal sounds (such as clearing the throat, spitting, hoarseness, or deep sighs) that could also mirror their own ill-health mood or feelings.

How people remember things could present a potential weakness of the studies, and patients in the first study, the time span from diagnosis to interview varied from 4 months to 14 years. It is known that the memory can change, but people always remember the critical incidences that occur and being stricken with cancer is an extremely traumatic experience accompanied by feelings that your whole existence is threatened (cf. Carnevali & Reiner, 1990). Flanagan (1954) asserted that the authenticity of data collected via the critical incident technique is very high since the participants narrate real, critical events from life. Research shows that it is easier to remember negative incidents since often they are experienced as more intense and distinct than positive incidents.

7. Conclusions

The aims of the studies have been to reach a deeper understanding of living with HNC and to identify the experiences that patients felt promoted their health and well-being. It further conveys the patients' experiences of care and contact with health professionals, and examines whether these encounters could increase patients' feelings of better health and well-being.

- The deeper understanding of 35 patients' everyday life with HNC was expressed as living on a virtual rollercoaster, with many 'ups and downs', i.e. interpreted as living in captivity, day and night, because of the symptoms. However, when searching and finding inner strength, patients could experience better health and well-being, and this could generate strong beliefs in the future.
- The patients' inner strength potentially enhanced their will to live, to handle their situation, and to be open towards continuing with a changed life.
- Emotional support and good interpersonal relationships with next of kin was important, 24 hours a day, i.e. someone who could ameliorate the 'downs' and supporting the 'ups'. Other findings reflected the concern that patients have for the strained life situation of their loved ones, and the changes in emotional and sexual relationships experienced by the women interviewed.
- The patients' gained a sense of strength not only from nature, but also from hobbies and activities that enhanced their control and power over everyday life.
- Some patients experienced vulnerability and psychological stress, e.g. due to changed appearance, transformed eating and speaking ability, and the inconvenience of being in a dependent position.
- Some patients' felt that barriers hindered their access to health care. In particular, they found it difficult to make initial contact with health professionals working on the front line. An important finding in this context is that many patients felt they were not being respected or believed when telling their illness history.
- The patients' had feelings of exposure and vulnerability in encounters with health professionals. Health professionals' views of mankind, roles, and behaviours (e.g. body language) could either strengthen or weaken the patients' health and well-being. The findings correspond to those from other cancer research.
- The patients' had different strength to handle their altered life situations. However, the findings highlight that nearly every patient felt, at times, lost and abandoned in health care during their long-term illness trajectory, especially before and after the treatment phase.
- Participation in patient organisations and courses (e.g. learning to live with cancer) was found to be valuable in lessening the patients' isolation.

- Learning and practising self-care seemed to lessen patients' dependency and increase their autonomy and self-worth.

8. Implications for health promotion

The findings seem to confirm that health promotion is not something that is done *for* or *to* people; it is done *with* people, either as individuals or in groups. This correspond with the basic principles in health promotion that is participation, partnership, empowerment, equity, holism, inter-sector cooperation, sustainability, and the use of multi-strategy approaches are (cf. Nutbeam, 1998). These principles are regularly updated, since health is shaped by individual factors and the physical, social, economic, and political contexts in which people live. For example, needs assessment, evidence-based health promotion, and self-efficacy are new terms added to the mix. Beliefs in the latter, i.e. self-efficacy, determine how people feel, think, motivate themselves, and behave. In other words, it is the effort people expend and how long they persist in the face of disadvantage and adversity.

In health care, patients need easy access, coordination, continuity, support from trained professionals and psychosocial rehabilitation in a patient-centred organisation. Supportive clinics could give patients, and their next of kin, long-term emotional, psychological, and practical support throughout the life-threatening and lengthy illness trajectory of HNC. Positive human encounters could help counterbalance the patients' unequal position in health care and strengthen patients' activity, participation, and co-operation, e.g. in smoking or alcohol cessation.

Maybe health care and health professionals need to place greater focus on salutogenic approaches, and receive further education in the bottom-up approach that starts from the patient's individual strengths and health resources. Such an approach would put patients in a better position to choose what they want to discuss and share, and ultimately could help empower them to achieve their defined health goals. The Shifting Perspectives Model of Chronic Illness could be useful and evaluate in this context since the model seems to be suitable of its elements of both the wellness and illness perspectives.

The findings could indicate that there is a need of greater support for the more vulnerable patients who live alone without nearby next of kin or friends and who experience severe emotional and existential confinement. Patient organisations that give a voice to this group of patients in society also need to be supported.

There appears to be a need to improve communication strategies and devices to facilitate patients' contact with the care system. Such strategies would include continuing education in communication for health professionals working with HNC care. Co-operation needs to improve between patient organisations, health professionals, and politicians in efforts to enhance economic, social, and health security. It includes support to help patients continue working and to meet needs for long-term rehabilitation.

Health care services need to take a greater interest in making cultural activities, arts, music, libraries, cafés, etc. accessible to patients. Greater interest and action is needed to create healthy care environments for everyone who visits a care facility or is hospitalised. This includes easy access and comprehensive planning that takes into account secluded, quiet, relaxing rooms and views of parks and green spaces for patients and their next of kin.

9. Further research

Health and health promotion is an integral part of nursing, and maybe the findings in the studies could be valuable in nursing and oncology practice; in rehabilitation and in palliative care. Conceivably these findings could be a starting point for further research in this important and demanding field. More qualitative studies could be done in this area to heightening awareness and create a dialogue about the concept of health promotion in HNC. For example, more research needs to address the salutogenic factors that promote feelings of better health and well-being and generate strength and power for patients in a vulnerable and dependent position. More research is needed to explore whether spiritual growth promotes feelings of better health and well-being in people with HNC.

More research should focus on the next of kin's perspectives on what promotes health and well-being and what gives them strength in their 24-hour emotional support. Further gender research needs to investigate emotional and sexual relationships between couples, especially from the woman's perspective. Other research from the perspective of health professionals should investigate what promotes their health and well-being and what gives them strength and power in their daily work as they encounter HNC patients and the next of kin.

Further research into new technologies and specific communicative devices in this care context could facilitate patients' contacts with others. Also, the working situation of patients and the impact of long-term, post-treatment side effects, e.g. eating and communication problems need further scientific investigation.

More quantitative studies could be done when testing hypothesis for example: Is there an association between patients with HNC that have experiences better health and well-being and being treated by nurses trained in bottom up approaches. However, an important issue is how we as researcher might influence health professionals to implement research results in practical settings qualitative or quantitative. For example by applying in clinical practice the knowledge gained from evidence-based research into clinical health practice such as the of Sense of Coherence studies (cf. Langius et al, 1995; Antonovsky, 1996) and Quality of life studies (Aarstad, 2008) and the use of a holistic needs assessment e.g. the Patients Concerns Inventory [PCI] (Rogers et al. 2009).

10. References

Aarstad, A.K.H. (2008). *Psychosocial factors and health related quality of life in former head and neck cancer patients.* Quality of life and Head and Neck cancer. [Dissertation], University of Bergen, ISBN 978-82-308-0657-9, Bergen

Adell, R., Svensson, B., & Bågenholm, T. (2008). Dental rehabilitation in 101 primarily reconstructed jaws after segmental resections – Possibilities and problems. An 18-

year study. *Journal of Cranio- Maxillofacial Surgery*, Vol.36, No.7, (October), pp. 395-402

Allison, P.J. (2002). Alcohol consumption is associated with improved health related Quality of life in head and neck cancer patients. *Oral Oncology*, Vol.38, No.1, (January), pp. 81- 86

Antonovsky, A. (1987). *Unraveling the Mystery of Health: How people manage stress and stay well*. Jossey-Bass Publishers, ISBN 978-1555420284, San Francisco

Antonovsky, A. (1996). The salutogenic model as a theory to guide health promotion. *Health Promotion International*, Vol. 11, No. 1, pp. 11-18, 19.08.2011. Retrieved from: <http://heapro.oxfordjournals.org/content/11/1/11.full.pdf+html>

Baxter, LA. (1991). Content Analysis. In: *Studying Interpersonal Interaction*. Montgomery BM & Duck S. Ed, Guildford, ISBN 0-89862-290-5 , New York, pp. 239-254

Beaglehole, R., & Bonita, R. (2001). *Public Health at Crossroads- achievements and prospects*. University Press, ISBN 0-521-58665-8, Cambridge

Berg, B. L. (2004). *Qualitative Research Methods for the Social Sciences* (5th Ed.). Allyn & Bacon, ISBN 0-205-31 847-9, Boston

Berg, G.V., Sarvimaki, A., & Hedelin, B. (2006). Hospitalized older peoples´ views of healthand health promotion. *International Journal of Older People Nursing*, Vol.1, No. 1, (March), pp. 25- 33

Bjorklund, M., & Fridlund, B. (1999). Cancer patients´ experiences of nurses´ behaviour and health promotion activities: A Critical Incident Analysis. *European Journal of Cancer Care*, Vol.8, No.4, (December), pp. 204-212

Björklund, M, Sarvimäki, A., & Berg, A. (2008). Health promotion and empowerment fromthe perspective of individuals living with head and neck cancer. *European Journal of Oncology Nursing*, Vol.12, No.1, (February), pp. 26-34

Björklund, M., Sarvimäki, A., & Berg, A. (2009). Health promoting contacts as encountered by individuals with head and neck cancer. *Journal of Nursing and Healthcare of Chronic Illness*, Vol.1, No.3, (September), pp. 261-268

Björklund, M. (2010). *Living with head and neck cancer – A health promotion perspective- a qualitative study*. [Dissertation], Nordic School of Public Health 2010:8, ISBN 978-85721-93-1, ISSN 0283-1961, Göteborg, 19.08.2011. Retrieved from: < http://www.nhv.se/upload/dokument/forskning/Publikationer/DrPH-avhandlingar/Margereth_Bj%C3%B6rklund_Avhandlingen_f%C3%B6r_hemsidan_101028.pdf>

Björklund, M., Sarvimäki, A. & Berg A. (2010). Living with head and neck cancer – A profile of captivity. *Journal of Nursing and Healthcare of Chronic Illness*, Vol.2, No.1, (March), pp. 22-31

Carnevali, D.L., & Reiner, A.C. (1990). *The Cancer Experience: Nursing Diagnosis and Management*. Lippincott Company, ISBN 0-397-54726-9, Philadelphia

Dossey, B.M., Keegan, L., & Guzwwetta, C.E. (2000). *Holistic Nursing A Handbook for Practice* (3rd ed.). Aspen Publication, ISBN 0-8342-1629-9, Gaithersburg

Dropkin, M.J. (1999). Body image and quality of life after head and neck cancer surgery. *Cancer Practice*, Vol.7, No.6, (November-December), pp. 309-313

Dropkin, M.J. (2001). Anxiety, coping strategies, and coping behaviours in patients undergoing head and neck cancer surgery. *Cancer Nursing*, Vol.24, No.2, (April), pp. 143-148

Feber, T. (2000). *Head and Neck Oncology Nursing*. Whurr Publishers Ltd, ISBN 1-86156-147-4, London

Flanagan J. C. (1954). The critical incident technique. *Psychological Bulletin* , Vol.51, No.4, (July), pp. 327-358

Frenkel, E., Arye, B., Carlson, C., & Sierpina, V. (2008) Integrating complementary and alternative medicine into conventional primary care: the patient perspective. EXPLORE: *The Journal of Science and Healing*, Vol.4, No.3, (May), pp. 178-186

Grahn, G., Danielson, M., & Ulander, K. (1999). Learning to live with cancer in European countries. *Cancer Nursing*, Vol.22, No.1, (February), 79-84

Halldórsdóttir, S., & Hamrin, E. (1997). Caring and uncaring encounters within nursing and health care from the cancer patient's perspective. *Cancer Nursing*, Vol.20, No.2, (April), pp. 120-128

Hodges, L.J. & Humphris, G.M. (2009). Fear of recurrence and psychological distress in head and neck cancer patients and their carers. *Psycho-Oncology*, Vol.18, No.8, (August), pp. 841-848

Hover-Kramer, D. (2002). *Healing Touch: A Guidebook for Practitioners* (2nd ed.). Delmar, ISBN 978-0-7668-2519-2, Albany

Hök, J. (2009). *Use of complementary and alternative medicine in the context of cancer. Perspectives on exceptional experiences*. [Dissertation], Karolinska Institutet, ISBN 978-91-7409-412-1, Stockholm, 19.08.2011. Retrieved from: <http://publications.ki.se/jspui/bitstream/10616/39202/1/thesis.pdf>

Kvale, S. (1996). *InterViews - An Introduction to Qualitative Research Interviewing*. SAGE publications, ISBN 0-8039-5819-6, Thousand Oaks

IOM (Institute of Medicine). (2000). National Academy of Sciences, Committee on Quality of Care in America. *Crossing the Quality Chasm*. National Academy Press, ISBN9780309072809, Washington, 19.08.2011. Retrieved from: <http://www.nap.edu/openbook.php?isbn=0309072808>

Langius, A. (1995) *Quality of Life in a Group of patients with Oral and Pharyngeal Cancer. Sense ofCoherence, Functional Status and Well-being*. [Dissertation], Karolinska Institute, ISBN 91-628-1474-5, Stockholm

Larsson, M. (2006). Eating problems in patients with head and neck cancer treated with radiotherapy. Needs, problems and support during the trajectory of care. [Dissertation], Karlstad University Studies 2006:7, ISBN 91-7063-038-0, Karlstad, 19.08.2011. Retrieved from: <http://www.google.se/search?sourceid=chrome&ie=UTF-8&q=Eating+problems+in+patients+with+head+and+neck+cancer+treated+with+radiotherapy.+Needs%2C+problems+and+support+during+the+trajectory+of+care.>

Leddy, S.K. (2003). *Integrative Health Promotion Conceptual Bases for Nursing Practice*. Slack incorporated, ISBN 1-55642-587-2, Thorafare

Lindenfield, G. (1996). *Tro på dig själv*. [Self-esteem]. ISBN 91-23-01582-9. Liber-Hermods, Malmö (In Swedish).

McCreaddie, M, Payne, S & Frogatt, K (2010). Ensnared by positivity: A constructive perspective on 'being positive' in cancer care. *European Journal of Oncology Nursing*, Vol.14, No.4, (September), pp. 283-290

McLane, L., Jones, K., Lydiatt, W., Lydiatt, D., & Richards, A. (2003). Taking away the fear: a grounded theory study of cooperative care in the treatment of head and neck cancer. *Psycho-Oncology*, Vol.12, No.5, (July-August), pp. 474-490

Mok, E, Martinson, I., & Wong, T.K.S. (2004). Individual empowerment among Chinese cancer patients in Hong Kong. *Western Journal of Nursing Research*, Vol.26, No.1, pp. 59-75

Mok, E, Wong, F., & Wong, D. (2010). The meaning of spirituality and spiritual care amongthe Hong Kong Chinese terminal ill. *Journal of Advanced Nursing*, Vol.66, No.2, (February), pp. 360-370

Molassiotis, A, Ozden, G, Platin, N, Scott, J.A, Pud, P., Fernandez-Ortega, P., et al. (2006). Complementary/alternative medicine use in patients with head and neck cancers in Europe. *European Journal of Cancer Care*, Vol. 15, No.1, (March), pp. 19-24

NCCDPHP (National Center for Chronic Disease Prevention and Health Promotion) (2010). 19.08.2011. Retrieved from: <http://www.cdc.gov/nccdphp/about.htm>

NIPH (National Institute of Public Health). (2005). Stockholm, Sweden. *Towards More Health Promoting Health and Medical Care*. 19.08.2011. Retrieved from: <http://www.fhi.se/PageFiles/4413/r200455towardsmorehealthpromoting0503.pdf?epslanguage=sv>

NNF (Northern Nurses Federation). (2003) Ethical guidelines for nursing research in the Nordic countries. *Vård i Norden: Nordic Journals of Nursing Research*, Vol. 23, No.4, pp. 1-19, 19.08.2011. Retrieved from: <http://www.sykepleien.no/ikbViewer/Content/337889/SSNs%20etiske%20retningslinjer.pdf>

Nordenfelt, L. (1995). *On the Nature of Health: An Action-Theoretic Approach* (2nd ed.). Kluwer Academic Publisher, ISBN 9780792333692, Dordrecht

Nordenfelt, L. (2007). The concept of health and illness revisited. *Medicine, Health Care and Philosophy*, Vol.10, No.1, pp. 5-10

Nutbeam, D. (1998). Health promotion glossary. *Health Promotion International*, Vol.13, No.4, pp. 349-364, 19.08.2011. Retrieved from: <http://www.bvsde.paho.org/bvsacd/cd26/promocion/v13n4/349.pdf>

Näsman, A., Attner, P., Hammerstedt, L., Du, J., Eriksson, M., Giraud, G., et al., (2009). Incidence of human papilloma virus (HPV) positive tonsillar carcinoma in Stockholm, Sweden: An epidemic of viral-induced carcinoma? *International Journal of Cancer*, Vol. 125, No.2, (July), pp. 362-366

Paterson, B. L. (2001). The shifting perspectives model of chronic illness. *Journal of Nursing Scholarship*, Vol.33, No.1, (March), pp. 21-26

Paterson, B. L. (2003). The Koala has Claws: Applications of the Shifting Perspectives Model in Research of Chronic Illness. *Qualitative Health Research*, Vol.13, No.7, (September), pp. 987-994

Pender, N. J. (1996). *Health Promotion in Nursing Practice*. Pretince Hall, ISBN 978-0-8385-3659-9, Upper Saddle River

Polit, D.F., & Beck, C.T. (2008). *Nursing Research: Generating and Assessing Evidence for Nursing Practice* (8th Ed.). Lippincott Williams & Wilkins, ISBN 978-0-7817-9468-8, Philadelphia

Richardson, J. (2002). Health promotion in palliative care: the patients' perception of therapeutic interaction with palliative nurse in the primary care setting. *Journal of Advanced Nursing*, Vol.40, No.4, (November), pp. 432-440

Rogers, S.N., El-Sheikha, J., & Lowe, D. (2009). The development of a Patients Concerns Inventory (PCI) to help reveal patients concerns in the head and neck clinic. *Oral Oncology*. Vol. 45, No. 7, (July), pp. 555-561

Rumsey, N., Clarke, A., White, P., Wyn-Williams, M., & Garlick, W. (2004). Altered body image: appearance-related concerns of people with visible disfigurement. *Journal of Advanced Nursing*, Vol.48, No.5, (December), pp. 443-453

Semple, C.J., Dunwoody, L., Kernohan, W. G., McCaughan, E., & Sullivan, K. (2008). Changes and challenges to patients 'lifestyle patterns following treatment for head and neck cancer. *Journal of Advanced Nursing*, Vol.63, No.1, (July), pp. 85-93

Siegel, B.S. (1990). Exceptional patients live long and live well. *Maryland Medical Journal*, Vol. 39, No.2, (February), pp. 181-182.

Sharp, L. (2006). Aspects of nursing care for patients with head and neck cancer receiving radiation therapy. [Dissertation], Karolinska Institutet, ISBN 91-7140-619-0, Stockholm, 19.08.2011. Retrieved from: <http://publications.ki.se/jspui/bitstream/10616/38757/1/thesis.pdf>

Vickery, L.E.; Latchford, G.; Hewison, J.; Bellew, M. & Feber, T. (2003). The impact of headand neck cancer and facial disfigurement on the quality of life of patients and their partners. *Head & Neck*, Vol.25, No.4, (April), pp. 289-296

Thorne, S.; Reimer Kirkham, S. & MacDonald-Emes, J. (1997). Interpretative description: A non -categorical qualitative alternative for developing nursing knowledge. *Research in Nursing & Health*, Vol.20, pp. 169-177. 19.08.2011. Retrieved from: <http://onlinelibrary.wiley.com/doi/10.1002/(SICI)1098-240X(199704)20:2%3C169::AID-NUR9%3E3.0.CO;2-I/pdf>

Thorne, S., & Paterson B. L. (1998). Shifting images of chronic illness. *Image*, Vol.30, No.2, (June), pp. 173-178

Thorne, S.; Reimer Kirkham, S. & and O'Flynn-Magee, K. (2004). The Analytic Challenge inInterpretive Description. *International Journal of Qualitative Methods*, Vol.3, No.1, (April), pp. 1-21. 19.08.2011. Retrieved from: <http://www.ualberta.ca/~iiqm/backissues/3_1/pdf/thorneetal.pdf>

Thorne, S. (2006). Patient-Provider Communication in chronic illness: a health promotion window of opportunity. *Family & Community Health*, Vol.29, No.1, (Jan-Mar), pp. 4-11

Tones K, & Tilford S. (1994). *Health Education: Effectiveness, Efficiency and Equity*.2nd Ed. Chapman and Hall, ISBN 0-7487-4527-0, London

Trillin, A.S. (1981). Of dragons and gardens peas: a cancer patients talks to doctors. *NewEngland Journal of Medicine* Vol.304, No.12, (March), pp. 699- 701

Turpin, M, Dallos, R., Owen, R., & Thomas, M. (2008). The meaning and impact of head andneck cancer: an interpretative phenomenological and repertory grid analysis. *Journal of Constructivist Psychology*, Vol.22, No.1, (January), pp. 24- 54

Vickery, L.E.; Latchford, G.; Hewison, J.; Bellew, M. & Feber, T. (2003). The impact of headand neck cancer and facial disfigurement on the quality of life of patients and their partners. *Head & Neck*, Vol.25, No.4, (April), pp. 289-296

Wells, M. (1998). The hidden experience of radiotherapy to the head and neck: a qualitative study of patients after completion of treatment. *Journal of Advanced Nursing*, Vol.28, No.4, (October), pp. 840- 848

WHO. (1986). *Ottawa Charter for Health Promotion*, 19.08.2011. Retrieved from: <http://www.who.int/healthpromotion/conferences/previous/ottawa/en/>

WHO (World Health Organization). (2002). *Traditional Medicine Strategy*, 19.08.2011. Retrieved from: <http://www.who.int/medicines/publications/traditionalpolicy/en/index.html>

WMA (World Medical Association). (2004). *Declaration of Helsinki - Ethical Principles for Medical Research involving Human Subjects*. 19.08.2011. Retrieved from: >http://www.wma.net/en/30publications/10policies/b3/index.html<

Young, L.E., & Hayes, V. (2002). *Transforming Health Promotion Practice Concepts, Issues, and Applications*. Davis Company, ISBN 0-8036-0814-4, Philadelphia

Permissions

The contributors of this book come from diverse backgrounds, making this book a truly international effort. This book will bring forth new frontiers with its revolutionizing research information and detailed analysis of the nascent developments around the world.

We would like to thank Mark Agulnik, MD, for lending his expertise to make the book truly unique. He has played a crucial role in the development of this book. Without his invaluable contribution this book wouldn't have been possible. He has made vital efforts to compile up to date information on the varied aspects of this subject to make this book a valuable addition to the collection of many professionals and students.

This book was conceptualized with the vision of imparting up-to-date information and advanced data in this field. To ensure the same, a matchless editorial board was set up. Every individual on the board went through rigorous rounds of assessment to prove their worth. After which they invested a large part of their time researching and compiling the most relevant data for our readers. Conferences and sessions were held from time to time between the editorial board and the contributing authors to present the data in the most comprehensible form. The editorial team has worked tirelessly to provide valuable and valid information to help people across the globe.

Every chapter published in this book has been scrutinized by our experts. Their significance has been extensively debated. The topics covered herein carry significant findings which will fuel the growth of the discipline. They may even be implemented as practical applications or may be referred to as a beginning point for another development.

The editorial board has been involved in producing this book since its inception. They have spent rigorous hours researching and exploring the diverse topics which have resulted in the successful publishing of this book. They have passed on their knowledge of decades through this book. To expedite this challenging task, the publisher supported the team at every step. A small team of assistant editors was also appointed to further simplify the editing procedure and attain best results for the readers.

Our editorial team has been hand-picked from every corner of the world. Their multi-ethnicity adds dynamic inputs to the discussions which result in innovative outcomes. These outcomes are then further discussed with the researchers and contributors who give their valuable feedback and opinion regarding the same. The feedback is then collaborated with the researches and they are edited in a comprehensive manner to aid the understanding of the subject.

Apart from the editorial board, the designing team has also invested a significant amount of their time in understanding the subject and creating the most relevant covers. They scrutinized every image to scout for the most suitable representation of the subject and create an appropriate cover for the book.

The publishing team has been involved in this book since its early stages. They were actively engaged in every process, be it collecting the data, connecting with the contributors or procuring relevant information. The team has been an ardent support to the editorial, designing and production team. Their endless efforts to recruit the best for this project, has resulted in the accomplishment of this book. They are a veteran in the field of academics and their pool of knowledge is as vast as their experience in printing. Their expertise and guidance has proved useful at every step. Their uncompromising quality standards have made this book an exceptional effort. Their encouragement from time to time has been an inspiration for everyone.

The publisher and the editorial board hope that this book will prove to be a valuable piece of knowledge for researchers, students, practitioners and scholars across the globe.

List of Contributors

Valentina Krstevska
Department of Head and Neck Cancer, University Clinic of Radiotherapy and Oncology, Skopje, Republic of Macedonia

Mala Bukar Sandabe, Hamman Garandawa and Abdullahi Isa
Department of ENT University of Maiduguri, Teaching Hospital, Nigeria

Federica Ganci, Andrea Sacconi, Valentina Manciocco, Renato Covello, Giuseppe Spriano, Giulia Fontemaggi and Giovanni Blandino
Regina Elena Cancer Institute, Italy

Mehmet Gunduz
Departments of Medical Genetics, Turkey
Otolaryngology Head and Neck Surgery, Turkey
Department of Otolaryngology Head and Neck Surgery, Faculty of Medicine, Wakayama Medical University, Wakayama, Japan

Esra Gunduz
Departments of Medical Genetics, Turkey

Levent Beder and Noboru Yamanaka
Department of Otolaryngology Head and Neck Surgery, Faculty of Medicine, Wakayama Medical University, Wakayama, Japan

Ramazan Yigitoglu
Medical Biochemistry, Turkey

Bunyamin Isik
Family Medicine, Faculty of Medicine, Fatih University, Ankara, Turkey

Yuh Baba
Department of Otolaryngology, Ohtawara Red Cross Hospital, Ohtawara, Japan
National Institute of Sensory Organs, National Tokyo Medical Center, Tokyo, Japan
Department of Oral Function and Molecular Biology, Ohu University, Misumido Tomita-machi Koriyama, Japan

Masato Fujii and Yutaka Tokumaru
National Institute of Sensory Organs, National Tokyo Medical Center, Tokyo, Japan

Yasumasa Kato
Department of Oral Function and Molecular Biology, Ohu University, Misumido Tomita-machi Koriyama, Japan

Sittichai Koontongkaew
Faculty of Dentistry, Thammasat University, Pathumthani, Thailand
Medicinal Herb Research Unit, Thammasat University, Pathumthani, Thailand

Kantima Leelahavanichkul
Faculty of Dentistry, Thammasat University, Pathumthani, Thailand

Jared Knol
Department of Medicine, Feinberg School of Medicine, Northwestern University, Chicago, Illinois, USA

Tiffany King
Division of Hematology/Oncology, Northwestern Medical Faculty Foundation, Chicago, Illinois, USA

Mark Agulnik
Division of Hematology/Oncology, Department of Medicine, Feinberg School of Medicine, Northwestern University, Robert H. Lurie Comprehensive Cancer Center, Chicago, Illinois USA

Putipun Puataweepong
Ramathibodi Hospital, Mahidol University, Thailand

Ritesh Rathore
Roger Williams Medical Center, Boston University School of Medicine, USA

Krzysztof Szyfter
Institute of Human Genetics, Polish Academy of Sciences, Poznań, Poland
Dept. of Otolaryngology and Laryngological Oncology, K. Marcinkowski, University of Medical Sciences, Poznań, Poland

Marcin Szaumkessel
Institute of Human Genetics, Polish Academy of Sciences, Poznań, Poland

Wojciech Gawęcki
Dept. of Otolaryngology and Laryngological Oncology, K. Marcinkowski, University of Medical Sciences, Poznań, Poland

Loredana G. Marcu
Department of Medical Physics, Royal Adelaide Hospital, Australia
School of Chemistry and Physics, University of Adelaide, Australia
Faculty of Science, University of Oradea, Romania

Eric Yeoh
Department of Radiation Oncology, Royal Adelaide Hospital, Australia
School of Medicine, University of Adelaide, Australia

Yueh-Bih Tang Chen and Shih-Heng Chen
National Taiwan University Hospital, Taipei, Taiwan

Hung-Chi Chen
China Medical University Hospital, Taichung, Taiwan

Mutsumi Okazaki
Department of Plastic and Reconstructive Surgery, Graduate School, Tokyo Medical and Dental University, Tokyo, Japan

Sneha Mantri
Hitkarini Dental College and Hospital, Jabalpur, India

Zafrulla Khan
James Graham Brown Cancer Center Louisville, Kentucky, USA

Kate Reid and Carol Dealey
University Hospital Birmingham NHS Foundation Trust, United Kingdom
University of Birmingham, United Kingdom

Derek Farrell
University of Birmingham, United Kingdom

Ping-Yi Kuo and John E Williams
Royal Marsden Hospital Foundation NHS Trust, United Kingdom

Margereth Björklund
Kristianstad University, Sweden